Effects of Probiotics, Prebiotics, and Postbiotics on Human Health

Guest Editors

Katerina Kotzampassi
George Stavrou

MDPI

Basel • Beijing • Wuhan • Barcelona • Belgrade • Novi Sad • Cluj • Manchester

Guest Editors
Katerina Kotzampassi
Department of Surgery
Aristotle University of Thessaloniki
Thessaloniki
Greece

George Stavrou
Department of General Surgery
Addenbrooke's Hospital
Cambridge
UK

Editorial Office
MDPI AG
Grosspeteranlage 5
4052 Basel, Switzerland

This is a reprint of the Special Issue, published open access by the journal *Nutrients* (ISSN 2072-6643), freely accessible at: https://www.mdpi.com/journal/nutrients/special_issues/1374DXS50R.

For citation purposes, cite each article independently as indicated on the article page online and as indicated below:

Lastname, A.A.; Lastname, B.B. Article Title. *Journal Name* **Year**, *Volume Number*, Page Range.

ISBN 978-3-7258-7635-8 (Hbk)
ISBN 978-3-7258-7636-5 (PDF)
https://doi.org/10.3390/books978-3-7258-7636-5

Contents

nutrients

MDPI

Editorial

The Expanding Role of Probiotics in Human Health

George Stavrou [1,*] and Katerina Kotzampassi [2,*]

1 1st Surgical Department, 417 NIMTS (Army Share Fund) Hospital, 11521 Athens, Greece
2 Department of Surgery, Aristotle University of Thessaloniki, 54636 Thessaloniki, Greece
* Correspondence: stavgd@gmail.com (G.S.); kakothe@yahoo.com (K.K.)

Since the 1990s, it has been widely documented that probiotics, either alone or in combination with prebiotic supplements, play a vital role in host health and disease management. However, at present, with increased knowledge of their specific actions, i.e., antioxidant and immunomodulatory actions and enhancement of epithelial barrier function—most likely driven through the modulation of the local microbiota—and their beneficial effects in disease prevention and treatment, a significant proportion of experimental research, in addition to hundreds of clinical applications, is currently focusing on their use [1,2].

The word "probiotics" tends to be automatically linked to the gut microbiota; however, almost all scientists today recognize that the gut, despite being the oldest recognized and perhaps even central "host" organ, is not unique [1]; other sites, including the oral cavity, the lungs, the urinary tract/bladder, and the skin microbiota, are also recognized and crucially implicated both in local and remote-organ disease [3–6]. Postbiotics, recently defined as "inanimate microorganisms and/or their components that confer a health benefit on the host", were used as cosmetics for the enhancement of skin health long before they were renamed postbiotics [7]. Moreover, they have traditionally been used in immunocompromised patients rather than as live probiotics, eliminating the theoretical risk of bacteremia induction while also exerting equally positive effects. Prebiotics, being the physical background for bacterial growth, were defined 30 years ago as "non-digestible food ingredients that beneficially affect the host, by selectively stimulating the growth and/or activity of one or a limited number of bacteria already resident in the colon" [2,8,9].

The growing belief that diseases of any type and body system—from atopic dermatitis to neurodegenerative disorders—are related to the destruction of the related microbiome has led to the hypothesis that, by modulating the local microbiome through a probiotic formula, disease can be prevented or even cured. Thus, the human microbiome has emerged as a central focus in medical research, revealing intricate connections between the composition of the microbiota (and not exclusively of the gut) and systemic health. The symbiotic relationship between the microbiota and the host affects metabolic functions, immune responses, and neurological processes through the gut–brain axis and even reproductive and dermatological health.

With growing evidence supporting the impact of beneficial bacteria, alone or with prebiotics, or alternatively postbiotics, on specific mechanisms of human biology and the two-way communication of local microbiomes via the nervous system, there is increasing interest in harnessing these bacterial elements both to prevent and treat illness and sustain and improve health.

The exceptional collection of both research articles and reviews in this Special Issue delves into the diverse applications of microbiome-modulating interventions, providing insights into their physiological and clinical implications.

 https://doi.org/10.3390/nu17071116

One of the key areas of investigation in this issue is metabolic health and chronic disease management. Liu et al. [10] present a meta-analysis of *Akkermansia muciniphila*, a new-generation probiotic, known for its beneficial effects in preventing the onset of type-2 diabetes and obesity through the promotion of the gut production of short-chain fatty acids—thus improving insulin resistance and the host metabolism—along with the stimulation of beneficial gut bacteria, such as *Bifidobacteria*. The authors emphasize that *A. muciniphila* treatment significantly reduces fasting blood glucose levels, by improving glucose tolerance and increasing blood insulin levels, thus being effective in preventing type 2 diabetes in animals, while significantly reducing the increase in body weight by 10.4%. Jang et al. [11] contribute to this argument with their study on *Lactobacillus delbrueckii* subsp. lactis CKDB001, aimed at demonstrating, in a murine model of high-fat diet-induced obesity, its capacity to counteract metabolic disturbances. The study results highlight improvements in insulin sensitivity, reductions in serum triglycerides and hepatic lipid accumulation, and the alleviation of metabolic dysfunction-associated steatotic liver disease. In the same manner, Zhang et al. [12], in a clinical trial, examine the beneficial effects of *Weizmannia coagulans* BC99 in long-term alcohol consumers. Patients randomized to a *W. coagulans* BC99 group for 60 days demonstrated, compared to the placebo, improvements in hepatic enzyme profiles and anti-inflammatory factors, in addition to an increased abundance of *Muribaculaceae*, considered the key factor in alleviating alcohol-induced liver damage in long-term alcohol consumers. The potential of *W. coagulans* to promote gut–liver axis homeostasis could have further implications for managing hepatic disorders in general.

Expanding beyond metabolic conditions, López-Yerena et al. [13] review papers on the cardiovascular benefits exerted by probiotics, emphasizing the potential mechanisms through which specific strains may lower cholesterol, reduce inflammation, and improve endothelial function. Their findings focus on the impact of probiotics on major cardiovascular risk factors, such as hypertension, type 2 diabetes mellitus, metabolic syndrome, and hypercholesterolemia, and thus their use for the secondary prevention of coronary artery disease, acknowledging them as adjunct "therapies" in cardiovascular disease prevention. However, further interpretation of their properties, in terms of the optimal strains, dosage, and treatment duration, in addition to the influence of genus and the delivery vehicle, is required.

The role of probiotics in immune function and gastrointestinal health is another important topic. Wada et al. [14], in their innovative clinical study, investigate the immunomodulatory properties of *Lactobacillus helveticus* GCL1815, which optimally prevents the onset of systemic and local common cold symptoms in healthy adults. Their findings clearly indicate that *L. helveticus* GCL1815 enhances the response to viruses by activating two distinct dendritic cell pathways: significantly increasing the expression of [i] CD86 and HLA-DR in plasmacytoid dendritic cells from the fourth week of intake and [ii] the expression of HLA-DR in type 1 conventional dendritic cells at 8 weeks of intake, while also maintaining stable levels of CD86 in type 1 conventional dendritic cells, which otherwise decrease in the placebo. In the same vein, Naghibi et al. [15], in a randomized, double-blind controlled trial, evaluate the effects of the postbiotic *Bifidobacterium longum* CECT 7347 in healthy adults with mild-to-moderate gastrointestinal symptoms. Although minimal improvement was observed in gastrointestinal symptoms per se and visceral sensitivity tests, 8 weeks of treatment with this probiotic seems to promote gut health by increasing the abundance of butyrate-producing bacteria (mainly *Faecalibacterium* and *Anaerobutyricum*) while maintaining fecal calprotectin levels and reducing serum cholesterol levels. Additionally, Matar et al. [16] provide a comprehensive review of the intestinal barrier and its permeability by analyzing the harmful effects of specific food ingredients, the impact of altered permeability in pre-clinical models and human diseases, and the role of the microbiome and epigenomics in controlling epithelial barrier function. The authors then focus on the possibility of restoring gut integrity using beneficial microbiota interventions, emphasizing the interplay between probiotics, together with their active metabolites, and other secreted compounds, and the tight junction proteins in intestinal epithelial cells, which are crucial for preventing systemic inflammation and metabolic endotoxemia.

Stachelska et al. [17] analyze the health-promoting properties of probiotic bacteria linked to fermented milk beverages, emphasizing their role in preventing lifestyle-related diseases. In their study, the authors detail the modifications occurring in the intestinal microbiota that lead—through various mechanisms—to the strengthening of the immune system and the prevention of the diseases of modern life, i.e., obesity, diabetes, and possibly cancer. However, all of these conditions/diseases seem to be closely linked to one vicious cycle or another, influenced by independent parameters. This new direction in personalized medicine is gaining exceptional traction in probiota research as well. These results evidence the importance of screening across multiple age groups separately to provide details on how therapeutics impact the microbiome and, consequently, human health. Firrman et al. [18] highlight the influence of age in shaping the gut microbiome, with the dominant taxa together with their metabolites changing over a person's lifetime, making it important to screen individuals in each age group to determine how therapeutics—in the present case, the human milk oligosaccharide 2′-fucosyllactose—as above, impact the microbiome and, consequently, human health.

Beyond the traditional domains of gut and metabolic health, this Special Issue also explores the expanding applications of beneficial bacteria research in reproductive medicine. Raimundo et al. [19] present a retrospective analysis of *Ligilactobacillus salivarius* PS11610, assessing its potential role as a one-month oral pretreatment in enhancing in-vitro fertilization success rates, particularly in the frozen embryo transfer group. Although the quality of embryos was lower than in the placebo group, there was an increase in the number of live births and biochemical pregnancy rates. However, further research in this field is required, including the possibility of topical application.

Lastly, in the field of dermatology/cosmetology science, Park et al. [20] examine the protective effects of *Limosilactobacillus fermentum* MG5368 and *Lactiplantibacillus plantarum* MG989 in UVB-induced skin damage. Their experimental study, conducted on both HaCaT cells and hairless mice, provides evidence that these two probiotic strains have the potential to be utilized as probiotic-based skin anti-photoaging formulations, since they can equally contribute to the promotion of collagen synthesis and hyaluronic acid restoration and thus maintain skin elasticity while inhibiting wrinkle formation.

To comply with regulation for the characterization of a microorganism as a specific probiotic strain, the pro- or postbiotics incorporated into a cosmetic regime should be both genetically and phenotypically defined. Based on this assumption, Theodorou et al. [21] analyze 14 published clinical trials and discuss the beneficial effects of those cosmeceuticals—fulfilling the above criteria—applied to volunteers with healthy skin. Their analysis emphasizes the growing consumer interest in microbiome-based skincare products and highlights the trend toward personalized skin care, which may lead to genomic sequencing and metabolomics to tailor probiotic and postbiotic treatments to individual skin microbiomes.

Collectively, these studies illustrate the growing recognition of the microbiome as a fundamental determinant of human health. As research continues to unravel the complex interactions between beneficial bacteria and host physiology—either as a generalized interface, as with the gut–brain axis, or at a local level, as with the skin microbiome—in health and disease, the field of medicine in the future will increasingly integrate microbiome-targeted strategies. It is our hope that this Special Issue will serve as a valuable resource, inspiring further exploration into the transformative potential of the human microbiome(s) in both preventive and therapeutic contexts.

Author Contributions: Both authors equally contributed to the Editorial. All authors have read and agreed to the published version of the manuscript.

Funding: The authors declare that no funding was received for the publication of this Editorial.

Institutional Review Board Statement: Not applicable.

Informed Consent Statement: Not applicable.

Conflicts of Interest: The authors declare no conflicts of interest.

References

1. Fuller, R. Probiotics in human medicine. *Gut* **1991**, *32*, 439–442. [PubMed]
2. Hill, C.; Guarner, F.; Reid, G.; Gibson, G.R.; Merenstein, D.J.; Pot, B.; Morelli, L.; Canani, R.B.; Flint, H.J.; Salminen, S.; et al. Expert consensus document. The International Scientific Association for Probiotics and Prebiotics consensus statement on the scope and appropriate use of the term probiotic. *Nat. Rev. Gastroenterol. Hepatol.* **2014**, *11*, 506–514. [PubMed]
3. Grice, E.A.; Segre, J.A. The skin microbiome. *Nat. Rev. Microbiol.* **2011**, *9*, 244–253. [PubMed]
4. Beck, J.M.; Young, V.B.; Huffnagle, G.B. The microbiome of the lung. *Transl. Res.* **2012**, *160*, 258–266.
5. Dharmarathne, G.; Kazi, S.; King, S.; Jayasinghe, T.N. The Bidirectional Relationship Between Cardiovascular Medications and Oral and Gut Microbiome Health: A Comprehensive Review. *Microorganisms* **2024**, *12*, 2246. [CrossRef] [PubMed]
6. Dalvi, H.; De Nisco, N.J. The evolving world of the urinary microbiome. *Curr. Opin. Urol.* **2024**, *34*, 422–427. [CrossRef] [PubMed]
7. Salminen, S.; Collado, M.C.; Endo, A.; Hill, C.; Lebeer, S.; Quigley, E.M.M.; Sanders, M.E.; Shamir, R.; Swann, J.R.; Szajewska, H.; et al. The International Scientific Association of Probiotics and Prebiotics (ISAPP) consensus statement on the definition and scope of postbiotics. *Nat. Rev. Gastroenterol. Hepatol.* **2021**, *18*, 649–667. [PubMed]
8. Gibson, G.R.; Hutkins, R.; Sanders, M.E.; Prescott, S.L.; Reimer, R.A.; Salminen, S.J.; Scott, K.; Stanton, C.; Swanson, K.S.; Cani, P.D.; et al. Expert consensus document: The International Scientific Association for Probiotics and Prebiotics (ISAPP) consensus statement on the definition and scope of prebiotics. *Nat. Rev. Gastroenterol. Hepatol.* **2017**, *14*, 491–502. [PubMed]
9. Gibson, G.R.; Roberfroid, M.B. Dietary modulation of the human colonic microbiota: Introducing the concept of prebiotics. *J. Nutr.* **1995**, *125*, 1401–1412.
10. Liu, E.; Ji, X.; Zhou, K. *Akkermansia muciniphila* for the Prevention of Type 2 Diabetes and Obesity: A Meta-Analysis of Animal Studies. *Nutrients* **2024**, *16*, 3440. [CrossRef]
11. Jang, H.; Joung, H.; Chu, J.; Cho, M.; Kim, Y.W.; Kim, K.H.; Shin, C.H.; Lee, J.; Ha, J.H. *Lactobacillus delbrueckii* subsp. lactis CKDB001 Ameliorates Metabolic Complications in High-Fat Diet-Induced Obese Mice. *Nutrients* **2024**, *16*, 4260. [PubMed]
12. Zhang, J.; Li, C.; Duan, M.; Qu, Z.; Wang, Y.; Dong, Y.; Wu, Y.; Fang, S.; Gu, S. The Improvement Effects of *Weizmannia coagulans* BC99 on Liver Function and Gut Microbiota of Long-Term Alcohol Drinkers: A Randomized Double-Blind Clinical Trial. *Nutrients* **2025**, *17*, 320. [CrossRef] [PubMed]
13. López-Yerena, A.; de Santisteban Villaplana, V.; Badimon, L.; Vilahur, G.; Padro, T. Probiotics: A Potential Strategy for Preventing and Managing Cardiovascular Disease. *Nutrients* **2024**, *17*, 52. [CrossRef] [PubMed]
14. Wada, H.; Mawatari, T.; Saito, Y.; Azuma, N.; Iwama, Y. Lactobacillus helveticus Induces Two Types of Dendritic Cell Activation and Effectively Suppresses Onset of the Common Cold: A Randomized, Double-Blind, Placebo-Controlled Trial. *Nutrients* **2024**, *17*, 101. [CrossRef]
15. Naghibi, M.; Pont-Beltran, A.; Lamelas, A.; Llobregat, L.; Martinez-Blanch, J.F.; Rojas, A.; Álvarez, B.; López Plaza, B.; Arcos Castellanos, L.; Chenoll, E.; et al. Effect of Postbiotic *Bifidobacterium longum* CECT 7347 on Gastrointestinal Symptoms, Serum Biochemistry, and Intestinal Microbiota in Healthy Adults: A Randomised, Parallel, Double-Blind, Placebo-Controlled Pilot Study. *Nutrients* **2024**, *16*, 3952. [CrossRef] [PubMed]
16. Matar, A.; Damianos, J.A.; Jencks, K.J.; Camilleri, M. Intestinal Barrier Impairment, Preservation, and Repair: An Update. *Nutrients* **2024**, *16*, 3494. [CrossRef] [PubMed]
17. Stachelska, M.A.; Karpiński, P.; Kruszewski, B. Health-Promoting and Functional Properties of Fermented Milk Beverages with Probiotic Bacteria in the Prevention of Civilization Diseases. *Nutrients* **2024**, *17*, 9. [CrossRef]
18. Firrman, J.; Deyaert, S.; Mahalak, K.K.; Liu, L.; Baudot, A.; Joossens, M.; Poppe, J.; Cameron, S.J.S.; Van den Abbeele, P. The Bifidogenic Effect of 2'Fucosyllactose Is Driven by Age-Specific Bifidobacterium Species, Demonstrating Age as an Important Factor for Gut Microbiome Targeted Precision Medicine. *Nutrients* **2024**, *17*, 151. [CrossRef] [PubMed]
19. Raimundo, M.; Rodrigues, P.; Esteban, S.; Espinosa-Martos, I.; Jiménez, E. *Ligilactobacillus salivarius* PS11610 Enhances the Fertilization Success of IVF: A Preliminary Retrospective Analysis. *Nutrients* **2025**, *17*, 410. [CrossRef]

20. Park, J.Y.; Lee, J.Y.; Hong, S.; Heo, H.; Lee, H.; Kim, Y.G.; Kim, B.K.; Choi, S.I.; Lee, J. *Limosilactobacillus fermentum* MG5368 and *Lactiplantibacillus plantarum* MG989 Regulates Skin Health in UVB-Induced HaCaT Cells and Hairless Mice Model. *Nutrients* **2024**, *16*, 4083. [CrossRef] [PubMed]
21. Theodorou, I.M.; Kapoukranidou, D.; Theodorou, M.; Tsetis, J.K.; Menni, A.E.; Tzikos, G.; Bareka, S.; Shrewsbury, A.; Stavrou, G.; Kotzampassi, K. Cosmeceuticals: A Review of Clinical Studies Claiming to Contain Specific, Well-Characterized Strains of Probiotics or Postbiotics. *Nutrients* **2024**, *16*, 2526. [CrossRef]

nutrients

MDPI

Article

The Positive Effect of *Akkermansia muciniphila* postbiotics on the Glycolipid Metabolism of *Caenorhabditis elegans* Induced by High-Glucose Diet

Zhongqin Wu [1,2,3], Ke Li [1,3], Aixing Hou [1,3], Yuanliang Wang [1,3] and Zongjun Li [1,3,*]

1 Hunan Province Key Laboratory of Food Science and Biotechnology, College of Food Science and Technology, Hunan Agricultural University, Changsha 410128, China; hnwuzhongqin@163.com (Z.W.); wangyuanliang@hunau.edu.cn (Y.W.)
2 School of Pharmaceutical and Bioengineering, Hunan Chemical Vocational Technology College, Zhuzhou 412000, China
3 National Research Center of Engineering Technology for Utilization of Functional Ingredients from Botanicals, Changsha 410128, China
* Correspondence: hnlizongjun@163.com; Tel.: +86-731-84635215

Abstract: Background: Glycolipid metabolism is essential for maintaining metabolic homeostasis. As a new postbiotic, pasteurized *Akkermansia muciniphila* (P-AKK) is important for the regulation of immunity and metabolism. Objectives: This study aimed to evaluate the effects of P-AKK on glycolipid metabolism in *Caenorhabditis elegans* fed a high glucose diet. Results: We discovered that feeding nematodes P-AKK improved their healthy lifespan when fed a high-glucose diet. Furthermore, P-AKK contributes to reducing the accumulation of glucose, advanced glycation end products, and lipids and maintains a better physiological state. In addition, P-AKK improved the composition of free fatty acids and decreased the total free fatty acid content of *C. elegans*. Transcriptome sequencing analysis revealed that P-AKK induced significant enrichment of carbohydrate, oxidative phosphorylation, and fatty acid metabolism pathways. These significantly enriched biological processes were closely related to glucose and lipid metabolism. Among them, P-AKK activated the β-oxidation of fatty acids while inhibiting the de novo synthesis of fatty acids to regulate fatty acid metabolism. Conclusions: The administration of P-AKK positively affected the body phenotypes of *C. elegans* under high glucose conditions. P-AKK mitigated the fat accumulation induced by a high-glucose diet by regulating key metabolic enzymes, including acyl-CoA synthetase and stearoyl-CoA desaturase.

Keywords: *Akkermansia muciniphila*; postbiotics; *Caenorhabditis elegans*; healthy lifespan; glucolipid metabolism; high-glucose diet

1. Introduction

In recent years, Western eating habits, which are rich in meat and refined sugar, have gradually begun to prevail in China. The narrative must shift away from individual choice to structural factors, as more than half of the global population will be living with overweight or obesity by 2035 if current trends continue, and more than 1.3 billion people worldwide will have diabetes by 2050 [1]. Overconsumption of sugar causes most new cases, fueled by changes in obesity and dietary risk. Therefore, we must pay more attention to diet and health.

The intestine plays a vital role in nutrient digestion and absorption, especially by gut microorganisms. Moreover, the intestinal microbiota is susceptible to dietary nutrients, which subsequently influence metabolic levels in a beneficial manner [2,3]. A study reported that a modified dietary structure has a positive effect on lipid metabolism in obese mice because the abundance of *Akkermansia*, *Lactobacillus*, and other beneficial microbes increases in the gut [4]. *Akkermansia muciniphila* is a promising probiotic candidate that promotes metabolic balance. Compared with individuals with normal glucose tolerance, the abundance of *Akkermansia muciniphila* in the fecal samples of patients with prediabetes was lower, suggesting that there may be a negative correlation between them [5]. In addition, because diabetes and obesity are related to intestinal permeability and low-grade inflammation, *Akkermansia muciniphila* inhibits the occurrence of disease by promoting intestinal microbial diversity and intestinal health by improving healthy mucous layer circulation [6,7]. Even *Akkermansia muciniphila* is expected to become the next generation of probiotics, similar to *Lactobacillus* and *Bifidobacteria*. Dietary probiotic interventions are currently popular means of regulating dietary patterns. For example, oral administration of *Lactobacillus plantarum* Q16 inhibited metabolic disorders of the gut microbiota and improved fat and energy metabolism in mice fed a high-fat diet [8]. Plovier et al. first showed that pasteurized *Akkermansia muciniphila* (P-AKK) augments its beneficial effects on obesity and insulin resistance in HFD-fed mice and that Amuc_1100, a thermostable outer-membrane protein of *A. muciniphila*, recapitulates most of these effects [9,10]. This suggests that *A. muciniphila* retains its biological activity at pasteurization temperatures and exerts beneficial effects. However, it is unclear how P-AKK, as a novel postbiotic, regulates host physiological pathways such as fat distribution and energy homeostasis.

Caenorhabditis elegans is a model organism that feeds on *Escherichia coli* OP50. Bacteria provide essential nutrients for the growth and development of nematodes. Therefore, the *Caenorhabditis elegans* model allows direct changes in the bacterial diet to be used to study its effects on host physiology. In this study, *Caenorhabditis elegans* fed a high-glucose diet was used to investigate the effects of P-AKK on the glycolipid metabolism pathways. Accordingly, we tested the lifespan, glycolipid metabolism-related markers, and behavioral phenotypes of *C. elegans*. To further elucidate the positive effects of P-AKK on glycolipid metabolism, we conducted RNA sequencing and quantitative real-time polymerase chain reaction (PCR) analysis of differentially expressed genes (DEGs) in *C. elegans* induced by P-AKK.

2. Materials and Methods

2.1. Bacterial Culture Conditions and Strains

Akkermansia muciniphila (ATCC BAA-835) was obtained from the American Type Culture Collection (ATCC). The culture and enrichment of *A. muciniphila* and *Escherichia coli* OP50 were performed as described previously [11]. P-AKK was prepared as described previously [12]. Briefly, the *A. muciniphila* concentrate was pasteurized for 30 min at 70 °C. It was then immediately stored at −80 °C until use.

Caenorhabditis elegans and *Escherichia coli* OP50 were originally obtained from the Caenorhabditis Genetics Center (University of Minnesota, MN, USA). N2 Bristol was used as the wild-type strain. *Escherichia coli* OP50 was used as a standard food for *C. elegans*. P-AKK was used as a test food source for *C. elegans*. To explore the physiological changes caused by nematodes under different dietary patterns, nematodes were divided into OP50 and OP50 with 2% glucose, P-AKK, and P-AKK with 2% glucose groups. *C. elegans* were synchronized and normally fed to the L4 stage and then treated with *E. coli* OP50 or P-AKK for 24 h to reach adulthood on nematode growth medium plates with or without glucose.

A high-glucose diet culture plate [13]: Peptone-free modified nematode growth medium (mNGM) was autoclaved at 121 °C for 20 min and then cooled in a 55 °C water bath for 15 min. Glucose water (the final concentration of glucose was 2%) and FUdR (final concentration of 0.12 mM) were added before pouring.

Normal diet culture plates were arranged according to the standardized mNGM protocol without the addition of additional glucose.

2.2. Lifespan Assay

Worms at the L4 stage were transferred to the corresponding treatment plate, and this time was denoted as day 0. For the first seven days, the worms were transferred to fresh mNGM every day, after which they were transferred once per week for the remainder of the experiment to maintain a sufficient food source. Worms were scored daily by strong light exposure or mechanical stimulation with a platinum wire until all animals died. Worms that did not respond were scored as dead. The experiments were performed in triplicate with 20 $\pm$ 5 nematodes per plate. Statistical analysis of lifespan data was performed using Kaplan–Meier analysis.

2.3. Healthy Lifespan: Body Bends/Movements on mNGM Plates

L4 late larvae were transplanted into experimental plates and cultured for 24 h. At this time, the nematodes were 4 days old. Body bend frequency and movement status of 4-, 6-, 8-, 10-, and 12-day-old nematodes were determined.

The body bends and movement of *C. elegans* were defined according to previous methods [14,15].

2.4. Biochemical Assay

For each group, worms were washed from the plates with M9 buffer and transferred to fresh tubes. The worms were then homogenized using an ultrasonic cell crusher. After centrifugation at 8000$\times$ g for 10 min, the supernatants were used for subsequent assays.

Advanced glycosylation end product (AGE) levels were measured according to the manufacturer's instructions (Shanghai Zcibio Technology Co., Ltd., Shanghai, China). Glucose and triglyceride (TG) contents were measured according to the manufacturer's instructions (Solarbio Science and Technology Co., Ltd., Beijing, China), and the protein concentration was quantified using a BCA Protein Assay Kit (Nanjing Jiancheng Bioengineering Institute, Nanjing, China).

2.5. Oil Red O (ORO) Staining of Adipose Tissue

Fat accumulation in *C. elegans* was detected by ORO staining according to a previously described protocol [16]. The ORO stock solution was diluted with deionized water to 60% (v/v) and filtered through a 0.22 µM filter to remove impurities. Nematodes in different groups were completely washed with M9 buffer. Next, 600 µL of 40% isopropanol was used to fix nematodes. Subsequently, the samples were centrifuged at 560$\times$ g for 1 min to obtain *C. elegans*, which was stained with 600 µL of ORO solution for 2 h. After dyeing, the supernatant was removed by centrifugation, and excess floating color was removed by washing with M9 buffer. Cells were photographed under a microscope (Nikon Eclipse E100). The experiments were performed in triplicate. Ten nematodes in each experimental group were photographed. Images were analyzed using the ImageJ 1.52a version software (National Institutes of Health, Bethesda, MD, USA).

2.6. Measurement of Reactive Oxygen Species (ROS)

The assay was performed according to a previously described protocol with slight modifications [17]. Nematodes were collected 24 h after the intervention and completely washed with M9 buffer. The worms were transferred to 0.5 mL M9 buffer containing 5 µM H_2DCFDA and preincubated in protection from light for 3 h at 20 °C. Then, 200 µL per well of M9 buffer with the probe and nematodes (1000 worms) was added to a 96-well plate, and the results were read using a fluorescence microplate reader (Thermo Scientific™ Multiskan™ FC, Waltham, MA, USA) at an excitation wavelength of 485 nm and an emission filter of 535 nm. The quantified ROS levels were expressed as an increase in fluorescence in 2 h.

2.7. Antioxidant Enzyme Assay

Catalase (CAT), glutathione peroxidase (GSH-Px), and superoxide dismutase (SOD) activities were assayed using commercially available kits (Solarbio Science and Technology Co., Ltd., Beijing, China) and were processed according to the manufacturer's instructions. A BCA protein assay kit was used to quantify the protein concentrations in the homogenates of worms.

2.8. Free Fatty Acid Composition Analysis

Total free fatty acids were extracted and methylated as previously described [18]. Fatty acid methyl esters were then injected for gas chromatography/mass spectrometry analysis using an HP-5MS column (30 m × 0.25 mm × 0.25 μm) with helium as the carrier gas. The injector temperature was maintained at 250 °C. The initial temperature was 60 °C, which was increased to 150 °C at 15 °C/min, held for 3 min, increased from 5 °C/min to 195 °C for 5 min, increased from 6 °C/min to 230 °C for 3 min, and finally increased to 260 °C at 3 °C/min. The composition of fatty acids of *C. elegans* was identified by comparing the retention time and mass spectra with the commercial 37-component fatty acid methyl ester mixed standard. The desaturation index was calculated as the ratio of palmitoleic acid to palmitic acid or oleic acid to stearic acid [19].

2.9. Transcriptome Sequencing

Total RNA was extracted using TRIzol reagent at 4 °C, and the quality of the RNA was assessed using NanoDrop™ 2000 (Thermo Fisher Scientific, MA, USA) and RNase-free agarose gel electrophoresis. Total RNA from each sample was subjected to Illumina NovaSeq 6000 (Shanghai Majorbio Biopharm Technology Co., Ltd.) (Shanghai, China). Single-end and paired-end RNA-seq libraries were prepared following Illumina protocols.

The reads obtained from the sequencing machines were subjected to the following processes: filtering of clean reads, alignment with ribosomal RNA, alignment with the reference genome, and quantification of gene abundance. Finally, RNA differential expression analysis was performed using the DESeq2 software between two different groups and by Edger between two samples. Genes with a false discovery rate (FDR) < 0.05 and an absolute fold change ≥ 2 were differentially expressed.

All differentially expressed genes were mapped to Gene Ontology (GO) terms in the Gene Ontology database (http://www.geneontology.org/, accessed on 3 March 2022), and Kyoto Encyclopedia of Genes and Genomes (KEGG) pathway enrichment analyses were subsequently performed to identify significant pathways. The calculated *p*-value was subjected to FDR correction, with FDR ≤ 0.05, as the threshold.

2.10. Quantitative Real-Time PCR

After 24 h of intervention, the nematodes in each group were collected and cleaned using M9 buffer. The main DEGs were validated using real-time quantitative reverse-transcription PCR. Real-time PCR was performed using a HiScript II Q RT SuperMix Kit (Enzyme Biotech Co., Ltd., Beijing, China), and Power SYBR Green PCR Master Mix (Enzyme Biotech Co., Ltd., Beijing, China) was used to perform cDNA synthesis and quantitative PCR according to the manufacturer's protocols. Gene expression levels were calculated using the $2^{-\Delta\Delta CT}$ method and were normalized to β-actin expression [20]. The primer sequences used for qPCR are listed in the Supplementary Material S1.

2.11. Data Analysis

Data are expressed as the mean ± standard deviation. Graphs were generated using Prism 8.0.1 (GraphPad Software, San Diego, CA, USA). The results were analyzed using IBM SPSS Statistics software (version 25.0; IBM, Chicago, IL, USA), followed by one-way analysis of variance (ANOVAs) with Duncan tests for post hoc comparisons among groups. Statistical significance was set at $p < 0.05$. Statistical analysis of variance between two groups was performed using the Student's t-test. Differences were considered significant at $p < 0.05$ (*) and $p < 0.01$ levels (**). mRNA-seq analysis was performed using the online Majorbio Cloud Platform (www.majorbio.com, accessed on 1 December 2022).

3. Results

3.1. Healthy Lifespan of Nematodes Affected by P-AKK Under High Glucose Conditions

The healthy lifespan of nematodes includes the average lifespan, movement speed, and motility status. The results showed that the average lifespan of the OP50 + Glu group was 20.21% shorter than that of the OP50 group. However, the average lifespan of nematodes in the P-AKK group was similar to that of nematodes in the P-AKK + Glu group. However, the average life expectancy of the P-AKK + Glu group was 14.09% longer than that of the OP50 + Glu group. In addition, the longest lifespan of nematodes in the P-AKK + Glu group was 24 days, which was close to that of normally fed nematodes (Figure 1A, Table 1). Hence, the above results suggest that feeding on OP50 could not change the high glucose-induced shortening of the average lifespan of nematodes, but feeding on P-AKK helped to protect the normal lifespan of nematodes.

Table 1. Lifespans of nematodes subjected to different types of bacterial treatments.

Group	Number of Worms	Mean Lifespan (Days)	Maximum Lifespan (Days)	Median (Days)
OP50	63	14.94 ± 0.58 a	23	15.5
OP50 + Glu	68	11.92 ± 0.69 b	19	14.0
P-AKK	68	13.78 ± 0.81 ab	27	14.0
P-AKK + Glu	63	13.60 ± 0.78 ab	24	16.0

Note: Means with different letters in the same column are significantly different ($p < 0.05$).

Motricity is an important indicator of a healthy lifespan, and the exercise speed gradually decreases with increasing nematode age. In all groups, the speed of nematode movement was negatively correlated with age, and physical exercise was slower. The proportion of spontaneous movement of nematodes fed a high-glucose diet was lower, but the proportion of sinusoidal movement of nematodes fed P-AKK was always greater than that of nematodes fed OP50 at different ages (Figure 1B,C). This shows that P-AKK helps to maintain the healthy lifespan of nematodes.

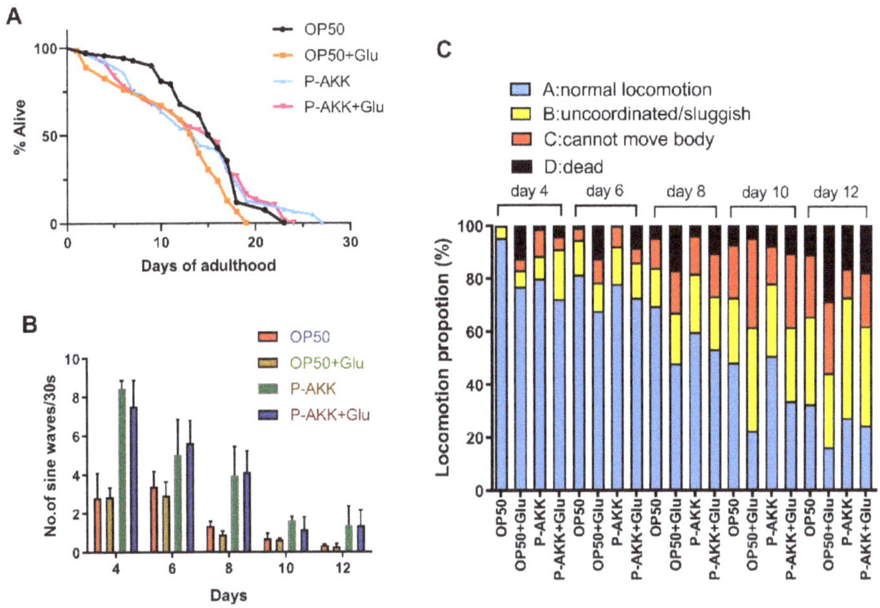

Figure 1. Effect of P-AKK on the healthy lifespan of nematodes under high glucose conditions. (**A**) Lifespan of nematodes (N = 3). (**B**) Nematode body bend frequency There were 10 worms in each group and the experiments were independently repeated three times. (**C**) Movement status of the nematodes. There were 10 worms in each group, and the experiments were independently repeated three times.

3.2. Effects of P-AKK on Biomarkers of Glucose and Lipid Metabolism in Nematodes Under High Glucose Conditions

Glucose is the main energy source and metabolic intermediate of animal cell metabolism; nevertheless, the long-term intake of large amounts of glucose harms cell and tissue function. Excessive carbohydrate intake activates several lipogenic enzymes in the body, leading to lipid metabolism disorders and obesity [21,22]. An imbalance in glucose metabolism leads to the long-term accumulation of methylglyoxal-derived AGEs and the production of ROS in the mitochondria, thus inducing cytotoxicity [23]. Therefore, the glucose, AGEs, and triglyceride contents were measured in nematodes fed a high-glucose diet.

Compared to the OP50 group, the high-glucose diet significantly increased the intracellular glucose concentration, induced the accumulation of AGEs, and increased the triglyceride content in the OP50 + Glu group ($p < 0.05$). The obese phenotype of nematodes was induced by high glucose levels under the OP50 diet. However, the storage of glucose and TG in nematodes fed with P-AKK was lower than that in nematodes fed with OP50. Compared to the OP50 + Glu group, the accumulation of glucose, AGEs, and TG in the P-AKK + Glu group decreased by 36.07%, 14.59%, and 59.33%, respectively ($p < 0.05$) (Figure 2A–C). Moreover, using Oil Red O staining to visualize the lipid droplet distribution in nematodes, it was found that the lipid droplets in nematodes were distributed at a high density in a high-glucose environment, and the number of lipid droplets in P-AKK-fed nematodes was lower than that in nematodes fed OP50 (Figure 2E). These results are consistent with the fat quantification results of Oil Red O staining (Figure 2D).

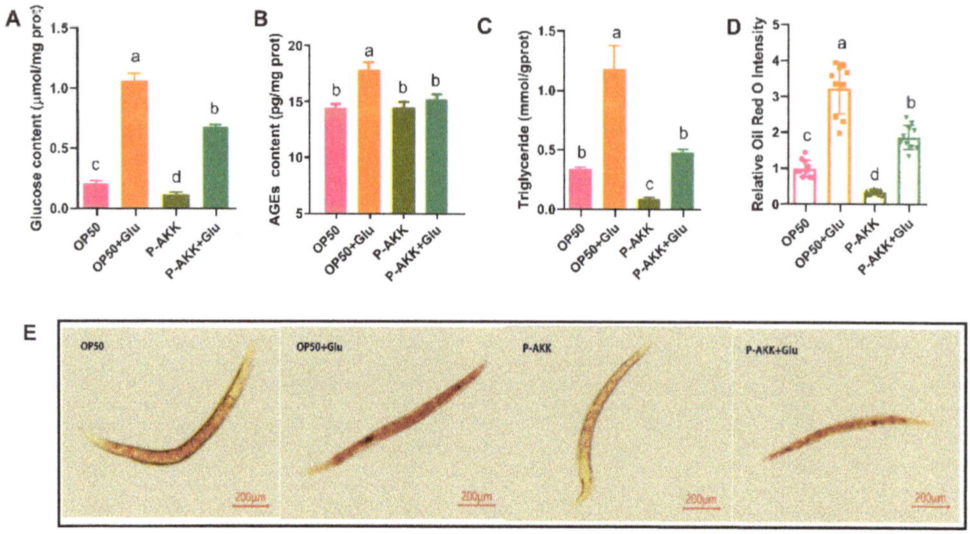

Figure 2. Effect of P-AKK dietary patterns on glucose and lipid accumulation in nematodes. (**A**) Glucose content in nematodes (N = 3); (**B**) AGE content in nematodes (N = 3); (**C**) triglyceride content in nematodes (N = 3); (**D**) quantification of fat content in nematodes stained with Oil Red O using ImageJ. There were 10 worms in each group, and the experiments were independently repeated three times. (**E**) Fat distribution in the nematodes stained with Oil Red O; the scale bar is 200 μm. The results are expressed as the mean ± SD, and *p*-values were calculated using Duncan's test. Different lowercase letters above the bar graphs represent significant differences between groups ($p < 0.05$).

3.3. P-AKK Changed the Level of Free Fatty Acids in Nematodes

The fatty acid composition of the nematodes was dominated by 16-, 18-, and 20-carbon chains. For example, palmitoleic acid (C16:1) and oleic acid (C18:1) are essential substrates for triglyceride biosynthesis [24]. Fatty acid composition is closely related to fat accumulation; therefore, changes in free fatty acids in nematodes were evaluated.

As shown in Figure 3, compared to those in the OP50 group, the contents of SFAs, MUFAs, and PUFAs were significantly higher in the OP50 + Glu group, and the total fatty acid content was also significantly higher ($p < 0.05$). Among them, C16:1 and C18:1 were significantly increased in the OP50 + Glu group and were 8.37 and 1.52 times greater than those in the OP50 group, respectively ($p < 0.05$, Figure 3A). The desaturation index C16:1/C16:0 ratio in the OP50 + Glu group was 2.75-fold higher than that of the OP50 group (Figure 3D). High glucose levels increased the substrate concentration for TG synthesis and promoted the conversion of palmitic acid to palmitic acid, which was helpful for the synthesis and accumulation of TG. Compared with the OP50 diet, feeding P-AKK changed the composition of free fatty acids in nematodes. Even in a high-sugar diet, consuming P-AKK maintained the contents of SFA, MUFA, PUFA, and total free fatty acids in nematodes at a reduced level (Figure 3B,C). The desaturation indices C16:1/C16:0 and C18:1/C18:0 decreased significantly in the P-AKK + Glu group, by 72.18% and 55.93% ($p < 0.05$), respectively, compared with those in the OP50 + Glu group (Figure 3D).

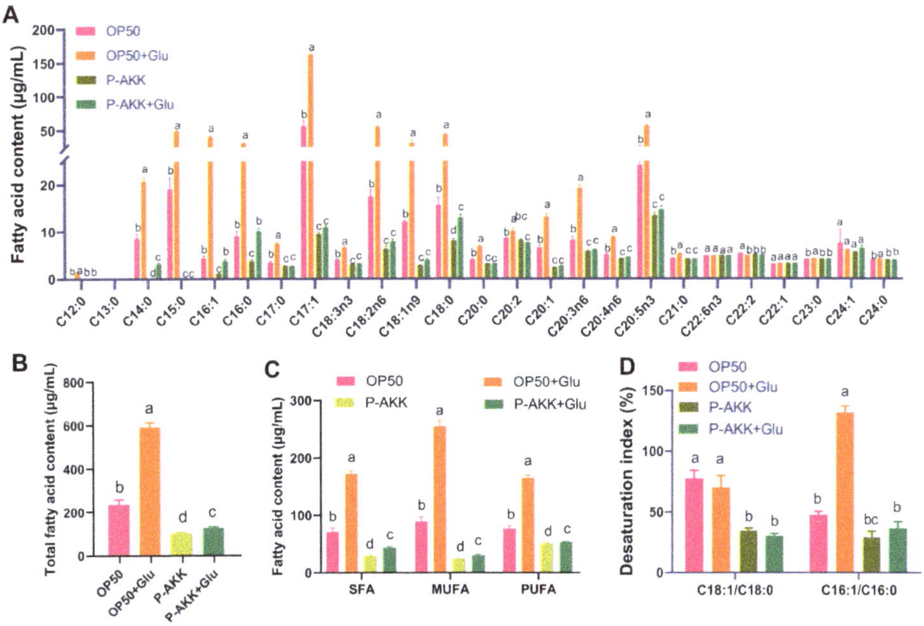

Figure 3. Effects of P-AKK on the free fatty acid composition of nematodes under high glucose conditions. (**A**) The free fatty acid content of nematodes (N = 3); (**B**) total free fatty acid content of nematodes (N = 3); (**C**) SFA, MUFA, and PUFA contents of nematodes (N = 3); (**D**) the desaturation index of nematodes (N = 3). The results are expressed as mean ± SD, and p-values were calculated using Duncan's test. Significant differences between groups are indicated by different letters ($p < 0.05$).

3.4. Effects of P-AKK on the Intracellular ROS Level of Nematodes Under High Glucose Conditions

Adipose factors induce ROS production and oxidative stress, which causes lipid membrane oxidation and leads to the gradual accumulation of fat [25,26]. Thus, mitochondrial dysfunction directly affects the efficiency of glucose and lipid metabolism; however, restoring mitochondrial activity may be beneficial for preventing obesity [27].

Intracellular ROS levels were evaluated using the fluorescent probe, H_2DCFDA. Based on OP50 dietary patterns, a high-glucose diet induces ROS accumulation in nematodes. However, when the nematode was fed P-AKK, the amount of ROS in the body was low, even under high glucose conditions, and the intracellular ROS level was consistent with the normal level. Additionally, compared with the OP50 + Glu group, the ROS level in the P-AKK + Glu group decreased by 17.67% (Figure 4). The results showed that P-AKK reduced intracellular ROS levels in nematodes fed a high-glucose diet.

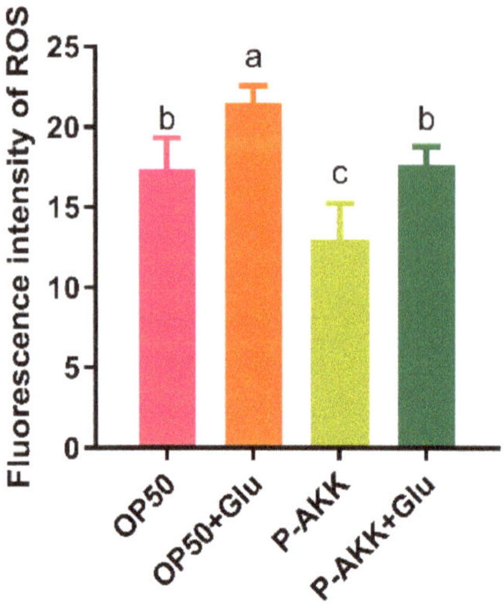

Figure 4. Effect of P-AKK on ROS levels in nematodes. The results are expressed as mean ± SD (N = 3,1,000 worms in each independent experiment), and p-values were calculated using Duncan's test. Significant differences between groups are indicated by different letters (a–c) ($p < 0.05$).

3.5. Effects of P-AKK on the Antioxidant Activity of Nematodes Under High Glucose

Figure 5 results showed that compared with the OP50 group, the CAT activity significantly increased by 25.79%, and the SOD activity significantly increased by 72.75%, but the GSH-Px activity decreased in the OP50 + Glu group ($p < 0.05$). OP50 intake may induce oxidative stress and lead to a secondary increase in CAT activity in nematodes fed a high-glucose diet. However, the CAT activity of nematodes fed P-AKK did not change significantly, even under a high-glucose diet, which could not stimulate oxidative stress. Moreover, the CAT activity of nematodes in the P-AKK + Glu group was lower than that in the OP50 + Glu group, but the GSH-Px activity significantly increased ($p < 0.05$). Therefore, P-AKK may suppress oxidative stress by decreasing CAT activity and enhancing GSH-Px activity in worms.

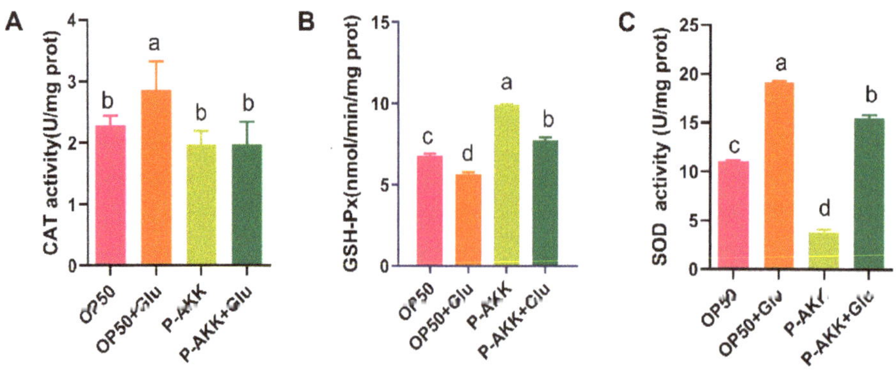

Figure 5. Levels of antioxidant enzymes in nematodes. (**A**) CAT activity level (N = 3); (**B**) GSH-PX activity level (N = 3); and (**C**) SOD activity level (N = 3). The results are expressed as the mean ± SD, and p-values were calculated by Duncan's test. Significant differences between groups are expressed by different letters ($p < 0.05$).

3.6. Effects of P-AKK on Lipid Metabolism in Nematodes According to Gene Expression Profiles Under High Glucose Conditions

3.6.1. Identification of DEGs

Based on the phenotypic data from the above experiments, high-throughput sequencing was used for the systematic analysis of gene expression to further understand the physiological effects and mechanisms of different dietary patterns on nematodes. A rigorous comparison at adjusted $p \leq 0.05$ and log2FC fold change ≥ 2 was performed to identify the number of DEGs for different groups (Figure 6). Through pairwise comparison, it was found that there were 2234 DEGs in the OP50 + Glu group compared with the OP50 group, of which 787 genes were downregulated and 1447 genes were upregulated. Compared to those in the OP50 + Glu group, there were 3300 DEGs in the P-AKK + Glu group, of which 1454 genes were downregulated and 1846 genes were upregulated. A total of 644 DEGs were obtained in the P-AKK + Glu group compared to the P-AKK group, of which 410 genes were downregulated and 234 genes were upregulated. These results indicated that feeding P-AKK significantly influenced the transcription of genes related to high glucose levels in nematodes.

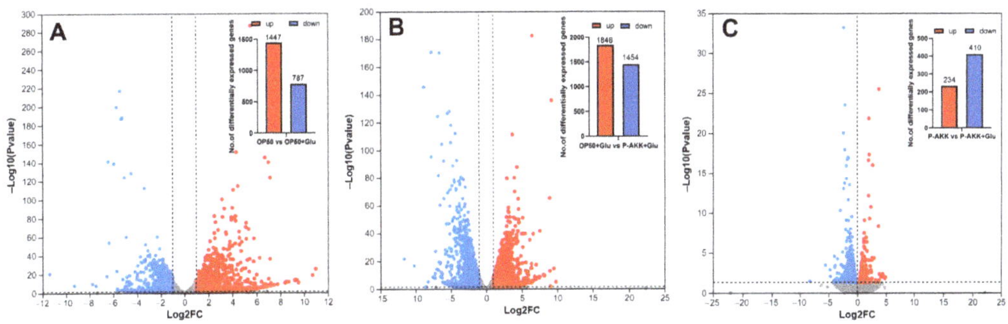

Figure 6. Scatter plot and statistical chart of differentially expressed genes in nematodes in different treatment groups. (**A**) OP50 vs. OP50 + Glu, (**B**) OP50 + Glu vs. P-AKK + Glu, (**C**) P-AKK vs. P-AKK + Glu. Note: The abscissa is the difference in the expression of the gene/transcript between the two samples; that is, the expression of the treatment sample was divided by the expression of the control sample, and the ordinate is the statistical test value of the difference in gene expression, namely, the p-value (N = 3).

Using iPath3.0 software (http://pathways.embl.de, accessed on 3 March 2022) to visually analyze the metabolic pathways associated with these DEGs, we determined which metabolic pathway was most affected. The results showed that the metabolic pathway was mainly involved in lipid and carbohydrate metabolism (Supplementary Material S2). This may be related to nematode feeding with high glucose levels, which induce a positive response to carbohydrate and lipid metabolism.

3.6.2. Functional Prediction of DEGs Induced by P-AKK in the High-Glucose Diet

To explore the physiological regulatory effects of P-AKK on nematodes fed a high-glucose diet, pairwise comparisons were made between the P-AKK + Glu group and the OP50 + Glu group. The corresponding functional set information was obtained from the Gene Ontology (GO) database, and the importance of this functional set to DEGs was calculated. Figure 7 shows the top 20 ranked GO terms for the DEGs. Carbohydrate metabolism had the strongest degree of enrichment, followed by oxidative phosphorylation and fatty acid metabolism. These significantly enriched biological processes were closely related to glucose and lipid metabolism, indicating that P-AKK ingestion by nematodes significantly affected the biological processes of energy metabolism.

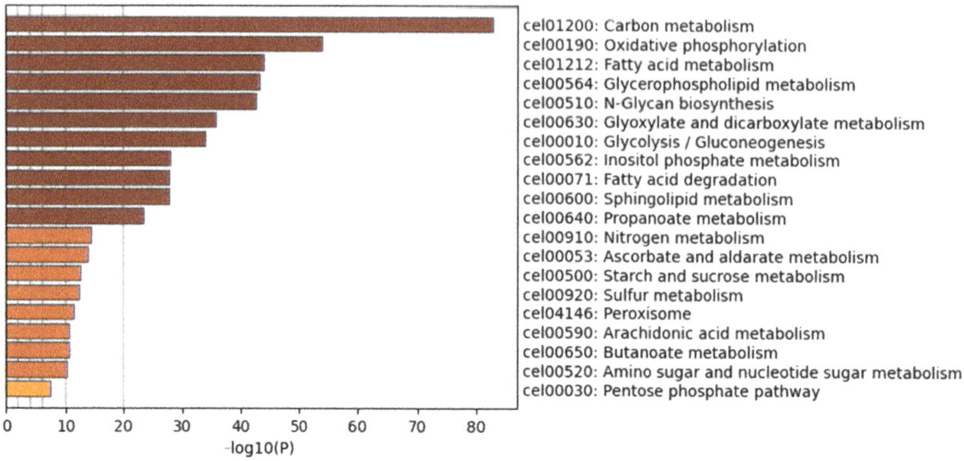

Figure 7. Histogram of the top 20 ranked GO terms of DEGs.

3.6.3. KEGG Pathway Analysis

Pathway analysis helps elucidate the biological functions of genes. By analyzing the KEGG pathways of the DEGs between the two groups, 266 typical pathways of significant enrichment were identified, of which 90 pathways showed the most significant difference ($p < 0.01$). Figure 8 shows the first 20 pathways of significant enrichment using a bubble chart. The results showed that the metabolic pathway of oxidative phosphorylation had the highest enrichment degree (enrichment factor of 0.97), followed by the TCA cycle pathway (enrichment factor of 0.95). In addition, the pathways of glycerol phospholipid metabolism, glycolysis/gluconeogenesis, fatty acid degradation, glyoxylic acid and dicarboxylic acid metabolism, and pyruvate metabolism were also significantly enriched, and these pathways were directly related to glucose and lipid metabolism. Among these pathways, P-AKK upregulated the glycolysis/gluconeogenesis pathway, glyoxylate and dicarboxylate metabolism pathway, and fatty acid degradation pathway, and downregulated the citrate cycle and fatty acid biosynthesis (Supplementary Material S3). Consequently, it can be speculated that one underlying mechanism by which P-AKK improves high-glucose-induced glycolipid metabolism is the regulation of dietary energy intake.

3.7. qPCR Validation of Differentially Expressed Genes

To verify the changes in key genes regulated by P-AKK, several DEGs, including *pmt-1*, *lipl-4*, *sodh-1*, *ech-8*, *icl-1*, *elo-6*, *fat-7*, *acox-3*, *hacd-1*, and *acs-2*, were selected for qPCR verification. These detection results were consistent with those of RNA-seq. Compared with that in OP50 + Glu, *fat-7* gene expression significantly decreased by 74.79%, *acs-2* gene expression significantly increased by 12.08 times, *lipl-4* gene expression increased by 20.05-fold, *icl-1* gene expression increased by 46.18-fold, and *acox-3* gene expression increased by 13.59-fold ($p < 0.01$, Figure 9). These results were in accordance with those of the phenotype experiments.

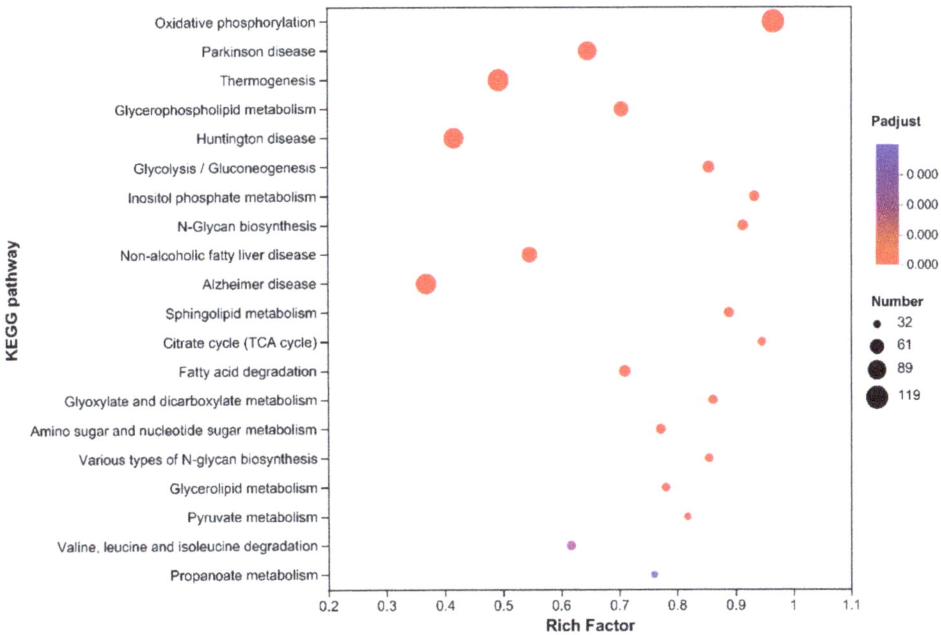

Figure 8. Bubble diagram of KEGG pathways.

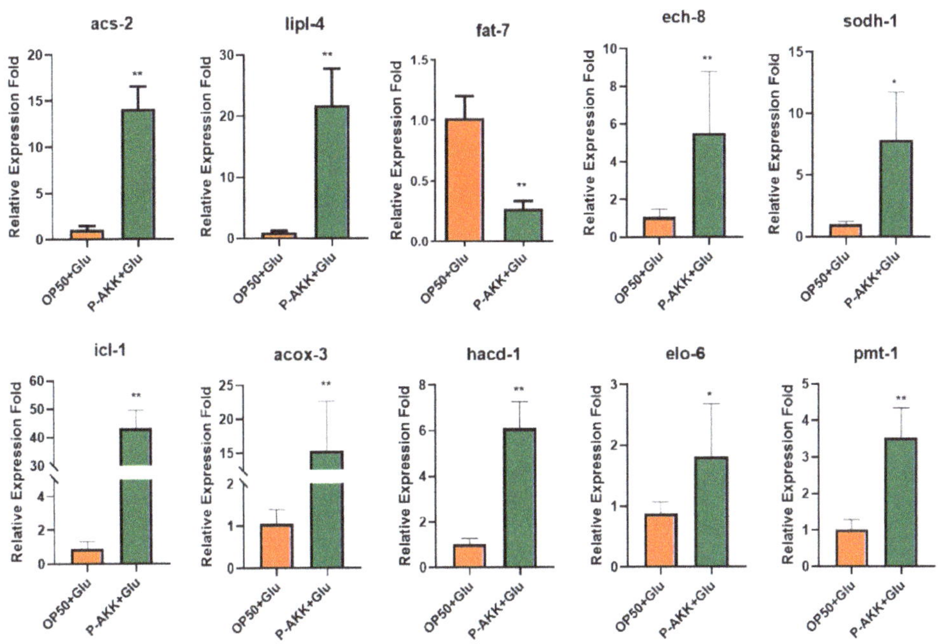

Figure 9. Effects of P-AKK on DEGs in *C. elegans* fed a high-glucose diet (n = 3). All data are expressed as mean ± standard deviation relative to the OP50 + Glu group. * $p < 0.05$, ** $p < 0.01$.

4. Discussion

In the present study, nematodes fed P-AKK exhibited better physiological phenotypes. The P-AKK diet improved the lifespan and mobility of *C. elegans* induced by a high-glucose diet. In addition, P-AKK intake regulated intracellular glucose concentration and AGE accumulation in a high-glucose diet, especially by decreasing triglyceride content and fat distribution density. Using RNA-seq to determine the whole gene expression profile of *C. elegans*, we found that feeding nematodes P-AKK significantly affected lipid metabolism by regulating the glucose metabolism pathway. Unlike our prior work demonstrating the nutritional adequacy of P-AKK under a standard diet [11], the current study establishes its therapeutic potential in counteracting glucose-induced metabolic dysregulation.

A diet of P-AKK is more beneficial to the healthy lifespan of *C. elegans*. In *C. elegans*, high glucose levels play a harmful role by increasing ROS production, TG accumulation, and AGE formation [28]. The lifespan of nematodes is shortened, and the level of oxidative stress increases after exposure to high concentrations of glucose [29]. In this study, the lifespan of nematodes fed P-AKK did not decrease in response to high glucose, and P-AKK protected them from a healthy lifespan (including motoricity) in a high-glucose environment. Furthermore, P-AKK reduced ROS levels and cytotoxicity by enhancing the activity of GSH-PX. ROS can easily cause DNA damage, and the accumulation of damage accelerates aging and affects healthy lifespan. Nevertheless, P-AKK can enhance the motoricity of nematodes to increase metabolic flux and the activity of antioxidant enzymes to eliminate excessive ROS and reduce the damage caused by a high-glucose diet. This explanation is supported by Xiong et al. [30]. It functions similar to oral *Pediococcus acidilactici* in that it decreases ROS levels, increases nematode longevity, and indirectly regulates lipid metabolism in vivo [31]. As a result, P-AKK consumption in nematodes benefits their healthy lifespan by preventing mitochondrial dysfunction and enhancing cell metabolic flux.

The P-AKK diet improved the glucose and lipid metabolism in nematodes. Excessive dietary sugar has been reported to weaken the insulin sensitivity of cells, resulting in a decrease in glucose uptake and an increase in glucose concentration in systemic circulation, whereas hyperglycemia induces protein glycosylation and causes cytotoxicity, which has a negative effect on protein, tissue, and organ function [32]. However, the intake of P-AKK helps nematodes to inhibit the stress toxicity of glucose and the cytotoxicity of AGEs under a high-glucose diet. This may be related to a decrease in glucose absorption by P-AKK [33]. Excessive glucose intake may upset the balance of fatty acids in the body, resulting in metabolic and cellular changes [34]. In this study, high glucose induced an overall increase in free fatty acids in nematodes and promoted the transformation of palmitic acid to palmitic acid, resulting in the accumulation of TG. However, the dietary intake of P-AKK could improve this high-glucose response, inhibit fatty acid desaturation, and reduce nematode fat accumulation. The quantitative results of Oil Red O staining also supported this conclusion.

According to the results of RNA-seq analysis, P-AKK not only has a regulatory effect on the carbohydrate metabolism pathway but also significantly affects the transcription of genes involved in lipid metabolism. P-AKK upregulated pathways involved in fatty acid degradation and glyoxylate and dicarboxylate metabolism and downregulated the de novo fat synthesis pathway. Therefore, it was speculated that P-AKK enhanced cell metabolic activity and significantly regulated lipid metabolism. P-AKK decreased the level of ROS and upregulated the fatty acid degradation pathway, which caused nematodes to maintain very low-fat storage, which may be related to fatty acid β-oxidation. In this study, nematode feeding on P-AKK significantly promoted the transcription of *lipl-4* and *acs-2* genes in the biological process of fatty acid β-oxidation under high-glucose conditions.

Lipl-4 encodes lipase, and increased lipase expression indicates increased lipid hydrolysis. In addition, LIPL-4 lipases mediate specific lysosomal signals and induce redox reactions in nematode mitochondria, thereby reducing lipid storage [35]. *Acs-2,* which encodes a fatty acid CoA synthetase, is the key target that induces fatty acid β-oxidation, and its upregulated expression could indicate enhanced fatty acid β-oxidation. Therefore, the synergistic effect of *lipl-4* and *acs-2* contributes to β-oxidation of fatty acids in nematodes. Additionally, the overexpression of *acs-2* causes *C. elegans* to be in a low-fat state [36]. Moreover, P-AKK significantly upregulated genes downstream of fatty acid β-oxidation, such as *ech-8* and *sodh-1,* indicating that P-AKK promotes the fatty acid β-oxidation pathway. Additionally, P-AKK significantly downregulated *fat-7* expression. *Fat-7* encodes stearoyl-CoA desaturase (SCD), which is the key enzyme for the conversion of palmitic acid and stearic acid to palmitic acid and oleic acid, respectively [37]. Glucose generates palmitic acid during lipid de novo synthesis and then upregulates SCD, causing palmitic acid to generate palmitoleic acid. This may be one of the mechanisms by which carbohydrate intake leads to an increase in palmitoleic acid in the body [38]. Therefore, we speculate that to counteract the excessive fat storage caused by a high-glucose diet, P-AKK may improve the health of nematodes by enhancing their ability to exercise, promoting β-oxidation of fatty acids, and maintaining a low-energy state. Another assumption is that there is a difference in the energy metabolism between OP50 and inactivated AKK because of the metabolic cycle capacity of living bacteria. The eating pattern of P-AKK is similar to that of a low-calorie diet, in which foods contain fewer calories while ensuring adequate dietary intake. Overall, the intake of P-AKK by nematodes is a healthier dietary mode that helps nematodes to stay low in fat. However, these speculations require further investigation.

5. Conclusions

In summary, the administration of P-AKK had a positive effect on the body phenotypes of *C. elegans* under high glucose conditions. Consumption of P-AKK enhanced motor activity, which decreased with age and protected the healthy lifespan of nematodes fed a high-glucose diet. P-AKK has strong metabolic activity and decreases the accumulation of glucose, AGEs, and TG in vivo. These effects result from a combination of key enzymes involved in fatty acid synthesis and oxidation processes. Among these, acyl-CoA synthetase and stearoyl-CoA desaturase play significant roles. Thus, P-AKK may be a potential postbiotic that can be used as a dietary supplement to change the dietary structure and improve fatty acid metabolism.

Supplementary Materials: The following supporting information can be downloaded at: https://www.mdpi.com/article/10.3390/nu17060976/s1, Supplementary Material S1 Primer sequences. Supplementary Material S2. Metabolic pathway map of the nematodes. Supplementary Material S3. P-AKK + Glu and OP50 + Glu groups pairwise compared differential genes in the glucose and lipid metabolism pathways. All authors have read and agreed to the published version of the manuscript.

Author Contributions: Conceptualization, Z.W.; Methodology, Z.W.; Software, A.H.; Formal analysis, Z.W.; Investigation, Z.W.; Resources, K.L.; Data curation, K.L. and Y.W.; Writing—original draft, Z.W.; Writing—review & editing, Z.L.; Visualization, A.H. and Y.W.; Supervision, Z.L.; Funding acquisition, Z.L. All authors have read and agreed to the published version of the manuscript.

Funding: This research was supported by "Hunan Natural Science Foundation Program" (Project No.2025JJ80342), and "Project support of the Hunan Province Agricultural Industry Technology System (2022-67)" funded by the Hunan Provincial Science and Technology Department, China.

Institutional Review Board Statement: Not applicable to this study.

Informed Consent Statement: Not applicable to this study.

Data Availability Statement: The authors confirm that the data supporting the findings of this study are available in the article and its Supplementary Materials.

Conflicts of Interest: The authors declare that they have no conflicts of interest.

References

1. Ladher, N.; Hinton, R.; Veitch, E. Challenges of obesity and type 2 diabetes require more attention to food environment. *BMJ* **2023**, *383*, p2269. [CrossRef]
2. Turnbaugh, P.J.; Ridaura, V.K.; Faith, J.J.; Rey, F.E.; Knight, R.; Gordon, J.I. The Effect of Diet on the Human Gut Microbiome: A Metagenomic Analysis in Humanized Gnotobiotic Mice. *Sci. Transl. Med.* **2009**, *1*, 6ra14. [CrossRef] [PubMed]
3. Zhou, Y.; Lu, H.; Zhao, S.; Yan, B.; Wang, H.; Zhou, X.; Xiao, Y. The beneficial effects of Tartary buckwheat (Fagopyrum tataricum Gaertn.) on diet-induced obesity in mice are related to the modulation of gut microbiota composition. *Food Sci. Hum. Wellness* **2023**, *12*, 1323–1330. [CrossRef]
4. Hussain, K.; Yang, Y.; Wang, J.; Bian, H.; Lei, X.; Chen, J.; Li, Q.; Wang, L.; Zhong, Q.; Fang, X. Comparative study on the weight loss and lipid metabolism by tea polyphenols in diet induced obese C57BL/6J pseudo germ free and conventionalized mice. *Food Sci. Hum. Wellness* **2022**, *11*, 697–710. [CrossRef]
5. Zhang, X.; Shen, D.; Fang, Z.; Jie, Z.; Qiu, X.; Zhang, C.; Chen, Y.; Ji, L. Human Gut Microbiota Changes Reveal the Progression of Glucose Intolerance. *PLoS ONE* **2013**, *8*, e71108. [CrossRef]
6. Reunanen, J.; Kainulainen, V.; Huuskonen, L.; Ottman, N.; Belzer, C.; Huhtinen, H.; de Vos, W.M.; Satokari, R. *Akkermansia muciniphila* Adheres to Enterocytes and Strengthens the Integrity of the Epithelial Cell Layer. *Appl. Env. Microbiol.* **2015**, *81*, 3655–3662. [CrossRef]
7. Rg, A.; Envelope, E.; Envelope, M.; Wmhl, D.; Mao, B.; Ma, E.; Myf, G.; Hk, B.; Rh, A.; Sb, H. The metabolic, protective, and immune functions of *Akkermansia muciniphila*. *Microbiol. Res.* **2023**, *266*, 127245. [CrossRef]
8. Tang, C.; Zhou, W.; Shan, M.; Lu, Z.; Lu, Y. Yogurt-derived *Lactobacillus plantarum* Q16 alleviated high-fat diet-induced non-alcoholic fatty liver disease in mice. *Food Sci. Hum. Wellness* **2022**, *11*, 1428–1439. [CrossRef]
9. Plovier, H.; Everard, A.; Druart, C.; Depommier, C.; Van Hul, M.; Geurts, L.; Chilloux, J.; Ottman, N.; Duparc, T.; Lichtenstein, L.; et al. A purified membrane protein from *Akkermansia muciniphila* or the pasteurized bacterium improves metabolism in obese and diabetic mice. *Nat. Med.* **2017**, *23*, 107–113. [CrossRef]
10. Wang, L.J.; Tang, L.; Feng, Y.M.; Zhao, S.Y.; Han, M.; Zhang, C.; Yuan, G.H.; Zhu, J.; Cao, S.Y.; Wu, Q.; et al. A purified membrane protein from *Akkermansia muciniphila* or the pasteurised bacterium blunts colitis associated tumourigenesis by modulation of CD8+T cells in mice. *Gut* **2020**, *69*, 1988–1997. [CrossRef]
11. Wu, Z.; Xiao, Y.; Zhou, F.; Chen, J.; Chen, X.; Hou, A.; Wang, Y.; Li, Z. Pasteurized *Akkermansia muciniphila* Reduces Fat Accumulation via nhr-49-Mediated Nuclear Hormone Signaling Pathway in *Caenorhabditis elegans*. *Molecules* **2022**, *27*, 6159. [CrossRef] [PubMed]
12. Liu, J.; Liu, H.; Liu, H.; Teng, Y.; Qin, N.; Ren, X.; Xia, X. Live and pasteurized *Akkermansia muciniphila* decrease susceptibility to Salmonella Typhimurium infection in mice. *J. Adv. Res.* **2023**, *52*, 89–102. [CrossRef] [PubMed]
13. Lee, D.; Jeong, D.E.; Son, H.G.; Yamaoka, Y.; Lee, S.J.V. SREBP and MDT-15 protect *C. elegans* from glucose-induced accelerated aging by preventing accumulation of saturated fat. *Genes. Dev.* **2015**, *29*, 2490–2503. [CrossRef] [PubMed]
14. Kwon, G.; Lee, J.; Lim, Y.H. Dairy Propionibacterium extends the mean lifespan of *Caenorhabditis elegans* via activation of the innate immune system. *Sci. Rep.* **2016**, *6*, 31713. [CrossRef]
15. Bai, J.; Zhu, Y.; Li, J.; Zhang, Y.; Dong, Y.; Xiao, X. Effects of Bitter Melon Saponin on the Glucose and Lipid Metabolism in HepG2 Cell and *C. elegans*. *J. Food Qual.* **2020**, *2020*, 8860356. [CrossRef]
16. Zhao, L.; Wu, B.; Liang, S.; Min, D.; Jiang, H. Insight of Silkworm Pupa Oil Regulating Oxidative Stress and Lipid Metabolism in *Caenorhabditis elegans*. *Foods* **2022**, *11*, 4084. [CrossRef]
17. Carranza, A.D.V.; Saragusti, A.; Chiabrando, G.A.; Carrari, F.; Asis, R. Effects of chlorogenic acid on thermal stress tolerance in *C. elegans* via HIF-1, HSF-1 and autophagy. *Phytomedicine* **2020**, *66*, 153132. [CrossRef]
18. Gu, M.; Werlinger, P.; Cho, J.-H.; Jang, N.; Choi, S.S.; Suh, J.-W.; Cheng, J. Lactobacillus pentosus MJM60383 Inhibits Lipid Accumulation in Caenorhabditis elegans Induced by Enterobacter cloacae and Glucose. *Int. J. Mol. Sci.* **2023**, *24*, 280. [CrossRef]
19. Yue, Y.; Shen, P.; Chang, A.L.; Qi, W.; Kim, K.H.; Kim, D.; Park, Y. trans-Trismethoxy resveratrol decreased fat accumulation dependent on *fat-6* and *fat-7* in *Caenorhabditis elegans*. *Food Funct.* **2019**, *10*, 4966–4974. [CrossRef]
20. Xiao, X.; Tan, C.; Sun, X.; Zhao, Y.; Zhou, X. Fermented Barley β-lucan Regulates Fat Deposition in *Caenorhabditis elegans*. *J. Sci. Food Agric.* **2020**, *100*, 3408–3417. [CrossRef]
21. Marcela, S.-G.; Martha, R.C.; Escalona-Cardoso, G.N.; Norma, P.C. Evaluation of Hypoglycemic and Genotoxic Effect of Polyphenolic Bark Extract from Quercus sideroxyla. *Evid. -Based Complement. Altern. Med.* **2016**, *2016*, 4032618. [CrossRef]

22. Mota, M.; Banini, B.A.; Cazanave, S.C.; Sanyal, A.J. Molecular mechanisms of lipotoxicity and glucotoxicity in nonalcoholic fatty liver disease. *Metabolism* **2016**, *65*, 1049–1061. [CrossRef] [PubMed]
23. Richard, J.P. Mechanism for the formation of methylglyoxal from triosephosphates. *Biochem. Soc. Trans.* **1993**, *21*, 549–553. [CrossRef] [PubMed]
24. Srinivasan, S. Regulation of body fat in *Caenorhabditis elegans*. *Annu. Rev. Physiol.* **2015**, *77*, 161–178. [CrossRef]
25. Fernández-Sánchez, A.; Madrigal-Santillán, E.; Bautista, M.; Esquivel-Soto, J.; Morales-González, Á.; Esquivel-Chirino, C.; Durante-Montiel, I.; Sánchez-Rivera, G.; Valadez-Vega, C.; Morales-González, J. Inflammation, Oxidative Stress, and Obesity. *Int. J. Mol. Sci.* **2011**, *12*, 3117–3132. [CrossRef]
26. Ahmad, S. Oxidative stress from environmental pollutants. *Arch. Insect Biochem. Physiol.* **1995**, *29*, 135–157. [CrossRef]
27. Laurent, D.; Yerby, B.; Deacon, R.; Gao, J. Diet-induced modulation of mitochondrial activity in rat muscle. *Am. J. Physiol. Endocrinol. Metab.* **2007**, *293*, E1169–E1177. [CrossRef]
28. Mondoux, M.A.; Love, D.C.; Ghosh, S.K.; Fukushige, T.; Bond, M.; Weerasinghe, G.R.; Hanover, J.A.; Krause, M.W. O-Linked-N-Acetylglucosamine Cycling and Insulin Signaling Are Required for the Glucose Stress Response in *Caenorhabditis Elegans*. *Genet* **2011**, *188*, 369–382. [CrossRef]
29. Zhu, G.; Yin, F.; Wang, L.; Wei, W.; Jiang, L.; Qin, J. Modeling type 2 diabetes-like hyperglycemia in *C. elegans* on a microdevice. *Integr. Biol.* **2016**, *8*, 30–38. [CrossRef]
30. Xiong, L.-G.; Pan, L.-Y.; Gong, Y.-S.; Huang, J.-A.; Liu, Z.-H. Fuzhuan Tea protects *Caenorhabditis elegans* from glucose and advanced glycation end products via distinct pathways. *J. Funct. Foods* **2019**, *59*, 148–155. [CrossRef]
31. Hu, R.; Zhang, Y.; Qian, W.; Leng, Y.; Long, Y.; Liu, X.; Li, J.; Wan, X.; Wei, X. Pediococcus acidilactici Promotes the Longevity of *C. elegans* by Regulating the Insulin/IGF-1 and JNK/MAPK Signaling, Fat Accumulation and Chloride Ion. *Front. Nutr.* **2022**, *9*, 821685. [CrossRef] [PubMed]
32. Svensk, E.; Devkota, R.; Stahlman, M.; Ranji, P.; Rauthan, M.; Magnusson, F.; Hammarsten, S.; Johansson, M.; Boren, J.; Pilon, M. *Caenorhabditis elegans* PAQR-2 and IGLR-2 Protect against Glucose Toxicity by Modulating Membrane Lipid Composition. *PLoS Genet.* **2016**, *12*, e1005982. [CrossRef]
33. Depommier, C.; Van Hul, M.; Everard, A.; Delzenne, N.M.; De Vos, W.M.; Cani, P.D. Pasteurized *Akkermansia muciniphila* increases whole-body energy expenditure and fecal energy excretion in diet-induced obese mice. *Gut Microbes* **2020**, *11*, 1231–1245. [CrossRef] [PubMed]
34. Garcia, A.M.; Ladage, M.L.; Dumesnil, D.R.; Zaman, K.; Shulaev, V.; Azad, R.K.; Padilla, P.A. Glucose induces sensitivity to oxygen deprivation and modulates insulin/IGF-1 signaling and lipid biosynthesis in *Caenorhabditis elegans*. *Genetics* **2015**, *200*, 167–184. [CrossRef]
35. Ramachandran, P.V.; Savini, M.; Folick, A.K.; Hu, K.; Wang, M.C. Lysosomal Signaling Promotes Longevity by Adjusting Mitochondrial Activity. *Dev. Cell* **2019**, *48*, 685–696. [CrossRef]
36. Zhou, X.; Li, J.; Zhang, X.; Zhang, C.; Bai, J.; Zhao, Y.; Zhu, Y.; Zhang, J.; Xiao, X. Bisphenol S promotes fat storage in multiple generations of *Caenorhabditis elegans* in a daf-16/nhr-49 dependent manner. *Comp. Biochem. Physiol. C Toxicol. Pharmacol.* **2021**, *250*, 109175. [CrossRef]
37. He, B.; Zhang, J.; Wang, Y.; Li, Y.; Zou, X.; Liang, B. Identification of cytochrome *b5* CYTB-5.1 and CYTB-5.2 in *C. elegans*; evidence for differential regulation of SCD. *Biochim. Biophys. Acta* **2017**, *1863*, 235–246. [CrossRef]
38. Landry, F.; Chan, C.C.; Huang, Z.; Leclair, G.; Bateman, K. Plasma-based approach to measure target engagement for liver-targeting stearoyl-CoA desaturase 1 inhibitors. *J. Lipid Res.* **2011**, *52*, 1494–1499. [CrossRef]

nutrients MDPI

Article

Psychobiotics Ameliorate Depression and Anxiety Status in Surgical Oncology Patients: Results from the *ProDeCa* Study

Georgios Tzikos [1], Eleni Chamalidou [2], Dimitra Christopoulou [1], Aikaterini Apostolopoulou [3], Sofia Gkarmiri [3], Marianthi Pertsikapa [3], Alexandra-Eleftheria Menni [1], Ioannis M. Theodorou [4], George Stavrou [5], Nektaria-Dimitra Doutsini [1], Anne D. Shrewsbury [1], Theodosios Papavramidis [1], Joulia K. Tsetis [6], Helen Theodorou [7], Anastasia Konsta [8] and Katerina Kotzampassi [1,*]

1 Department of Surgery, Aristotle University of Thessaloniki, 54636 Thessaloniki, Greece; gtziko@auth.gr (G.T.); dimitraxristopoulou9@gmail.com (D.C.); alexmenn@auth.gr (A.-E.M.); nektariadout@gmail.com (N.-D.D.); a_shrewsbury@yahoo.com (A.D.S.); tpapavra@auth.gr (T.P.)
2 Outpatient Surgical Oncology Unit, Chemotherapy Department, AHEPA University Hospital, Aristotle University of Thessaloniki, 54636 Thessaloniki, Greece; eleniham@gmail.com
3 Department of Emergency Medicine, AHEPA University Hospital, Aristotle University of Thessaloniki, 54636 Thessaloniki, Greece; aapostod@auth.gr (A.A.); sgkarmi@auth.gr (S.G.); marianpertsis@gmail.com (M.P.)
4 Hellenic Institute for the Study of Sepsis (HISS), 11528 Athens, Greece; itheodorou@med.uoa.gr
5 Department of Surgery, 417 NIMTS (Army Share Fund Hospital), 11521 Athens, Greece; stavgd@gmail.com
6 Uni-Pharma S.A., 14564 Athens, Greece; jtsetis@uni-pharma.gr
7 Department of Sociology, School of Social Sciences, University of Crete, 74100 Rethymno, Greece; psy5057@psy.soc.uoc.gr
8 First Department of Psychiatry, "Papageorgiou" General Hospital of Thessaloniki, Aristotle University of Thessaloniki, 54124 Thessaloniki, Greece; konstaa@auth.gr
* Correspondence: kakothe@yahoo.com

Abstract: Background: Psychological disorders are prevalent in patients having undergone gastrointestinal cancer surgery, and their emotional status may further deteriorate during subsequent chemotherapy. Psychobiotics are specific probiotics that have the unique characteristics of producing neuroactive substances that are thought to act on the brain–gut axis. The aim of the present study was to evaluate the benefits of a psychobiotic formula on depression and anxiety status, as well as on perceived stress, versus a placebo in patients on a chemotherapy course following gastrointestinal surgery for cancer. **Patients**: The enrolled patients, allocated to the psychobiotic and placebo groups, were assessed by means of these psychometric tests: Beck's Depression Inventory and the Hamilton Depression Rating 17-item Scale for depression; the General Anxiety Disorder-7 for anxiety; and the Perceived Stress Scale-14 Item for perceived stress at three time-points: upon allocation [T1], after one month of treatment [T2], and two months thereafter [T3]. **Results**: In total, 266 patients were included. One month of psychobiotic treatment improved [i] depression status by 60.4% [48 depressed patients at T1, reduced to 16 at T3]; [ii] anxiety by 57.0% [72 patients at T1, 26 at T3]; and [iii] stress by 60.4% [42 at T1, 14 at T3]. The placebo-treated patients experienced a deterioration in all parameters studied, i.e., depression increased by 62.9%, anxiety by 39.7%, and stress by 142.5%. **Conclusions**: Based on these findings, it can be recognized that psychobiotic treatment has great potential for every patient at risk of suffering from depression, anxiety, or stress during the course of surgery/chemotherapy for gastrointestinal cancer.

Keywords: psychobiotics; depression; anxiety; insomnia; perceived stress; surgical oncology; chemotherapy; gastrointestinal cancer

1. Introduction

Cancer diagnosis is a stressful situation that could be life-changing. Diagnosing cancer initially provokes feelings of anger, "why me", and anxiety, "what to do, now and from here on". Then, emotional turmoil follows, such as worry, sadness, nervousness, hopelessness, and loss of interest in daily activities [1–3]. Although surgery, and [neo]-adjuvant chemo-radiotherapy—of any type—are now considered, in general, as effective treatments, many other co-factors are involved: [a] the primary disease site; [b] the cancer stage and prognosis; [c] the treatment modalities; [d] the fear of disease progression and recurrence; and [e] malnutrition and/or sarcopenia. In the case of life-threatening cancers, along with loss of the autonomy, the sense of uncertainty, acute loss of perspective on life, sense of isolation, poor quality of life, fear of pain and adverse outcomes, and, particularly, the fear of death are also involved [2–6].

To those general negative emotional feelings, some cancer types add their discrete morbidity and some specific psychological issues: anorectal surgeries may involve permanent or temporary stoma, diarrhea and incontinence [7–9], gastric surgeries, reflux, dysphagia, eating restrictions, dyspnea, heartburn, and malnutrition [10]. Head and neck cancers commonly involve tracheostomy and, therefore, loss of voice and communication, and loss of taste and smell, as well as the inability to chew and enjoy eating and drinking [11–13]. Finally, complications related to adjuvant therapy may include nausea, vomiting, diarrhea [14–16], hair loss, fatigue, insomnia, and cognitive impairment after chemotherapy [17,18]. Long treatment periods, repeated hospitalizations due the side-effects of chemotherapy, and prolonged unemployment, in combination with low income [19], a low educational level, and parameters of gender, marital status, and religion, can all affect the psyche of cancer patients [14].

In the cases where the emotional burden exceeds a patient's ability to cope, specific psychiatric syndromes, such as prolonged stress, anxiety, and depressive disorders, may arise and are, in fact, relatively common [20]. Basak et al. [21] examined the prediction of anxiety and depression following abdominal surgery for cancer and revealed a rate of 31% to 56%, respectively, at the time of hospital discharge. Other studies have shown similar results of 30% to 40% [4,22,23]. When the Hospital Anxiety and Depression Scale (HADS) score was applied to a total of 200 gastric cancer patients scheduled for extended gastrectomies, a prevalence of 33.5% vs. 10.0% [$p < 0.001$], a HADS-anxiety score of 7.4 ± 3.8 vs. 4.7 ± 2.8, [$p < 0.001$], and a HADS-depression score of 6.9 ± 3.5 vs. 4.2 ± 2.6, [$p < 0.001$] in relation to healthy controls were reported [10]. Among all the cancer sufferers, the gastric cancer patients had the highest rate of mixed anxiety/depression symptoms [24]. Similarly, in anorectal cancer patients, depression and anxiety was positively correlated with persistent diarrhea and other gastrointestinal symptoms [7], while the fear of incontinence [8] or of odor from a stoma interfered with social functioning, thus increasing their psychological distress [9]. According to Purkayastha et al. [25], the prevalence rate for depression is three-fold higher in the cancer population in relation to the healthy population, and those at risk of suicide increased 2.5-fold [26]. Finally, in a study of 263 cancer patients [19] who were undergoing chemotherapy, fatigue, insomnia, anxiety, and depression were found to be positively correlated to each other and negatively correlated with the quality of life [$p < 0.001$], with the highest impact relating to depression.

Among 106 rectal cancer patients receiving neoadjuvant chemoradiation, 42% experienced acute toxicities and 24.5% late toxicities [27]. The data also suggest that cancer itself, along with chemotherapy and radiotherapy treatments, is implicated in persisting modifications of inflammatory setpoints through the epigenetic effects of genes related to inflammatory signaling pathways [11], leading to the activation of the neuroimmune response [28,29] through the hypothalamic–pituitary–adrenal (HPA) axis, and, thus, is linked to increased stress and neuro-psychiatric conditions [28,30–32]. It is also well known that depression and anxiety are the result of the inappropriate production of serotonin, dopamine, norepinephrine, and other neurotransmitters that are critical for proper mood functioning [28–30,33]. On the other hand, the increased expression of free radicals and of the pro-inflammatory cytokines by the cancer and the interventions for its treatment affect the microbiome composition and diversity [33–35], which is well known to be involved in mood disorders [30,36] through the nervous, neuroendocrine, and immune systems [33,37–39].

Psychobiotics, a specified group of probiotics, the name of which stands for probiotics that support mental health benefits in patients suffering from psychiatric illness, have been one of the most discussed interventions since their introduction by Ted Dyan and John Cryan in 2013 [40,41]. They have the unique characteristics of producing and delivering neuroactive substances such as gamma-aminobutyric acid and serotonin, which act on the brain–gut axis [42,43], and they generally exert beneficial effects on stress, anxiety, depression, insomnia, and other psychopathological disorders [44–46] by modifying the disturbed microbiome abundance [41,47].

In the present prospective, double-blind, and randomized trial, we decided to evaluate a probiotic formulation containing bacteria with well-recognized "psychobiotic properties" relating to mood performance in patients on a course of chemotherapy following gastrointestinal surgery for cancer by means of standard psychometric assessment tools. Our primary target was to evaluate depression status changes pre- and post-treatment and two months thereafter; the secondary outcomes were to estimate changes in anxiety, perceived stress, and sleeping disorders at the same time-points versus placebo treatment.

2. Materials and Methods

This was a randomized, double-blind, and placebo-controlled trial performed on patients undergoing chemotherapy who had previously been operated on for gastrointestinal cancer. This study, abbreviated to '*ProDeCa*' [PRObiotics for DEpression in CAncer] was conducted in the First Surgical Department of the AHEPA University Hospital of Thessaloniki, Greece, in collaboration with the Outpatient Surgical Oncology Unit, Chemotherapy Department, of the same institution, and started in November 2023.

2.1. Ethical Considerations

The study protocol was approved by the Ethics Committee of the AHEPA University Hospital of Thessaloniki, Greece (Scientific Council of the AHEPA Hospital, 313/4 July 2023), and was prospectively registered with ClinicalTrials.gov (NCT 06496438).

Written and oral informed consent was obtained from all eligible participants, and they were assured that they could withdraw from the study at any time.

2.2. Inclusion and Exclusion Criteria

All potential participants were assessed for eligibility.

Inclusion criteria included [i] being aged between 18 to 85 years; [ii] being able to understand the instructions associated with the study and to answer the questionnaires independently; [iii] being able to provide written consent, and being willing to comply with study requirements, namely completing questionnaires and not taking any other probiotic supplement for the 3-month duration of the study; and [iv] being on chemotherapy for gastrointestinal cancer after having been operated on.

Exclusion criteria included [i] being diagnosed for any psychiatric or neurological disorder or being on any antidepressant treatment, or having a history of a suicide attempt; [ii] already taking any type of probiotics, apart from yoghurt; [iii] study protocol violation, namely receiving less than 90% of the treatment, verified by the number of psychobiotics or placebo sachets returned; and [iv] already participating in another clinical trial.

2.3. Study Design and Participants

Patients were randomly assigned in a 1:1 ratio to receive either the psychobiotic regime or a placebo according to a computer-based table generated online [randomizer.org] under the supervision of the oncologist [E.C.], who was not further involved in the study process and data assessment. Randomization remained absolutely blinded to all other study coordinators. All participants received 4 packages—for the 4-week treatment—each containing 14 sachets of psychobiotics or placebo for the 7 days, and were instructed to take 1 sachet twice a day, diluted in a glass of tap water, two hours after eating. Sachets were identical in packaging, appearance, consistency, and solubility in drinking water, as well as in taste and smell—thanks to the kind preparation and donation of Uni-Pharma SA, Athens, Greece—thus, distinguishing between the placebo and the psychobiotics was impossible for both patient and physician.

A patient who forgot to take a dose could take it later the same day, or otherwise return the sachet at the follow-up appointment after treatment termination. A telephone-call the day before this appointment was made as a reminder. This was completed in order to exclude any patient who had not taken at least 90% of the doses. Additionally, in the middle of the treatment month, all patients were contacted either by phone or seen personally at their next chemotherapy appointment for a rough out-of-protocol communication. This contact, by the same physician who conducted the initial interview, aimed to confirm that the patients were taking the sachets and not experiencing any difficulties.

Finally, patients who only presented for the second psychometric assessment and who took more than the 90% of the doses of treatment, that is, at least 50 doses, were further evaluated.

2.4. Treatment Regimes

The psychobiotic formula consisted of 4 bacteria: *Bifidobacterium animalis* subsp. *lactis* LMG P-21384 [BS01] [2.50×10^{10} cfu/dose], *Bifidobacterium breve* DSM 16604 [BR03] [1.00×10^{10} cfu/dose], *Bifidobacterium longum* DSM 16603 [BL04] [8.00×10^{9} cfu/dose], and *Lacticaseibacillus rhamnosus* ATCC 53103 [GG] [4.50×10^{10} cfu/dose] to ensure a minimum microbial viable count of 1×10^{9} cfu/dose at the end of its shelf-life. The placebo contained Sorbitol, Steviol glycosides, Polyethylene Glycol 6000, and lemon–grapefruit flavors.

2.5. Participants' Psychometric Assessment

Patients eligible to participate were contacted by a physician while waiting in the daycare center for their chemotherapy. This physician handed out paper and pencil versions of the assessment questionnaires, but was blinded to any individual's group allocation. If necessary, patients could be helped by the physician, who could read out the questions and/or write down the dictated answers. Additionally, he/she collected patients' demographics [age, gender, marital status, education level, yearly income, type of health insurance] and anthropometrics [body weight, height, and weight loss], as well as a short medical history relating to habits [smoking, alcohol, and sedative use] and a short history relating to the present disease: tumor location and invasiveness and co-morbidity indices (Charlson Comorbidity Index) as well as common side-effects of chemotherapy such as hair loss, diarrhea, vomiting, and chemotherapy temporary discontinuation due to hematologic profile disturbances.

Participants completed the questionnaires under the supervision of the same physician (to encourage a sense of familiarity) at all three defined time-points: at the first contact, upon joining the trial [T1]; 30 days thereafter, just after treatment termination [T2]; and two months thereafter, a total of 3 months from the first contact [T3].

2.6. Psychometric Tools Used

All the participants were evaluated at these three time-points by means of standardized psychometric questionnaires, which had been officially translated and validated in the Greek language by others in the past [48–50]. For the evaluation of the depression status, Beck's Depression Inventory, 2nd Edition [BDI-II] [51], and the Hamilton Depression Rating 17-item Scale [HDRS] [52] were used. BDI-II is a self-report instrument first introduced by Beck et al. in 1961 and updated by him in 1996, the design of which was based on observations of attitudes and symptoms experienced mainly by patients with depression and, less frequently, by non-depressed individuals. The HDRS is a multi-dimensional tool for detecting a broad spectrum of clinical features associated with depression; it is considered a gold standard in depression studies and one of the most widely used observer-rated measures for the clinical evaluation of depression in clinical trials, with this version including 17 items serving as the standard. Anxiety was assessed by means of the General Anxiety Disorder-7 [GAD-7], which is a reliable and valid self-administered questionnaire developed by Spitzer et al. [53], evaluating generalized anxiety disorder symptomatology. Finally, the Perceived Stress Scale-14 Item [PSS-14] was used to evaluate patient's stress status. The PSS-14 was introduced to assess stress from a psychological perspective, aiming to evaluate the degree to which individuals perceive situations in their life as excessively stressful relative to their ability to cope. It was first proposed by Cohen et al. in 1983 [54], and since then it has become the world's most commonly used psychological instrument to measure perceived stress.

2.7. Sample Size Calculation and Power Analysis

A sample size calculation using the statistical program G*Power [Version 3] was performed based on bibliographic data on the prevalence of depression in cancer patients assessed with standard psychometric tools. Assuming that the overall prevalence of depression in patients with gastrointestinal cancer is up to 30% [55], independently of its severity, and by using a cut-off score of $\leq$7 [56] on the HDRS for discrimination between depressed and non-depressed participants, we hypothesized that the tested treatment should reduce the prevalence of depression in the participants by 50% based on the available literature [57] [i.e., the rate of depression in the psychobiotic group should decrease from 30% to 15% after treatment]. Based on these assumptions, we calculated that, for designing a superior trial with 80% power and a type I error rate of $\alpha = 0.05$, a sample size of 120 patients per study-arm would be required [58]. Given the close monitoring of participants in this trial, we did not expect a dropout rate higher than 10% per arm; thus, we aimed for a total enrollment of 264 patients [132 patients in each arm].

An Intent-to-Treat (ITT) analysis approach was followed. The ITT method ensures that all patients who were initially randomized into the study, regardless of whether they completed the treatment or not, were included in the final analysis. One key advantage of ITT is that it preserves the benefits of randomization, helping to prevent bias that could arise from differential drop-outs between groups. This approach also enhances the generalizability of the results, as it reflects the real-world scenario where not all patients adhere to the treatment protocol. Additionally, ITT is considered a conservative analysis, as it tends to underestimate the true effects of the clinical intervention by including participants who may not have fully complied with the study protocol. As a result, it helps to avoid the potential overestimation of treatment effects that might occur if only those who completed the study were analyzed. By using ITT, we aimed to provide a more accurate and reliable estimate of the treatment's effectiveness in a broader real-world context.

2.8. Data Collection and Statistical Analysis

All data collected were initially stored safely in a Microsoft Excel [Microsoft Office Professional Plus 2019] spreadsheet. The two investigators [G.T. and D.C.] responsible for entering data were both blinded regarding the patients' randomization. Then, an .sav file was created for the purpose of editing by the statistician using the statistical software. Statistical analysis was conducted using the Statistical Package for Social Science (SPSS® 25.0, IBM Corporation, Armonk, NY, USA for Windows®/Apple Mac®), with the level of statistical significance set at 0.05.

The normality of the data distribution was assessed by performing the Kolmogorov–Smirnov test, given the fact that each group had more than 50 participants. For continuous variables, the results were reported as means ± standard deviation (SD) or as median and its accompanied interquartile range (IQR) when normality was either assumed or not, respectively. Categorical variables were presented as percentages. Student's *t*-test or Wilcoxon test was performed in order for the means or medians, respectively, to be compared between the two independent groups at each evaluation. Moreover, repeated measures ANOVA or the Friedman test were used in order for the means or medians, respectively, to be compared between the three consecutive assessments within the same group. Regarding categorical data, statistically significant differences were detected by means of the Chi-square test. The McNemar test was used to determine whether there were differences in the dichotomous dependent variables between the two related groups. Moreover, the Risk Ratios (RRs) were calculated.

3. Results

3.1. Participant Characteristics

Four hundred and fifty-two patients on chemotherapy were initially screened for eligibility to enter the *ProDeCa* study. Full details of participants are reported in the CONSORT Flow Diagram [Figure 1]. Of the 452 candidates, 132 were ineligible, and 25 were not interested; the remaining 295 were initially enrolled and were randomized into the psychobiotics or placebo groups. Within the month of treatment there were three deaths, while another 26 participants returned more than six sachets/doses and were excluded from further assessment. Thus, a total of 266 participants [178 males, 88 females] remained for further analysis. According to protocol, participants should have completed at least the first two sets of questionnaires, that is, before [T1] and after treatment [T2], to finally be included.

Participant characteristics relating to demographics and anthropometrics, including habits, are summarized in Table 1A. It is of interest to note that more than 60% of the participants were married, had an under-diploma educational level, and a mid-level income of 10,000 to 30,000 euros. Table 1B summarizes information relating to medical history, the tumor location and invasiveness, the co-morbidity indices, and the side-effects of chemotherapy.

Overall, 21 [rate 15.9%] and 18 [rate 13.4%] patients in the psychobiotic and placebo groups, respectively, were lost at the 3-month follow up [T3]; these losses are analyzed to 4 and 3 deaths, 3 and 5 reoperations, 4 and 3 terminations of chemotherapy sessions, 2 and 4 refusals to complete the third course of questionnaires, and, finally, 8 and 3 continuations of the psychobiotic treatment with the commercially available product who were, thus, considered to be violating the protocol. We need to explain that this small number of patients [n = 11, still blinded], being very satisfied with their psychological improvement, asked for the name of the commercially available product in order to continue taking it. For ethical reasons, we did not feel able to refuse, although it would mean losing them to our study. Thus, the psychobiotics group at T3 had 111 patients instead of 132 and the placebo group had 116 instead of 134. When presenting the number of patients at T3, we insert a second number in parenthesis: this number represents the missing data extrapolated to the total number of patients.

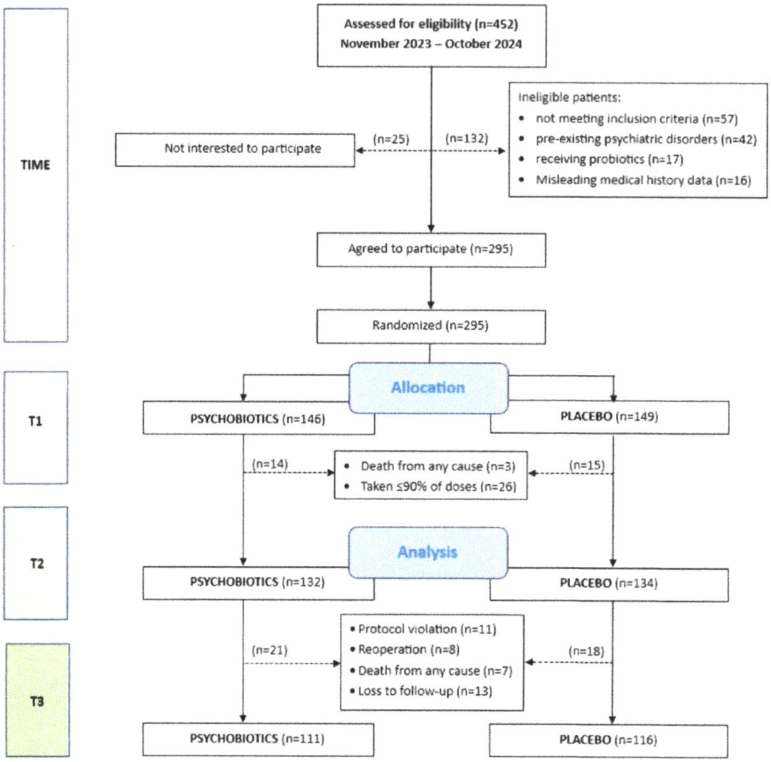

Figure 1. CONSORT flow diagram.

Table 1. (A). Participants' baseline demographics, anthropometrics, and habits. (B). Patients' baseline characteristics related to tumor location and invasiveness, co-morbidity indices, and the side-effects of chemotherapy.

(A)			
	Psychobiotics	**Placebo**	***p*-Value**
Number of patients	132	134	
Age (years) *	69.5 (17.0)	65.0 (15.0)	0.061
Gender (Male/Female)	88/44	90/44	0.931
Weight (kg) **	74.8 (14.9)	74.9 (18.0)	0.754
Height (cm) **	170.7 (8.2)	170.4 (9.0)	0.856
BMI (kg/m^2) **	25.7 (4.8)	25.9 (4.8)	0.816
Weight Loss (Yes/No)	104/28	96/38	0.177
Marital Status			
Free	22	22	0.265
Married	84	90	
Divorced/Widow/er	14/12	6/16	

Table 1. *Cont.*

(A)			
	Psychobiotics	**Placebo**	***p*-Value**
Education			
Basic	30	35	0.401
Secondary	70	60	
University	32	39	
Income			
EUR < 10 K	42	41	0.263
EUR 10–30 K	84	80	
EUR > 30 K	6	13	
Health Insurance			
Public/None	120/11	117/4	0.297
Private	2	2	
Both	4	11	
Habits			
Smoking (Yes/No)	54/78	46/88	0.395
Alcohol (Yes/No)	16/116	26/108	0.103
Sedatives (Yes/No)	32/100	24/110	0.205
(B)			
	Psychobiotics	**Placebo**	***p*-Value**
Number of patients	132	134	
Tumor Location			
Gastric	32	33	0.232
Large Bowel	65	64	
Rectum	24	27	
Pancreas	11	10	
Disease stage			
Stage I	16	15	0.571
Stage II	58	54	
Stage III	46	51	
Stage IV	12	14	
Charlson Comorbidity Index *	5.0 (1.0)	5.0 (1.0)	0.212
Side-effects of chemotherapy			
Diarrhea (Y/N)	34/98	37/97	0.732
Vomiting (Y/N)	17/115	21/113	0.515
Chemo—temporary discont. (Y/N)	17/115	14/120	0.382
Hair Loss (Y/N)	13/119	12/122	0.803

(A): * Data presented as median and interquartile range [IQR], or ** as mean ± standard deviation. Age was assessed by means of Mann–Whitney U test, anthropometric data [weight, height, BMI] by Student's *t*-test for intendent samples, and all other parameters by the Chi-square test. (B): * Data presented as median and interquartile range [IQR], Charlson Comorbidity Index was assessed by means of Mann–Whitney U test, and all other parameters by the Chi-square test.

3.2. Psychobiotics Downregulate Depression Status

From the total of 266 patients enrolled in the study, both BDI-II and HDRS psychometric tests revealed a total of 48 and 51 subjects out of the 266 studied [rates 36.4% and 38.1%, respectively] to be suffering from depression at different degrees of severity, with the male-to-female ratio being 2.8:1. Table S1 summarizes the depressed versus non-depressed patient characteristics in the psychobiotic and placebo groups; there is no significant difference between the two groups, so no parameter could be considered as a predisposing factor.

Since the BDI-II and HDRS psychometric tests have almost the same results, we decided from this point onwards to use only the results derived from the HDRS test. Thus, 99 depressed patients were allocated to the psychobiotic group [n = 48, in a ratio of 1:1.8

against the non-depressed] and to the placebo group [n = 51, in a ratio of 1:1.6 against the non-depressed].

Psychobiotics were found to significantly ameliorate the depression status of patients versus placebo treatment. Handling the result as a dichotomous variable [depressed and non-depressed, independently of the severity], there were 48 depressed individuals in the psychobiotics group at baseline [T1]; their number reduced progressively to 22 at the end of the treatment month [T2], and to 16 at the third-month follow-up [T3]. In other words, psychobiotic treatment switched 26 out of the 48 depressed patients into the non-depress status at T2, and then an additional 6 patients at T3, thus changing the ratio of non-depressed to depressed from 48 to 16 [relative improvement of 60.4%]. The RR at T2 was 0.18 (95% CI: 0.10–0.31), meaning that the risk of remaining depressed after psychobiotic treatment was 18% of the risk in the placebo group. At T3, the RR was 0.10 (95% CI: 0.05- 0.19). The opposite was the case in the placebo group, where the initial 51 depressed individuals increased to 71 [T2] and then to 73 [T3] [Table 2].

Table 2. Psychobiotics improve depression status: the number of non-depressed participants (HDRS) progressively increased, whereas for those taking a placebo, it decreased.

	Psychobiotics			Placebo		
Patients	T1 *	T2 [a]	T3 [b]	T1 **, ‡	T2	T3
Non-Depressed	84	110	95 (113)	83	63	43 (50)
Depressed	48	22	16 (19)	51	71	73 (84)
total number	132	132	111 (132)	134	134	116 (134)

* $p < 0.001$ between T1 and T2, and T1 and T3 within the same group (Mc Nemar test); ** $p = 0.002$ between T1 and T2 within the same group (Mc Nemar test); ‡ $p < 0.001$ between T1 and T3 within the placebo group (Mc Nemar test); [a] and [b] $p < 0.001$ between psychobiotics and placebo at T2 and T3 (Chi-square test). Parentheses represent the missing data, extrapolated to the total number of patients.

The discrete fluctuations in depressed patient numbers according to the severity of depression over the time-period and according to treatment or otherwise [placebo], expressed in percentages, are shown in Figure 2.

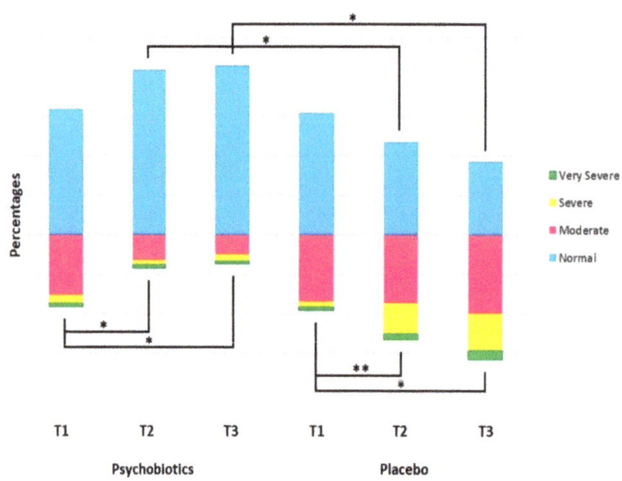

Figure 2. Distribution of participants according to depression status [HDRS scores: 0–7: Normal; 8–18: Moderate; 19–22: Severe; 23–50: Very Severe] in each group and at each time-point [T1: before treatment; T2: at treatment termination, one month; T3: at three months]. Data presented as percentages. Comparisons within the same group were made by means of McNemar test and between groups at each time-point by Chi-square test; * $p < 0.001$; ** $p < 0.010$.

3.3. *Psychobiotics Improve Sleep Quality*

By separately analyzing the questions relating to sleep quality and disorders of the BDI-II [question 16] and HDRS [questions Q4, Q5, Q6] tests, we studied the cases of insomnia and sleep quality in a dichotomous manner. To the question 'I can sleep as well as usual', the answers Yes/No were equal 1:1 at T1, while at T3 it improved (the Yeses) to 1.8:1 in the psychobiotics group, but fell to 0.9:1 in the placebo group. Regarding insomnia, the answers No/Yes for the 'Insomnia early in the night', meaning difficulty falling asleep, were 1:0.8 at T1 and improved to 3.6:1 in the psychobiotics group at T3. For the placebo, the ratio was 1:1 at T1 and deteriorated to 0.3:1 at T3. For the answer No/Yes for the 'Insomnia middle of the night', meaning waking during the night or being restless during the night, the ratio 0.7:1 in the psychobiotics group at T1 improved to 2:1 at T3. Correspondingly, for the placebo, it was 0.8:1 and 0.7:1, respectively.

Finally, for the answer No/Yes for the 'Insomnia early hours of the morning', meaning waking in the early hours in the morning and being unable to fall asleep again, the ratio was 1:0.9 at T1 and improved to 2.9:1 and 1.2:1, which slightly deteriorated to 1:1 at T3 in the psychobiotics and placebo groups, respectively. A detailed illustration of these changes over time is also added in Figure 3.

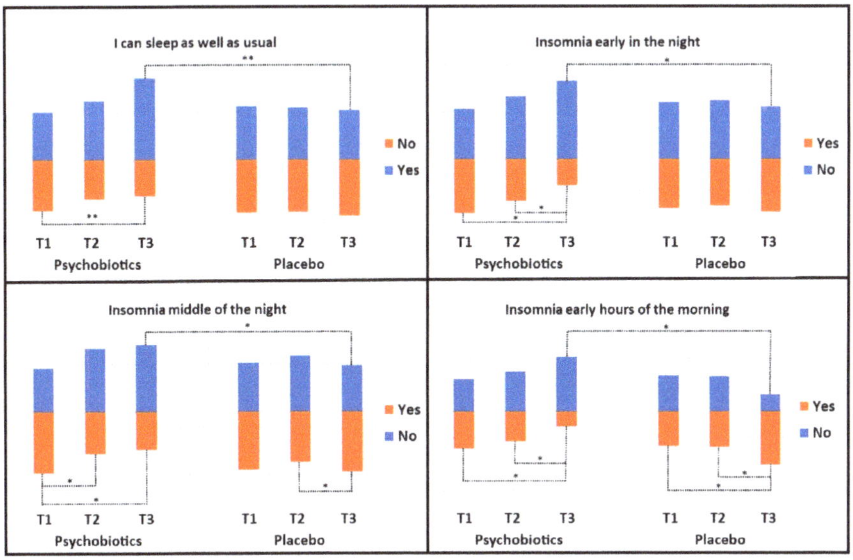

Figure 3. Distribution of participants according to dichotomous classification of sleeping disorders [yes or no] in each group and at each time-point: T1: before treatment; T2: at treatment termination, one month; T3: at three months. Data presented as percentages. Comparisons within the same group were made by means of McNemar test and between groups at each time-point by Chi-square test; * $p < 0.001$; ** $p < 0.05$.

3.4. *Psychobiotics Improve Anxiety Status*

The assessment of anxiety was made using the GAD-7 scale questionnaire. To discriminate between individuals with and without anxiety in a dichotomous manner, the validated cut-off value of ≥8 was used; half of the participants [n = 138, rate 51.9%] were experiencing anxiety. These were equally distributed between the psychobiotics group [n = 72, rate 54.5%] and the placebo group [n = 66, rate 49.2%]. Regarding age, gender, socioeconomic status, and education level, there was no clear difference between the anxiety and non-anxiety individuals [data not presented].

Psychobiotics were found to significantly improve anxiety: 54.5% of the treatment group [72 patients] at baseline was reduced to 36.4% [n = 48] after a month of taking psychobiotics and then further to 23.4% [n = 26 in a total of 111 patients presenting for follow-up] at the third month, that is, two months after treatment termination [relative improvement of 57.0%]. The RR at T2 and T3 was 0.30 (95% CI: 0.18–0.49) and 0.13 (95% CI: 0.07–0.24), respectively. However, the anxiety rates for the placebo group were found to progressively increase [relative deterioration of 39.7%]: 49.2% [n = 66 participants out of 132] at T1, 65.7% [n = 88 out of 132] at T2, and 69.8% [n = 81 out of the 116 who presented for follow-up at 3 months] at T3, respectively [Table 3].

Table 3. Psychobiotics improve anxiety status: the number of non-anxious participants (GAD-7 score) progressively increased in the psychobiotics group, whereas for those taking the placebo, it decreased.

	Psychobiotics			**Placebo**		
Patients	T1 *, ‡, **	T2 **, a	T3 b	T1 †	T2	T3
Non-Anxious	60	84	85 (101)	68	46	35 (40)
Anxious	72	48	26 (31)	66	88	81 (94)
total number	132	132	111 (132)	134	134	116 (134)

Comparisons within the same group were made by means of McNemar test: * $p < 0.001$ between T1 and T3 within the same group; ‡ $p = 0.009$ between T1 and T2 within the same group; ** $p = 0.002$ between T1 and T3 within the same group; † $p < 0.001$ between T1 and T3 within the same group. Comparisons between groups at each time-point were made by Chi-square test: [a] and [b] $p < 0.001$ between psychobiotics and placebo at T2 and T3. Parentheses represent the missing data extrapolated to the total number of patients.

The analysis of patients according to anxiety severity and consequent changes in relation to treatment or placebo over time are depicted in Figure 4.

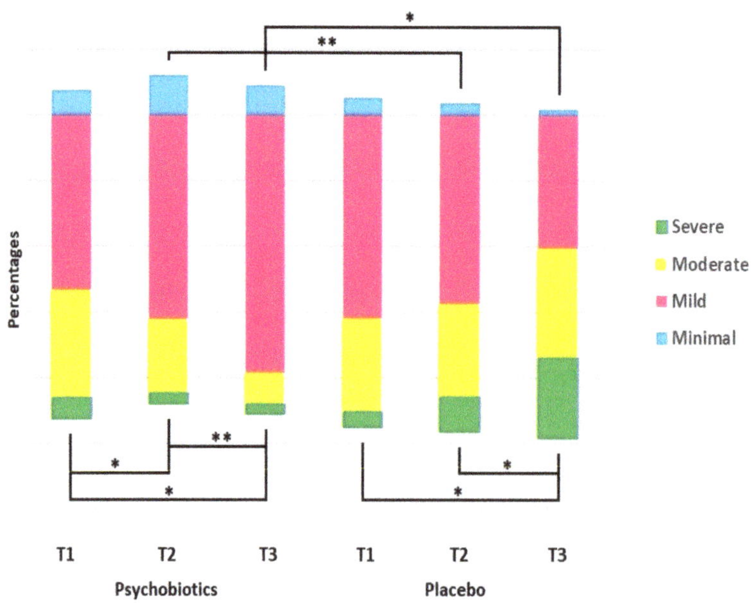

Figure 4. Distribution of participants according to severity of anxiety [GAD-7 scores: 0–4: Minimal Anxiety; 5–9: Mild Anxiety; 10–14: Moderate Anxiety; >15: Severe Anxiety] in each group and at each time-point: T1: before treatment; T2: at treatment termination, one month; T3: at three months. Data presented as percentages. Comparisons within the same group were made by means of McNemar test and between groups at each time-point by Chi-square test; * $p < 0.001$; ** $p < 0.010$.

3.5. Psychobiotics Improve Perceived Stress

For the assessment of stress, the PSS-14 was used, with scores ranging from 0 to 56. Low stress is characterized by scores between 0 and 18, which applied to 71 patients out of the 266 [rate 26.7%]. These 'low-stress' individuals were almost equally [$p = 0.536$] divided between the psychobiotics [n = 33] and placebo [n = 38] groups. After taking psychobiotics, the number of 'low-stress' participants increased to 49 [at T2] and 59 [at T3], while the placebo group had a decrease in the initial number from 38 to 24 [at T2] and then to 22 [at T3]. In other words, psychobiotics almost doubled the percentage of low-stress individuals from 33.3% to 53.1% [at T3] [$p < 0.001$], while for those taking the placebo, it decreased from 28.3% to 18.9% [at T3] [$p = 0.043$]. The results of the analysis of participants according to the PSS-14 score into three stress status levels [low, moderate, and high] at each time-point and for each treatment group are illustrated in Figure 5.

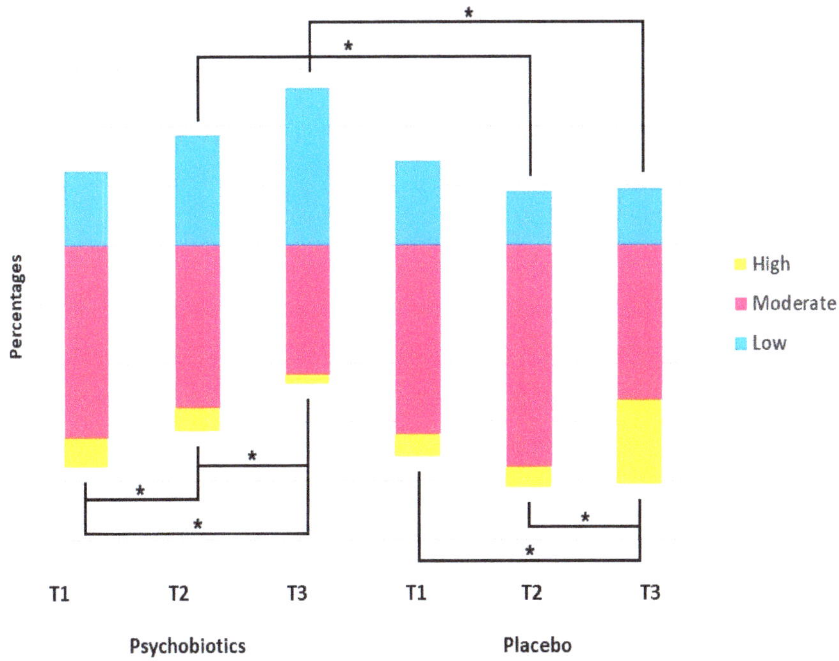

Figure 5. Distribution of participants according to stress status [PSS-14 scores: 0–18: Low Stress; 19–37: Moderate Stress; 38–56: High Stress] at each time-point and for each treatment group. T1: before treatment; T2: at treatment termination, one month; T3: at three months. Data are presented as percentages. Comparisons within the same group were made by means of McNemar test and between groups at each time-point by Chi-square test; * $p < 0.001$.

When the cut-off value of ≥28 [59] was used to simply dichotomize participants into No/Yes stress, the number of stressed patients taking psychobiotics was 42 [at T1], 27 [at T2], and 14 [at T3], presenting a significant decline [$p = 0.001$] in relation to the placebo-treated patients [relative improvement of 60.4%]. The RR at T2 and T3 was 0.51 (95% CI: 0.29–0.89) and 0.06 (95% CI: 0.03–0.12), respectively. For placebo-treated patients, stress progressively increased from 38 at T1 to 45 at T2 and then to 81 at T3 [$p < 0.001$] [relative deterioration of 142.5%], Table 4.

Table 4. Psychobiotics improve stress status. The number of non-stressed patients (based on PSS-14 score, cut-off value of 28) progressively increased, whereas for those taking the placebo, it decreased.

	Psychobiotics			Placebo		
Patients	**T1 *, ****	**T2 *, a**	**T3 **, b**	**T1 *****	**T2 *****	**T3**
Non-Stressed	90	105	97 (115)	96	89	35 (40)
Stressed	42	27	14 (17)	38	45	81 (94)
Total number	132	132	111 (132)	134	134	116 (134)

Comparisons within the same group were made by means of *McNemar test*: * $p = 0.001$ between T1 and T2 and T2 and T3 within the same group; ** $p < 0.001$ between T1 and T3 within the same group; *** $p < 0.001$ between T2 and T3 and T1 and T3 within the same group. Comparisons between groups at each time-point were made by Chi-square test: [a] $p = 0.016$ between psychobiotics and placebo at T2; [b] $p < 0.001$ between psychobiotics and placebo at T3. Parentheses represent the missing data extrapolated to the total number of patients.

4. Discussion

In the present study, we clearly accept the ability of this psychobiotic formula to downregulate the stress, anxiety, and depression status of patients undergoing complementary chemotherapy after a radical dissection for gastrointestinal cancer. Moreover, our encouraging results—in terms of emotion and mood status enhancement—are further reinforced by the negative findings in the placebo group: this group, consisting of patients who received placebo treatment, was found, as expected, to have a negative improvement on the psychometric parameters studied. This group had no psychological support apart from the "placebo effect", if such an effect really exists. However, according to the position statement on antidepressants issued by the Royal College of Psychiatrists, an improvement in depression symptoms is achieved at a rate of 50% to 65% for those patients receiving an antidepressant, and 25% to 30% for those taking a placebo [60].

Psychobiotics are defined as the probiotics which, when taken in adequate quantities, exert a health benefit on patients suffering from psychiatric illness by means of their unique characteristics of producing and delivering neuroactive substances which can influence the complex bidirectional microbiota–gut–brain axis [61]. The recognition of the involvement of gut bacteria in mood control led to the idea of manipulating the gut microbiota to produce benefits for brain function. From this point of view, the term 'psychobiotic' expresses any exogenous intervention that leads to a bacterially mediated impact on the brain [62]. An early study, almost the first, reporting the distinct impact of probiotic administration at behavioral, neural, and microbiome levels at the same time in healthy volunteers was that of Bagga et al. [63]. The authors revealed—by means of functional MRI—that a 4-week probiotic formula taken by healthy adults was directly related to changes in brain activation patterns, showing a significant difference in brain activity in the cingulum, precuneus, inferior parietal lobule, thalamus, and para-hippocampal gyrus. Additionally, the subtle modifications in the gut microbiome profile as well as behavioral improvements in memory and decision-making processes, especially in the context of emotions, triggered future investigations into the role of probiotics in the context of major depression and stress disorders [64].

Today, it is well known that gut bacteria communicate with the central nervous system by triggering the vagus nerve by producing antigens recruiting inflammatory cells, and by entero-endocrine signaling from the intestinal epithelial cells [65–67], to regulate neuroinflammation, neurogenesis, neurotransmission, and neuroendocrine signaling, by means of producing or being involved in the induction of neurotrophic factors and neurotransmitters, including γ-aminobutyric acid, dopamine, serotonin, glutamate, and the brain-derived neurotrophic factor (BDNF). All of these play a crucial role in governing the neural excitatory–inhibitory balance, mood, cognitive functions, learning and memory processes, and sleep disorders, among others [68,69]. On this basis, it has been suggested that the modification of gut microbiota may have translational applications in the modulation or even treatment of neuropsychiatric illnesses [39,70–72].

Experimental and clinical studies of bacteria with psychotropic effects—namely psychobiotics—have tended to concentrate on those belonging to the Bifidobacterium and Lactobacillus families. This does not, however, exclude other species, less studied as yet, such as *Escherichia coli Nissle* 1917, *Akkermansia muciniphila*, *Faecalibacterium prausnitzii*, and *Clostridium butyricum* [73]. In the present study, a psychobiotic formula containing *Bifidobacterium animalis* subsp. *lactis* LMG P-21384 [BS01], *Bifidobacterium breve* DSM 16604 [BR03], *Bifidobacterium longum* DSM 16603 [BL04], and *Lacticaseibacillus rhamnosus* ATCC 53103 [GG] at a concentration of 1×10^9 cfu/dose was used. These four probiotics are part of a commercially available formula also containing magnesium and saffron [LactoLevure® ProbioMood, Uni-Pharma, SA, Athens, Greece], well known for their antidepressant properties [74] and marketed for 'people with an anxious lifestyle, who often suffer from symptoms such as low mood or fatigue as a result of stress'. Since the research in psychobiotics covers only a short period of 10 years, it is evident that studies should investigate new species or strains, rather than repeat the use of the same ones, which means that extended research on particular bacteria is rather limited.

Regarding the bacteria included in the formula we used, we know the following: in a previous study, the same four-probiotic formula was used in concentrations which differed to ours, and it was found to increase *Bifidobacteria* counts and, thus, to improve sleep quality, general fatigue, anxiety, and cognitive symptoms [75]. *B. animalis* subsp. *lactis* LMG P-21384 [or *B. lactis* BS01] is known for its action in preventing and/or treating inflammatory processes—major surgery for cancer being such a serious process—by means of the highly effectively immune stimulation of the polarization of monocyte/macrophage subpopulations. Additionally, it was found to significantly mitigate oxidative stress [76], while *B. lactis* BS01 (2×10^9 cfu) and *L. acidophilus* LA02 were tested, prophylactically, in 50 healthy females to investigate whether it would exert benefits in cognitive functioning [77].

B. breve DSM 16604 [BR03] was found—by means of HPLC coupled with mass spectrometry—to have the ability to secrete high concentrations of acetic acid in the culture supernatant [78]. Although its exact role has not yet been fully demonstrated, it is known that it is widely effective in ameliorating obesity-associated insulin sensitivity by directly or indirectly modulating the local concentration of short-chain fatty acids [SCFAs] [79]. In addition to all the other well-known beneficial effects, like the maintenance of gut barrier integrity, the SCFAs have an impact on the production of neurotransmitters in the brain. Acetate has been documented to increase the hypothalamic levels of g-aminobutyric acid [GABA] and lactate in vivo, while in vitro studies have shown that it modulates serotonin levels by regulating the expression of tph1, which encodes tryptophan 5-hydroxylase 1, the enzyme necessary for serotonin production [80,81]. Another study showed the effects of *B. breve* BR03 along with *S. thermophilus* FP4 on stressed athletes, undergoing periods of intense training; the catabolism of tryptophan via kynurenine seems to play an important role in alleviating the transient suppression of the immune function due to prolonged intense exercise [82]. Thus, a 3-week treatment prior to muscle-damaging exercise may assist in performance recovery, reducing the inflammation subsequent to strenuous exercise [83]. Benefits were also reported for the improvement in the aerobic capacity of male soccer players [84].

B. longum DSM 16603 [BL04], along with *L. fermentum* LF16, *L. rhamnosus* LR06, and *L. plantarum* LP01, exerts a significant improvement in mood status, with a reduction in depression, anger, and fatigue, as well as an improvement in sleep quality; the effect was maintained 3 weeks after washing-out treatment [85]. Similarly, BL04 [along with *L. rhamnosus* HN001 and *B. infantis* Bi-26], given to children with an autism spectrum disorder [86], was reported to improve atypical emotional behavior and neurological dysfunction [87].

L. rhamnosus ATCC 53103 [LGG] is one of the most widely used probiotic strains in the world, and the health-promoting effects of this bacterium have been well documented in clinical and animal studies [88–90]. The oral administration of LGG alters autonomic neurotransmission, including adrenal sympathetic nerve activity, gastric vagal nerve activity, and cutaneous arterial sympathetic activity, in a dose- and strain-dependent manner [91]. It was also found that LGG positively influences hippocampal neuronal viability, along with synaptic and functional development, as well as the regulation of neuronal BDNF protein, when added to a hippocampal neuron culture [92]. Cryan's group, who are working on the established rat model of maternal separation for early-life stress induction, which is known to result in depression-like behaviors in adulthood [93], initially found a differentiation of the gut microbiota versus control rats, suggesting a mechanistic role for the microbiota–gut–brain axis. They then fed the rats with LGG, with or without prebiotics, and found that those who received LGG plus prebiotics exhibited a reduction in anxiety-like behavior and hippocampal-dependent learning due to alterations to the hippocampal mRNA expression of genes related to stress circuitry, anxiety, and learning [94]. In a rat model of Celiac disease, the brain-derived neurotrophic factor [BDNF]—known to act as the bridge between immune activation and the nervous system's adaptive response—was found decreased, which was associated with psychiatric comorbidities; ten days of treatment of rats with LGG [10^9 CFU/day] was found to positively affect BDNF levels [91]. Furthermore, LGG was found to be the major contributor to the induction of neurotrophic factors and the downregulation of monoamine oxidase B in relation to *B. animalis lactis* (BB-12) and *L. acidophilus* (LA-5). Regarding the mechanism of action, it seems clear that these specific probiotics can rescue the dopaminergic neurons by means of increasing butyrate production and, thus, increasing neurotrophic factors [95]. Finally, it was found that LGG secretes high concentrations of acetic acid [78], which has already been analyzed in relation to *B. breve* DSM 16604 [BR03].

In the present study, we used two different tools to identify and evaluate depressed individuals: the Beck's Depression Inventory [BDI] [51] and the Hamilton Depression Rating Scale [HDRS] [52]. We found a total of 48 and 51 subjects out of the 266 studied [rates 36.4% and 38.1%, respectively] suffering from depression of differing degrees of severity. This rate is, to some degree, consistent with the current bibliography; depression is estimated to affect approximately 25% of cancer patients, five times more than the general population [96]. Mitchell et al. [97] referred to percentages ranging from 4% to 60% in oncological, hematological, and palliative care patients, while Massie [98] to a rate of 38% for major depression and of 58% for depression spectrum syndromes. In 200 Chinese patients with gastric cancer, the prevalence was 33.5%, analyzed into 9.0%, 41.8%, and 49.3% in respect to severe, moderate, and mild depression [10]. In advanced colon cancer patients in Brazil, the prevalence of depression was 44.3% and of anxiety 25.7%, while 52.9% of patients had both [99]. In China, on the other hand, prevalence was only 11% for depression and 29% for anxiety [100]. Reported variances are due to differences in stage and tumor site, but should always take into consideration the emotions of individuals, which may relate to the geographical background, and the higher rates generally conform towards the end of a patient's life [101]. Our patients, although extroverted characters as typical of Mediterranean origin, were found to have a rather high prevalence of depression. Another point, however, is that our study deals with cancer patients being diagnosed with cancer, which was the first hit; being operated on for the cancer, which usually left externally visible changes on their bodies, i.e., long surgical incision scars and external stomas, which was the second hit; and then undertaking the long process of a chemotherapy course, which, besides the tissue destruction itself, can additionally have severe adverse effects [102], which was the third hit.

Despite all these negative impacts, it is of interest to underline the significant amelioration in depression status in the group who received psychobiotics versus the controls: at baseline [T1], there were 48 depressed individuals in the psychobiotics group and 51 in the control group. After the month on psychobiotics, the number of depressed patients was highly significantly decreased [from 48 to 22] and patients moved to a less severe status, while no suicide cases were identified in either group. Kamimura et al. [101], in 109 cancer patients assessed by psychometric questionnaires three times before finishing chemotherapy, found that their scores were the highest on commencing chemotherapy and declined thereafter. However, in 100 breast cancer females, the pre-chemotherapy depression severity was at a minimum level, but after the onset of therapy, it significantly increased [18]. This is consistent with our findings, since the placebo-treated group presented with a progressive increase in the number of depressed individuals, mainly due to the significant side-effects, i.e., diarrhea, hair loss, etc., negatively affecting quality of life and/or the prolongation [34,103] or the non-response to treatment [104]. Furthermore, it is known that patients receiving chemotherapy sessions with a short-term free interval and for a long period are considered to be more susceptible to systemic inflammations, perhaps due to the incomplete recovery of microbiota between treatments, and which could also contribute to increased depression symptoms [34].

Today, it is well known that psychobiotic supplementation significantly alleviates mood disorders due to its ability to produce tryptophan, assisting in serotonin synthesis by the host [105–109]. These positive effects of psychobiotic bacteria, mainly bifidobacteria, have been observed not only in depressed individuals, but also in healthy individuals: 4 weeks of *B. longum* W23 and W52 was found to reduce negative thoughts related to sad mood [110]. Similarly, in a 12-week clinical study of 32 volunteers self-defined as "non-stressed", the administration of a symbiotic formula containing *B. animalis* subsp. *lactis* and *L. paracasei* HII01, as well as galacto- and fructo-oligosaccharides, was found to significantly reduce tryptophan levels, while increasing, among other things, the amount of acetate and propionate [111]. Zhang et al. [112], in a recent meta-analysis of 13 studies, confirmed that the manipulation of the gut microbiota by the appropriate bacteria, namely psychobiotics, could become the new approach to treating patients with mild to moderate depression. However, it is of interest that studies in which the percentage of females was under 70% reported a larger reduction in depression scores, and in our study, the male-to-female ratio was 3:1 [73 males: 26 females] against 1.7:1 in the non-depressed. In another meta-analysis of 10 RCTs dealing with the effects of psychobiotics versus placebo in patients suffering Major Depressive Disorder, the authors conclude that psychobiotics have great potential in treating depression, with the results positively correlating with treatment duration, but no ideal specific strain, dosage, or treatment duration currently stand out [41].

The pathophysiology of depression in relation to gut microbiota was recently reconfirmed. *Bifidobacterium* and *Lactobacillus* counts estimated in fecal samples revealed significantly lower *Bifidobacterium* and a trend of lower *Lactobacillus* counts in patients with depression versus controls [113]. A meta-analysis involving 1519 individuals experiencing depression, anxiety, and other psychiatric disorders revealed consistent differences in gut microbiota diversity. Those with depression had reduced levels of the anti-inflammatory bacteria *Faecalibacterium* and *Coprococcus*, and increased levels of pro-inflammatory molecules in relation to healthy controls, thus suggesting that depression is characterized by a depletion of bacteria producing anti-inflammatory compounds like SCFAs, and, simultaneously, by an enrichment of pro-inflammatory microbial genera [114,115], implicated, among others things, in the modulation of tryptophan metabolism [116].

Biologically, inflammation has been extensively discussed for its association with depression in patients with medical illness, and is especially relevant to cancer, since many aspects of cancer induce inflammation. Apart from the cancer itself, all related manipulations—surgery, chemotherapy, radiotherapy, immunotherapy—which induce significant tissue damage and destruction also result in excess inflammation [101]. Inflammatory cytokines and other molecules can drive immunological alterations in the brain [11], and can affect the activity of the HPA axis, as well as every aspect of the metabolism of monoamines, including serotonin, norepinephrine, and dopamine, all crucial in the regulation of mood [33,117], and thus leading to anxiety, depression, and other psychiatric disorders [118].

Among the disorders related to depression is insomnia, although it is now considered as separate entity. Indicative of its seriousness is that the HDRS questionnaire dedicates 3 out of the 17 items to insomnia [and two to anxiety], while all other parameters of depression have 1 question each. Half of our participants, based on the question of the BDI-II test 'I can sleep as well as usual', were found to suffer from insomnia. However, when their 'yes' was analyzed based on the questions of the HDRS, that is, insomnia early or in the middle of the night or the next morning, we recognized that a small number of patients experienced at least one type. By taking psychobiotics, the ratio yes/no for the question 'I can sleep as well as usual' improved from 1:1 to 1.8:1. This became much better for the 'early in the night insomnia': no/yes from 1:0.8 at T1, which improved to 3.6:1 at T3; for the 'middle of the night', from 0.7:1 to 2:1; and for the 'early hours in the morning', from 1:0.9 to 2.9:1.

However, placebo-treated participants exhibited a deterioration, probably related to the progress of the cancer and its complications, as well as the increase in the severity of depression, anxiety, and perceived stress. Sixty anxious students took *L. plantarum* JYLP-326 or a placebo twice a day for three weeks. Insomnia was significantly decreased in the probiotic group, while it was marginally increased in the placebo group at the end of treatment, with the severity of insomnia being bidirectionally associated with anxiety and depression [3,119]. In the same manner, the *B. breve* CCFM1025 was found to improve sleep quality by enhancing stress-induced insomnia patients' subjective sleep quality and reducing sleep disturbance [particularly early waking at night], along with a more pronounced reduction in stress markers in relation to controls [120]. According to Haarhuis et al. [121], neural, endocrine, and immune pathways, as well as clock gene regulation, are involved in the sleep-promoting and wakefulness-promoting effects of psychobiotics. Additionally, besides their direct effects, beneficial microbiota can also influence these processes via the production of SCFAs. Two out of the four psychobiotics used in our study are documented to produce SCFAs, *B. breve* BR03 and *L. rhamnosus* [LGG], while *B. longum* BL04 have previously been confirmed to have positive effects on sleep disorders [85].

Regarding anxiety, in the present study, we identified more than half of our patients as suffering from anxiety according to the diagnosis made by the GAD-7 scale questionnaire [53,122]. In more detail, and by using $\geq$8 as the cut-off point, there were 72 out of 132 patients [rate 54.5%] in the treatment group and 66 out of 134 [rate 49.2%] in the placebo group. Anxiety in general is considered as a "normal" potentially adaptive psychological reaction in cases deemed to be life-threatening; but, it becomes a clinical issue when it is dominant and overarching and severity and/or duration surpass the normal expectations [2,24]. Then, it may become a generalized anxiety disorder, manifested by psychological arousal symptoms, such as sleeplessness, restlessness, and muscle tension, along with excessive worry [123]. Pandey et al. [14] splits anxiety into four types: situational anxiety, disease-related anxiety, treatment-related anxiety, and as an exacerbation of pre-treatment anxiety disorder.

Several studies have reported a prevalence of between 12% and 25% or even over 40% in oncological patients undergoing surgery [20,22–24]; anxiety is likely to be higher because of additional fears of the unknown, of response to tumor surgery, pain, loss of control over the situation, dysfunction, alienation, loss of autonomy, increased rates of complications and, thus, hospital readmissions, and perhaps of the perspective of life or even death [3,4,124]. Harms J et al. [3] reported a rate as high as 56% of mild or moderate anxiety in such a group of 101 patients, although the authors do comment that anxiety levels do not behave statically but dynamically during the perioperative course and are therefore less predictable. This ratio is closer to that of our study cohort; it must not be forgotten, however, that our subjects were chemotherapy patients who had already been subjected to gastrointestinal surgery a short time before. Although chemotherapy alone is considered to cause less anxiety than oncological surgery [3,125], the combination of the processes in sequence, and taking into consideration that chemotherapy is an intense and cyclic treatment associated with a number of side-effects [14], having a dramatic impact on patient mood should be considered probable.

As with depression, anxiety is generally more common in females, in patients older than 35 years, and in those of low socioeconomic status and of low education level [21,126]. However, a recent meta-analysis of 6317 cancer patients reported the opposite: males experienced significantly higher levels of anxiety than females, while the opposite was the case for depression [127]. In our patients, the male-to-female ratio was found to be almost equal. The reason for the gender difference could be attributable to the males having different perceptions and coping strategies to females for dealing with the 'accident' of cancer and the subsequent surgery. The female anxiety response could be exacerbated by their social role in the family network or the partnership [3], although, ultimately, how any individual responds will relate to their individual inherent predisposition to handle the disease condition they face [20,128,129].

Psychobiotics were found to significantly improve anxiety: 54.5% of those anxious in the treatment group [72 patients] at baseline was reduced to 36.4% after a month of receiving psychobiotics, and then further to 23.4% at the third month, that is, two months after treatment discontinuation. The rates for the controls, however, were 49.2%, 65.7%, and 69.8%, respectively, clearly highlighting the benefits psychobiotics. One could negatively comment on the gradual increase in anxiety rates in the placebo group, since the literature indicates that patients were more anxious at baseline and gain greater psychological stability later [130]. However, this can be easily explained by the extension in the number of chemotherapy sessions, by possible complications, by increasing frailty and the loss of muscle mass, and generally of the poor quality of life.

Along with anxiety and depression, participants were found to live in chronic stress following cancer diagnosis, and subsequence treatments trigger many additional stressors, such as fear of death, interruption of life plans, changes in body image and self-esteem, and changes in social role and lifestyle [131]. Stress, even at a low level, induces excessive corticosterone and adrenocorticotropic release [132], which, although beneficial in the short term by helping the body to fight the stress trigger, when continuous, it can suppress the effects of the acute response and lead to low-grade inflammation [133]. Stress as a chronic condition is considered capable of changing neuronal morphology, suppressing neural proliferation, and reducing synaptic plasticity and neuron firing properties. Finally, it may lead to a reduction in the volume of the hippocampus with, as a consequence, the disturbance of memory, learning, and cognitive functions related to the hippocampus [134].

A considerable proportion of our patients reported perceived stress during chemotherapy, as assessed by the PSS-14 score, used to evaluate the degree to which situations in the participant's life within the last month are appraised as stressful: 42 out of the 132 in the psychobiotic group and 38 out of 134 in the placebo group. At the end of the 3-month study, psychobiotics were found to have ameliorated stress, so that only 14 participants remained stressed. In the placebo-treated group, however, the 38 stressed participants increased to 81 at T3. In a clinical study [107], 45 healthy adults were allocated to a psychobiotic or control diet for 4 weeks. The psychobiotic diet resulted in a 32% reduction in perceived stress, the higher the adherence, the stronger the decrease, compared to only 17% with the control diet. In parallel, the psychobiotic diet induced significant changes in 40 specific fecal lipids as well as in urinary tryptophan metabolites. Restraint stress in adulthood in rats subjected to maternal separation in the first 10 days after birth resulted in exaggerated corticosterone plasma levels and increased stress-induced visceral sensitivity; LGG treatment improved beta diversity, while 41 genes in the spinal cord were downregulated after treatment, 12 of which were associated with stress, pain, or both [94].

This study has some limitations: first of all, we were not able to evaluate biological samples from the participants. It would have been very useful to have measured cortisol in saliva and tryptophan metabolites and/or microbiota in feces. Unfortunately, this was not possible due to the likelihood of refusal of a large percentage of participants. Second, we could have had double the number of participants; however, we thought it preferable to restrict the study to patients with gastrointestinal cancers in order to gain homogeneity, since a laparotomy and its possible complications is possibly the most stressful forerunner following chemotherapy. Third, treatment lasted only a month, although antidepressant formulas are classically given for 3 months to achieve some positive effects. We took this risk, although we had found only one study which mentioned the beneficial effects of psychobiotics lasting for 3 weeks after washing-out treatment [85]. Relative to this is the short—3 months only—follow-up. However, we are dealing with patients suffering from cancer and, thus, this would likely be impossible, taking into consideration that, within two months, from T2 measurement to T3, we lost 39 participants. Fourth, since depression is related—in many cases—to feeding refusal and, thus, to malnutrition and/or sarcopenia, one could comment that our participants should had been nutritionally assessed before recruitment. However, the main point of this study was to evaluate the beneficial effect of psychobiotics on depressed individuals, their depression status depending on their "disease" and other co-factors, including cancer-related malnutrition and frailty, and not to relate depression with any poor nutritional status. Fifth, one could comment that the dose of psychobiotics given is low [four bacteria at a concentration of 1×10^9 cfu/dose, twice a day] based on the principle 'as many strains/as high doses as possible' [121]. Finally, another suggestion could be to split the participants into four subgroups and treat each one with one of the strains used to determine their effectiveness. This has a logical background, but ignores all the synergic effects of the four psychobiotics, two of which are known to release SCFAs too.

5. Conclusions

Our findings from this ProDeCa study strongly suggest that, in patients on a course of chemotherapy following gastrointestinal surgery for cancer, depression and anxiety, as well as perceived stress and sleep disorders, are a severe burden. More than half of the study population had at least one of these psychiatric disorders, diagnosed by the use of standard psychometric assessment tools, and which, in most of the cases, had remained otherwise undiagnosed. Psychobiotics taken twice a day for a month affected a highly significant improvement in all parameters, in parallel with a significant decline in the placebo group, as the 3-month study period progressed. Our results suggest the benefit of early assessment and psychobiotic support in oncological patients, even before surgery. However, further research is required both to elucidate in depth the specific mechanisms and to test the reproduction of results in different carcinoma groups or produce better results in relation to different concentrations of psychobiotics or to different strains. We are already working to this end.

Supplementary Materials: The following supporting information can be downloaded at: https://www.mdpi.com/article/10.3390/nu17050857/s1, Table S1: Baseline characteristics based on depression status within the same group.

Author Contributions: Conceptualization, J.K.T., H.T., A.K. and K.K.; Data curation, G.T., D.C. and H.T.; Formal analysis, G.T.; Investigation, A.A., S.G., M.P., A.-E.M. and I.M.T.; Methodology, G.T. and G.S.; Project administration, A.K. and K.K.; Resources, E.C., S.G., T.P. and J.K.T.; Software, G.T. and D.C.; Supervision, A.K. and K.K.; Validation, M.P., A.-E.M., I.M.T., G.S. and N.-D.D.; Visualization, A.D.S. and K.K.; Writing—review and editing, G.T. and G.S. All authors have read and agreed to the published version of the manuscript.

Funding: This research received no external funding.

Institutional Review Board Statement: The study was conducted in accordance with the Declaration of Helsinki and approved by the Ethics Committee of the AHEPA University Hospital of Thessaloniki, Greece (Scientific Council of the AHEPA Hospital, 313, 4 July 2023).

Informed Consent Statement: Informed consent was obtained from all subjects involved in the study.

Data Availability Statement: The data that support the findings of this study are available on request from the corresponding author K.K.

Acknowledgments: We would like to thank the Pharmaceutical Company Uni-Pharma, SA, Athens, Greece, for the kind donation of psychobiotics.

Conflicts of Interest: Author Joulia K. Tsetis was employed by the company Uni-Pharma S.A. The remaining authors declare that the research was conducted in the absence of any commercial or financial relationships that could be construed as a potential conflict of interest.

Abbreviations

The following abbreviations are used in this manuscript:

HDRS	Hamilton Depression Rating 17-item Scale
BDI-II	Beck's Depression Inventory, 2nd Edition
GAD-7	General Anxiety Disorder-7
PSS-14	Perceived Stress Scale-14 Item
SCFA	Short-chain fatty acids

References

1. Rades, D.; Al-Salool, A.; Yu, N.Y.; Bartscht, T. Emotional Distress Prior to Chemoradiation for Rectal or Anal Cancer. *In Vivo* **2023**, *37*, 1205–1210. [CrossRef] [PubMed]
2. Grassi, L.; Caruso, R.; Riba, M.B.; Lloyd-Williams, M.; Kissane, D.; Rodin, G.; McFarland, D.; Campos-Ródenas, R.; Zachariae, R.; Santini, D.; et al. Anxiety and depression in adult cancer patients: ESMO Clinical Practice Guideline. *ESMO Open* **2023**, *8*, 101155. [CrossRef]
3. Harms, J.; Kunzmann, B.; Bredereke, J.; Harms, L.; Jungbluth, T.; Zimmermann, T. Anxiety in patients with gastrointestinal cancer undergoing primary surgery. *J. Cancer Res. Clin. Oncol.* **2023**, *149*, 8191–8200. [CrossRef] [PubMed]
4. Jawaid, M.; Mushtaq, A.; Mukhtar, S.; Khan, Z. Preoperative anxiety before elective surgery. *Neurosciences* **2007**, *12*, 145–148.
5. Simard, S.; Thewes, B.; Humphris, G.; Dixon, M.; Hayden, C.; Mireskandari, S.; Ozakinci, G. Fear of cancer recurrence in adult cancer survivors: A systematic review of quantitative studies. *J. Cancer Surviv.* **2013**, *7*, 300–322. [CrossRef]
6. Mitchell, A.J.; Ferguson, D.W.; Gill, J.; Paul, J.; Symonds, P. Depression and anxiety in long-term cancer survivors compared with spouses and healthy controls: A systematic review and meta-analysis. *Lancet Oncol.* **2013**, *14*, 721–732. [CrossRef] [PubMed]

7. Benedict, C.; Rodriguez, V.M.; Carter, J.; Temple, L.; Nelson, C.; DuHamel, K. Investigation of body image as a mediator of the effects of bowel and GI symptoms on psychological distress in female survivors of rectal and anal cancer. *Support. Care Cancer* **2016**, *24*, 1795–1802. [CrossRef]
8. Desnoo, L.; Faithfull, S. A qualitative study of anterior resection syndrome: The experiences of cancer survivors who have undergone resection surgery. *Eur. J. Cancer Care* **2006**, *15*, 244–251. [CrossRef]
9. Chambers, S.K.; Meng, X.; Youl, P.; Aitken, J.; Dunn, J.; Baade, P. A five-year prospective study of quality of life after colorectal cancer. *Qual. Life Res.* **2012**, *21*, 1551–1564. [CrossRef] [PubMed]
10. Han, L. Prevalence, risk factors and prognostic role of anxiety and depression in surgical gastric cancer patients. *Transl. Cancer Res.* **2020**, *9*, 1371–1383. [CrossRef] [PubMed]
11. McFarland, D.C.; Riba, M.; Grassi, L. Clinical Implications of Cancer Related Inflammation and Depression: A Critical Review. *Clin. Pract. Epidemiol. Ment. Health* **2021**, *17*, 287–294. [CrossRef]
12. Katz, M.R.; Irish, J.C.; Devins, G.M.; Rodin, G.M.; Gullane, P.J. Psychosocial adjustment in head and neck cancer: The impact of disfigurement, gender and social support. *Head Neck* **2003**, *25*, 103–112. [CrossRef]
13. Bonafede, M.; d'Errico, A.; Rugarli, S.; Mensi, C.; Miligi, L.; Calisti, R.; Della Gatta, R.; Piro, S.; Melis, P.; Vasselli, D.; et al. The psychological impact of diagnosis of sinonasal, nasopharyngeal, and laryngeal cancers: A systematic review. *Front. Psychol.* **2024**, *15*, 1355186. [CrossRef] [PubMed]
14. Pandey, M.; Sarita, G.P.; Devi, N.; Thomas, B.C.; Hussain, B.M.; Krishnan, R. Distress, anxiety, and depression in cancer patients undergoing chemotherapy. *World J. Surg. Oncol.* **2006**, *4*, 68. [CrossRef] [PubMed]
15. Magee, D.E.; Hird, A.E.; Klaassen, Z.; Sridhar, S.S.; Nam, R.K.; Wallis, C.J.D.; Kulkarni, G.S. Adverse event profile for immunotherapy agents compared with chemotherapy in solid organ tumors: A systematic review and meta-analysis of randomized clinical trials. *Ann. Oncol.* **2020**, *31*, 50–60. [CrossRef]
16. Retornaz, F.; Guillem, O.; Rousseau, F.; Morvan, F.; Rinaldi, Y.; Nahon, S.; Castagna, C.; Boulahssass, R.; Grino, M.; Gholam, D. Predicting Chemotherapy Toxicity and Death in Older Adults with Colon Cancer: Results of MOST Study. *Oncologist* **2020**, *25*, e85–e93. [CrossRef]
17. Ahles, T.A.; Saykin, A.J.; McDonald, B.C.; Furstenberg, C.T.; Cole, B.F.; Hanscom, B.S.; Mulrooney, T.J.; Schwartz, G.N.; Kaufman, P.A. Cognitive function in breast cancer patients prior to adjuvant treatment. *Breast Cancer Res. Treat.* **2008**, *110*, 143–152. [CrossRef] [PubMed]
18. Hormozi, M.; Hashemi, S.M.; Shahraki, S. Investigating Relationship between Pre- and Post-Chemotherapy Cognitive Performance with Levels of Depression and Anxiety in Breast Cancer Patients: A Cross-Sectional Study. *Asian Pac. J. Cancer Prev.* **2019**, *20*, 3831–3837. [CrossRef]
19. Redeker, N.S.; Lev, E.L.; Ruggiero, J. Insomnia, fatigue, anxiety, depression, and quality of life of cancer patients undergoing chemotherapy. *Sch. Inq. Nurs. Pract.* **2000**, *14*, 275–290; discussion 291–278. [CrossRef]
20. Moldes-Moro, R.; de Dios-Duarte, M.J. Colorectal Cancer Surgery: Influence of Psychosocial Factors. *Cancers* **2023**, *15*, 4140. [CrossRef]
21. Basak, F.; Hasbahceci, M.; Guner, S.; Sisik, A.; Acar, A.; Yucel, M.; Kilic, A.; Bas, G. Prediction of anxiety and depression in general surgery inpatients: A prospective cohort study of 200 consecutive patients. *Int. J. Surg.* **2015**, *23*, 18–22. [CrossRef]
22. Caumo, W.; Schmidt, A.P.; Schneider, C.N.; Bergmann, J.; Iwamoto, C.W.; Bandeira, D.; Ferreira, M.B. Risk factors for preoperative anxiety in adults. *Acta Anaesthesiol. Scand.* **2001**, *45*, 298–307. [CrossRef] [PubMed]
23. Teunissen, S.C.; Wesker, W.; Kruitwagen, C.; de Haes, H.C.; Voest, E.E.; de Graeff, A. Symptom prevalence in patients with incurable cancer: A systematic review. *J. Pain Symptom Manag.* **2007**, *34*, 94–104. [CrossRef]
24. Brintzenhofe-Szoc, K.M.; Levin, T.T.; Li, Y.; Kissane, D.W.; Zabora, J.R. Mixed anxiety/depression symptoms in a large cancer cohort: Prevalence by cancer type. *Psychosomatics* **2009**, *50*, 383–391. [CrossRef] [PubMed]
25. Purkayastha, D.; Venkateswaran, C.; Nayar, K.; Unnikrishnan, U.G. Prevalence of Depression in Breast Cancer Patients and its Association with their Quality of Life: A Cross-sectional Observational Study. *Indian J. Palliat. Care* **2017**, *23*, 268–273. [PubMed]
26. Currier, M.B.; Nemeroff, C.B. Depression as a risk factor for cancer: From pathophysiological advances to treatment implications. *Annu. Rev. Med.* **2014**, *65*, 203–221. [CrossRef] [PubMed]
27. Chomicki, S.; Chapet, S.; Drifa, M.; Ouaissi, M.; Bourlier, P.; Debbi, K.; Loganadane, G.; Calais, G. Outcomes and Side Effects of Preoperative Chemoradiotherapy for Locally Advanced Upper Rectal Cancer. *Anticancer Res.* **2022**, *42*, 4833–4840. [CrossRef] [PubMed]
28. Bajic, J.E.; Johnston, I.N.; Howarth, G.S.; Hutchinson, M.R. From the Bottom-Up: Chemotherapy and Gut-Brain Axis Dysregulation. *Front. Behav. Neurosci.* **2018**, *12*, 104. [CrossRef] [PubMed]
29. Loman, B.R.; Jordan, K.R.; Haynes, B.; Bailey, M.T.; Pyter, L.M. Chemotherapy-induced neuroinflammation is associated with disrupted colonic and bacterial homeostasis in female mice. *Sci. Rep.* **2019**, *9*, 16490. [CrossRef] [PubMed]
30. Petra, A.I.; Panagiotidou, S.; Hatziagelaki, E.; Stewart, J.M.; Conti, P.; Theoharides, T.C. Gut-Microbiota-Brain Axis and Its Effect on Neuropsychiatric Disorders with Suspected Immune Dysregulation. *Clin. Ther.* **2015**, *37*, 984–995. [CrossRef]

31. Marsland, A.L.; Gianaros, P.J.; Kuan, D.C.; Sheu, L.K.; Krajina, K.; Manuck, S.B. Brain morphology links systemic inflammation to cognitive function in midlife adults. *Brain Behav. Immun.* **2015**, *48*, 195–204. [CrossRef]
32. Seruga, B.; Zhang, H.; Bernstein, L.J.; Tannock, I.F. Cytokines and their relationship to the symptoms and outcome of cancer. *Nat. Rev. Cancer* **2008**, *8*, 887–899. [CrossRef] [PubMed]
33. Miller, A.H.; Raison, C.L. The role of inflammation in depression: From evolutionary imperative to modern treatment target. *Nat. Rev. Immunol.* **2016**, *16*, 22–34. [CrossRef] [PubMed]
34. Bilenduke, E.; Sterrett, J.D.; Ranby, K.W.; Borges, V.F.; Grigsby, J.; Carr, A.L.; Kilbourn, K.; Lowry, C.A. Impacts of breast cancer and chemotherapy on gut microbiome, cognitive functioning, and mood relative to healthy controls. *Sci. Rep.* **2022**, *12*, 19547. [CrossRef] [PubMed]
35. Montassier, E.; Gastinne, T.; Vangay, P.; Al-Ghalith, G.A.; Bruley des Varannes, S.; Massart, S.; Moreau, P.; Potel, G.; de La Cochetière, M.F.; Batard, E.; et al. Chemotherapy-driven dysbiosis in the intestinal microbiome. *Aliment. Pharmacol. Ther.* **2015**, *42*, 515–528. [CrossRef] [PubMed]
36. Valles-Colomer, M.; Falony, G.; Darzi, Y.; Tigchelaar, E.F.; Wang, J.; Tito, R.Y.; Schiweck, C.; Kurilshikov, A.; Joossens, M.; Wijmenga, C.; et al. The neuroactive potential of the human gut microbiota in quality of life and depression. *Nat. Microbiol.* **2019**, *4*, 623–632. [CrossRef]
37. Jordan, K.R.; Loman, B.R.; Bailey, M.T.; Pyter, L.M. Gut microbiota-immune-brain interactions in chemotherapy-associated behavioral comorbidities. *Cancer* **2018**, *124*, 3990–3999. [CrossRef] [PubMed]
38. Flux, M.C.; Lowry, C.A. Finding intestinal fortitude: Integrating the microbiome into a holistic view of depression mechanisms, treatment, and resilience. *Neurobiol. Dis.* **2020**, *135*, 104578. [CrossRef]
39. Kelly, J.R.; Borre, Y.; O'Brien, C.; Patterson, E.; El Aidy, S.; Deane, J.; Kennedy, P.J.; Beers, S.; Scott, K.; Moloney, G.; et al. Transferring the blues: Depression-associated gut microbiota induces neurobehavioural changes in the rat. *J. Psychiatr. Res.* **2016**, *82*, 109–118. [CrossRef]
40. Dinan, T.G.; Stanton, C.; Cryan, J.F. Psychobiotics: A novel class of psychotropic. *Biol. Psychiatry* **2013**, *74*, 720–726. [CrossRef] [PubMed]
41. Misera, A.; Liśkiewicz, P.; Łoniewski, I.; Skonieczna-Żydecka, K.; Samochowiec, J. Effect of Psychobiotics on Psychometric Tests and Inflammatory Markers in Major Depressive Disorder: Meta-Analysis of Randomized Controlled Trials with Meta-Regression. *Pharmaceuticals* **2021**, *14*, 952. [CrossRef] [PubMed]
42. Sanada, K.; Nakajima, S.; Kurokawa, S.; Barceló-Soler, A.; Ikuse, D.; Hirata, A.; Yoshizawa, A.; Tomizawa, Y.; Salas-Valero, M.; Noda, Y.; et al. Gut microbiota and major depressive disorder: A systematic review and meta-analysis. *J. Affect. Disord.* **2020**, *266*, 1–13. [CrossRef] [PubMed]
43. Ma, Q.; Xing, C.; Long, W.; Wang, H.Y.; Liu, Q.; Wang, R.F. Impact of microbiota on central nervous system and neurological diseases: The gut-brain axis. *J. Neuroinflamm.* **2019**, *16*, 53. [CrossRef] [PubMed]
44. Wauters, L.; Van Oudenhove, L.; Accarie, A.; Geboers, K.; Geysen, H.; Toth, J.; Luypaerts, A.; Verbeke, K.; Smokvina, T.; Raes, J.; et al. *Lactobacillus rhamnosus* CNCM I-3690 decreases subjective academic stress in healthy adults: A randomized placebo-controlled trial. *Gut Microbes* **2022**, *14*, 2031695. [CrossRef]
45. Messaoudi, M.; Lalonde, R.; Violle, N.; Javelot, H.; Desor, D.; Nejdi, A.; Bisson, J.F.; Rougeot, C.; Pichelin, M.; Cazaubiel, M.; et al. Assessment of psychotropic-like properties of a probiotic formulation (*Lactobacillus helveticus* R0052 and *Bifidobacterium longum* R0175) in rats and human subjects. *Br. J. Nutr.* **2011**, *105*, 755–764. [CrossRef]
46. Le Morvan de Sequeira, C.; Hengstberger, C.; Enck, P.; Mack, I. Effect of Probiotics on Psychiatric Symptoms and Central Nervous System Functions in Human Health and Disease: A Systematic Review and Meta-Analysis. *Nutrients* **2022**, *14*, 621. [CrossRef] [PubMed]
47. Mörkl, S.; Butler, M.I.; Holl, A.; Cryan, J.F.; Dinan, T.G. Probiotics and the Microbiota-Gut-Brain Axis: Focus on Psychiatry. *Curr. Nutr. Rep.* **2020**, *9*, 171–182. [CrossRef]
48. Mystakidou, K.; Tsilika, E.; Parpa, E.; Smyrniotis, V.; Galanos, A.; Vlahos, L. Beck Depression Inventory: Exploring its psychometric properties in a palliative care population of advanced cancer patients. *Eur. J. Cancer Care* **2007**, *16*, 244–250. [CrossRef] [PubMed]
49. Vogazianos, P.; Motrico, E.; Domínguez-Salas, S.; Christoforou, A.; Hadjigeorgiou, E. Validation of the generalized anxiety disorder screener (GAD-7) in Cypriot pregnant and postpartum women. *BMC Pregnancy Childbirth* **2022**, *22*, 841. [CrossRef] [PubMed]
50. Katsarou, A.; Panagiotakos, D.; Zafeiropoulou, A.; Vryonis, M.; Skoularigis, I.; Tryposkiadis, F.; Papageorgiou, C. Validation of a Greek version of PSS-14; a global measure of perceived stress. *Cent. Eur. J. Public Health* **2012**, *20*, 104–109. [CrossRef] [PubMed]
51. Beck, A.T.; Steer, R.A.; Brown, G. Beck depression inventory—II. *Psychol. Assess.* **1996**, *67*, 588–597.
52. Hamilton, M. A rating scale for depression. *J. Neurol. Neurosurg. Psychiatry* **1960**, *23*, 56–62. [CrossRef] [PubMed]
53. Spitzer, R.L.; Kroenke, K.; Williams, J.B.; Löwe, B. A brief measure for assessing generalized anxiety disorder: The GAD-7. *Arch. Intern. Med.* **2006**, *166*, 1092–1097. [CrossRef] [PubMed]

54. Cohen, S.; Kamarck, T.; Mermelstein, R. A global measure of perceived stress. *J. Health Soc. Behav.* **1983**, *24*, 385–396. [CrossRef] [PubMed]
55. Krebber, A.M.; Buffart, L.M.; Kleijn, G.; Riepma, I.C.; de Bree, R.; Leemans, C.R.; Becker, A.; Brug, J.; van Straten, A.; Cuijpers, P.; et al. Prevalence of depression in cancer patients: A meta-analysis of diagnostic interviews and self-report instruments. *Psychooncology* **2014**, *23*, 121–130. [CrossRef] [PubMed]
56. Zimmerman, M.; Martinez, J.H.; Young, D.; Chelminski, I.; Dalrymple, K. Severity classification on the Hamilton Depression Rating Scale. *J. Affect. Disord.* **2013**, *150*, 384–388. [CrossRef]
57. Zhang, X.; Chen, S.; Zhang, M.; Ren, F.; Ren, Y.; Li, Y.; Liu, N.; Zhang, Y.; Zhang, Q.; Wang, R. Effects of Fermented Milk Containing *Lacticaseibacillus paracasei* Strain Shirota on Constipation in Patients with Depression: A Randomized, Double-Blind, Placebo-Controlled Trial. *Nutrients* **2021**, *13*, 2238. [CrossRef]
58. Kane, S. Sample Size Calculator. Available online: https://clincalc.com/stats/samplesize.aspx (accessed on 19 June 2023).
59. Shah, M.; Hasan, S.; Malik, S.; Sreeramareddy, C.T. Perceived stress, sources and severity of stress among medical undergraduates in a Pakistani medical school. *BMC Med. Educ.* **2010**, *10*, 2. [CrossRef]
60. Royal College of Psychiatrists. Position Statement on Antidepressants and Depression. 2019. Available online: https://www.rcpsych.ac.uk/docs/default-source/improving-care/better-mh-policy/position-statements/ps04_19---antidepressants-and-depression.pdf (accessed on 4 November 2024).
61. Margolis, K.G.; Cryan, J.F.; Mayer, E.A. The Microbiota-Gut-Brain Axis: From Motility to Mood. *Gastroenterology* **2021**, *160*, 1486–1501. [CrossRef] [PubMed]
62. Sarkar, A.; Lehto, S.M.; Harty, S.; Dinan, T.G.; Cryan, J.F.; Burnet, P.W.J. Psychobiotics and the Manipulation of Bacteria-Gut-Brain Signals. *Trends Neurosci.* **2016**, *39*, 763–781. [CrossRef]
63. Bagga, D.; Reichert, J.L.; Koschutnig, K.; Aigner, C.S.; Holzer, P.; Koskinen, K.; Moissl-Eichinger, C.; Schöpf, V. Probiotics drive gut microbiome triggering emotional brain signatures. *Gut Microbes* **2018**, *9*, 486–496. [CrossRef]
64. Bagga, D.; Aigner, C.S.; Reichert, J.L.; Cecchetto, C.; Fischmeister, F.P.S.; Holzer, P.; Moissl-Eichinger, C.; Schöpf, V. Influence of 4-week multi-strain probiotic administration on resting-state functional connectivity in healthy volunteers. *Eur. J. Nutr.* **2019**, *58*, 1821–1827. [CrossRef] [PubMed]
65. Wang, H.X.; Wang, Y.P. Gut Microbiota-brain Axis. *Chin. Med. J.* **2016**, *129*, 2373–2380. [CrossRef]
66. Dicks, L.M.T. Our Mental Health Is Determined by an Intrinsic Interplay between the Central Nervous System, Enteric Nerves, and Gut Microbiota. *Int. J. Mol. Sci.* **2023**, *25*, 38. [CrossRef]
67. Dicks, L.M.T. Gut Bacteria and Neurotransmitters. *Microorganisms* **2022**, *10*, 1838. [CrossRef] [PubMed]
68. Cheng, L.H.; Liu, Y.W.; Wu, C.C.; Wang, S.; Tsai, Y.C. Psychobiotics in mental health, neurodegenerative and neurodevelopmental disorders. *J. Food Drug Anal.* **2019**, *27*, 632–648. [CrossRef]
69. Wang, H.; Lee, I.S.; Braun, C.; Enck, P. Effect of Probiotics on Central Nervous System Functions in Animals and Humans: A Systematic Review. *J. Neurogastroenterol. Motil.* **2016**, *22*, 589–605. [CrossRef] [PubMed]
70. Cryan, J.; Dinan, T. Microbiota and neuroimmune signalling—Metchnikoff to microglia. *Nat. Rev. Gastroenterol. Hepatol.* **2015**, *12*, 494–496. [CrossRef] [PubMed]
71. Desbonnet, L.; Clarke, G.; Shanahan, F.; Dinan, T.G.; Cryan, J.F. Microbiota is essential for social development in the mouse. *Mol. Psychiatry* **2014**, *19*, 146–148. [CrossRef]
72. Hsiao, E.Y.; McBride, S.W.; Hsien, S.; Sharon, G.; Hyde, E.R.; McCue, T.; Codelli, J.A.; Chow, J.; Reisman, S.E.; Petrosino, J.F.; et al. Microbiota modulate behavioral and physiological abnormalities associated with neurodevelopmental disorders. *Cell* **2013**, *155*, 1451–1463. [CrossRef]
73. Dziedzic, A.; Maciak, K.; Bliźniewska-Kowalska, K.; Gałecka, M.; Kobierecka, W.; Saluk, J. The Power of Psychobiotics in Depression: A Modern Approach through the Microbiota–Gut–Brain Axis: A Literature Review. *Nutrients* **2024**, *16*, 1054. [CrossRef] [PubMed]
74. Chen, C.; Zheng, Z.; Gao, K.; Fan, Q.; Li, Y.; Chen, S. Prophylactic effects of supplementation of a combination of Lactobacillus lactis WHH2078 and saffron on depressive-like behaviors in mice exposed to chronic stress. *J. Food Sci.* **2024**, *89*, 5912–5927. [CrossRef] [PubMed]
75. Wallis, A.; Ball, M.; Butt, H.; Lewis, D.P.; McKechnie, S.; Paull, P.; Jaa-Kwee, A.; Bruck, D. Open-label pilot for treatment targeting gut dysbiosis in myalgic encephalomyelitis/chronic fatigue syndrome: Neuropsychological symptoms and sex comparisons. *J. Transl. Med.* **2018**, *16*, 24. [CrossRef] [PubMed]
76. Mogna, L.; Amoruso, A.; Pane, M.; Nicola, S.; Allesina, S.; Deidda, F. Micronized Cells of the Probiotic Strain *Bifidobacterium lactis* BS01 Activate Monocyte Polarization: A New Approach. *J. Clin. Gastroenterol.* **2018**, *52* (Suppl. S1), S57–S61. [CrossRef] [PubMed]
77. Czajeczny, D.; Kabzińska, K.; Wójciak, R.W. Effects of *Bifidobacterium Lactis* BS01 and *Lactobacillus Acidophilus* LA02 on cognitive functioning in healthy women. *Appl. Neuropsychol. Adult* **2023**, *30*, 552–560. [CrossRef] [PubMed]

78. Calvigioni, M.; Bertolini, A.; Codini, S.; Mazzantini, D.; Panattoni, A.; Massimino, M.; Celandroni, F.; Zucchi, R.; Saba, A.; Ghelardi, E. HPLC-MS-MS quantification of short-chain fatty acids actively secreted by probiotic strains. *Front. Microbiol.* **2023**, *14*, 1124144. [CrossRef]
79. Solito, A.; Bozzi Cionci, N.; Calgaro, M.; Caputo, M.; Vannini, L.; Hasballa, I.; Archero, F.; Giglione, E.; Ricotti, R.; Walker, G.E.; et al. Supplementation with *Bifidobacterium breve* BR03 and B632 strains improved insulin sensitivity in children and adolescents with obesity in a cross-over, randomized double-blind placebo-controlled trial. *Clin. Nutr.* **2021**, *40*, 4585–4594. [CrossRef] [PubMed]
80. Reigstad, C.S.; Salmonson, C.E.; Rainey, J.F., 3rd; Szurszewski, J.H.; Linden, D.R.; Sonnenburg, J.L.; Farrugia, G.; Kashyap, P.C. Gut microbes promote colonic serotonin production through an effect of short-chain fatty acids on enterochromaffin cells. *FASEB J.* **2015**, *29*, 1395–1403. [CrossRef] [PubMed]
81. Mudaliar, S.B.; Poojary, S.S.; Bharath Prasad, A.S.; Mazumder, N. Probiotics and Paraprobiotics: Effects on Microbiota-Gut-Brain Axis and Their Consequent Potential in Neuropsychiatric Therapy. *Probiot. Antimicrob. Proteins* **2024**, *16*, 1440–1464. [CrossRef]
82. Strasser, B.; Geiger, D.; Schauer, M.; Gostner, J.M.; Gatterer, H.; Burtscher, M.; Fuchs, D. Probiotic Supplements Beneficially Affect Tryptophan-Kynurenine Metabolism and Reduce the Incidence of Upper Respiratory Tract Infections in Trained Athletes: A Randomized, Double-Blinded, Placebo-Controlled Trial. *Nutrients* **2016**, *8*, 752. [CrossRef] [PubMed]
83. Jäger, R.; Purpura, M.; Stone, J.D.; Turner, S.M.; Anzalone, A.J.; Eimerbrink, M.J.; Pane, M.; Amoruso, A.; Rowlands, D.S.; Oliver, J.M. Probiotic *Streptococcus thermophilus* FP4 and *Bifidobacterium breve* BR03 Supplementation Attenuates Performance and Range-of-Motion Decrements Following Muscle Damaging Exercise. *Nutrients* **2016**, *8*, 642. [CrossRef]
84. Imanian, B.; Hemmatinafar, M.; Daryanoosh, F.; Koureshfard, N.; Sadeghi, R.; Niknam, A.; Rezaei, R.; Qashqaei, A. The effect of probiotics and casein supplementation on aerobic capacity parameters of male soccer players. *J. Int. Soc. Sports Nutr.* **2024**, *21*, 2382165. [CrossRef] [PubMed]
85. Marotta, A.; Sarno, E.; Del Casale, A.; Pane, M.; Mogna, L.; Amoruso, A.; Felis, G.E.; Fiorio, M. Effects of Probiotics on Cognitive Reactivity, Mood, and Sleep Quality. *Front. Psychiatry* **2019**, *10*, 164. [CrossRef]
86. Mitrea, L.; Nemeş, S.A.; Szabo, K.; Teleky, B.E.; Vodnar, D.C. Guts Imbalance Imbalances the Brain: A Review of Gut Microbiota Association with Neurological and Psychiatric Disorders. *Front. Med.* **2022**, *9*, 813204. [CrossRef]
87. Cocean, A.M.; Vodnar, D.C. Exploring the gut-brain Axis: Potential therapeutic impact of Psychobiotics on mental health. *Prog. Neuropsychopharmacol. Biol. Psychiatry* **2024**, *134*, 111073. [CrossRef] [PubMed]
88. Smiljanic, K.; Pesic, V.; Mladenovic Djordjevic, A.; Pavkovic, Z.; Brkic, M.; Ruzdijic, S.; Kanazir, S. Long-term dietary restriction differentially affects the expression of BDNF and its receptors in the cortex and hippocampus of middle-aged and aged male rats. *Biogerontology* **2015**, *16*, 71–83. [CrossRef] [PubMed]
89. Drago, S.; El Asmar, R.; Di Pierro, M.; Grazia Clemente, M.; Tripathi, A.; Sapone, A.; Thakar, M.; Iacono, G.; Carroccio, A.; D'Agate, C.; et al. Gliadin, zonulin and gut permeability: Effects on celiac and non-celiac intestinal mucosa and intestinal cell lines. *Scand. J. Gastroenterol.* **2006**, *41*, 408–419. [CrossRef] [PubMed]
90. Orlando, A.; Linsalata, M.; Bianco, G.; Notarnicola, M.; D'Attoma, B.; Scavo, M.P.; Tafaro, A.; Russo, F. *Lactobacillus rhamnosus* GG Protects the Epithelial Barrier of Wistar Rats from the Pepsin-Trypsin-Digested Gliadin (PTG)-Induced Enteropathy. *Nutrients* **2018**, *10*, 1698. [CrossRef]
91. Orlando, A.; Chimienti, G.; Lezza, A.M.S.; Pesce, V.; Gigante, I.; D'Attoma, B.; Russo, F. *Lactobacillus Rhamnosus* GG Affects the BDNF System in Brain Samples of Wistar Rats with Pepsin-Trypsin-Digested Gliadin (PTG)-Induced Enteropathy. *Nutrients* **2020**, *12*, 629. [CrossRef] [PubMed]
92. Cheng, R.; Xu, T.; Zhang, Y.; Wang, F.; Zhao, L.; Jiang, Y.; He, F. *Lactobacillus rhamnosus* GG and *Bifidobacterium bifidum* TMC3115 Can Affect Development of Hippocampal Neurons Cultured In Vitro in a Strain-Dependent Manner. *Probiot. Antimicrob. Proteins* **2020**, *12*, 589–599. [CrossRef] [PubMed]
93. Desbonnet, L.; Garrett, L.; Clarke, G.; Kiely, B.; Cryan, J.F.; Dinan, T.G. Effects of the probiotic *Bifidobacterium infantis* in the maternal separation model of depression. *Neuroscience* **2010**, *170*, 1179–1188. [CrossRef] [PubMed]
94. McVey Neufeld, K.A.; O'Mahony, S.M.; Hoban, A.E.; Waworuntu, R.V.; Berg, B.M.; Dinan, T.G.; Cryan, J.F. Neurobehavioural effects of *Lactobacillus rhamnosus* GG alone and in combination with prebiotics polydextrose and galactooligosaccharide in male rats exposed to early-life stress. *Nutr. Neurosci.* **2019**, *22*, 425–434. [CrossRef] [PubMed]
95. Srivastav, S.; Neupane, S.; Bhurtel, S.; Katila, N.; Maharjan, S.; Choi, H.; Hong, J.T.; Choi, D.Y. Probiotics mixture increases butyrate, and subsequently rescues the nigral dopaminergic neurons from MPTP and rotenone-induced neurotoxicity. *J. Nutr. Biochem.* **2019**, *69*, 73–86. [CrossRef]
96. Hartung, T.J.; Brähler, E.; Faller, H.; Härter, M.; Hinz, A.; Johansen, C.; Keller, M.; Koch, U.; Schulz, H.; Weis, J.; et al. The risk of being depressed is significantly higher in cancer patients than in the general population: Prevalence and severity of depressive symptoms across major cancer types. *Eur. J. Cancer* **2017**, *72*, 46–53. [CrossRef] [PubMed]

97. Mitchell, A.J.; Chan, M.; Bhatti, H.; Halton, M.; Grassi, L.; Johansen, C.; Meader, N. Prevalence of depression, anxiety, and adjustment disorder in oncological, haematological, and palliative-care settings: A meta-analysis of 94 interview-based studies. *Lancet Oncol.* **2011**, *12*, 160–174. [CrossRef] [PubMed]
98. Massie, M.J. Prevalence of depression in patients with cancer. *J. Natl. Cancer Inst. Monogr.* **2004**, *2004*, 57–71. [CrossRef] [PubMed]
99. Gontijo Garcia, G.S.; Meira, K.C.; de Souza, A.H.; Guimarães, N.S. Anxiety and depression disorders in oncological patients under palliative care at a hospital service: A cross-sectional study. *BMC Palliat. Care* **2023**, *22*, 116. [CrossRef]
100. He, Y.; Pang, Y.; Su, Z.; Zhou, Y.; Wang, Y.; Lu, Y.; Jiang, Y.; Han, X.; Song, L.; Wang, L.; et al. Symptom burden, psychological distress, and symptom management status in hospitalized patients with advanced cancer: A multicenter study in China. *ESMO Open* **2022**, *7*, 100595. [CrossRef] [PubMed]
101. Kamimura, K.; Haga, H.; Wada, T.; Aoyama, M.; Ito, R.; Minami, J.; Uchitsubo, T.; Saijo, Y. Changes in Psychological Condition during Cancer Chemotherapy. *Asian Pac. J. Cancer Prev.* **2024**, *25*, 2475–2481. [CrossRef] [PubMed]
102. Breen, S.J.; Baravelli, C.M.; Schofield, P.E.; Jefford, M.; Yates, P.M.; Aranda, S.K. Is symptom burden a predictor of anxiety and depression in patients with cancer about to commence chemotherapy? *Med. J. Aust.* **2009**, *190*, S99–S104. [CrossRef]
103. Peng, J.; Cheng, D. The effectiveness of therapeutic artmaking on depression, anxiety, quality of life, and psychological distress in cancer patients on chemotherapy: A systematic review of the literature. *Support. Care Cancer* **2024**, *32*, 245. [CrossRef] [PubMed]
104. Vyas, D.; Laput, G.; Vyas, A.K. Chemotherapy-enhanced inflammation may lead to the failure of therapy and metastasis. *Onco Targets Ther.* **2014**, *7*, 1015–1023. [CrossRef]
105. O'Mahony, S.M.; Clarke, G.; Borre, Y.E.; Dinan, T.G.; Cryan, J.F. Serotonin, tryptophan metabolism and the brain-gut-microbiome axis. *Behav. Brain Res.* **2015**, *277*, 32–48. [CrossRef] [PubMed]
106. Magalhães-Guedes, K.T. Psychobiotic Therapy: Method to Reinforce the Immune System. *Clin. Psychopharmacol. Neurosci.* **2022**, *20*, 17–25. [CrossRef]
107. Berding, K.; Bastiaanssen, T.F.S.; Moloney, G.M.; Boscaini, S.; Strain, C.R.; Anesi, A.; Long-Smith, C.; Mattivi, F.; Stanton, C.; Clarke, G.; et al. Feed your microbes to deal with stress: A psychobiotic diet impacts microbial stability and perceived stress in a healthy adult population. *Mol. Psychiatry* **2023**, *28*, 601–610. [CrossRef] [PubMed]
108. Lee, Y.S.; Kim, T.Y.; Kim, Y.; Lee, S.H.; Kim, S.; Kang, S.W.; Yang, J.Y.; Baek, I.J.; Sung, Y.H.; Park, Y.Y.; et al. Microbiota-Derived Lactate Accelerates Intestinal Stem-Cell-Mediated Epithelial Development. *Cell Host Microbe* **2018**, *24*, 833–846.E6. [CrossRef] [PubMed]
109. Akkasheh, G.; Kashani-Poor, Z.; Tajadadi-Ebrahimi, M.; Jafari, P.; Akbari, H.; Taghizadeh, M.; Memarzadeh, M.; Asemi, Z.; Esmaillzadeh, A. Clinical and metabolic response to probiotic administration in patients with major depressive disorder: A randomized, double-blind, placebo-controlled trial. *Nutrition* **2015**, *32*, 315–320. [CrossRef] [PubMed]
110. Steenbergen, L.; Sellaro, R.; van Hemert, S.; Bosch, J.A.; Colzato, L.S. A randomized controlled trial to test the effect of multispecies probiotics on cognitive reactivity to sad mood. *Brain Behav. Immun.* **2015**, *48*, 258–264. [CrossRef] [PubMed]
111. Patterson, A.M.; Mulder, I.E.; Travis, A.J.; Lan, A.; Cerf-Bensussan, N.; Gaboriau-Routhiau, V.; Garden, K.; Logan, E.; Delday, M.I.; Coutts, A.G.P.; et al. Human Gut Symbiont Roseburia hominis Promotes and Regulates Innate Immunity. *Front. Immunol.* **2017**, *8*, 1166. [CrossRef]
112. Zhang, Q.; Chen, B.; Zhang, J.; Dong, J.; Ma, J.; Zhang, Y.; Jin, K.; Lu, J. Effect of prebiotics, probiotics, synbiotics on depression: Results from a meta-analysis. *BMC Psychiatry* **2023**, *23*, 477. [CrossRef]
113. Aizawa, E.; Tsuji, H.; Asahara, T.; Takahashi, T.; Teraishi, T.; Yoshida, S.; Ota, M.; Koga, N.; Hattori, K.; Kunugi, H. Possible association of *Bifidobacterium* and *Lactobacillus* in the gut microbiota of patients with major depressive disorder. *J. Affect. Disord.* **2016**, *202*, 254–257. [CrossRef] [PubMed]
114. Nikolova, V.L.; Smith, M.R.B.; Hall, L.J.; Cleare, A.J.; Stone, J.M.; Young, A.H. Perturbations in Gut Microbiota Composition in Psychiatric Disorders: A Review and Meta-analysis. *JAMA Psychiatry* **2021**, *78*, 1343–1354. [CrossRef]
115. Donoso, F.; Cryan, J.F.; Olavarría-Ramírez, L.; Nolan, Y.M.; Clarke, G. Inflammation, Lifestyle Factors, and the Microbiome-Gut-Brain Axis: Relevance to Depression and Antidepressant Action. *Clin. Pharmacol. Ther.* **2023**, *113*, 246–259. [CrossRef] [PubMed]
116. Tian, P.; Chen, Y.; Zhu, H.; Wang, L.; Qian, X.; Zou, R.; Zhao, J.; Zhang, H.; Qian, L.; Wang, Q.; et al. *Bifidobacterium breve* CCFM1025 attenuates major depression disorder via regulating gut microbiome and tryptophan metabolism: A randomized clinical trial. *Brain Behav. Immun.* **2022**, *100*, 233–241. [CrossRef] [PubMed]
117. Haroon, E.; Raison, C.L.; Miller, A.H. Psychoneuroimmunology meets neuropsychopharmacology: Translational implications of the impact of inflammation on behavior. *Neuropsychopharmacology* **2012**, *37*, 137–162. [CrossRef]
118. Rudzki, L.; Ostrowska, L.; Pawlak, D.; Małus, A.; Pawlak, K.; Waszkiewicz, N.; Szulc, A. Probiotic *Lactobacillus Plantarum* 299v decreases kynurenine concentration and improves cognitive functions in patients with major depression: A double-blind, randomized, placebo controlled study. *Psychoneuroendocrinology* **2019**, *100*, 213–222. [CrossRef] [PubMed]

119. Zhu, R.; Fang, Y.; Li, H.; Liu, Y.; Wei, J.; Zhang, S.; Wang, L.; Fan, R.; Wang, L.; Li, S.; et al. Psychobiotic *Lactobacillus plantarum* JYLP-326 relieves anxiety, depression, and insomnia symptoms in test anxious college via modulating the gut microbiota and its metabolism. *Front. Immunol.* **2023**, *14*, 1158137. [CrossRef]
120. Lan, Y.; Lu, J.; Qiao, G.; Mao, X.; Zhao, J.; Wang, G.; Tian, P.; Chen, W. *Bifidobacterium breve* CCFM1025 Improves Sleep Quality via Regulating the Activity of the HPA Axis: A Randomized Clinical Trial. *Nutrients* **2023**, *15*, 4700. [CrossRef] [PubMed]
121. Haarhuis, J.E.; Kardinaal, A.; Kortman, G.A.M. Probiotics, prebiotics and postbiotics for better sleep quality: A narrative review. *Benef. Microbes* **2022**, *13*, 169–182. [CrossRef] [PubMed]
122. Esser, P.; Hartung, T.J.; Friedrich, M.; Johansen, C.; Wittchen, H.U.; Faller, H.; Koch, U.; Härter, M.; Keller, M.; Schulz, H.; et al. The Generalized Anxiety Disorder Screener (GAD-7) and the anxiety module of the Hospital and Depression Scale (HADS-A) as screening tools for generalized anxiety disorder among cancer patients. *Psychooncology* **2018**, *27*, 1509–1516. [CrossRef] [PubMed]
123. Peng, J.; Yuan, S.; Wei, Z.; Liu, C.; Li, K.; Wei, X.; Yuan, S.Q.; Guo, Z.; Wu, L.; Feng, T.; et al. Temporal network of experience sampling methodology identifies sleep disturbance as a central symptom in generalized anxiety disorder. *BMC Psychiatry* **2024**, *24*, 241. [CrossRef]
124. Stark, D.; Kiely, M.; Smith, A.; Velikova, G.; House, A.; Selby, P. Anxiety disorders in cancer patients: Their nature, associations, and relation to quality of life. *J. Clin. Oncol.* **2002**, *20*, 3137–3148. [CrossRef] [PubMed]
125. Truong, D.V.; Bui, Q.T.T.; Nguyen, D.T.; Moore, J. Anxiety Among Inpatients with Cancer: Findings From a Hospital-Based Cross-Sectional Study in Vietnam. *Cancer Control* **2019**, *26*, 1073274819864641. [CrossRef] [PubMed]
126. Rassoulian, A.; Gaiger, A.; Loeffler-Stastka, H. Gender Differences in Psychosocial, Religious, and Spiritual Aspects in Coping: A Cross-Sectional Study with Cancer Patients. *Womens Health Rep.* **2021**, *2*, 464–472. [CrossRef] [PubMed]
127. Vitale, E.; Halemani, K.; Shetty, A.; Chang, Y.C.; Hu, W.Y.; Massafra, R.; Moretti, A. Sex Differences in Anxiety and Depression Conditions among Cancer Patients: A Systematic Review and Meta-Analysis. *Cancers* **2024**, *16*, 1969. [CrossRef]
128. Hasan, E.M.; Calma, C.L.; Tudor, A.; Oancea, C.; Tudorache, V.; Petrache, I.A.; Tudorache, E.; Papava, I. Coping, Anxiety, and Pain Intensity in Patients Requiring Thoracic Surgery. *J. Pers. Med.* **2021**, *11*, 1221. [CrossRef] [PubMed]
129. Rand, K.L.; Cripe, L.D.; Monahan, P.O.; Tong, Y.; Schmidt, K.; Rawl, S.M. Illness appraisal, religious coping, and psychological responses in men with advanced cancer. *Support. Care Cancer* **2012**, *20*, 1719–1728. [CrossRef]
130. Hinz, A.; Krauss, O.; Stolzenburg, J.U.; Schwalenberg, T.; Michalski, D.; Schwarz, R. Anxiety and depression in patients with prostate cancer and other urogenital cancer: A longitudinal study. *Urol. Oncol.* **2009**, *27*, 367–372. [CrossRef]
131. Pasquini, M.; Biondi, M. Depression in cancer patients: A critical review. *Clin. Pract. Epidemiol. Ment. Health* **2007**, *3*, 2. [CrossRef]
132. Wei, P.; Keller, C.; Li, L. Neuropeptides in gut-brain axis and their influence on host immunity and stress. *Comput. Struct. Biotechnol. J.* **2020**, *18*, 843–851. [CrossRef]
133. McEwen, B.S. Neurobiological and Systemic Effects of Chronic Stress. *Chronic Stress* **2017**, *1*, 2470547017692328. [CrossRef] [PubMed]
134. Kim, E.J.; Pellman, B.; Kim, J.J. Stress effects on the hippocampus: A critical review. *Learn. Mem.* **2015**, *22*, 411–416. [CrossRef] [PubMed]

nutrients

MDPI

Article

Five-Day Treatment with *B. licheniformis* Along with Classical Vancomycin Treatment Was Effective in Preserving Gut Microbiota in Patients with *Clostridioides difficile* Infection

Tae-Geun Gweon [1,2], Sang-Bum Kang [1,3], Soo-Young Na [1,4], Dong Jun Oh [5], Sang Wook Kim [6], Geom Seog Seo [7,*] and Joo Young Cho [8,*]

1 Department of Internal Medicine, College of Medicine, The Catholic University of Korea, Seoul 02812, Republic of Korea; gweontae@naver.com (T.-G.G.); sangucsd@gmail.com (S.-B.K.); sktndud@hanmail.net (S.-Y.N.)
2 Department of Internal Medicine, Bucheon St. Mary's Hospital, College of Medicine, The Catholic University of Korea, Bucheon 14662, Republic of Korea
3 Department of Internal Medicine, Daejeon St. Mary's Hospital, College of Medicine, The Catholic University of Korea, Daejeon 34943, Republic of Korea
4 Department of Internal Medicine, Incheon St. Mary's Hospital, College of Medicine, The Catholic University of Korea, Incheon 21431, Republic of Korea
5 Department of Internal Medicine, Dongguk University Ilsan Hospital, Goyang 10326, Republic of Korea; mileo31@naver.com
6 Department of Internal Medicine, Jeonbuk National University Hospital, Jeonju 54907, Republic of Korea; clickm@jbnu.ac.kr
7 Department of Internal Medicine, Digestive Disease Research Institute, Wonkwang University Hospital, Iksan 54538, Republic of Korea
8 Department of Internal Medicine, Cha Medical Center Gangnam, Seoul 06135, Republic of Korea
* Correspondence: medsgs@wonkwang.ac.kr (G.S.S.); cjy6695@naver.com (J.Y.C.); Tel.: +82-63-859-2565 (G.S.S.); +82-10-9496-6695 (J.Y.C.); Fax: +82-63-855-2025 (G.S.S.)

Abstract: Background/Objectives: *Clostridioides difficile* infection (CDI) is an important nosocomial diarrheal disease. The benefits of the probiotic *Bacillus licheniformis* (*B. licheniformis*) in the preservation of intestinal microbiota have not been studied in patients with CDI to date. Therefore, we aimed to investigate the efficacy of *B. licheniformis* in preserving the intestinal microbiota in patients with CDI. **Methods:** A multicenter, randomized, placebo-controlled trial was carried out at six academic centers in Korea. Individuals diagnosed with mild to moderate CDI were included in this trial. CDI was treated with vancomycin 125 mg four times daily for two weeks. Along with vancomycin, *B. licheniformis* was administered for five days in this study, while a placebo was given to the placebo group. Microbiome analysis was performed before and five days after administering vancomycin and *B. licheniformis* or placebo, using 16S rRNA amplicon sequencing. Alpha and beta diversity was compared between the two groups. **Results:** A total of 35 participants were finally included in this study, with 16 in the study group and 19 in the placebo group. The alpha diversity was similar in both groups before CDI treatment. After five days of the administration of vancomycin and *B. licheniformis* or placebo, alpha diversity did not decrease in the study group (Chao1 index, $p = 0.665$; observed features, $p = 0.692$). In contrast, alpha diversity decreased in the placebo group (Chao1 index, $p = 0.011$; observed features, $p = 0.011$). Beta diversity did not differ between the two groups. **Conclusions:** The addition of *B. licheniformis* to vancomycin was effective in preserving gut microbiota in patients with CDI.

Keywords: *Clostridioides difficile* infection; *Bacillus licheniformis*; probiotic; microbiota

1. Introduction

Clostridioides difficile infection (CDI) is an important nosocomial diarrheal disease caused by the disruption of intestinal microbiota (dysbiosis) [1]. Antimicrobial use, chronic inflammation, and chronic diseases contribute to dysbiosis [2]. CDI is related to longer hospital stays and increased medical costs [3,4]. In the US, CDI is associated with roughly 500,000 infections, and mortality is reported at 30,000 deaths annually [5,6]. In the past, the incidence of CDI was lower in Asian countries compared to Western countries [7]. However, recent studies have shown that the incidence of CDI is increasing in Eastern countries [8,9].

CDI is regarded as a high-risk factor for post-infectious irritable bowel syndrome (IBS) [10], which is complicated in approximately 20% of patients with CDI [11]. The restoration of the disrupted intestinal microbiota is essential for recovery in patients with CDI [12]. Dysbiosis is related to CDI recurrence and the development of post-infectious IBS [13,14].

Fecal microbiota transplantation (FMT) is recommended as standard treatment for recurrent or refractory CDI [15–18]. Furthermore, dysbiosis can be restored after FMT [19]. Although various novel products have been developed for FMT to date [20], there is a potential for adverse events, including the transmission of pathogens [21].

Probiotics have emerged as an effective option for modulating human immunity [22] and can be used to restore the disrupted intestinal microbiota in various diseases. Probiotics have also been investigated for the treatment of CDI. A meta-analysis of randomized controlled trials (RCTs) reported that probiotic treatment effectively decolonizes *C. difficile* [23]. Another systematic review and meta-analysis showed a modest effect of probiotics for preventing recurrent CDI [24]. However, the number of patients that needed treatment was 42 in that review.

Bacillus licheniformis (*B. licheniformis*) is a Gram-positive spore-forming anaerobic bacterium. Spore-based probiotics have the ability to withstand acid in the stomach and can survive in the intestines [25,26]. The benefits of *B. licheniformis* have been investigated in various diseases, including colitis, infectious diarrhea, metabolic diseases, and cardiovascular disease [27]. In an animal study, *B. licheniformis* attenuated dextran sulfate sodium-induced colitis's disrupted intestinal barrier integrity [28]. However, the efficacy of *B. licheniformis* in preserving the intestinal microbiota has not yet been studied in patients with CDI. It is important to identify new probiotics for the treatment of CDI.

In this multicenter trial, we investigated the efficacy of *B. licheniformis* on the intestinal microbiota using microbiome analysis in patients with CDI.

2. Methods

This was a multicenter, double-blinded RCT. Adults, aged ≥18 years, who were diagnosed with mild to moderate CDI were eligible for inclusion. CDI was diagnosed when the patients passed loose stools at least three times a day and tested positive for toxins [9]. The exclusion criteria were as follows: (1) recurrent CDI, (2) inflammatory bowel disease, (3) a history of immunosuppressive agent use or chemotherapy, (4) the use of probiotics three months prior to inclusion, and (5) inability to discontinue causative antibiotics for CDI at the time of inclusion. A toxin assay was performed using a Wampole™ C. DIFF QUIK CHEK COMPLETE™ (TechLab, Blacksburg, VA, USA).

After obtaining informed consent, the study participants were randomized into the study and placebo groups. *B. licheniformis* 250 mg or placebo three times per day was administered for five days in the study and placebo groups, respectively. The placebo, which contained starch as its main component, was designed to match the study drug in color and shape. CDI treatment was performed using 125 mg of vancomycin four times per day for both groups. Enrollment was performed between July 2021 and December 2022 at six academic hospitals in Korea: Bucheon St. Mary's Hospital, Incheon St. Mary's Hospital, Daejeon St. Mary's Hospital, Wonkwang University Hospital, Jeonbuk National University Hospital, and Dongguk University Ilsan Hospital. The institutional review boards of the participating hospitals approved the study protocol.

2.1. Microbiome Analysis

Microbiome analysis was performed before and five days after the administration of vancomycin and *B. licheniformis* or placebo. The stool was collected from the study participants, and at least 1 g was stored in a THERAbiome stool kit (THERAGEN Health, Seongnam, Republic of Korea). Using the sampling kit, the stool microbiome was preserved at room temperature for up to 65 days after collection [29]. The stool kit was delivered to each hospital within three days of collection. The participating hospitals then sent the stool kits to Theragen Bio (Seongnam, Republic of Korea) every week.

The protocol for microbiome analysis was described previously [29,30]. Metagenomic DNA was extracted from stool samples using QIAmp (Qiagen, Germany). Long-read metagenomic sequencing was performed using MiSeq software (version 4.0) (Illumina, CA, USA). The V3–V4 region of microbial 16S rRNA genes was targeted.

Alpha diversity, beta diversity, and microbial species were compared between the two groups using 16S rRNA amplicon sequencing [30]. Alpha diversity was compared using the Shannon, Simpson, and Chao 1 indices and the observed features. Beta diversity was investigated using UniFrac analysis. Bacterial 16S rRNA sequencing data were analyzed using the QIIME2 bioinformatics pipeline (http://qiime2.org, accessed on 26 September 2022).

The primary endpoint of this study was microbial changes after five days of treatment. Patient characteristics, stool frequency, and form measured using the Bristol stool scale (BSS); CDI treatment results; and adverse events during the trial were investigated. The participants were followed up for two months after inclusion.

2.2. Statistical Analysis

This was a pilot study. We planned to include 40 patients with CDI (20 patients per group). The alpha and beta diversities of the two groups were compared using the Kruskal–Wallis test. Continuous data were presented as means or medians, as appropriate for clinical data. The Mann–Whitney U-test was used for continuous variables. The chi-square and Fisher's exact tests were used for binary outcomes, as appropriate. Statistical analyses were performed using R software (version 4.3).

3. Results

The 40 participants were randomized in a 1:1 ratio. After excluding 5 participants (withdrawal of informed consent, $n = 2$; improper collection of stool samples, $n = 3$), 35 participants (study group, $n = 16$; placebo, $n = 19$) were finally included. The demographic characteristics of the study participants are presented in Table 1. Age, sex, body mass index, admission status, duration of antibiotic use, stool form, and stool frequency were comparable between the two groups.

3.1. Microbiome Analysis at Randomization

The alpha diversity measured at randomization was comparable between the two groups (Chao 1 index, $p = 0.337$; observed features, $p = 0.290$; Shannon index, $p = 0.832$; Simpson index, $p = 0.806$; Figure 1).

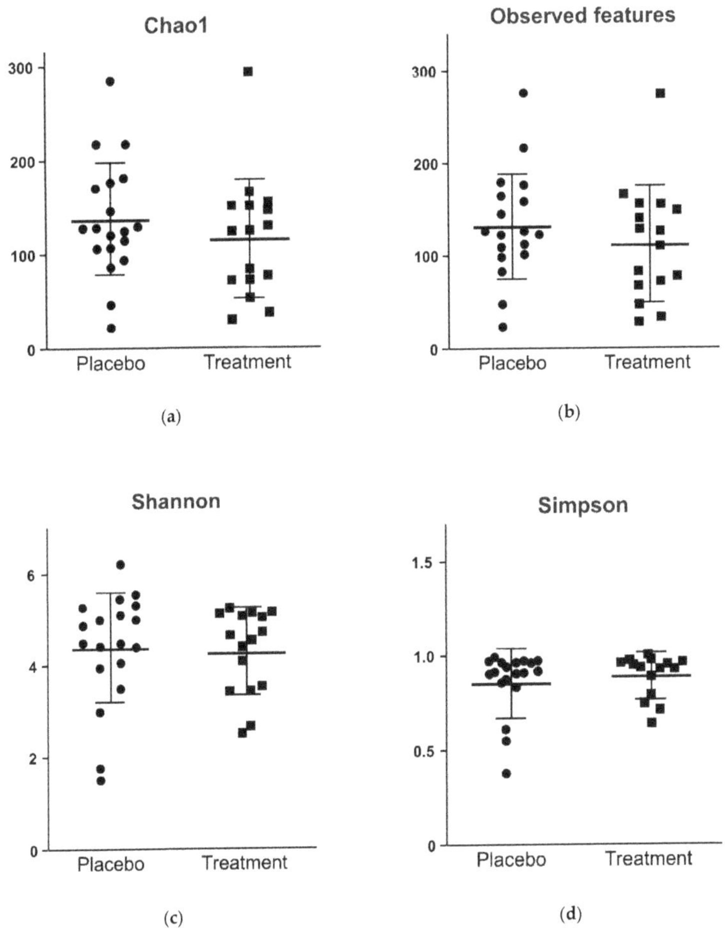

Figure 1. Comparison of alpha diversity between probiotic and placebo groups at randomization. Alpha diversities measured using Chao1 index, $p = 0.337$ (**a**); observed features, $p = 0.290$ (**b**); Shannon diversity index, $p = 0.832$ (**c**); and Simpson diversity index, $p = 0.806$ (**d**), are comparable between the two groups.

Table 1. Baseline characteristics.

Characteristics	**Probiotic (n = 16)**	**Placebo (n = 19)**	p
Age, median (IQR)	70.5 (60.5, 78.0)	62.0 (54.5, 72.0)	0.226
Male, n (%)	7 (43.8%)	5 (26.3%)	0.468
Body mass index, median (IQR)	23.3 (19.3, 25.3)	23.1 (20.6, 25.8)	0.441
Inpatient, n (%)	14 (87.5%)	17 (89.5%)	1.000
Duration of antibiotic treatment, n (%)			1.000
≥2 weeks	4 (25.0%)	5 (26.3%)	
<2 weeks	12 (75.0%)	14 (73.7%)	
Smoking, n (%)			0.677
Current or ex-smoker	4 (25.0%)	3 (15.8%)	
Non-smoker	12 (75.0%)	16 (84.2%)	
Alcohol use, n (%)			0.379
Yes	4 (25.0%)	2 (10.5%)	
<1/month	12 (75.0%)	17 (89.5%)	

Table 1. *Cont.*

Characteristics	Probiotic (n = 16)	Placebo (n = 19)	p
BSS, n (%)			1.000
Type 6	9 (56.2%)	10 (52.6%)	
Type 7	7 (43.8%)	9 (47.4%)	
Stool frequency, number/day (%)			0.152
3	13 (81.2%)	10 (52.6%)	
≥4	3 (18.8%)	9 (47.4%)	

IQR, interquartile range; BSS, Bristol stool scale.

3.2. Microbiome Analysis at Five Days After Treatment

The results of the microbiome analysis five days after treatment are presented in Figure 2. In the study group, alpha diversity did not decrease after five days of the administration of the study drug and vancomycin (Chao1 index, p = 0.665; observed features, p = 0.692; Shannon index, p = 0.287; Simpson index, p = 0.361; Figure 2).

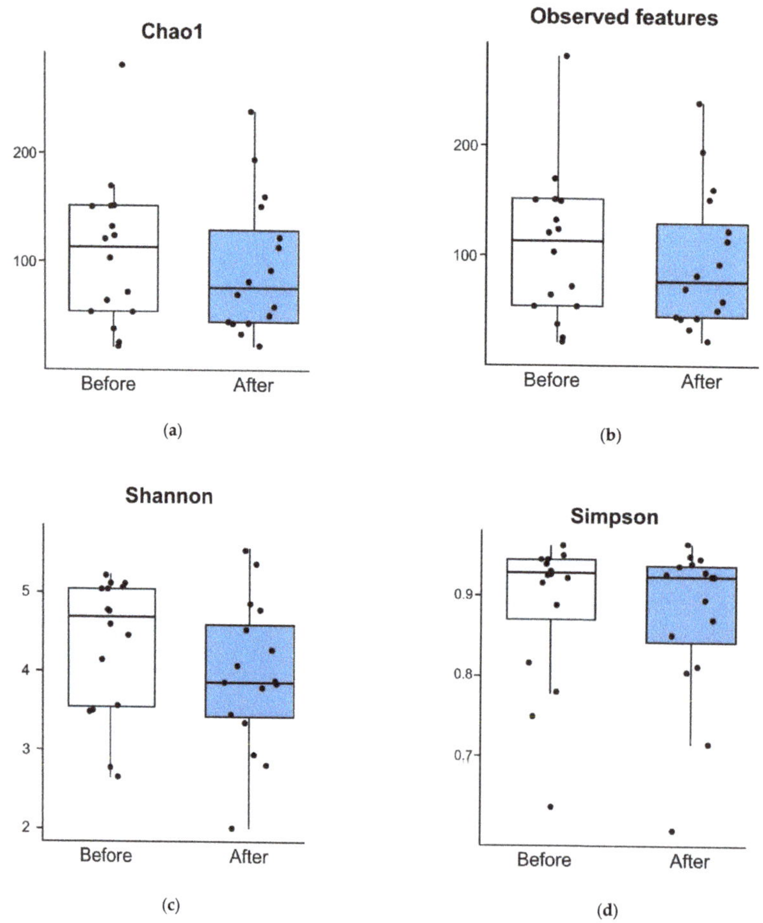

Figure 2. Comparison of alpha diversity for probiotic group between before and five days after treatment. Alpha diversities measured using Chao1 index (p = 0.665) (**a**), observed features (p = 0.692) (**b**), Shannon diversity index (p = 0.287) (**c**), and Simpson diversity index (p = 0.806) (**d**) are comparable before and after treatment.

However, in the placebo group, alpha diversity significantly decreased five days after treatment (Chao1 index, $p = 0.011$; observed features, $p = 0.011$; Figure 3a,b). The alpha diversity measured using the Shannon ($p = 0.138$, Figure 3c) and Simpson ($p = 0.311$, Figure 3d) indices was similar before and after treatment in the placebo group.

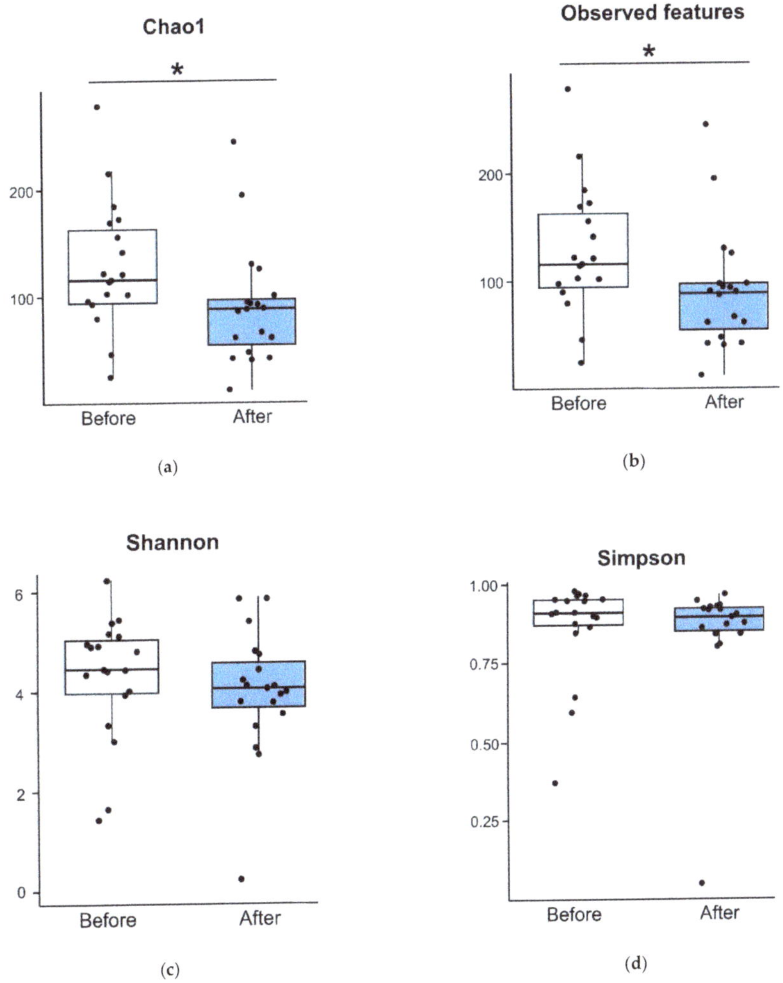

Figure 3. Comparison of alpha diversity for placebo group between before and five days after treatment. Alpha diversity measured using Chao1 index ($p = 0.011$) (**a**) and observed features ($p = 0.011$) (**b**) are decreased five days after treatment. However, alpha diversities measured using Shannon ($p = 0.138$) (**c**) and Simpson ($p = 0.311$) (**d**) diversity indices are comparable. * Statistically significant.

Beta diversity after treatment, measured using weighted UniFrac, differed from that before treatment in the study ($p = 0.001$, Figure 4a) and placebo ($p = 0.002$, Figure 4b) groups. However, beta diversity did not differ between the placebo and study groups (Figure 4c).

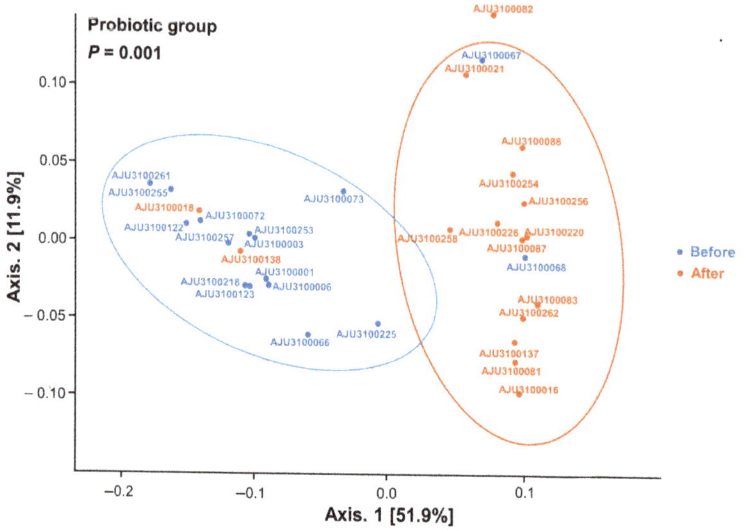

(**a**)

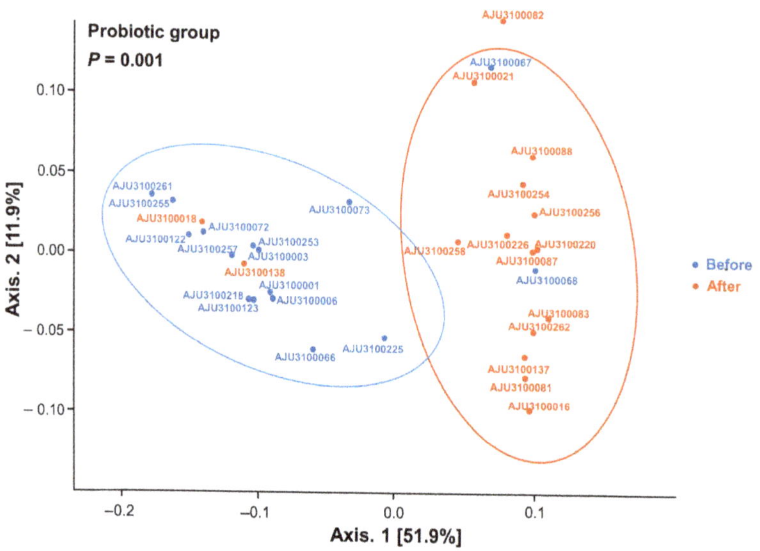

(**b**)

Figure 4. *Cont.*

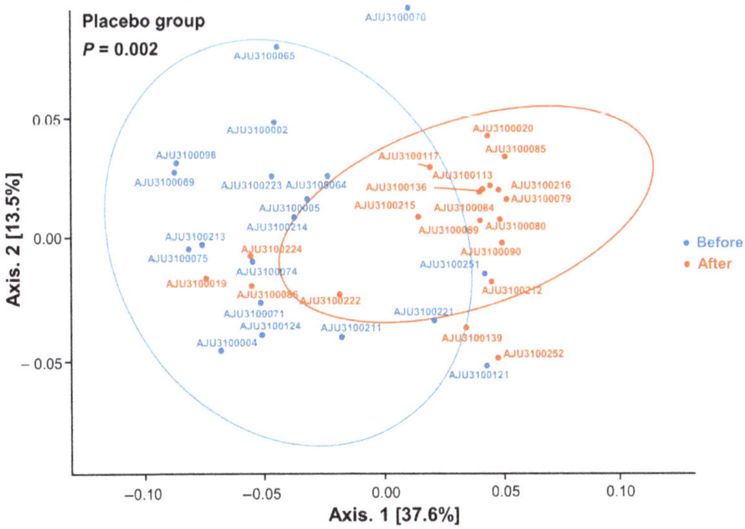

(c)

Figure 4. Comparison of beta diversity. Beta diversity differs between before and five days after treatment in probiotic group (p = 0.001) (**a**). Beta diversity differs between before and five days after treatment in placebo group (p = 0.002) (**b**). Beta diversity is comparable between probiotic and placebo groups (**c**).

3.3. Treatment Results

All patients were cured after two weeks of vancomycin treatment. No adverse events occurred during treatment. Stool form and the frequency of defecation did not differ between the two groups. Five days after treatment, 65.7% and 51.4% of participants showed an improvement in stool type (from BSS type 6 and 7 to type 3–5) and frequency (from $\geq$3/day to 1–2/day), respectively (Table 2).

Table 2. Stool characteristics at 5 days after treatment.

Characteristics	Probiotic (n = 16)	Placebo (n = 19)	p
BSS, n (%)			0.713
Type 3, 4, 5	10 (62.5)	13 (68.4)	
Type 6, 7	6 (37.5)	6 (31.6)	
Stool frequency, n (%)			0.947
1–2/day	8 (50.0%)	10 (52.6%)	
3–4/day	5 (31.2%)	5 (26.3%)	
$\geq$5/day	3 (18.8%)	4 (21.1%)	

BSS, Bristol stool scale

4. Discussion

In this pilot study, a combination of the probiotic *B. licheniformis* and vancomycin showed positive efficacy in preserving the intestinal microbiota in patients with CDI during the early stages of this disease. In the placebo group, alpha diversity was measured using the Chao1 index, and the observed features decreased after five days of treatment. However, the alpha diversity measured using all diversity indices did not decrease in the probiotic group.

The benefits of probiotics have been investigated in clinical practice, where the temporal disruption of the intestinal microbiota was implicated, such as *Helicobacter pylori*

(*H. pylori*) eradication or bowel preparation. The addition of a probiotic supplement was effective in restoring beneficial microbiota during *H. pylori* eradication using bismuth quadruple therapy [31]. In another study, the efficacy of probiotic treatment during bowel preparation was investigated. Probiotics have shown positive effects on preserving intestinal microbiota and decreasing mild abdominal pain after bowel preparation [32].

The use of probiotics in patients with CDI is still controversial [33]. The American Gastroenterological Association guidelines suggest only four types of probiotics for preventing CDI in patients receiving antibiotic treatment [34]. In this study, *B. licheniformis* was used as a supplement for CDI treatment because this strain has not been investigated to date for the treatment of CDI. In our study, we excluded those who could not cease causative antibiotics for CDI at the time of inclusion because the continuous use of antibiotics is related to the deleterious effects of probiotics. Although the cessation of causative antibiotics is recommended in guidelines [15,35], it is challenging to cease them in cases where the index infection is not controlled. To date, the proper duration of probiotic treatment has not been determined. We hypothesized that dysbiosis was the most severe at the time of CDI diagnosis due to recent antibiotic treatment and diarrhea. Thus, in this study, probiotic *B. licheniformis* was prescribed for five days in the early stages of CDI. Although stool frequency and form improved five days after vancomycin treatment, alpha diversity in the placebo group decreased compared to the baseline at randomization, as measured using the Chao1 index and observed features representing microbial richness. However, the evenness of microbial diversity measured using the Shannon and Simpson indices did not differ before treatment and five days after treatment in both groups. The *B. licheniformis* probiotic was partly effective in preserving microbial richness during the early stages of CDI. In this study, beta diversity differed before and after the administration of the probiotic and placebo, along with vancomycin, for the two groups. However, beta diversity did not differ between the two groups after completing the *B. licheniformis* probiotic and placebo. This finding suggests that the overall structure of the microbial community in the probiotic group was similar to that of the placebo group. The addition of a single strain did not affect the compositional change in the microbial structure.

The recurrence rate of CDI is estimated to be approximately 20% [36]. Dysbiosis is more severe in patients with recurrent CDI than in those with primary CDI [12]. Therefore, the preservation of the intestinal microbiota is important for treating CDI. It is acknowledged that maintaining microbial diversity is associated with preventing recurrence. The mechanisms underlying the efficacy of probiotics in treating CDI have also been investigated. One study reported that the engineered probiotic *E. coli* Nissel 1917 limited the germination of endospores of *C. difficile* and thereby the growth of *C. difficile* [37]. Another study suggested that the probiotic *Bacillus amyloliquefaciens* showed an anti-CDI effect by synthesizing extracellular antimicrobial compounds [38]. However, these studies were performed using animal models. The health benefits of the *B. licheniformis* probiotic have been linked to the modulation of the intestinal microbiota, anti-inflammatory activity, and improvement in the lipid profile. However, these effects have not yet been investigated in patients with CDI.

This study has several limitations. First, although CDI treatment is recommended for 10–14 days, microbial analysis was not performed at the time of treatment completion. We investigated the effects of probiotics in the early stages of treatment (five days after treatment). Second, a long-term follow-up was not performed. Consequently, it remains unclear whether the beneficial effects of probiotic supplementation observed five days post-CDI treatment persist over an extended period. Third, the mechanism of action of *B. licheniformis* in patients with CDI was not investigated. Fourth, the sample size was small and was not calculated. Because this was a pilot study, the sample size could not be calculated. Fifth, a detailed analysis investigating the specific taxa affected by probiotic was not performed.

5. Conclusions

In conclusion, the addition of *B. licheniformis* helped preserve microbial richness in patients with CDI during the early stages of treatment. However, our study has several limitations, including a small sample size and short-term follow-up. Future studies are needed to investigate the long-term effects of probiotic treatment and to reveal the mechanisms of probiotic treatment in patients with CDI. The effects of this strain on CDI recurrence should be investigated in future large-scale studies.

Author Contributions: Conceptualization: G.S.S. and J.Y.C.; Methodology: S.W.K., D.J.O. and S.-Y.N.; Formal analysis: T.-G.G. and S.-B.K.; Writing: T.-G.G.; Review and Editing: G.S.S. and J.Y.C. All authors have read and agreed to the published version of the manuscript.

Funding: This research was funded by Aju Pharm (Seoul, Republic of Korea; 20AAD40401).

Institutional Review Board Statement: This study was conducted in accordance with the Declaration of Helsinki and approved by the Institutional Review Board (or Ethics Committee) of Bucheon St. Mary's Hospital, HC21MIDI0005, on 7 May 2021; Daejeon St. Mary's Hospital, DC21MIDI0079, on 27 December 2021; Incheon St. Mary's Hospital, OC21MIDI0003, on 24 May 2021; Dongguk University Ilsan hospital, DUIH IRB No. 2020-12-016, on 16 February 2021; Jeonbuk National University Hospital, 2021-11-019, on 7 January 2022; and Wonkwang University Hospital, WKUH2020-11-002, on 14 December 2020.

Informed Consent Statement: Informed consent was obtained from all participants at the time of inclusion.

Data Availability Statement: The data presented in this study are available on request from the corresponding author due to privacy policies.

Acknowledgments: We gratefully thank nurses, study coordinators, and study participants for their support during this study.

Conflicts of Interest: The authors declare no conflicts of interest.

Abbreviations

The following abbreviations are used in this manuscript:

CDI	*Clostridioides difficile* infection
IBS	Irritable bowel syndrome
FMT	Fecal microbiota transplantation
RCT	Randomized controlled trial
BSS	Bristol stool scale

References

1. Ananthakrishnan, A.N. *Clostridium difficile* infection: Epidemiology, risk factors and management. *Nat. Rev. Gastroenterol. Hepatol.* **2011**, *8*, 17–26. [CrossRef] [PubMed]
2. Winter, S.E.; Bäumler, A.J. Gut dysbiosis: Ecological causes and causative effects on human disease. *Proc. Natl. Acad. Sci. USA* **2023**, *120*, e2316579120. [CrossRef] [PubMed]
3. Lessa, F.C.; Mu, Y.; Bamberg, W.M.; Beldavs, Z.G.; Dumyati, G.K.; Dunn, J.R.; Farley, M.M.; Holzbauer, S.M.; Meek, J.I.; Phipps, E.C.; et al. Burden of *Clostridium difficile* infection in the United States. *N. Engl. J. Med.* **2015**, *372*, 825–834. [CrossRef] [PubMed]
4. Baek, J.; Choi, I.; Cho, Y.; Kim, J.; Lee, Y.; Kim, M.; Kim, K.; Cho, Y.-S. Clinical characteristics and outcomes of *Clostridioides difficile* infection in the intensive care unit: A KASID multi-centre study. *J. Hosp. Infect.* **2023**, *139*, 106–112. [CrossRef]

5. Guh, A.Y.; Mu, Y.; Winston, L.G.; Johnston, H.; Olson, D.; Farley, M.M.; Wilson, L.E.; Holzbauer, S.M.; Phipps, E.C.; Dumyati, G.K.; et al. Trends in U.S. Burden of *Clostridioides difficile* Infection and Outcomes. *N. Engl. J. Med.* **2020**, *382*, 1320–1330. [CrossRef]
6. Feuerstadt, P.; Theriault, N.; Tillotson, G. The burden of CDI in the United States: A multifactorial challenge. *BMC Infect. Dis.* **2023**, *23*, 132. [CrossRef]
7. Collins, D.A.; Hawkey, P.M.; Riley, T.V. Epidemiology of *Clostridium difficile* infection in Asia. *Antimicrob. Resist. Infect. Control* **2013**, *2*, 21. [CrossRef]
8. Borren, N.Z.; Ghadermarzi, S.; Hutfless, S.; Ananthakrishnan, A.N. The emergence of *Clostridium difficile* infection in Asia: A systematic review and meta-analysis of incidence and impact. *PLoS ONE* **2017**, *12*, e0176797. [CrossRef]
9. Kim, J.; Myung, R.; Kim, B.; Kim, J.; Kim, T.; Lee, M.S.; Kim, U.J.; Park, D.W.; Kim, Y.S.; Lee, C.S.; et al. Incidence of *Clostridioides difficile* Infections in Republic of Korea: A Prospective Study with Active Surveillance vs. National Data From Health Insurance Review & Assessment Service. *J. Korean Med. Sci.* **2024**, *39*, e118.
10. Wadhwa, A.; Al Nahhas, M.F.; Dierkhising, R.A.; Patel, R.; Kashyap, P.; Pardi, D.S.; Khanna, S.; Grover, M. High risk of post-infectious irritable bowel syndrome in patients with *Clostridium difficile* infection. *Aliment. Pharmacol. Ther.* **2016**, *44*, 576–582. [CrossRef]
11. Saha, S.M.; Sehgal, K.M.; Singh, S.M.; Grover, M.M.; Pardi, D.; Khanna, S.M. Postinfection Irritable Bowel Syndrome Following *Clostridioides difficile* Infection: A Systematic-review and Meta-analysis. *J. Clin. Gastroenterol.* **2022**, *56*, e84–e93. [CrossRef] [PubMed]
12. Gonzales-Luna, A.J.; Carlson, T.J.; Garey, K.W. Gut microbiota changes associated with Clostridioides difficile infection and its various treatment strategies. *Gut Microbes* **2023**, *15*, 2223345. [CrossRef] [PubMed]
13. Kelly, C.R.; Allegretti, J.R. Review Article: Gastroenterology and *Clostridium difficile* Infection: Past, Present, and Future. *Clin. Infect. Dis.* **2023**, *77*, S463–S470. [CrossRef] [PubMed]
14. Jalanka, J.; Salonen, A.; Fuentes, S.; de Vos, W.M. Microbial signatures in post-infectious irritable bowel syndrome–toward patient stratification for improved diagnostics and treatment. *Gut Microbes* **2015**, *6*, 364–369. [CrossRef]
15. Johnson, S.; Lavergne, V.; Skinner, A.M.; Gonzales-Luna, A.J.; Garey, K.W.; Kelly, C.P.; Wilcox, M.H. Clinical Practice Guideline by the Infectious Diseases Society of America (IDSA) and Society for Healthcare Epidemiology of America (SHEA): 2021 Focused Update Guidelines on Management of *Clostridioides difficile* Infection in Adults. *Clin. Infect. Dis.* **2021**, *73*, 755–757. [CrossRef]
16. Gweon, T.-G.; Lee, Y.J.; Kim, K.O.; Yim, S.K.; Soh, J.S.; Kim, S.Y.; Park, J.J.; Shin, S.Y.; Lee, T.H.; Choi, C.H.; et al. Clinical Practice Guidelines for Fecal Microbiota Transplantation in Korea. *J. Neurogastroenterol. Motil.* **2022**, *28*, 28–42. [CrossRef]
17. Lee, C.H.; Steiner, T.; Petrof, E.O.; Smieja, M.; Roscoe, D.; Nematallah, A.; Weese, J.S.; Collins, S.; Moayyedi, P.; Crowther, M.; et al. Frozen vs Fresh Fecal Microbiota Transplantation and Clinical Resolution of Diarrhea in Patients with Recurrent *Clostridium difficile* Infection: A Randomized Clinical Trial. *JAMA* **2016**, *315*, 142–149. [CrossRef]
18. Gweon, T.-G.; Kim, J.; Lim, C.-H.; Park, J.M.; Lee, D.-G.; Lee, I.S.; Cho, Y.-S.; Kim, S.W.; Choi, M.-G. Fecal Microbiota Transplantation Using Upper Gastrointestinal Tract for the Treatment of Refractory or Severe Complicated *Clostridium difficile* Infection in Elderly Patients in Poor Medical Condition: The First Study in an Asian Country. *Gastroenterol. Res. Pract.* **2016**, *2016*, 2687605. [CrossRef]
19. Kao, D.; Roach, B.; Silva, M.; Beck, P.; Rioux, K.; Kaplan, G.G.; Chang, H.J.; Coward, S.; Goodman, K.J.; Xu, H.; et al. Effect of Oral Capsule- vs Colonoscopy-Delivered Fecal Microbiota Transplantation on Recurrent *Clostridium difficile* Infection: A Randomized Clinical Trial. *JAMA* **2017**, *318*, 1985–1993. [CrossRef]
20. Gweon, T.G.; Na, S.Y. Next Generation Fecal Microbiota Transplantation. *Clin. Endosc.* **2021**, *54*, 152–156. [CrossRef]
21. Park, S.Y.; Seo, G.S. Fecal Microbiota Transplantation: Is It Safe? *Clin. Endosc.* **2021**, *54*, 157–160. [CrossRef] [PubMed]
22. Wang, X.; Zhang, P.; Zhang, X. Probiotics Regulate Gut Microbiota: An Effective Method to Improve Immunity. *Molecules* **2021**, *26*, 6076. [CrossRef] [PubMed]
23. Rahman, N.; Barua, N.; Tin, M.C.; Dharmaratne, P.; Wong, S.H.; Ip, M. The use of probiotics and prebiotics in decolonizing pathogenic bacteria from the gut; a systematic review and meta-analysis of clinical outcomes. *Gut Microbes* **2024**, *16*, 2356279. [CrossRef] [PubMed]
24. Goldenberg, J.Z.; Yap, C.; Lytvyn, L.; Lo, C.K.F.; Beardsley, J.; Mertz, D.; Johnston, B.C. Probiotics for the prevention of Clostridium difficile-associated diarrhea in adults and children. *Cochrane Database Syst. Rev.* **2017**, *12*, Cd006095. [CrossRef]
25. Hong, H.A.; To, E.; Fakhry, S.; Baccigalupi, L.; Ricca, E.; Cutting, S.M. Defining the natural habitat of *Bacillus* spore-formers. *Res. Microbiol.* **2009**, *160*, 375–379. [CrossRef]
26. Cutting, S.M. *Bacillus* probiotics. *Food Microbiol.* **2011**, *28*, 214–220. [CrossRef]
27. Ramirez-Olea, H.; Reyes-Ballesteros, B.; Chavez-Santoscoy, R.A. Potential application of the probiotic *Bacillus licheniformis* as an adjuvant in the treatment of diseases in humans and animals: A systematic review. *Front. Microbiol.* **2022**, *13*, 993451. [CrossRef]
28. Li, Y.; Liu, M.; Zhou, J.; Hou, B.; Su, X.; Liu, Z.; Yuan, J. *Bacillus licheniformis* Zhengchangsheng® attenuates DSS-induced colitis and modulates the gut microbiota in mice. *Benef. Microbes* **2019**, *10*, 543–553. [CrossRef]

29. Park, C.; Yun, K.E.; Chu, J.M.; Lee, J.Y.; Hong, C.P.; Nam, Y.D.; Jeong, J.; Han, K.; Ahn, Y.J. Performance comparison of fecal preservative and stock solutions for gut microbiome storage at room temperature. *J. Microbiol.* **2020**, *58*, 703–710. [CrossRef]
30. Jeong, J.; Yun, K.; Mun, S.; Chung, W.-H.; Choi, S.-Y.; Nam, Y.-D.; Lim, M.Y.; Hong, C.P.; Park, C.; Ahn, Y.J.; et al. The effect of taxonomic classification by full-length 16S rRNA sequencing with a synthetic long-read technology. *Sci. Rep.* **2021**, *11*, 1727. [CrossRef]
31. Tang, B.; Tang, L.; Huang, C.; Tian, C.; Chen, L.; He, Z.; Yang, G.; Zuo, L.; Zhao, G.; Liu, E.; et al. The Effect of Probiotics Supplementation on Gut Microbiota After Helicobacter pylori Eradication: A Multicenter Randomized Controlled Trial. *Infect. Dis. Ther.* **2021**, *10*, 317–333. [CrossRef] [PubMed]
32. Son, D.; Choi, Y.J.; Son, M.Y.; Moon, W.; Park, S.J.; Lim, S.; Kim, J.H. Benefits of Probiotic Pretreatment on the Gut Microbiota and Minor Complications after Bowel Preparation for Colonoscopy: A Randomized Double-Blind, Placebo-Controlled Pilot Trial. *Nutrients* **2023**, *15*, 1141. [CrossRef] [PubMed]
33. McFarland, L.V.; Kullar, R.; Johnson, S.; Sniffen, J.C.; Woolard, K.; Goldstein, E.J. Why Do ACG and AGA Guidelines Differ for the Use of Probiotics and the Prevention of CDI? *Am. J. Gastroenterol.* **2022**, *117*, 501. [CrossRef]
34. Su, G.L.; Ko, C.W.; Bercik, P.; Falck-Ytter, Y.; Sultan, S.; Weizman, A.V.; Morgan, R.L. AGA Clinical Practice Guidelines on the Role of Probiotics in the Management of Gastrointestinal Disorders. *Gastroenterology* **2020**, *159*, 697–705. [CrossRef] [PubMed]
35. van Prehn, J.; Reigadas, E.; Vogelzang, E.H.; Bouza, E.; Hristea, A.; Guery, B.; Krutova, M.; Norén, T.; Allerberger, F.; Coia, J.E.; et al. European Society of Clinical Microbiology and Infectious Diseases: 2021 update on the treatment guidance document for *Clostridioides difficile* infection in adults. *Clin. Microbiol. Infect.* **2021**, *27* (Suppl. 2), S1–S21. [CrossRef]
36. McCollum, D.L.; Rodriguez, J.M. Detection, treatment, and prevention of *Clostridium difficile* infection. *Clin. Gastroenterol. Hepatol.* **2012**, *10*, 581–592. [CrossRef]
37. Koh, E.; Hwang, I.Y.; Lee, H.L.; De Sotto, R.; Lee, J.W.J.; Lee, Y.S.; March, J.C.; Chang, M.W. Engineering probiotics to inhibit *Clostridioides difficile* infection by dynamic regulation of intestinal metabolism. *Nat. Commun.* **2022**, *13*, 3834. [CrossRef]
38. Islam, I.; Seo, H.; Redwan, A.; Kim, S.; Lee, S.; Siddiquee, M.; Song, H.-Y. In Vitro and In Vivo Anti-*Clostridioides difficile* Effect of a Probiotic *Bacillus amyloliquefaciens* Strain. *J. Microbiol. Biotechnol.* **2022**, *32*, 46–55. [CrossRef]

nutrients

MDPI

Article

Ligilactobacillus salivarius PS11610 Enhances the Fertilization Success of IVF: A Preliminary Retrospective Analysis

Miguel Raimundo [1,*], Patrícia Rodrigues [2], Sergio Esteban [3], Irene Espinosa-Martos [3] and Esther Jiménez [3]

1 NOVA National School of Public Health, NOVA University Lisbon, 1600-560 Lisbon, Portugal
2 School of Psychology and Life Sciences, Lusófona University Lisbon, 1749-024 Lisbon, Portugal; patricia.rodrigues@ulusofona.pt
3 Probisearch SLU, 28760 Tres Cantos, Spain; sergio.esteban@probisearch.com (S.E.); irene.espinosa@probisearch.com (I.E.-M.); esther.jimenez@probisearch.com (E.J.)
* Correspondence: jmm.raimundo@ensp.unl.pt

Abstract: Background/Objectives: Infertility affects couples at reproductive age, with *in vitro* fertilization (IVF) being the most effective treatment. Success rates of IVF are influenced by several factors, including a healthy female reproductive system microbiome, which can improve implantation rates and pregnancy outcomes. This study evaluated the impact of *Ligilactobacillus salivarius* PS11610 on IVF outcomes. This strain showed antimicrobial activity against pathogens related to dysbiosis, commonly observed in women undergoing assisted reproductive treatment. Results: The administration of *L. salivarius* PS11610 at a dose of 1×10^9 CFU every 12 h for at least one month before IVF procedures, particularly in the frozen embryo transfer (FET) group, appears to enhance the success rate of IVF. IVF procedures without embryo transfer showed no significant differences between the groups. However, there were statistically significant differences in the quality of embryos, specifically in category 2, which were higher in the group without *L. salivarius* PS11610 supplementation ($p = 0.042$). Similar results were seen in the IVF with embryo transfer group, where the quality of embryos in categories 2 and 3 was higher in the group without *L. salivarius* PS11610 ($p = 0.019$ and $p = 0.05$, respectively). IVF with FET showed notable improvements, where intake of *L. salivarius* PS11610 was associated with a significant increase in live birth infants (26.4% with *L. salivarius* PS11610 vs. 17.9% without, $p = 0.034$) and higher biochemical pregnancy rates (42.6% vs. 34%, $p = 0.071$). Conclusions: Despite some differences in embryo quality, the overall positive impact on pregnancy and birth outcomes highlights *L. salivarius* PS11610 as a promising supplement in assisted reproductive treatments.

Keywords: *in vitro* fertilization; probiotics; *Ligilactobacillus salivarius*; infertility

1. Introduction

Infertility is defined by the World Health Organization (WHO) as the failure to achieve a clinical pregnancy after 12 months of unprotected sexual intercourse and affects 15% of couples worldwide [1].

The associated causes are divided, almost equally between male, female, or combined failure, leaving approximately 15–30% of infertility to unknown causes, also referred to as idiopathic [2].

Many infertile couples seek treatment options, with *in vitro* fertilization (IVF) recognized as the most effective method [3,4]. However, success rates of IVF cycles only lead to pregnancy with a live birth in about 30–35% of women [5,6]. Several factors can influence the success rate, including the embryo's quality and the endometrium's receptivity, including the microbiota of female reproductive system [7,8].

Human microbiota, the community of microorganisms living inside and outside our body, is a good indicator of our health status [9]. Until recently, this microbiota was evaluated in the context of disease, but this view is changing. In the last decade, numerous publications have broken the old paradigm that considered the urogenital tract as sterile, demonstrating that microorganisms present in the urogenital tract represent 9% of the whole human microbiome [10–12]. A healthy urogenital microbiome improves implantation rate and pregnancy outcomes, whereas 40% of dysbiosis prevalence is observed in women under assisted reproductive treatment (ART) [5,13–15]. A healthy intestinal microbiome was reinforced by studies suggesting improvement in disease outcomes such as colorectal cancer, inflammatory bowel disease, pancreatic ductal adenocarcinoma, and post-fecal microbiota transplantation [16,17].

The female urogenital microbiota is characterized by low bacterial diversity and *Lactobacillus* genus predominance (>90%) [14,16,17], protecting against pathogens by producing lactic acid, lowering the vaginal pH. They also prevent pathogens from colonizing by blocking adhesion sites on epithelial cells and producing substances like bacteriocins and hydrogen peroxide (H_2O_2) [18–20]. Recently, Moreno and collaborators showed better implantation rates in *In Vitro* Fertilization (IVF) in women whose endometrial microbiota was dominated by *Lactobacillus* [14].

Bacterial vaginosis (BV) is the most common urogenital dysbiosis, or bacterial imbalance in women, where *Lactobacillus* is usually replaced by a plethora of pro-inflammatory microorganisms such as *Gardnerella vaginalis*, *Atopobium vaginae*, *Prevotella* spp., and *Veillonella* spp. [18,21,22]. Although some women may be asymptomatic, BV induce vaginal itching, pain, or vaginal secretions, which may lead to new infections, and most importantly to infertility, and preterm birth or miscarriage, if occurring in pregnant women [23–25].

The urogenital microbiome also plays an essential role in spermatogenesis, the absence of Lactobacilli and the increase in *Prevotella spp.* was associated with alterations in semen quality, and hence male fertility [26–29].

It has been shown that oral or vaginal treatment with *Lactobacillus,* restores vaginal microbiota [9,30–34]. However, the direct effect of this supplementation on fertility and the endometrial microbiome needs more studies [35]. In males, treatment with Lactobacillus, was shown to improve sperm quality in almost every parameters [36–38].

Despite the studies using probiotic-based treatments, diseases associated with male and female urogenital bacterial imbalance are mainly treated with antibiotic therapy [32,39].

Fertibiome® (Zinereo Pharma, Vigo, Spain) with *Ligilactobacillus salivarius* (formerly named *Lactobacillus salivarius*) PS11610 strain, is one of such probiotic treatments and it has shown its antimicrobial activity *in vitro* agains pathogens associated with bacterial imbalances of the female and male genital tract. In a pilot study, supplementation with *L. salivarius* PS11610 has shown to improve pregnancy and delivery rates by treating bacterial imbalance in 67% of couples [40–42].

The European Food Safety Authority (EFSA) has qualified *L. salivarius* as a microorganism with a Qualified Presumption of Safety (QPS) [43].

Considering the results obtained in the *in vitro* and *in vivo* trials, this study aimed to assess the impact of *L. salivarius* PS11610 on couples undergoing IVF treatments.

2. Materials and Methods

2.1. Study Population

Six hundred and ninety-four women aged 18 to 49 participated in their first IVF treatment, either with or without embryo transfer, at a fertility clinic in Lisbon, Portugal. This study was conducted over two one-year periods: from September 2021 to August 2022, during which no probiotic supplementation was administered, and from September 2022 to August 2023, when *L. salivarius* PS11610 (also identified as Fertibiome®) was included in the treatment protocol.

During the first period, women took only daily supplements prescribed by the gynecologist. During the second period, they took daily supplements prescribed by the gynecologist plus 1 capsule every 12 h of Fertibiome® (10^9 CFU of *L. salivarius* PS11610) for at least one month before the procedure.

The primary outcomes for women undergoing IVF in freeze-all cycles (no embryo transfer post oocyte collection) were the number of oocytes, number of frozen oocytes, number of fertilized oocytes, number and quality (1, 2, and 3, according to Istanbul Consensus classification) of embryos, number of frozen embryos, and number of blastocytes. For those women undergoing IVF with fresh embryo transfer, the primary outcomes were biochemical pregnancy (level of beta-hCG in blood > 5 and <50 IU/L), clinical pregnancy (value of beta-hCG in blood > 50 IU/L and ultrasound confirmation), miscarriage, and live births.

The data collected were oocyte origin (Own/Donor/Receiving Oocytes from the Partner (ROPA)), number of embryos transferred, biochemical pregnancy (No/Yes), clinical pregnancy (No/Yes), miscarriage (No/Yes), voluntary interruption of pregnancy (VIP) (No/Yes), ectopic pregnancy (No/Yes), heterotopic pregnancy (No/Yes), pregnancy type (Single/Multiple) and live birth (No/Yes).

In our study of IVF that does not involve embryo transfer, we gathered important data, which include: oocyte extraction procedure (Punction/Cryopreserved/Both), semen origin (Frozen Testicular Biopsy/Frozen/Donor/Fresh), fertilization procedure (IVF/Intracytoplasmic sperm injection (ICSI)), number of oocytes, number of cryopreserved oocytes, number of fertilized oocytes, number of embryos produced, number of blastocysts in each quality grade (1, 2, and 3), number of cryopreserved embryos, and number of blastocysts. In the IVF embryo transfer procedure, additional information was collected, including the following: the origin of oocytes (Fresh/Vitrified), the source of semen (Fresh/Frozen/Donor), the number of thawed embryos, the number of days from thawing to transfer, and the number of sacs.

These parameters were categorized based on their relevance to the procedure or the outcome, depending on the specific goals of the IVF process implemented (IVF without transfer, IVF with transfer, or IVF with frozen embryo transfer (FET).

2.2. Statistical Analysis

Data distribution was assessed using the Shapiro test, histograms, skewness, and kurtosis. Quantitative variables under normal distribution were summarized as mean ± standard deviation (SD), and comparisons between the two evaluated periods were assessed using a *t*-test. When data were not normally distributed, median and interquartile range (IQR) and the Kruskal–Wallis test were used. Qualitative variables were summarized using absolute and relative frequencies, and contingency tables were evaluated using the Chi-square test. Finally, multiple factor analysis (MFA) was used to summarize and visualize the relationship between characteristics and outcomes (quantitative and/or qualitative), considering the use of Fertibiome® as the stratification factor. Results were considered statistically significant when a *p*-value equal to or below 0.05 was obtained.

All the analyses were performed in RStudio 2022.12.0 + 353 "Elsbeth Geranium" Release (7d165dcfc1b6d300eb247738db2c7076234f6ef0, 3 December 2022) for Windows using R version 3.6.0 (26 April 2019)—"Planting of a Tree" Copyright (C) 2019 The R Foundation for Statistical Computing.

3. Results

3.1. IVF Without Embryo Transfer

From September 2021 to August 2023, a total of 148 cycles of IVF without embryo transfer were performed, of which 85 cases were without *L. salivarius* PS11610 and 63 with *L. salivarius* PS11610. The characteristics of the cycles are summarized in Table 1, and no differences between the two periods of time were found.

Table 1. Characteristics of IVF procedures without transfer cases during the evaluated periods.

	Without *L. salivarius* PS11610 (N = 85)	**With *L. salivarius* PS11610 (N = 63)**	***p*-Value *,‡**
Oocyte extraction Technique			
Both	2 (2.4%)	0 (0%)	0.702
Cryopreserved	3 (3.5%)	2 (3.2%)	
Punction	80 (94.1%)	61 (96.8%)	
Oocyte Origin			
Donor	6 (7.1%)	4 (6.3%)	1.000
Own	79 (92.9%)	59 (93.7%)	
ROPA	0 (0%)	0 (0%)	
Semen			
Frozen Testicular Biopsy	2 (2.4%)	4 (6.3%)	0.399
Frozen	2 (2.4%)	3 (4.8%)	
Donor	8 (9.4%)	3 (4.8%)	
Fresh	73 (85.9%)	52 (82.5%)	
Fertilization Procedure			
ICSI	50 (58.8%)	39 (61.9%)	0.492
IVF	35 (41.2%)	21 (33.3%)	
Subject Age			
Median (Q1–Q3)	37.00 (32.00–39.00)	34.00 (30.00–39.50)	0.219
Min–Max	20.00–45.00	22.00–45.00	

N, number of cases; ROPA, Receiving oocytes from the partner; ICSI, Intracytoplasmic sperm injection; IVF, *In vitro* fertilization. Qualitative variable results are expressed as absolute and relative frequencies (%, over the group margin). Missing values were considered in calculating the relative frequencies, although not evaluated in the comparison. Thus, they were excluded from the table. Quantitative variable results are expressed as median (1st–3rd quartile) and (minimum–maximum). * Kruskal–Wallis test. ‡ Chi-square test.

The procedure's outcomes are summarized in Table 2. No differences were found for oocyte extraction, preservation, or fertilization features. Further, the number of embryos obtained, and their quality were similar in both periods except for embryos of quality 2, which were higher without *L. salivarius* PS11610 (p = 0.042 and p = 0.028, respectively).

Table 2. Comparison of clinical outcomes obtained from IVF without transfer procedure in the evaluated periods.

	Without *L. salivarius* PS11610 (N = 85)	With *L. salivarius* PS11610 (N = 63)	*p*-Value *
No. of Oocytes			
Median (Q1–Q3) Min–Max	11.00 (5.00–20.00) 0.00–48.00	13.00 (6.50–22.00) 0.00–50.00	0.429
No. of Frozen Oocytes			
Median (Q1–Q3) Min–Max	0.00 (0.00–0.00) 0.00–0.00	0.00 (0.00–0.00) 0.00–4.00	0.099
No. Fertilized Oocytes			
Median (Q1–Q3) Min–Max	6.00 (2.00–12.00) 0.00–42.00	7.00 (3.00–11.50) 0.00–43.00	0.631
No. Embryo			
Median (Q1–Q3) Min–Max	6.00 (2.00–11.00) 0.00–38.00	7.00 (2.50–11.00) 0.00–35.00	0.510
No. Embryo Quality 1			
Median (Q1–Q3) Min–Max	2.00 (0.00–5.00) 0.00–24.00	2.00 (0.00–4.00) 0.00–17.00	0.692
No. Embryo Quality 2			
Median (Q1–Q3) Min–Max	0.00 (0.00–0.00) 0.00–9.00	0.00 (0.00–0.00) 0.00–5.00	0.042
No. Embryo Quality 3			
Median (Q1–Q3) Min–Max	0.00 (0.00–0.00) 0.00–1.00	0.00 (0.00–0.00) 0.00–0.00	0.133
No. Cryopreserved Embryos			
Median (Q1–Q3) Min–Max	3.00 (0.00–5.00) 0.00–24.00	2.00 (1.00–4.00) 0.00–14.00	0.522
No. Blastocysts			
Median (Q1–Q3) Min–Max	3.00 (0.00–7.00) 0.00–25.00	3.00 (1.00–7.50) 0.00–27.00	0.516

N, number of cases; IVF, *In vitro* fertilization. Results were also reported as median (1st–3rd quartile) and (minimum–maximum) values. * Kruskal–Wallis test.

3.2. IVF with Embryo Transfer

During the two evaluated periods, 76 cycles of IVF were performed, followed by embryo transfer: 44 without *L. salivarius* PS11610 and 32 with it. The characteristics of the cases are summarized in Table 3. Only embryos of quality 2 and 3 show some statistically significant differences between the two periods, with higher values in the period without using *L. salivarius* PS11610.

Regarding the outcomes, measured by biochemical (very early) and clinical (ultrasound confirmed) pregnancy, miscarriage, and live birth, as seen in Table 4, no statistically significant differences were found between with and without the intake of *L. salivarius* before IVF treatment (Table 4).

Table 3. Characteristics of IVF with transfer cases within the evaluated periods.

	Without *L. salivarius* PS11610 (N = 44)	**With *L. salivarius* PS11610 (N = 32)**	***p*-Value *,‡**
Oocyte extraction Technique			1.000
Both	1 (2.3%)	1 (3.1%)	
Cryopreserved	7 (15.9%)	5 (15.6%)	
Punction	36 (81.8%)	26 (81.3%)	
Oocyte Origin			0.868
Donor	5 (11.4%)	5 (15.6%)	
Own	38 (86.4%)	26 (81.3%)	
ROPA	1 (2.3%)	1 (3.1%)	
Semen			0.428
Frozen Testicular Biopsy	1 (2.3%)	2 (6.3%)	
Frozen	2 (4.5%)	3 (9.4%)	
Donor	2 (4.5%)	3 (9.4%)	
Fresh	39 (88.6%)	24 (75.0%)	
Fertilization Procedure			1.000
ICSI	32 (72.7%)	23 (71.9%)	
IVF	11 (25.0%)	9 (28.1%)	
Subject Age			
Median (Q1–Q3)	36.50 (33.00–41.00)	39.00 (34.75–43.00)	0.217
Min–Max	18.00–47.00	26.00–48.00	
No. of Oocytes			
Median (Q1–Q3)	7.00 (5.00–11.00)	6.50 (3.00–9.25)	0.493
Min–Max	0.00–47.00	1.00–27.00	
No. Oocytes Fertilized			
Median (Q1–Q3)	3.00 (2.00–4.25)	3.50 (1.00–7.00)	0.899
Min–Max	0.00–12.00	0.00–21.00	
No. Embryo			
Median (Q1–Q3)	3.00 (2.00–4.25)	3.50 (1.00–7.00)	0.702
Min–Max	0.00–11.00	0.00–17.00	
No, Embryo Quality 1			
Median (Q1–Q3)	1.00 (0.00–2.00)	1.00 (0.75–3.00)	0.167
Min–Max	0.00–9.00	0.00–7.00	
No. Embryo Quality 2			
Median (Q1–Q3)	0.00 (0.00–1.00)	0.00 (0.00–0.00)	0.013
Min–Max	0.00–4.00	0.00–2.00	
No. Embryo Quality 3			
Median (Q1–Q3)	0.00 (0.00–0.00)	0.00 (0.00–0.00)	0.050
Min–Max	0.00–2.00	0.00–0.00	
No. Transferred			
Median (Q1–Q3)	1.00 (1.00–1.00)	1.00 (0.00–1.00)	0.134
Min–Max	0.00–2.00	0.00–2.00	

Table 3. *Cont.*

	Without *L. salivarius* PS11610 (N = 44)	With *L. salivarius* PS11610 (N = 32)	*p*-Value *,‡
No. Cryopreserved Embryos			
Median (Q1–Q3)	0.00 (0.00–1.00)	0.00 (0.00–2.00)	0.618
Min–Max	0.00–9.00	0.00–7.00	
No. Blastocysts			
Median (Q1–Q3)	2.00 (1.00–3.00)	1.50 (0.00–3.25)	0.621
Min–Max	0.00–9.00	0.00–10.00	

N, number of cases; ROPA, Receiving oocytes from the partner; ICSI, Intracytoplasmic sperm injection; IVF, *In vitro* fertilization. The results of the qualitative variables are expressed as absolute and relative frequencies (%, over the group margin). Missing values were considered when calculating the relative frequencies, although they were not evaluated in the comparison. Thus, they were excluded from the table. The results of the quantitative variables are expressed as median (1st quartile–3rd quartile) and (minimum–maximum) values, which were also reported. * Kruskal–Wallis test. ‡ Chi-square test.

Table 4. Comparison of clinical outcomes obtained from IVF with transfer procedure in the evaluated periods.

	Without *L. salivarius* PS11610 (N = 44)	With *L. salivarius* PS11610 (N = 32)	*p*-Value ‡
Biochemical Pregnancy			1.000
No	28 (63.6%)	21 (65.6%)	
Yes	13 (29.5%)	11 (34.4%)	
Clinical Pregnancy			0.327
No	4 (9.1%)	1 (3.1%)	
Yes	9 (20.5%)	10 (31.3%)	
Miscarriage			0.350
No	5 (11.4%)	8 (25.0%)	
Yes	4 (9.1%)	2 (6.3%)	
Live births			0.350
No	4 (9.1%)	2 (6.3%)	
Yes	5 (11.4%)	8 (25.0%)	

N, number of cases. The results of qualitative variables are expressed as absolute and relative frequencies (%, over the group margin). Missing values were considered in calculating the relative frequencies, although they were not evaluated in the comparison; thus, they were excluded from the table. ‡ Chi-square test.

3.3. IVF with Frozen Embryo Transfer (FET)

A total of 470 cycles of FET were performed, with 235 cycles in each evaluated period. Table 5 summarizes the characteristics of the cases, showing the similarity between the two periods being assessed. Only the number of days between thawing and transfer showed statistically significant differences between both periods when it was analyzed as a numeric variable, and also if the discrete values were considered as the level of a factor, using the Fisher test or the mosaic plot (Table 5 and Figure 1, respectively).

Regarding the primary outcome, the number of live births was higher during the period where *L. salivarius* PS11610 was intake compared to the one that it was not (62 (26.4%) vs. 42 (17.9%), $p = 0.034$). Biochemical pregnancies refer to early pregnancies that can be confirmed through a blood test detecting pregnancy hormones. The pregnancy may not yet be visible on an ultrasound at this stage. Biochemical pregnancies were also higher with *L. salivarius* PS11610 intake. However, this difference was statistically significant only at the 90% confidence level (80 (34.0%)/100 (42.6%), $p = 0.071$) (Table 6).

In Figure 2, the number of live births according to age is represented in a mosaic plot, which includes the Pearson residuals distribution and the signification of the log regression model. It shows a higher live birth rate in women under 37-years-old when *L. salivarius* PS11610 is used ($p = 0.0016$).

Table 5. Characteristics of IVF with FET cases in the evaluated periods.

	Without *L. salivarius* PS11610 (N = 235)	With *L. salivarius* PS11610 (N = 235)	*p*-Value *,‡
Oocyte Origin			
Donor	28 (11.9%)	36 (15.3%)	0.291
Own	205 (87.2%)	194 (82.6%)	
ROPA	2 (0.9%)	5 (2.1%)	
Oocytes Type			
Fresh	216 (91.9%)	219 (93.2%)	0.726
Vitrified	19 (8.1%)	16 (6.8%)	
Semen			
Frozen Testicular Biopsy	1 (0.4%)	0 (0%)	0.350
Frozen	20 (8.5%)	16 (6.8%)	
Donor	8 (3.4%)	14 (6.0%)	
Fresh	206 (87.7%)	205 (87.2%)	
Subject Age			
Median (Q1–Q3)	37.00 (34.00–41.00)	37.00 (33.00–42.00)	0.831
Min–Max	20.00–50.00	16.00–49.00	
No. Thawed Embryos			
Median (Q1–Q3)	1.00 (1.00–2.00)	1.00 (1.00–1.00)	0.213
Min–Max	1.00–16.00	1.00–9.00	
No. Embryo Transfer			
Median (Q1–Q3)	1.00 (1.00–1.00)	1.00 (1.00–1.00)	0.270
Min–Max	0.00–2.00	0.00–2.00	
0	8 (3.4%)	6 (2.6%)	0.320
1	175 (74.5%)	189 (80.4%)	
2	52 (22.1%)	40 (17.0%)	
No. of Days from Thawing to Transfer			
Median (Q1–Q3)	5.00 (5.00–5.00)	5.00 (5.00–5.00)	0.030
Min–Max	2.00–7.00	2.00–6.00	
Missing	0 (0%)	2 (0.9%)	0.026
2	1 (0.4%)	2 (0.9%)	
3	22 (9.4%)	8 (3.4%)	
4	1 (0.4%)	0 (0%)	
5	174 (74.0%)	176 (74.9%)	
6	36 (15.3%)	47 (20.0%)	
7	1 (0.4%)	0 (0%)	

N, number of cases; ROPA, Receiving oocytes from the partner. The results of the qualitative variables are expressed as absolute and relative frequencies (%, over the group margin). Missing values were considered when calculating the relative frequencies, although they were not evaluated in the comparison. Thus, they were excluded from the table. The results of the quantitative variables are expressed as median (1st quartile–3rd quartile) and (minimum–maximum) values, which were also reported. * Kruskal–Wallis test. ‡ Chi-square test.

Table 6. Comparison of clinical outcomes obtained from the FET procedure in the evaluated periods.

	Without *L. salivarius* PS11610 (N = 235)	With *L. salivarius* PS11610 (N = 235)	*p*-Value ‡
Biochemical Pregnancy			
No	155 (66.0%)	135 (57.4%)	0.071
Yes	80 (34.0%)	100 (42.6%)	
Clinical Pregnancy			
No	170 (72.3%)	157 (66.8%)	0.229
Yes	65 (27.7%)	78 (33.2%)	
No. of sacs			
0	177 (75.3%)	166 (70.6%)	0.527
1	54 (23.0%)	63 (26.8%)	
2	4 (1.7%)	6 (2.6%)	
Miscarriage			
No	218 (92.8%)	219 (93.2%)	1.000
Yes	17 (7.2%)	16 (6.8%)	
VIP			
No	234 (99.6%)	235 (100%)	1.000
Yes	1 (0.4%)	0 (0%)	
Ectopic Pregnancy			
No	234 (99.6%)	235 (100%)	1.000
Yes	1 (0.4%)	0 (0%)	
Pregnancy Type			
Twins	2 (0.9%)	4 (1.7%)	1.000
Single	40 (17.0%)	58 (24.7%)	
Live Births			
No	193 (82.1%)	173 (73.6%)	0.034
Yes	42 (17.9%)	62 (26.4%)	

N, number of cases. The results of qualitative variables are expressed as absolute and relative frequencies (%, over the group margin). Missing values were considered in calculating the relative frequencies, although they were not evaluated in the comparison; thus, they were excluded from the table. ‡ Chi-square test.

This study's dataset of IVF cycles with FET was organized into four feature groups. These included three qualitative groups: *L. salivarius* PS11610, qualitative case characteristics, and outcome characteristics. Additionally, one quantitative group focused on the quantitative characteristics of the cases. This organization was carried out to facilitate a Multiple Factor Analysis (MFA). *L. salivarius* PS11610 was used to stratify the cases but not to calculate the dimensions. The first two dimensions of the MFA explain the 35% of the variability with eigenvalues greater than 1 (Figure 3A–C). In the factor map, the groups of characteristics trigger the separation between cases in the first dimension, and the outcomes trigger the second dimension (Figure 3A). Regarding individual maps, there is no clear separation between the 95% confidence ellipses of the cases from both periods (Figure 3B). Nevertheless, a separation between the 95% confidence ellipses of the stratification factor "intake of *L. salivarius* PS11610" is shown, and this separation is almost due to the 2nd Dim, triggered by the outcomes evaluated (Figure 3C).

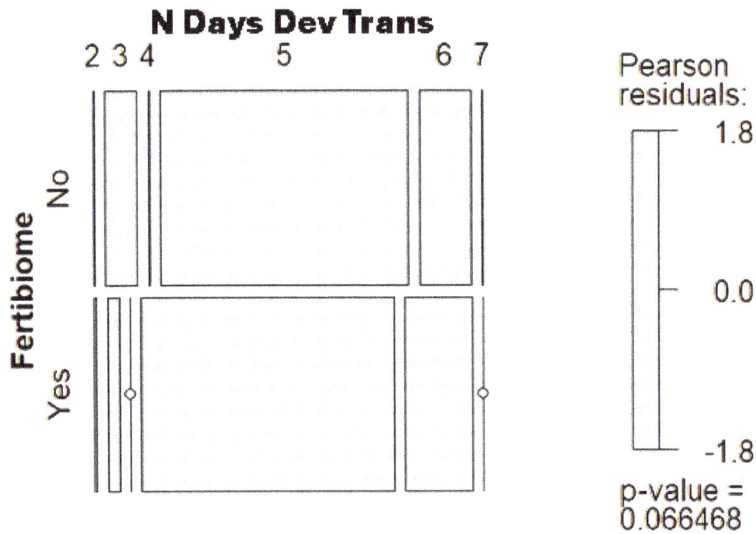

Figure 1. The mosaic chart of the distribution of the number of days from thawing to transfer, considering a multilevel factor, within both evaluated periods.

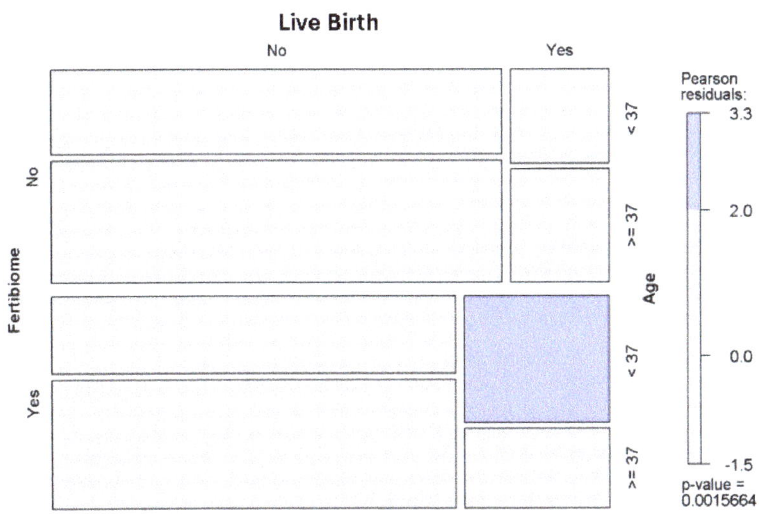

Figure 2. Mosaic chart of the distribution of live birth infants within the two evaluated periods according to age.

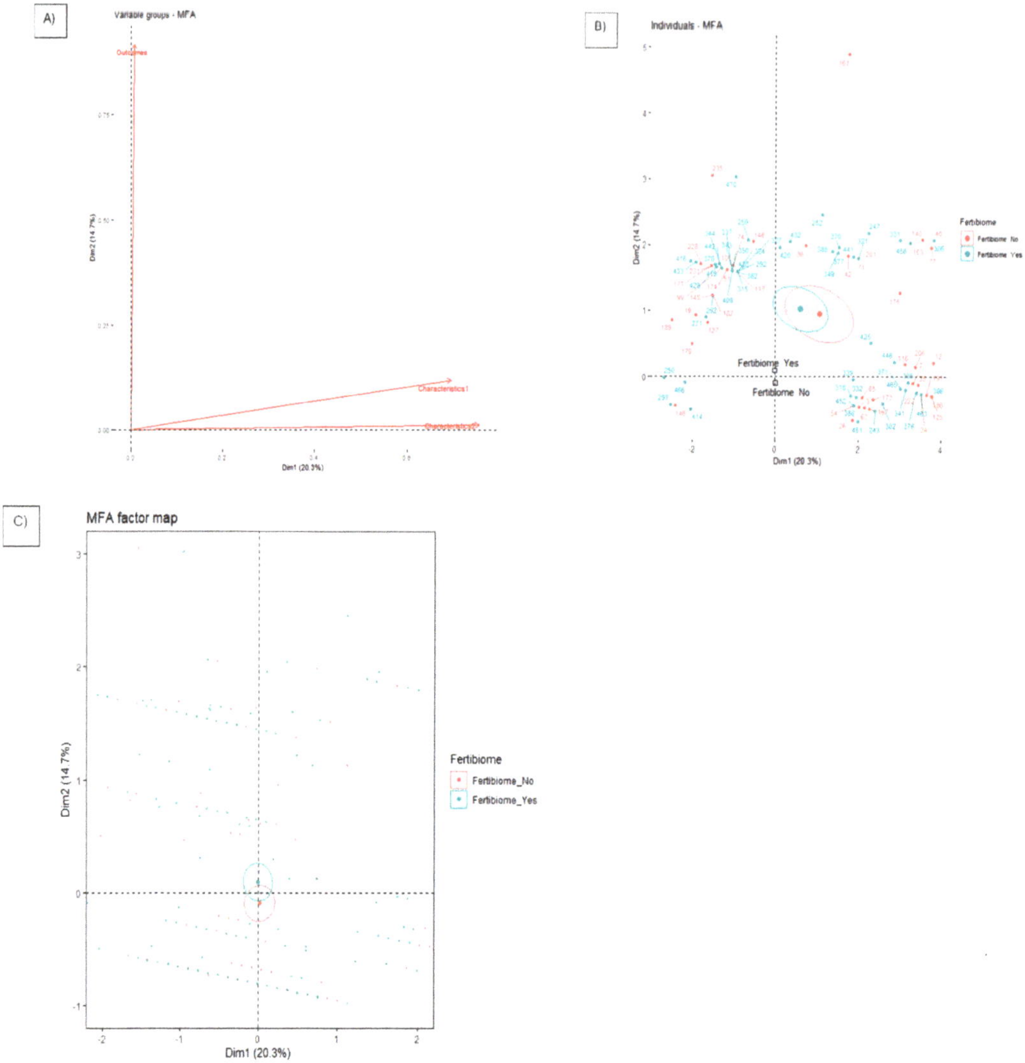

Figure 3. MFA chart of the groups of features represented with continuous arrows and labeled (**A**), MFA chart of the 95% confidence ellipses of the cases stratified by intake of *L. salivarius*—PS11610 (**B**), and MFA chart of the 95% confidence ellipses the stratified factor used (**C**) for the first two dimensions of the FET cases dataset.

4. Discussion

The current study evaluated the impact of *L. salivarius* PS11610 on IVF procedures outcomes. The findings were analyzed across three groups: IVF without embryo transfer, IVF with embryo transfer, and IVF with FET.

The analysis of IVF procedures without embryo transfer showed no significant differences between the groups with and without *L. salivarius* PS11610 regarding the number of oocytes, fertilized oocytes, and embryos obtained. However, there were statistically significant differences in the quality of embryos, specifically in category 2, which were higher in the group without *L. salivarius* PS11610 supplementation. This suggests that while *L. salivarius* PS11610 may not affect the number of embryos, it might influence certain aspects of embryo quality.

In the IVF with embryo transfer group, the characteristics of the cases and the primary outcomes were comparable between the two groups (with or without *L. salivarius* treatment). The quality of embryos in categories 2 and 3 was higher in the group without *L. salivarius* PS11610. Despite these differences in embryo quality, the overall outcomes did not show significant improvement with using *L. salivarius* PS11610, indicating that other factors might play a more critical role in the success of IVF with embryo transfer.

A similar study selected 17 couples for assisted reproduction treatment with confirmed urogenital dysbiosis and unknown or idiopathic infertility for a period of 6-month treatment with *L. salivarius* (1 dose every 12 h for females and 1 dose every 24 h for males), prior IVF procedures. Ultimately, *L. salivarius* PS11610 supplementation significantly improve the balance of the urogenital microbiome composition in male and female. Particularly, increasing Lactobacilli percentage in the vagina after 3 and 6 months of treatment. Moreover, the oral intake of *L. salivarius* PS11610 seemed to change the uterine microbiome and improve the general immunological profile of couples, becoming anti-inflammatory. The rates of pregnancy and delivery were also improved [42].

In a study by Sofia Väinämö et al., a beneficial effect of using *Lactobacillus crispatus* was observed in a couple who underwent IVF treatment and fresh embryo transfer [44]. In another study, the importance of a balanced microbiome to a successful IVF procedure was shown, when a cohort study of 84 women who underwent IVF cycles, only 8% of them with bacterial vaginosis, urogenital bacterial imbalance, were able to conceive compared with 40% of clinical pregnancy in women with balanced urogenital microbioma [45]. In a randomized controlled study, Isarin Thanaboonyawat et al. gave intravaginal supplements of *Lactobacillus acidophilus* for 6 days to infertile women significantly lowering the miscarriage rate in the study group compared to the control group, 9.5% and 19.1%, respectively [46].

The most notable findings were observed in the FET group, where the intake of *L. salivarius* PS11610 was associated with a significant increase in live birth (26.4% with *L. salivarius* PS11610 vs. 17.9% without, $p = 0.034$).

In another study, the cervicovaginal environment of women with reproductive failure (repetitive abortion, infertility of unknown origin) was assessed and compared to that of healthy fertile women. Daily oral administration of *L. salivarius* CECT5713 resulted in an overall successful pregnancy rate of 56%. The authors of this study emphasized how probiotics can influence important microbiological, biochemical, and immunological aspects in pregnant women. They concluded that *L. salivarius* could be a promising option for enhancing reproductive success in women experiencing reproductive challenges [47].

Additionally, the rate of biochemical pregnancies, defined as early pregnancies, confirmed by the levels of pregnancy hormones in the blood but not yet visible on an ultrasound, was higher in the *L. salivarius* PS11610 group, achieving statistical significance at a 90% confidence level ($p = 0.071$). This result suggested a positive impact of *L. salivarius* PS11610 on the success rates of FET procedures. In fact, in another study, Irollo AM. et al. showed that the treatment with probiotics and prebiotics in infertile women affected by acute or severe intestinal bacterial imbalance could influence the modulation of some mechanisms involved in embryo implantation [48].

The multiple factor analysis (MFA) further supported these findings by showing that the primary source of variability in the dataset was related to the outcomes rather than the characteristics of the cases. This indicates that the intake of *L. salivarius* PS11610 may enhance FET's success by improving pregnancy outcomes.

5. Conclusions

The administration of *L. salivarius* PS11610 at a dose of 1×10^9 CFU every 12 h at least 1 month before IVF procedures, particularly with FET, appears to enhance the success of these procedures. This enhancement is evidenced by increased live births and biochemical pregnancy rates. While some differences in embryo quality classification were noted, the overall positive impact on pregnancy and birth outcomes underscores the potential of *L. salivarius* PS11610 as a beneficial supplement in assisted reproductive treatments.

Additional research is necessary to investigate how *L. salivarius* PS11610 influences outcomes, particularly concerning its effects on the urogenital microbiome and the immune profiles of couples undergoing IVF. A controlled randomized trial is being prepared to enhance the robustness of findings and provide more conclusive insights.

Author Contributions: Conceptualization—M.R.; methodology—M.R., S.E., I.E.-M. and E.J.; software—S.E., I.E.-M. and E.J.; validation—M.R. and P.R.; formal analysis—I.E.-M.; investigation—P.R.; resources—M.R., P.R., S.E., I.E.-M. and E.J.; data curation—M.R., P.R., S.E., I.E.-M. and E.J.; writing—S.E., I.E.-M. and E.J.; review and editing—M.R. and P.R.; supervision—E.J. All authors have read and agreed to the published version of the manuscript.

Funding: This research received no external funding.

Institutional Review Board Statement: The study was conducted in accordance with the Declaration of Helsinki and approved by the Ethics Committee of School of Psychology and Life Sciences of Lusofona University—CEDIC (reference CEDIC-2023-3-14, approved on 4 October 2023) for studies involving humans.

Informed Consent Statement: Informed consent was obtained from all subjects involved in the study.

Data Availability Statement: The raw data supporting the conclusions of this article will be made available by the authors on request.

Conflicts of Interest: I.E.-M., E.J. and S.E. are Probisearch employees. Probisearch was involved in the interpretation of data, writing of the report, and the decision to submit the report for publication.

References

1. Zegers-Hochschild, F.; Adamson, G.D.; De Mouzon, J.; Ishihara, O.; Mansour, R.; Nygren, K.; Sullivan, E.; Vanderpoel, S. International Committee for Monitoring Assisted Reproductive Technology (ICMART) and the World Health Organization (WHO) revised glossary of ART terminology, 2009. *Fertil. Steril.* **2009**, *92*, 1520–1524. [CrossRef] [PubMed]
2. Quaas, A.; Dokras, A. Diagnosis and treatment of unexplained infertility. *Rev. Obstet. Gynecol.* **2008**, *1*, 69–76. [PubMed]
3. Elzeiny, H.; Garrett, C.; Toledo, M.; Stern, K.; McBain, J.; Baker, H.W.G. A randomised controlled trial of intra-uterine insemination versus in vitro fertilisation in patients with idiopathic or mild male infertility. *Aust. N. Z. J. Obstet. Gynaecol.* **2014**, *54*, 156–161. [CrossRef] [PubMed]
4. Cui, W. Mother or nothing: The agony of infertility. *Bull. World Health Organ.* **2010**, *88*, 881–882. [CrossRef] [PubMed]
5. Smith, A.D.A.C.; Tilling, K.; Nelson, S.M.; Lawlor, D.A. Live-Birth Rate Associated with Repeat In Vitro Fertilization Treatment Cycles. *JAMA* **2015**, *314*, 2654–2662. [CrossRef]
6. Høyer, S.; Kesmodel, U.S.; Aagaard, J. Conditional and cumulative live birth rates after blastocyst transfer. *Eur. J. Obstet. Gynecol. Reprod. Biol.* **2021**, *261*, 46–51. [CrossRef]
7. Koedooder, R.; Singer, M.; Schoenmakers, S.; Savelkoul, P.H.M.; Morré, S.A.; de Jonge, J.D.; Poort, L.; Cuypers, W.J.S.S.; Beckers, N.G.M.; Broekmans, F.J.M.; et al. The vaginal microbiome as a predictor for outcome of in vitro fertilization with or without intracytoplasmic sperm injection: A prospective study. *Hum. Reprod.* **2019**, *34*, 1042–1054. [CrossRef]
8. Macklon, N. Recurrent implantation failure is a pathology with a specific transcriptomic signature. *Fertil. Steril.* **2017**, *108*, 9–14. [CrossRef]
9. García-Velasco, J.A.; Menabrito, M.; Catalán, I.B. What fertility specialists should know about the vaginal microbiome: A review. *Reprod. Biomed. Online* **2017**, *35*, 103–112. [CrossRef]
10. The NIH HMP Working Group; Peterson, J.; Garges, S.; Giovanni, M.; McInnes, P.; Wang, L.; Schloss, J.A.; Bonazzi, V.; McEwen, J.E.; Wetterstrand, K.A.; et al. The NIH Human Microbiome Project. *Genome Res.* **2009**, *19*, 2317–2323. [CrossRef]

11. Baker, J.M.; Chase, D.M.; Herbst-Kralovetz, M.M. Uterine Microbiota: Residents, Tourists, or Invaders? *Front. Immunol.* **2018**, *9*, 208. [CrossRef] [PubMed]
12. Lundy, S.D.; Vij, S.C.; Rezk, A.H.; Cohen, J.A.; Bajic, P.; Ramasamy, R. The microbiome of the infertile male. *Curr. Opin. Urol.* **2020**, *30*, 355–362. [CrossRef] [PubMed]
13. Liversedge, N.H.; Turner, A.; Horner, P.J.; Keay, S.D.; Jenkins, J.M.; Hull, M.G.R. The influence of bacterial vaginosis on in-vitro fertilization and embryo implantation during assisted reproduction treatment. *Hum. Reprod.* **1999**, *14*, 2411–2415. [CrossRef]
14. Moreno, I.; Codoñer, F.M.; Vilella, F.; Valbuena, D.; Martinez-Blanch, J.F.; Jimenez-Almazán, J.; Alonso, R.; Alamá, P.; Remohí, J.; Pellicer, A.; et al. Evidence that the endometrial microbiota has an effect on implantation success or failure. *Am. J. Obstet. Gynecol.* **2016**, *215*, 684–703. [CrossRef]
15. Pelzer, E.S.; Allan, J.A.; Waterhouse, M.A.; Ross, T.; Beagley, K.W.; Knox, C.L. Microorganisms within Human Follicular Fluid: Effects on IVF. *PLoS ONE* **2013**, *8*, e59062. [CrossRef]
16. Boicean, A.; Ichim, C.; Todor, S.B.; Anderco, P.; Popa, M.L. The Importance of Microbiota and Fecal Microbiota Transplantation in Pancreatic Disorders. *Diagnostics* **2024**, *14*, 861. [CrossRef]
17. Brusnic, O.; Onisor, D.; Boicean, A.; Hasegan, A.; Ichim, C.; Guzun, A.; Chicea, R.; Todor, S.B.; Vintila, B.I.; Anderco, P.; et al. Fecal Microbiota Transplantation: Insights into Colon Carcinogenesis and Immune Regulation. *J. Clin. Med.* **2024**, *13*, 6578. [CrossRef]
18. Ravel, J.; Gajer, P.; Abdo, Z.; Schneider, G.M.; Koenig, S.S.K.; McCulle, S.L.; Karlebach, S.; Gorle, R.; Russell, J.; Tacket, C.O.; et al. Vaginal microbiome of reproductive-age women. *Proc. Natl. Acad. Sci. USA* **2011**, *108*, 4680–4687. [CrossRef]
19. Jakobsson, T.; Forsum, U. Changes in the predominant human Lactobacillus flora during in vitro fertilisation. *Ann. Clin. Microbiol. Antimicrob.* **2008**, *7*, 14. [CrossRef]
20. Tachedjian, G.; Aldunate, M.; Bradshaw, C.S.; Cone, R.A. The role of lactic acid production by probiotic Lactobacillus species in vaginal health. *Res. Microbiol.* **2017**, *168*, 782–792. [CrossRef]
21. Hawes, S.E.; Hillier, S.L.; Benedetti, J.; Stevens, C.E.; Koutsky, L.A.; Wolner-Hanssen, P.; Holmes, K.K. Hydrogen Peroxide--Producing Lactobacilli and Acquisition of Vaginal Infections. *J. Infect. Dis.* **1996**, *174*, 1058–1063. [CrossRef] [PubMed]
22. Aroutcheva, A.; Gariti, D.; Simon, M.; Shott, S.; Faro, J.; Simoes, J.A.; Gurguis, A.; Faro, S. Defense factors of vaginal lactobacilli. *Am. J. Obstet. Gynecol.* **2001**, *185*, 375–379. [CrossRef] [PubMed]
23. Sirota, I.; Zarek, S.; Segars, J. Potential Influence of the Microbiome on Infertility and Assisted Reproductive Technology. *Semin. Reprod. Med.* **2014**, *32*, 035–042. [CrossRef] [PubMed]
24. Onderdonk, A.B.; Delaney, M.L.; Fichorova, R.N. The Human Microbiome during Bacterial Vaginosis. *Clin. Microbiol. Rev.* **2016**, *29*, 223–238. [CrossRef]
25. Ralph, S.G.; Rutherford, A.J.; Wilson, J.D. Influence of bacterial vaginosis on conception and miscarriage in the first trimester: Cohort study. *BMJ* **1999**, *319*, 220–223. [CrossRef]
26. Leitich, H.; Bodner-Adler, B.; Brunbauer, M.; Kaider, A.; Egarter, C.; Husslein, P. Bacterial vaginosis as a risk factor for preterm delivery: A meta-analysis. *Am. J. Obstet. Gynecol.* **2003**, *189*, 139–147. [CrossRef]
27. Leitich, H.; Kiss, H. Asymptomatic bacterial vaginosis and intermediate flora as risk factors for adverse pregnancy outcome. *Best Pract. Res. Clin. Obstet. Gynaecol.* **2007**, *21*, 375–390. [CrossRef]
28. Baud, D.; Pattaroni, C.; Vulliemoz, N.; Castella, V.; Marsland, B.J.; Stojanov, M. Sperm Microbiota and Its Impact on Semen Parameters. *Front. Microbiol.* **2019**, *10*, 234. [CrossRef]
29. Farahani, L.; Tharakan, T.; Yap, T.; Ramsay, J.W.; Jayasena, C.N.; Minhas, S. The semen microbiome and its impact on sperm function and male fertility: A systematic review and meta-analysis. *Andrology* **2021**, *9*, 115–144. [CrossRef]
30. Monteiro, C.; Marques, P.I.; Cavadas, B.; Damião, I.; Almeida, V.; Barros, N.; Barros, A.; Carvalho, F.; Gomes, S.; Seixas, S. Characterization of microbiota in male infertility cases uncovers differences in seminal hyperviscosity and oligoasthenoteratozoospermia possibly correlated with increased prevalence of infectious bacteria. *Am. J. Reprod. Immunol.* **2018**, *79*, e12838. [CrossRef]
31. Weng, S.-L.; Chiu, C.-M.; Lin, F.-M.; Huang, W.-C.; Liang, C.; Yang, T.; Yang, T.-L.; Liu, C.-Y.; Wu, W.-Y.; Chang, Y.-A.; et al. Bacterial Communities in Semen from Men of Infertile Couples: Metagenomic Sequencing Reveals Relationships of Seminal Microbiota to Semen Quality. *PLoS ONE* **2014**, *9*, e110152. [CrossRef] [PubMed]
32. Anukam, K.; Osazuwa, E.; Ahonkhai, I.; Ngwu, M.; Osemene, G.; Bruce, A.W.; Reid, G. Augmentation of antimicrobial metronidazole therapy of bacterial vaginosis with oral probiotic Lactobacillus rhamnosus GR-1 and Lactobacillus reuteri RC-14: Randomized, double-blind, placebo controlled trial. *Microbes Infect.* **2006**, *8*, 1450–1454. [CrossRef] [PubMed]
33. Hilton, E.; Isenberg, H.D.; Alperstein, P.; France, K.; Borenstein, M.T. Ingestion of Yogurt Containing *Lactobacillus acidophilus* as Prophylaxis for Candidal Vaginitis. *Ann. Intern. Med.* **1992**, *116*, 353–357. [CrossRef]
34. Li, C.; Wang, T.; Li, Y.; Zhang, T.; Wang, Q.; He, J.; Wang, L.; Li, L.; Yang, N.; Fang, Y. Probiotics for the treatment of women with bacterial vaginosis: A systematic review and meta-analysis of randomized clinical trials. *Eur. J. Pharmacol.* **2019**, *864*, 172660. [CrossRef]
35. López-Moreno, A.; Aguilera, M. Probiotics Dietary Supplementation for Modulating Endocrine and Fertility Microbiota Dysbiosis. *Nutrients* **2020**, *12*, 757. [CrossRef]

36. Reid, G.; Bruce, A.W.; Fraser, N.; Heinemann, C.; Owen, J.; Henning, B. Oral probiotics can resolve urogenital infections. *FEMS Immunol. Med. Microbiol.* **2001**, *30*, 49–52. [CrossRef]
37. García-Velasco, J.A.; Budding, D.; Campe, H.; Malfertheiner, S.F.; Hamamah, S.; Santjohanser, C.; Schuppe-Koistinen, I.; Nielsen, H.S.; Vieira-Silva, S.; Laven, J. The reproductive microbiome—Clinical practice recommendations for fertility specialists. *Reprod. Biomed. Online* **2020**, *41*, 443–453. [CrossRef]
38. Helli, B.; Kavianpour, M.; Ghaedi, E.; Dadfar, M.; Haghighian, H.K. Probiotic effects on sperm parameters, oxidative stress index, inflammatory factors and sex hormones in infertile men. *Hum. Fertil.* **2022**, *25*, 499–507. [CrossRef]
39. Maretti, C.; Cavallini, G. The association of a probiotic with a prebiotic (Flortec, Bracco) to improve the quality/quantity of spermatozoa in infertile patients with idiopathic oligoasthenoteratospermia: A pilot study. *Andrology* **2017**, *5*, 439–444. [CrossRef]
40. Valcarce, D.G.; Genovés, S.; Riesco, M.F.; Martorell, P.; Herráez, M.P.; Ramón, D.; Robles, V. Probiotic administration improves sperm quality in asthenozoospermic human donors. *Benef. Microbes* **2017**, *8*, 193–206. [CrossRef]
41. Hamada, A.; Agarwal, A.; Sharma, R.; French, D.B.; Ragheb, A.; Sabanegh, E.S. Empirical Treatment of Low-level Leukocytospermia with Doxycycline in Male Infertility Patients. *Urology* **2011**, *78*, 1320–1325. [CrossRef] [PubMed]
42. Iniesta, S.; Esteban, S.; Armijo, Ó.; Lobo, S.; Manzano, S.; Espinosa, I.; Cárdenas, N.; Bartha, J.L.; Jiménez, E. *Ligilactobacillus salivarius* PS11610 exerts an effect on the microbial and immunological profile of couples suffering unknown infertility. *Am. J. Reprod. Immunol.* **2022**, *88*, e13552. [CrossRef]
43. The EU-FORA Programme; Villamar, V. Introduction. *EFSA J.* **2022**, *20*, e200402. [CrossRef]
44. Väinämö, S.; Saqib, S.; Kalliala, I.; Kervinen, K.; Luiro, K.; Niinimäki, M.; Halttunen-Nieminen, M.; Virtanen, S.; Nieminen, P.; Salonen, A.; et al. Longitudinal analysis of vaginal microbiota during IVF fresh embryo transfer and in early pregnancy. *Microbiol. Spectr.* **2023**, *11*, e0165023. [CrossRef]
45. Haahr, T.; Jensen, J.S.; Thomsen, L.; Duus, L.; Rygaard, K.; Humaidan, P. Abnormal vaginal microbiota may be associated with poor reproductive outcomes: A prospective study in IVF patients. *Hum. Reprod.* **2016**, *31*, 795–803. [CrossRef] [PubMed]
46. Thanaboonyawat, I.; Pothisan, S.; Petyim, S.; Laokirkkiat, P. Pregnancy outcomes after vaginal probiotic supplementation before frozen embryo transfer: A randomized controlled study. *Sci. Rep.* **2023**, *13*, 11892. [CrossRef]
47. Fernández, L.; Castro, I.; Arroyo, R.; Alba, C.; Beltrán, D.; Rodríguez, J.M. Application of Ligilactobacillus salivarius CECT5713 to Achieve Term Pregnancies in Women with Repetitive Abortion or Infertility of Unknown Origin by Microbiological and Immunological Modulation of the Vaginal Ecosystem. *Nutrients* **2021**, *13*, 162. [CrossRef]
48. Irollo, A.M.; Gangale, M.F.; Tartaglione, A.; Criscuolo, C.; Aiello, R.; Stortini, E.; Infante, V. Does probiotic and prebiotic treatement in ivf cycles of infertile women with intestinal dysbiosis, affect pregnancy rate? *J. Siena Acad. Sci.* **2018**, *9*. [CrossRef]

nutrients

MDPI

Article

The Improvement Effects of *Weizmannia coagulans* BC99 on Liver Function and Gut Microbiota of Long-Term Alcohol Drinkers: A Randomized Double-Blind Clinical Trial

Jie Zhang [1,2,†], Cheng Li [1,2,†], Mengyao Duan [1], Zhen Qu [1], Yi Wang [1], Yao Dong [3,4], Ying Wu [1,2], Shuguang Fang [3] and Shaobin Gu [1,2,5,*]

1 College of Food and Bioengineering, Henan University of Science and Technology, Luoyang 471000, China
2 Henan Engineering Research Center of Food Material, Henan University of Science and Technology, Luoyang 471023, China
3 Department of Research and Development, Wecare Probiotics Co., Ltd., Suzhou 215200, China
4 Germline Stem Cells and Microenvironment Lab, College of Animal Science and Technology, Nanjing Agricultural University, Nanjing 210095, China
5 Henan Engineering Research Center of Food Microbiology, Luoyang 471000, China
* Correspondence: shaobingu@haust.edu.cn
† These authors contributed equally to this work.

Abstract: Background/Objectives: With the improvement of living standards, alcoholic liver disease caused by long-term drinking has been a common multiple disease. Probiotic interventions may help mitigate liver damage caused by alcohol intake, but the mechanisms need more investigation. Methods: This study involved 70 long-term alcohol drinkers (18–65 years old, alcohol consumption $\geq$20 g/day, lasting for more than one year) who were randomly assigned to either the BC99 group or the placebo group. Two groups were given BC99 (3 g/day, 1×10^{10} CFU) or placebo (3 g/day) for 60 days, respectively. Before and after the intervention, blood routine indicators, liver function, renal function, inflammatory factors and intestinal flora were evaluated. Results: The results showed that intervention with *Weizmannia coagulans* BC99 reduced the levels of alanine aminotransferase, aspartate aminotransferase, glutamyl transpeptidase, serum total bilirubin, blood urea nitrogen, uric acid and 'blood urea nitrogen/creatinine'. *Weizmannia coagulans* BC99 also reduced the levels of pro-inflammatory factors TNF-α and IL-6 and increased the levels of anti-inflammatory factor IL-10. The results of intestinal flora analysis showed that *Weizmannia coagulans* BC99 regulated the imbalance of intestinal flora, increased the beneficial bacteria abundance (*Prevotella*, *Faecalibacterium* and *Roseburia*) and reduced the conditionally pathogenic bacteria abundance (*Escherichia-Shigella* and *Klebsiella*). Both LEfSe analysis and random forest analysis indicated that the increase in the abundance of *Muribaculaceae* induced by BC99 was a key factor in alleviating alcohol-induced liver damage. Conclusions: These findings demonstrate that *Weizmannia coagulans* BC99 has the potential to alleviate alcoholic liver injury and provide an effective strategy for liver protection in long-term drinkers.

Keywords: *Weizmannia coagulans* BC99; randomized controlled trial; alcoholic liver injury; gut microbiota; oxidative stress

1. Introduction

Alcohol is one of the most commonly abused drinks by modern people. Alcoholic liver disease (ALD) caused by long-term drinking has been a common multiple disease [1].

In recent years, with the improvement of living standards, the drinking amount of residents has been increasing, and the incidence of ALD in China and most developed countries in Europe and America has been increasing year by year. According to the epidemiological investigation report [2], alcohol has become the second leading cause of liver damage after viral hepatitis. Globally, ALD causes more than 3.3 million deaths every year, accounting for 5.1% of the global disease burden [3]. The progress of ALD is mainly related to the amount and duration of alcohol consumption. The symptoms of patients are mostly progressive or occult, initially presenting as fatty liver, which can progress to alcoholic hepatitis, liver fibrosis and even cirrhosis [4]. Severe alcoholism can induce extensive hepatocyte necrosis and even lead to liver failure, which seriously endangers human life [5]. Modern medical research has proved that the liver is the main metabolic organ for ethanol, and long-term excessive alcohol consumption will lead to the accumulation of ethanol and acetaldehyde in the liver, which will lead to ALD through various mechanisms, such as damaging lipid metabolism, aggravating inflammatory reaction and inducing fibrosis [6]. At present, lifestyle change including abstinence from alcohol and a healthy diet is still one of the main treatments for ALD patients. However, because of the heavy dependence on alcohol, most long-term drinkers have difficulty sticking to lifestyle changes. Therefore, how to adopt effective methods to protect the liver from alcohol damage has become a new idea to reduce the occurrence of ALD.

There is a close relationship between liver metabolism and intestinal flora [7]. Gut microbiota can regulate liver metabolic function, which is of great significance for maintaining human health. Long-term excessive alcohol consumption will lead to significant changes in the composition of gut microbiota, especially by inhibiting the growth of beneficial bacteria and promoting the overgrowth of pathogenic bacteria in intestine, thereby disrupting the gut microbiota and damaging the intestinal barrier function [8,9]. Modern medicine believes that the etiology of ALD is clear, but the pathogenesis is complex, which has not been fully explained. The treatment still focuses on anti-inflammatory mechanisms and liver protection, but this method has significant side effects, and the therapeutic effect cannot satisfy patients.

As living microorganisms, probiotics are believed to improve gastrointestinal health, lower cholesterol and blood pressure, improve immune function and reduce inflammation [10]. Previous studies have discussed the use of probiotics to improve intestinal health, showing their potential to restore intestinal microflora and enhance intestinal–liver signal transduction. *Bifidobacterium* and *Lactobacillus* are widely regarded as typical probiotics, and their therapeutic effects on alcoholic liver injury have been extensively studied. *Bifidobacterium lactis* TY-S01 helps maintain the integrity of the intestinal barrier and the balance of the intestinal flora, thereby reducing alcohol-induced liver injury [11]. Wang et al. [12] found that *Lactobacillus rhamnosus* suspension (containing live bacteria, LGG) can effectively treat alcohol-induced liver fat accumulation and liver injury in mice. In recent years, there has been a growing interest in *Bacillus* as a probiotic due to its high tolerance to adverse environments. There are some studies on improving liver function through *Bacillus* intervention. Lu et al. [13] showed that *Bacillus subtilis* had protective effects on alcohol induced liver injury in mice, indicating that probiotics also played a key role in alcoholism. *Weizmannia coagulans* BC99 probiotic has been reported to have the ability to relieve inflammation and oxidative stress, suggesting its potential in the treatment of alcoholic liver injury. Previous studies were carried out in vitro and in animals, but their effectiveness in relieving alcoholism and protecting the liver in the clinic has not been fully explored.

Therefore, in this study, a randomized, double-blind, placebo-controlled crossover study was conducted to evaluate the protective effects of *Weizmannia coagulans* BC99 on the livers of long-term drinkers. In addition to liver function indicators, the effects of *Weizmannia coagulans* BC99 on renal function, inflammatory factors and gut microbiota, and on the correlations among these characteristic indicators, were also be evaluated. This study can provide a more comprehensive scientific basis for the clinical application of *Weizmannia coagulans* BC99 in the prevention and treatment of alcoholic liver disease.

2. Materials and Methods

2.1. Study Subjects

A randomized, double-blind, placebo-controlled trial was conducted at Henan University of Science and Technology, Luoyang, China, from July 2024 to November 2024. The study protocol complies with the World Medical Association Declaration of Helsinki [14] and was approved by the Ethics Committee of the First Affiliated Hospital of Henan University of Science and Technology (NCT06607562, May, 2024). This study recruited 70 participants. All participants met the inclusion criteria: aged between 18–65 years old, with a long-term history of alcohol consumption (alcohol $\geq$ 20 g/day, lasting for more than 1 year, alcohol (g) = alcoholic beverage (mL) $\times$ alcohol content (%) $\times$ 0.8 (alcohol specific gravity)). People with basic diseases such as hepatitis, liver cirrhosis, hypertension and diabetes were not included in the recruitment. All participants were required to be informed of the research procedure and sign a written consent form before they could be included in the study.

2.2. Study Design

A total of 72 participants were recruited for screening in this study, with 70 eligible participants. Among them, 60 participants completed the entire experimental process. As shown in Figure 1, 70 eligible participants were randomly assigned into a placebo group or a probiotic group (35 participants in each group). Participants in the placebo group were daily treated with placebo (composed of 3 g maltodextrin) intervention, while participants in the probiotic group were daily treated with *Weizmannia coagulans* BC99 (3 g, 1 $\times$ 10^{10} CFU) probiotic intervention. The total duration of the study was 60 days, and participants were followed up and sampled on day 1 and day 60, respectively. During the intervention period, participants in each group were required to take the corresponding products daily and record any adverse reactions. After the intervention period was completed, the remaining products and empty packaging boxes were all recovered.

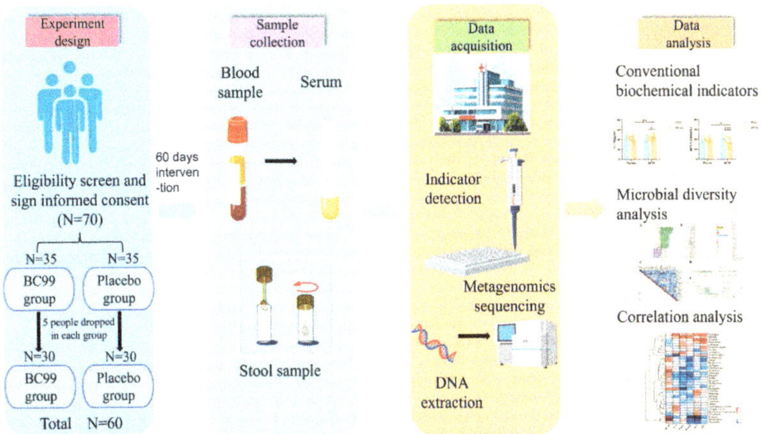

Figure 1. Flowchart of the study design.

2.3. Probiotic

Weizmannia coagulans BC99 was provided by Wecare Probiotics Co., Ltd., Suzhou, China. The entire development process of *Weizmannia coagulans* BC99 was carried out in an extremely professional production environment, with a 100,000 level GMP clean workshop and a constant temperature of 28 °C and humidity of 35%. At the same time, unique cell microencapsulation technology was used to ensure the stability and efficacy of *Weizmannia coagulans* BC99.

2.4. Collection and Determination of Blood Samples

Collection and biochemical determination of blood samples were conducted using clinical standard measurement methods after baseline abdominal blood collection and intervention for 60 days. Blood samples were collected for clinical chemical analysis after fasting for at least 10 h. Blood samples were centrifuged and the serum was stored at −80 °C before analysis. The liver and renal function indicators were measured using an automatic biochemical analyzer (KHB ZY-1280, Shanghai Kehua Biotechnology Co., Ltd., Shanghai, China). The inflammatory factor-related indicators including high-sensitive C-reactive protein (hs-CRP), tumor necrosis factor-α (TNF-α), interleukin-6 (IL-6) and interleukin-10 (IL-10) were measured using the commercial kit (Shanghai Hepeng Biotechnology Co., Ltd., Shanghai, China). The operation was carried out in strict accordance with the manufacturer's protocol.

2.5. Collection and Preparation of Fecal Samples

After fasting for at least 10 h, fresh fecal samples were collected and stored sterile at −80 °C for analysis.

2.6. Intestinal Microbiota Analysis

The genomic DNA of the sample was extracted using the MagPureSoil DNA LQ Kit (Magan, Aurora, ON, Canada). The operation was carried out in strict accordance with the instructions. The concentration of the extracted DNA was determined using Ultramicrospectrophotometer NanoDrop 2000 (Thermo Fisher Scientific, Waltham, MA, USA). The purity of the extracted DNA was determined by agarose gel electrophoresis. The extracted genomic DNA was stored at −20 °C before analysis. The 16S rRNA gene was amplified using the universal primers 343F (primer sequence, 5′-TACGGRAGGCAGCAG-3′) and 798R (primer sequence, 5′-AGGGTATCTAATCCT-3′). PCR amplification products were determined by agarose gel electrophoresis. After two rounds of PCR amplification, the sequencing was performed using the Illumina NovaSeq6000 sequencing platform of Shanghai Ouyi Biotechnology Co., Ltd. (Shanghai, China). After quality control analysis of sequencing data, representative sequences and ASV abundance tables were obtained. The QIIME2 (2020.11) software package was used to select the representative sequences for each ASV. All representative sequences were compared against the Silva (version 138) database and then annotated. Species annotation was analyzed using the q2-feature-classifier (2020.11) software. Diversity analysis and differential analysis were performed using the QIIME2 software and the ANOVA *t*-test statistical algorithm based on the R package (3.5.1), respectively. Differential analysis of species abundance profiles was conducted using LEfSe (1.0.0).

2.7. Statistical Analysis

SPSS 25.0 was used for statistical analysis [15]. The experimental data are presented as mean ± standard deviation. The confidence interval is 95%. For intergroup comparison, if the data conform to the assumptions of normal distribution and homogeneity of variance, the independent sample t-test was used. If not, the Mann–Whitney U test was used. For multiple group comparison, if the data conform to the assumptions of normal distribution and homogeneity of variance, one-way ANOVA was used. If not, the Kruskal–Wallis test was used. $p < 0.05$ indicates a difference, $p < 0.01$ indicates a significant difference and $p < 0.001$ indicates an extremely significant difference. Graphpad Prism 10.1.2 (www.graphpad.com) software was used to draw graphics.

3. Results

3.1. Baseline Characteristics

The baseline characteristics of the participants such as mean age, sex distribution, metabolic characteristics, liver function indicators and renal function indicators are shown in Table 1. The mean age of the participants in the placebo group and the BC99 group was 43.60 ± 11.31 years and 42.87 ± 11.15 years, respectively. There was no significant difference in age and sex distribution between the placebo group and the BC99 group. The baseline BMI values, which were 24.24 ± 2.89 kg/m^2 in placebo group and 24.87 ± 2.68 kg/m^2 in BC99 group, also did not exhibit a significant difference between the two groups. Furthermore, no significant differences were observed in liver function indicators or renal function indicators between the two groups.

Table 1. Baseline characteristics in the placebo group and BC99 group.

Projects	Placebo Group (n = 30)		BC99 Group (n = 30)		p Value
	Mean	SD	Mean	SD	
Age	43.60	11.31	42.87	11.15	0.801
Sex (M/F)	30/0		29/1		0.313
Metabolic characteristics					
Height (cm)	173.4	5.02	171.03	5.38	0.084
Weight (kg)	72.85	9.15	72.63	7.09	0.919
BMI (kg/m^2)	24.24	2.89	24.87	2.68	0.382
Liver function indicators					
ALT (U/L)	40.60	22.81	40.50	23.73	0.990
AST (U/L)	35.82	11.13	40.17	21.38	0.392
γ-GT (U/L)	60.79	22.49	61.08	51.06	0.979
TBil (μmol/L)	12.42	3.48	14.03	3.11	0.073
Renal function indicators					
BUN (mmol/L)	5.92	0.88	6.16	0.78	0.393
Cr (μmol/L)	73.67	10.20	70.41	10.20	0.325
UA (μmol/L)	393.67	75.41	406.74	71.13	0.500

Abbreviations: ALT, alanine aminotransferase; AST, aspartate aminotransferase; γ-GT, glutamyl transpeptidase; TBil, serum total bilirubin; BUN, blood urea nitrogen; Cr, creatinine; UA, uric acid.

3.2. Blood Routine Indicators

The blood routine indicators of the placebo group and BC99 group before and after 60 days of intervention were compared, and the results were shown in Table 2. There was no significant difference in blood routine indicators between the placebo group and the BC99 group before and after 60 days of intervention ($p > 0.05$).

Table 2. Comparison of blood routine indicators before and after intervention.

Projects	Placebo Group (n = 30)			BC99 Group (n = 30)		
	0 Day	60 Day	p-Value	0 Day	60 Day	p-Value
Neutrophils ($\times 10^9$/L)	3.08 ± 1.15	3.44 ± 1.42	0.277	3.04 ± 0.77	3.2 ± 0.75	0.429
Lymphocyte ($\times 10^9$/L)	1.99 ± 0.51	2.08 ± 0.66	0.558	1.99 ± 0.53	3.36 ± 5.94	0.213
Red blood cell ($\times 10^9$/L)	4.73 ± 0.80	4.48 ± 0.32	0.122	4.48 ± 0.42	4.36 ± 0.37	0.266
Hemoglobin (g/L)	136.83 ± 13.73	130.93 ± 11.06	0.072	141.67 ± 35.74	132.83 ± 10.90	0.201
Platelet ($\times 10^9$/L)	181.33 ± 52.43	170.40 ± 46.44	0.396	179.53 ± 50.24	172.16 ± 68.50	0.637

3.3. Liver Function Indicators

The differences in liver function indicators such as ALT, AST, TBil and γ-GT between the placebo group and the BC99 group after a 60-day intervention are shown in Figure 2. For the placebo group, there was no significant difference in the above indicators before and after the 60-day intervention. However, after 60 days of intervention in the BC99 group, three indicators, AST, TBil and γ-GT, showed significant decreases ($p < 0.01$, Figure 2B–D). Especially for AST and γ-GT, the unqualified rates of the two indicators were 34.78% and 30.43% before intervention, respectively, and all decreased to 0% after intervention. In addition, after 60 days of intervention, the ALT level in the BC99 group showed a decrease (Figure 2A), and the unqualified rates of the indicator decreased from 38.88% before intervention to 11.11% after intervention.

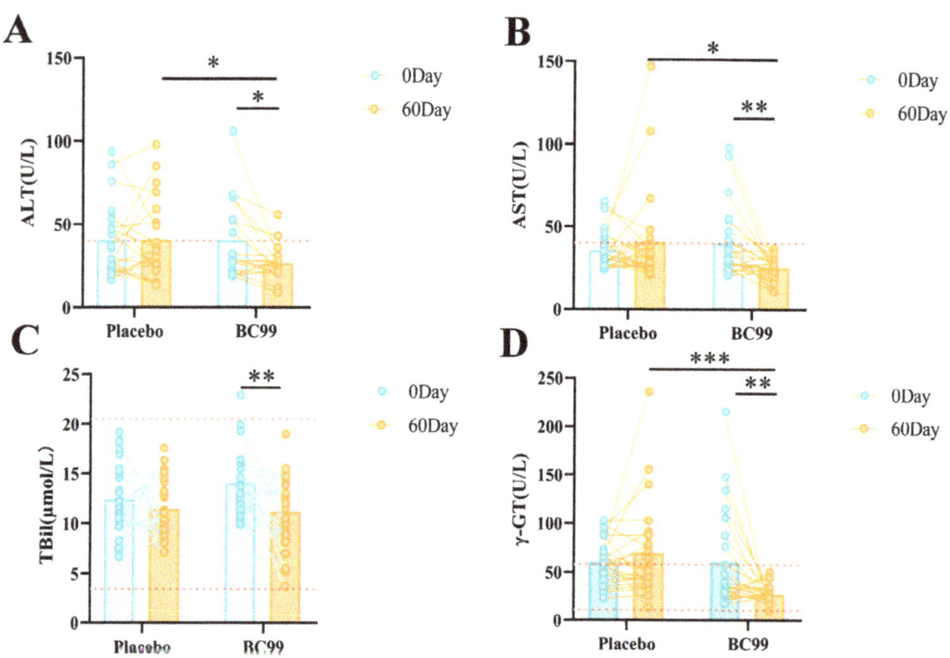

Figure 2. The regulatory effect of *Weizmannia coagulans* BC99 on liver function indicators. (**A**) The effect of BC99 on ALT. (**B**) The effect of BC99 on AST. (**C**) The effect of BC99 on TBil. (**D**) The effect of BC99 on γ-GT. * $p < 0.05$, ** $p < 0.01$, *** $p < 0.001$.

3.4. Renal Function Indicators

The differences in renal function indicators such as BUN, UA and Cr between the placebo group and the BC99 group after a 60-day intervention are shown in Table 3. There was no significant difference in renal function indicators before and after the 60-day intervention for the placebo group. After 60 days of intervention in the BC99 group, two indicators, BUN and UA, showed a significant decrease, while the Cr level did not change significantly. However, as it is shown in Figure 3, the "BUN/Cr" level significantly decreased. In clinical practice, "BUN/Cr" is commonly used to characterize acute renal injury, indicating the degree of damage to glomerular filtration function. In this study, after 60 days of intervention, the number of subjects with abnormal "BUN/Cr" in the BC99 group decreased from 14 to five, while there was no significant difference in the placebo group.

Table 3. Comparison of renal function indicators before and after intervention.

Projects	Placebo Group (n = 30)			BC99 Group (n = 30)		
	0 Day	60 Day	p-Value	0 Day	60 Day	p-Value
BUN (mmol/L)	5.92 ± 0.88	5.67 ± 0.87	0.366	6.16 ± 0.78	5.00 ± 0.98	<0.001
UA (μmol/L)	393.67 ± 75.41	375.11 ± 113.17	0.466	406.74 ± 71.13	365.99 ± 61.68	0.023
Cr (μmol/L)	73.67 ± 10.20	73.25 ± 11.04	0.902	70.41 ± 10.20	72.91 ± 9.12	0.431

Abbreviations: BUN, blood urea nitrogen; UA, uric acid; Cr, creatinine.

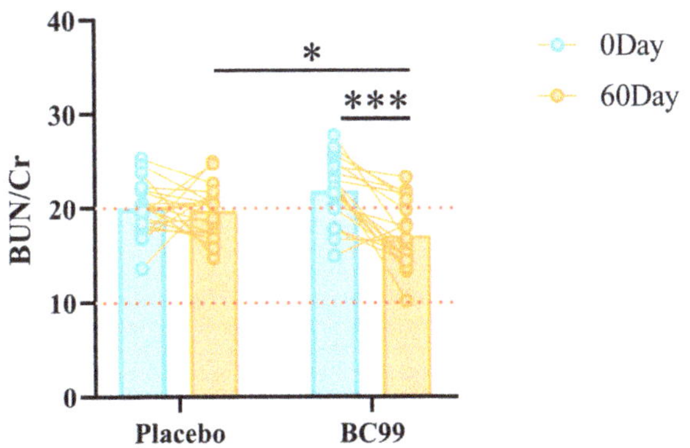

Figure 3. The regulatory effect of *Weizmannia coagulans* BC99 on "BUN (mg/dL)/Cr (mg/dL)". The conversion relationship between different units refers to Beeler [16]. * $p < 0.05$, *** $p < 0.001$. The two red dashed lines represent the range of clinical normal values for this indicator.

3.5. hs-CRP and Inflammatory Factors

In this study, the hs-CRP levels before and after 60 days of intervention were compared between the placebo group and the BC99 group. As shown in Figure 4A, there was no significant difference in the hs-CRP levels of the placebo group before and after 60 days of intervention, while the BC99 group showed a significant decrease in hs-CRP levels after 60 days of intervention, from 28.18 mg/L to 21.71 mg/L. As for the pro-inflammatory factors TNF-α and IL-6, they also showed a similar trend of change (Figure 4B,C). There was no significant change in these two indicators before and after intervention in the placebo group. However, in the BC99 group, after 60 days of intervention, the levels of both indicators showed a significant downward trend, especially IL-6, which decreased from 193.08 mg/mL before intervention to 156.21 mg/mL after intervention, a decrease of more than 30%. In addition, 23 subjects showed a decreasing trend in the IL-6 level, accounting for 76.67% of the total participants. Furthermore, as can be seen from Figure 4D, the anti-inflammatory factor IL-10 level in the BC99 group was significantly increased after 60 days of intervention, from 41.55 pg/mL to 45.34 pg/mL. In contrast, the IL-10 level in the placebo group decreased slightly, from 43.92 pg/mL before intervention to 41.47 pg/mL after intervention.

3.6. *Efficacy of BC99 on Gut Microbiota*

We further studied the effect of BC99 on the composition of the gut microbiota in long-term alcohol drinkers by using 16S rRNA gene sequencing of fecal samples. As shown in Figure 5A,B, the ace index evaluates the richness and evenness of species composition in the sample, and the observed species index indicates the number of species present in the sample. Compared with the placebo group, there were significant changes in the microbiota alpha diversity after intervention with BC99. Beta diversity is an indicator of the similarity in microbial community structure between samples. The diversity results based on NMDS analysis showed that the confidence ellipses between the two groups were not clearly separated, but some points of the BC99 group were distant from those of the placebo group, indicating that the intervention of BC99 had, to some extent, altered the gut microbiota structure (Figure 5C). The analysis of species structure adopts statistical methods and can obtain which dominant species are present in each sample at various levels (including domain, kingdom, phylum, class, order, family, genus, species, OTU, etc.), as well as the relative abundance of each dominant species. As shown in Figure 5D,E, the gut microbiota of the two groups included similar microbial community structures. At the phylum level, the gut microbiota was mainly composed of Firmicutes, Bacteroidota and Proteobacteria, accounting for over 90% of the human gut microbiota. Compared to the placebo group, the abundance of Firmicutes in the BC99 group increased while the abundance of Proteobacteria decreased. This indicated that the BC99 intervention significantly changed the gut microbiota at the phylum level in long-term alcohol drinkers. At the genus level, it was found that the most abundant genera in the gut microbiota of all groups were *Bacteroides*, *Prevotella*, *Faecalibacterium*, *Escherichia-Shigella*, *Klebsiella* and *Roseburia*. Compared to the placebo group, the BC99 group showed an increased abundance of *Prevotella*, *Faecalibacterium* and *Roseburia*, while the abundance of *Bacteroides*, *Escherichia-Shigella* and *Klebsiella* decreased.

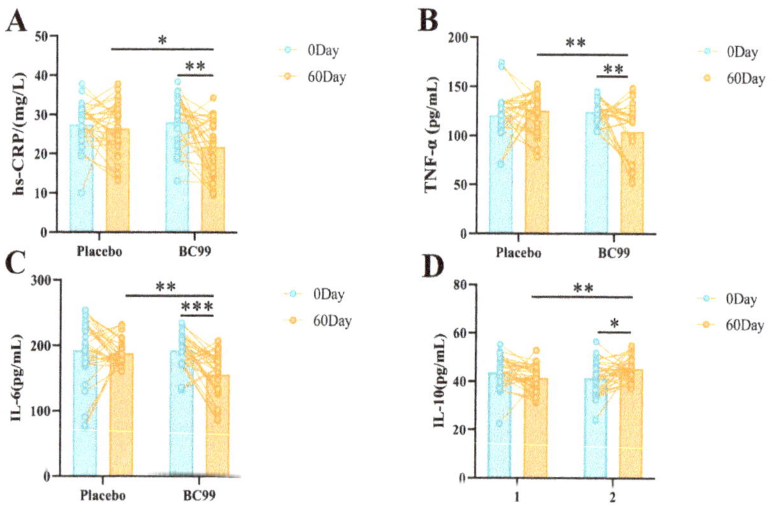

Figure 4. The regulatory effect of *Weizmannia coagulans* BC99 on hs-CRP (**A**) and inflammatory factors TNF-α (**B**), IL-6 (**C**) and IL-10 (**D**). * $p < 0.05$, ** $p < 0.01$, *** $p < 0.001$.

According to LEfSe analysis (Figure 6A), differentially abundant microbial communities in the BC99 intervention can be identified. In the placebo group, the differential strains were found to be *Morganella*, *Lachnospiraceae* UCG-010 and *Comamonas*. The enrichment of *Muribaculaceae*, *Anaerostipes*, *Streptococcus*, *Pseudomnas* and *Kosakonia* were found in the

BC99 group, and *Bacillus* was also detected in the BC99 group. These differential strains may be key strains in alleviating alcohol-induced damage in the BC99 group. To study the relationships among the microbiota, the present study conducted an analysis of microbial interactions (Figure 6C). The results showed that *Faecalibacterium* was significantly negatively correlated with *Escherichia-Shigella* and *Klebsiella*, and significantly positively correlated with *Roseburia* and *Lachnospiraceae* UCG-010. *Muribaculaceae* was significantly positively correlated with *Pseudomnas* and *Kosakonia*, while *Bacillus* was significantly negatively correlated with *Klebsiella*. It was also found that *Escherichia-Shigella* was significantly positively correlated with *Klebsiella*. This demonstrated that long-term alcohol consumption could lead to the mutual growth of conditionally pathogenic bacteria, while intervention with BC99 could synergistically increase the abundance of beneficial bacteria in the gut and suppress the growth of pathogenic bacteria. At the same time, random forest analysis was used to identify key species that could differentiate between groups. As shown in the Figure 6B, the most significantly important key strain was *Muribaculaceae*. This was also consistent with the conclusion of the LEfSe analysis, which indicated that *Muribaculaceae* may be the key strain for BC99 to alleviate alcohol damage.

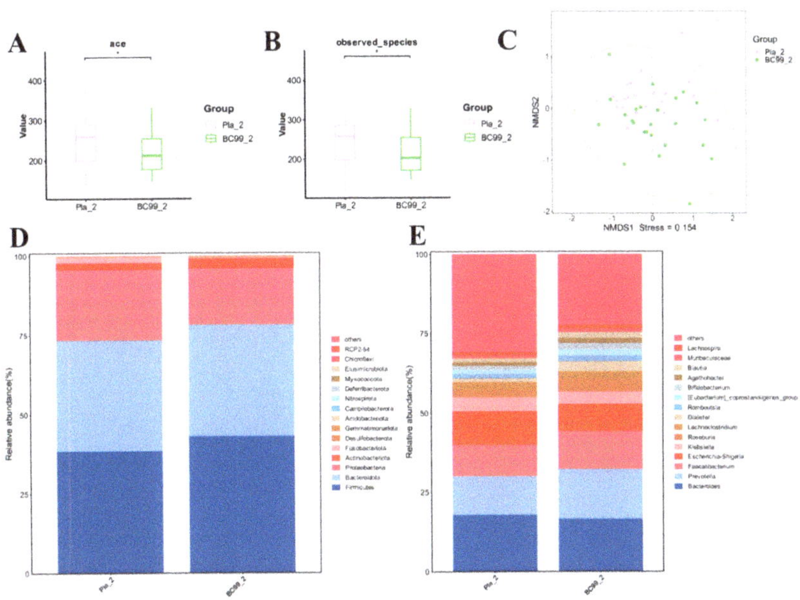

Figure 5. BC99 regulated the composition of gut microbiota. (**A**) ace indice; (**B**) observed indice; (**C**) NMDS analysis; (**D**) abundance of phylum-level flora; (**E**) abundance of genus-level flora. Pla_2 and BC99_2 represented samples from the placebo group and BC99 group after 60 days of intervention, respectively. * $p < 0.05$.

Based on marker gene sequences, microbial community functional analysis was carried out using PICRUSt (2.3.0b0) software and the KEGG database. The results are shown in Figure 6D,E. At the KEGG L2 classification level, there was a significant difference in one pathway related to the digestive system between the two groups. Further screening at the KEGG L3 level revealed five different pathways, including the Toll and Imd signaling pathways and pancreatic secretion.

3.7. Correlation Analysis

By performing correlation analysis between inflammatory factors and liver function indicators with the levels of intestinal microbiota, this study explored the key strains that alleviate liver damage in long-term drinkers. From Figure 7, it can be found that the differential strain *Klebsiella* in the placebo group was significantly positively correlated with the pro-inflammatory factor TNF-α. *Aeromonas* was significantly positively correlated with ALT and AST. This indicated a strong correlation between these strains and the body's inflammatory response and liver damage. Additionally, the differential strain *Anaerostipes* in the BC99 group was significantly negatively correlated with TNF-α and hs-CRP. *Muribaculaceae* and *Kosakonia* were significantly positively correlated with anti-inflammatory factors IL-10 and significantly negatively correlated with hs-CRP and ALT, indicating that they may be the key strains in BC99 to alleviate acute alcohol poisoning.

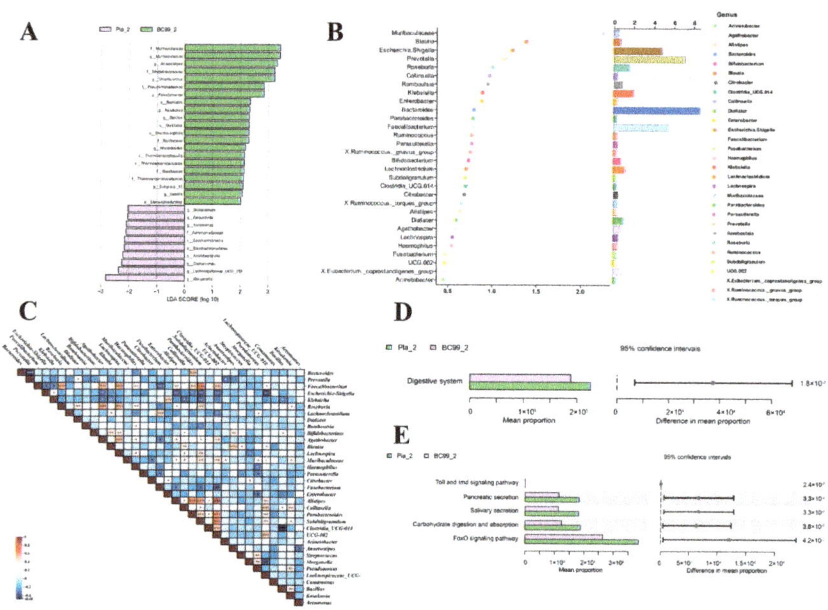

Figure 6. BC99 elevated the levels of beneficial bacteria while reducing the levels of pathogenic bacteria. (**A**) Analysis of differences in the microbial taxa by LEfSe; (**B**) random forest analysis; (**C**) analysis of flora interaction; (**D**) KEGG L2 metabolism pathway; (**E**) KEGG L3 metabolism pathway. Pla_2 and BC99_2 represented samples from the placebo group and BC99 group after 60 days of intervention, respectively. * $p < 0.05$, ** $p < 0.01$, *** $p < 0.001$.

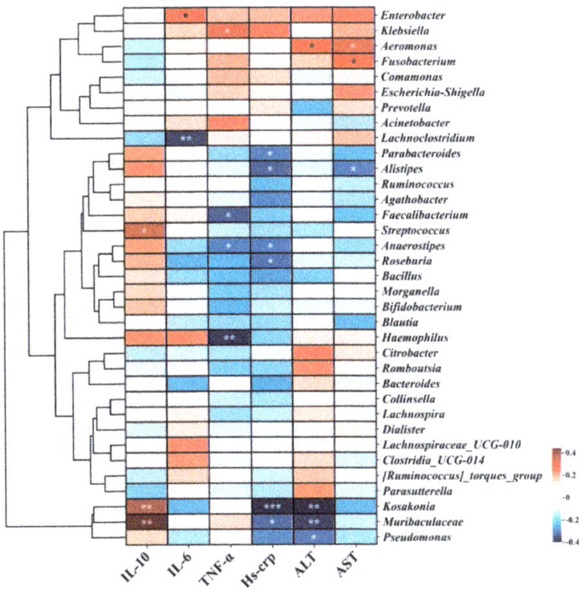

Figure 7. Correlation analysis of intestinal flora with inflammation and physiological indexes. * $p < 0.05$, ** $p < 0.01$, *** $p < 0.001$.

4. Discussion

Drinking has become a popular form of social entertainment for people. According to the survey, the incidence rate of alcoholic liver disease is increasing year by year worldwide [17]. Long-term alcoholism will not only cause liver fibrosis and fatty liver, but can also lead to cirrhosis, liver cancer and other diseases, in severe cases, that seriously threaten the physical health of people [18]. The mechanism of action of alcoholic liver injury is related to a variety of factors, including oxidative stress reaction, inflammatory signaling pathways, etc. [19,20]. At present, clinical methods for treating alcoholic liver injury include drug-assisted therapy and alcohol abstinence, but the efficacy is not outstanding, and adverse reactions often occur after drug intervention [21]. A growing body of research suggests that using probiotics to control the gut microbiota may be a potential way to protect the liver from alcohol damage. In this work, we investigated the improvement effect of BC99 on the physical functions of long-term alcohol drinkers, mainly including liver function, renal function, inflammatory factors and gut microbiota. The final results indicated that BC99 indeed played a good role in the above aspects.

The liver, as the main organ for alcohol metabolism, plays a crucial role in its normal function. The results in this study indicated that after intervention with BC99, subjects' liver function indicators including ALT, AST, TBil and γ-GT have significantly improved, demonstrating the good protective effect of BC99 on the liver. In addition, BC99 also significantly improved the renal function of the subjects, mainly reflected in the reduction in BUN, UA and BUN/Cr levels. Inflammatory factor analysis also confirmed the reliability of the above results. Hs-CRP is considered to be one of the most sensitive markers of inflammation. A large number of studies have shown that hs-CRP levels in alcohol-dependent patients were significantly higher than those in healthy individuals [22]. TNF-α is a pro-inflammatory cytokine mainly produced by macrophages and monocytes, which can lead to a series of problems such as hepatic steatosis, inflammatory cytokine infiltration and hepatocyte necrosis. Therefore, the reduction in the TNF-α level can effectively block the inflammatory pathway associated with liver injury and inhibit the development of liver disease [23]. As another typical pro-inflammatory factor, the release of IL-6 can induce local inflammatory responses in the body or liver [24]. Therefore, reducing the level of IL-6 can weaken local inflammation in the liver. As a typical anti-inflammatory factor, the effect of IL-10 is opposite to that of TNF-α and IL-6. IL-10 is an immunomodulatory cytokine produced primarily by Th2 cells and acts primarily through its receptors. It can not only down-regulate the inflammatory response by inhibiting the activation and proliferation of mononuclear macrophages, but also inhibit the synthesis and expression of inflammatory mediators IL-1, IL-6, IL-8 and TNF in mononuclear macrophages in a broad spectrum [25,26]. The occurrence of inflammatory response is usually closely related to the oxidative stress of the body. Animal experiments have shown that *Weizmannia coagulans* BC99 can increase the levels of superoxide dismutase (SOD) and glutathione (GSH), thereby enhancing the body's antioxidant capacity [27]. On one hand, this helps to resist oxidative stress caused by alcohol metabolism, and on the other hand, it can reduce the toxicity of drugs and chemicals, alleviate liver damage and slow down the progression of liver diseases [28].

In order to explore the mechanism by which *Weizmannia coagulans* BC99 alleviates liver damage in long-term drinkers, we further analyzed the gut microbiota. Through the analysis of microbial diversity, it was found that BC99 significantly altered microbial diversity, but the samples of the BC99 group were not completely separated from those of the placebo group, which may be related to factors such as intervention dosage and intervention time. Long-term alcohol consumption leads to a significant decrease in the relative abundance of the Firmicutes phylum [29] and a significant increase in the relative abundance of the Bacteroidetes phylum [30] in the gut, which is consistent with the results obtained in this study. Compared with the placebo group, the relative abundance of the Firmicutes phylum significantly increased in the BC99 group, while the relative abundance of the Bacteroidetes phylum decreased. At the taxonomic level, BC99 intervention reduced the relative abundance of *Escherichia-Shigella* and *Klebsiella*. In patients with alcoholic liver cirrhosis, the relative abundance of *Escherichia-Shigella* significantly increases and is associated with liver inflammation and fibrosis [31]. *Klebsiella*, a gram-negative bacterium, with increased abundance, can lead to liver cell damage and may further exacerbate liver injury by activating immune responses (such as the IFN-γ/STAT/IRF-1 signaling pathway) and the expression of inflammatory factors (such as TNF-α, IL-6) [32]. Meanwhile, intervention with BC99 increased the relative abundance of *Prevotella*, *Faecalibacterium* and *Roseburia*. Prevotella belongs to the Bacteroidetes phylum, and studies have shown a significantly decreased relative abundance in alcohol-induced liver injury mice [33], which is consistent with our clinical findings. In addition to assisting in the breakdown of proteins and carbohydrates, *Prevotella* can also produce short-chain fatty acids (SCFAs) [34]. SCFAs such as acetate and butyrate can protect the liver by enhancing intestinal barrier function. *Faecalibacterium* is a symbiotic bacterium that is believed to have anti-inflammatory properties and is an important producer of butyric acid, playing a significant role in the gut microbiota. The abundance of *Faecalibacterium* is usually reduced in ALD patients [35], consistent with the results of this study. *Roseburia*, through the production of SCFAs such as butyric acid, can regulate immune responses and inflammation. Studies have shown that supplementation of bacteria belonging to the *Roseburia* genus can improve alcohol-induced fatty liver in mice [36]. Lefse analysis was performed to analyze the key strains of bacteria responsible for alcohol-induced damage and the alleviation of damage by BC99. As shown in the Figure 6A, the most significant differential strain in the placebo group was *Morganella*. *Morganella* is a Gram-negative opportunistic pathogenic bacterium that is commonly found in the intestines of humans and other animals. It is an opportunistic pathogen that can cause various infections and induce a variety of diseases, including sepsis, liver abscess and central nervous system infections [37] when the host's immune system is compromised.

In the BC99 group, the most significant differential strain was *Muribaculaceae*. *Muribaculaceae* is a bacterial family in the order Bacteroidales. *Muribaculaceae* can produce SCFAs through endogenous (mucin glycans) and exogenous polysaccharides (dietary fiber) [38]. It is worth mentioning that more and more plant extracts such as polysaccharides and polyphenols have been proven to have health promoting effects. Zhang et al. found that *Artemisia argyi* polysaccharides can induce the body to produce a large amount of SCFAs to alleviate intestinal inflammation and gut microbiota imbalance [39]. Flavonoid-rich mulberry leaf extract has been reported to regulate lipid metabolism and intestinal microbiota disorders caused by a high-fat diet [40]. Therefore, combining probiotics with some plant supplements may achieve better effects [41]. In addition, the abundance of *Muribaculaceae* is negatively correlated with inflammatory factors in the serum, and it can inhibit the activation of CD8+ T cells, resisting immune stimulation, indicating its potential anti-inflammatory and immune-regulating functions [42]. The study of Zhang [43] can also prove that *Muribaculaceae* may have an anti-inflammatory effect, and thus, it has a certain protective effect against liver injury caused by alcohol. Furthermore, the key strain screened by the random forest analysis method was *Muribaculaceae*. Therefore, we have reason to speculate that *Muribaculaceae* may be the key strain in BC99 alleviating liver damage in long-term alcohol drinkers. The analysis of microbial interactions showed that beneficial bacteria and pathogenic bacteria have an antagonistic relationship. BC99 intervention increased the abundance of beneficial bacteria and reduced the abundance of pathogenic bacteria. BC99 intervention can reduce alcohol-induced liver injury by regulating intestinal flora structure and restoring microbial imbalance caused by long-term alcohol consumption.

By conducting PICRUSt functional prediction analysis on various microbial groups, it was found that the pathways at the KEGG L2 level were related to the digestive system. Alcohol can cause direct damage to the digestive system during its absorption process in the human body. Alcohol can increase intestinal permeability, leading to dysbiosis of the gut microbiota and the release of bacterial products, exacerbating inflammation in the body [27]. At the KEGG L3 level, the Toll and Imd signaling pathways mainly involve the activation of the innate immune system and the regulation of inflammatory responses. According to reports, TLR4 can promote the production of inflammatory factors (such as TNF-α and IL-1β) and affect the activation of hepatic stellate cells, thus exacerbating liver fibrosis and inflammatory reactions in alcohol-induced liver injury by activating Kupffer cells [44]. Long-term alcohol consumption can lead to excessive stimulation and increased secretion of pancreatic exocrine function. In addition, alcohol can also affect the response of pancreatic cells to cholecystokinin (CCK) and other stimuli, leading to abnormal pancreatic secretion function [45]. The specific role of carbohydrate digestion and absorption in alcoholic liver injury may be related to its impact on liver metabolism. For example, excessive intake of carbohydrates may lead to insulin resistance and endoplasmic reticulum stress, both of which are associated with an increased risk of alcoholic liver injury [46]. The FoxO signaling pathway plays a key role in oxidative stress and cell apoptosis. Among the FoxO family, FoxO3a, as a mitochondrial protein, regulates the levels of SOD messenger RNA and protein in response to oxidative stress, thereby maintaining mitochondrial homeostasis [47]. Based on the literature and previous research, it is speculated that BC99 may improve the digestive system and alleviate alcohol-induced damage by regulating the occurrence of inflammatory oxidative stress. This provides a basis for further exploration of the mechanism of action of BC99 in the treatment of alcohol-induced liver injury.

This study suggests that BC99 can alleviate alcoholic liver injury in long-term alcohol drinkers, and is more comprehensive compared to previous research. In addition to evaluating the improvement of liver function indicators through BC99 intervention, it also elaborated on regulating inflammatory factors, alleviating oxidative stress and regulating gut microbiota. However, additional research is needed to uncover which microbial groups or key metabolites are playing a role.

5. Conclusions

In summary, the findings in this study demonstrate that BC99 intervention can effectively improve liver function (ALT, AST, TBil and γ-GT) and renal function (BUN, UA, Cr and BUN/Cr) in long-term alcohol drinkers, and that it also has a good regulatory effect on inflammatory factors (hs-CRP, TNF-α, IL-6 and IL-10). The potential mechanism by which BC99 effectively regulates clinical indicators may be attributed to its impact on key gut microbiota genera (*Muribaculaceae*, *Prevotella*, *Faecalibacterium*, *Escherichia-Shigella*, *Klebsiella* and *Roseburia*). These results will provide scientific evidence that BC99 intervention can reduce the extent of damage to the liver caused by alcohol intake. Future research may focus on exploring the deeper mechanisms by which BC99 affects these key bacterial genera or metabolites.

Author Contributions: J.Z.: Data curation, Investigation, Methodology, Writing—original draft, Software, Writing—review and editing; C.L.: Data curation, Investigation, Writing—original draft, Software; M.D.: Investigation, Methodology, Data curation; Z.Q.: Resources, Software; Y.W. (Yi Wang): Investigation, Software; Y.D.: Investigation, Methodology; Y.W. (Ying Wu): Resources, Writing—review and editing; S.F.: Resources; S.G.: Project administration, Resources, Supervision, Validation. All authors have read and agreed to the published version of the manuscript.

Funding: This work was supported by Major Science and Technology Special Projects in Henan Province (No. 231100310200) and Key R&D Projects in Henan Province (No. 241111314200, No. 221111111400).

Institutional Review Board Statement: The study was conducted in accordance with the Declaration of Helsinki, and approved by the Ethics Committee of First Affiliated Hospital of Henan University of Science and Technology (NCT06607562 and 30 May 2024).

Informed Consent Statement: All participants provided written informed consent prior to study enrollment.

Data Availability Statement: The original contributions presented in the study are included in the article; further inquiries can be directed to the corresponding author.

Conflicts of Interest: Authors Yao Dong and Shuguang Fang were employed by the company Department of Research and Development, Wecare Probiotics Co., Ltd. The remaining authors declare that the research was conducted in the absence of any commercial or financial relationships that could be construed as a potential conflict of interest.

References

1. Xiao, C.; Zhou, F.; Zhao, M.; Su, G.; Sun, B. Chicken breast muscle hydrolysates ameliorate acute alcohol-induced liver injury in mice through alcohol dehydrogenase (ADH) activation and oxidative stress reduction. *Food Funct.* **2018**, *9*, 774–784. [CrossRef]
2. Gowing, L.R.; Ali, R.L.; Allsop, S.; Marsden, J.; Turf, E.E.; West, R.; Witton, J. Global statistics on addictive behaviours: 2014 status report. *Addiction* **2015**, *110*, 904–919. [CrossRef] [PubMed]
3. Liang, X.T.; Wang, Y.Y.; Hu, X.Y.; Wang, S.B. The Protective Effects of Water Extracts of Compound Turmeric Recipe on Acute Alcoholism: An Experimental Research Using a Mouse Model. *Evid. Based Complement. Alternat. Med.* **2021**, *2021*, 6641919. [CrossRef] [PubMed]
4. Xu, L.; Guo, W.; Dai, J.; Cheng, Y.; Chen, Y.; Liu, W.; Xu, J.; Su, W.; Zhang, X.; Wang, C.; et al. Hydrogen gas alleviates acute ethanol-induced hepatotoxicity in mice via modulating TLR4/9 innate immune signaling and pyroptosis. *Int. Immunopharmacol.* **2024**, *127*, 111399. [CrossRef]

5. Khanam, A.; Kottilil, S. Acute-on-Chronic Liver Failure: Pathophysiological Mechanisms and Management. *Front. Med.* **2021**, *8*, 752875. [CrossRef]
6. Abulikemu, A.; Zhao, X.; Xu, H.; Li, Y.; Ma, R.; Yao, Q.; Wang, J.; Sun, Z.; Li, Y.; Guo, C. Silica nanoparticles aggravated the metabolic associated fatty liver disease through disturbed amino acid and lipid metabolisms-mediated oxidative stress. *Redox Biol.* **2023**, *59*, 102569. [CrossRef]
7. Albillos, A.; de Gottardi, A.; Rescigno, M. The gut-liver axis in liver disease: Pathophysiological basis for therapy. *J. Hepatol.* **2020**, *72*, 558–577. [CrossRef]
8. Zhao, H.; Kong, L.; Shao, M.; Liu, J.; Sun, C.; Li, C.; Wang, Y.; Chai, X.; Wang, Y.; Zhang, Y.; et al. Protective effect of flavonoids extract of *Hippophae rhamnoides* L. on alcoholic fatty liver disease through regulating intestinal flora and inhibiting TAK1/p38MAPK/p65NF-κB pathway. *J. Ethnopharmacol.* **2022**, *292*, 115225. [CrossRef]
9. Giuffrè, M.; Campigotto, M.; Campisciano, G.; Comar, M.; Crocè, L.S. A story of liver and gut microbes: How does the intestinal flora affect liver disease? A review of the literature. *Am. J. Physiol. Gastrointest. Liver Physiol.* **2020**, *318*, G889–G906. [CrossRef] [PubMed]
10. Jones, A.W.; Jönsson, K.A. Between-subject and within-subject variations in the pharmacokinetics of ethanol. *Br. J. Clin. Pharmacol.* **1994**, *37*, 427–431. [CrossRef] [PubMed]
11. Shu, X.; Wang, J.; Zhao, L.; Wang, J.; Wang, P.; Zhang, F.; Wang, R. *Bifidobacterium lactis* TY-S01 protects against alcoholic liver injury in mice by regulating intestinal barrier function and gut microbiota. *Heliyon* **2023**, *9*, e17878. [CrossRef]
12. Wang, Y.; Kirpich, I.; Liu, Y.; Ma, Z.; Barve, S.; McClain, C.J.; Feng, W. *Lactobacillus rhamnosus* GG treatment potentiates intestinal hypoxia-inducible factor, promotes intestinal integrity and ameliorates alcohol-induced liver injury. *Am. J. Pathol.* **2011**, *179*, 2866–2875. [CrossRef] [PubMed]
13. Lu, J.; Zhu, X.; Zhang, C.; Lu, F.; Lu, Z.; Lu, Y. Co-expression of alcohol dehydrogenase and aldehyde dehydrogenase in *Bacillus subtilis* for alcohol detoxification. *Food Chem. Toxicol.* **2020**, *135*, 110890. [CrossRef] [PubMed]
14. World Medical Association (WMA). WMA Declaration of Helsinki—Ethical Principles for Medical Research Involving Human Participants. Available online: https://www.wma.net/policies-post/wma-declaration-of-helsinki/ (accessed on 31 October 2024).
15. IBM Corp. *IBM SPSS Statistics for Windows, Version 25.0*; Released 2017; IBM Corp.: Armonk, NY, USA, 2017.
16. Beeler, M.F. SI Units and the AJCP. *Am. J. Clin. Pathol.* **1987**, *87*, 140. [CrossRef]
17. Asrani, S.K.; Devarbhavi, H.; Eaton, J.; Kamath, P.S. Burden of liver diseases in the world. *J. Hepatol.* **2019**, *70*, 151–171. [CrossRef]
18. Lieber, C.S. Alcoholic fatty liver: Its pathogenesis and mechanism of progression to inflammation and fibrosis. *Alcohol* **2004**, *34*, 9–19. [CrossRef]
19. Galicia-Moreno, M.; Gutiérrez-Reyes, G. The role of oxidative stress in the development of alcoholic liver disease. *Rev. Gastroenterol. Mex.* **2014**, *79*, 135–144. [CrossRef]
20. Wen, B.; Zhang, C.; Zhou, J.; Zhang, Z.; Che, Q.; Cao, H.; Bai, Y.; Guo, J.; Su, Z. Targeted treatment of alcoholic liver disease based on inflammatory signalling pathways. *Pharmacol. Ther.* **2021**, *222*, 107752. [CrossRef]
21. Björnsson, H.K.; Björnsson, E.S. Drug-induced liver injury: Pathogenesis, epidemiology, clinical features, and practical management. *Eur. J. Intern. Med.* **2022**, *97*, 26–31. [CrossRef]
22. Grodin, E.N.; Meredith, L.R.; Burnette, E.M.; Miotto, K.; Irwin, M.R.; Ray, L.A. Baseline C-reactive protein levels are predictive of treatment response to a neuroimmune modulator in individuals with an alcohol use disorder: A preliminary study. *Am. J. Drug Alcohol Abus.* **2023**, *49*, 333–344. [CrossRef]
23. Vachliotis, I.D.; Polyzos, S.A. The Role of Tumor Necrosis Factor-Alpha in the Pathogenesis and Treatment of Nonalcoholic Fatty Liver Disease. *Curr. Obes. Rep.* **2023**, *12*, 191–206. [CrossRef]
24. Obeagu, E.; Muhimbura, E.; Kagenderezo, B.; Nakyeyune, S.; Obeagu, G. An Insight of Interleukin -6 and Fibrinogen: In Regulating the Immune System. *J. Biomed. Sci.* **2022**, *11*, 83.
25. Luo, Y.; Lin, H. Inflammation initiates a vicious cycle between obesity and nonalcoholic fatty liver disease. *Immun. Inflamm. Dis.* **2021**, *9*, 59–73. [CrossRef]
26. Nagata, K.; Nishiyama, C. IL-10 in Mast Cell-Mediated Immune Responses: Anti-Inflammatory and Proinflammatory Roles. *Int. J. Mol. Sci.* **2021**, *22*, 4972. [CrossRef] [PubMed]
27. Li, C.; Zhai, S.; Duan, M.; Cao, L.; Zhang, J.; Wang, Y.; Wu, Y.; Gu, S. *Weizmannia coagulans* BC99 Enhances Intestinal Barrier Function by Modulating Butyrate Formation to Alleviate Acute Alcohol Intoxication in Rats. *Nutrients* **2024**, *16*, 4142. [CrossRef]
28. Abdel-Daim, M.M.; Abo-El-Sooud, K.; Aleya, L.; Bungau, S.G.; Najda, A.; Saluja, R. Alleviation of drugs and chemicals toxicity: Biomedical value of antioxidants. *Oxid. Med. Cell. Longev.* **2019**, *2018*, 6276438. [CrossRef] [PubMed]
29. Huang, H.; Lin, Z.; Zeng, Y.; Lin, X.; Zhang, Y. Probiotic and glutamine treatments attenuate alcoholic liver disease in a rat model. *Exp. Ther. Med.* **2019**, *18*, 4733–4739. [CrossRef]
30. Lang, S.; Schnabl, B. Microbiota and Fatty Liver Disease-the Known, the Unknown, and the Future. *Cell Host Microbe* **2020**, *28*, 233–244. [CrossRef] [PubMed]

31. Baltazar-Díaz, T.A.; González-Hernández, L.A.; Aldana-Ledesma, J.M.; Peña-Rodríguez, M.; Vega-Magaña, A.N.; Zepeda-Morales, A.S.M.; López-Roa, R.I.; Del Toro-Arreola, S.; Martínez-López, E.; Salazar-Montes, A.M.; et al. *Escherichia/Shigella*, SCFAs, and Metabolic Pathways-The Triad That Orchestrates Intestinal Dysbiosis in Patients with Decompensated Alcoholic Cirrhosis from Western Mexico. *Microorganisms* **2022**, *10*, 1231. [CrossRef]
32. Lin, Y.C.; Lu, M.C.; Lin, C.; Chiang, M.K.; Jan, M.S.; Tang, H.L.; Liu, H.C.; Lin, W.L.; Huang, C.Y.; Chen, C.M.; et al. Activation of IFN-γ/STAT/IRF-1 in hepatic responses to *Klebsiella pneumoniae* infection. *PLoS ONE* **2013**, *8*, e79961. [CrossRef] [PubMed]
33. Fang, C.; Du, H.; Zheng, X.; Zhao, A.; Jia, W.; Xu, Y. Flavor compounds in fermented Chinese alcoholic beverage alter gut microbiota and attenuate ethanol-induced liver damages. *bioRxiv* **2018**. [CrossRef]
34. Mangalam, A.K.; Murray, J. Microbial monotherapy with *Prevotella histicola* for patients with multiple sclerosis. *Expert Rev. Neurother.* **2019**, *19*, 45–53. [CrossRef] [PubMed]
35. Jinato, T.; Anuntakarun, S.; Satthawiwat, N.; Chuaypen, N.; Tangkijvanich, P. Distinct alterations of gut microbiota between viral- and non-viral-related hepatocellular carcinoma. *Appl. Microbiol. Biotechnol.* **2024**, *108*, 34. [CrossRef]
36. Zhou, J.; Zhang, N.; Zhao, L.; Wu, W.; Zhang, L.; Zhou, F.; Li, J. Astragalus Polysaccharides and Saponins Alleviate Liver Injury and Regulate Gut Microbiota in Alcohol Liver Disease Mice. *Foods* **2021**, *10*, 2688. [CrossRef] [PubMed]
37. Kim, J.H.; Cho, C.R.; Um, T.H.; Rhu, J.Y.; Kim, E.S.; Jeong, J.W.; Lee, H.R. Morganella morganii sepsis with massive hemolysis. *J. Korean Med. Sci.* **2007**, *22*, 1082–1084. [CrossRef] [PubMed]
38. Zhu, Y.; Chen, B.; Zhang, X.; Akbar, M.T.; Wu, T.; Zhang, Y.; Zhi, L.; Shen, Q. Exploration of the *Muribaculaceae* Family in the Gut Microbiota: Diversity, Metabolism, and Function. *Nutrients* **2024**, *16*, 2660. [CrossRef]
39. Ning, E.J.; Sun, C.W.; Wang, X.F.; Chen, L.; Li, F.F.; Zhang, L.X.; Wang, L.P.; Ma, Y.N.; Zhu, J.; Li, X.; et al. *Artemisia argyi* polysaccharide alleviates intestinal inflammation and intestinal flora dysbiosis in lipopolysaccharide-treated mice. *Food Med. Homol.* **2024**, *1*, 9420008. [CrossRef]
40. Liu, Y.F.; Ling, N.; Zhang, B.; Chen, C.; Mo, X.N.; Cai, J.Y.; Tan, X.D.; Yu, Q.M. Flavonoid-rich mulberry leaf extract modulate lipid metabolism, antioxidant capacity, and gut microbiota in high-fat diet-induced obesity: Potential roles of FGF21 and SOCS2. *Food Med. Homol.* **2024**, *1*, 9420016. [CrossRef]
41. Behl, T.; Rocchetti, G.; Chadha, S.; Zengin, G.; Montesano, D. Phytochemicals from Plant Foods as Potential Source of Antiviral Agents: An Overview. *Pharmaceuticals* **2021**, *14*, 381. [CrossRef]
42. Wang, T.; Jia, Z.; An, C.; Ren, P.; Yang, Y.; Wang, W.; Su, L. The Protective Effect of Auricularia cornea var. Li. Polysaccharide on Alcoholic Liver Disease and Its Effect on Intestinal Microbiota. *Molecules* **2023**, *28*, 8003. [CrossRef]
43. Zhang, H.; Zuo, Y.; Zhao, H.; Zhao, H.; Wang, Y.; Zhang, X.; Zhang, J.; Wang, P.; Sun, L.; Zhang, H.; et al. Folic acid ameliorates alcohol-induced liver injury via gut-liver axis homeostasis. *Front. Nutr.* **2022**, *9*, 989311. [CrossRef] [PubMed]
44. Roh, Y.S.; Seki, E. Toll-like receptors in alcoholic liver disease, non-alcoholic steatohepatitis and carcinogenesis. *J. Gastroenterol. Hepatol.* **2013**, *28* (Suppl. S1), 38–42. [CrossRef] [PubMed]
45. Lugea, A.; Gong, J.; Nguyen, J.; Nieto, J.; French, S.W.; Pandol, S.J. Cholinergic mediation of alcohol-induced experimental pancreatitis. *Alcohol Clin. Exp. Res.* **2010**, *34*, 1768–1781. [CrossRef] [PubMed]
46. Tsukamoto, H.; Machida, K.; Dynnyk, A.; Mkrtchyan, H. "Second hit" models of alcoholic liver disease. *Semin. Liver Dis.* **2009**, *29*, 178–187. [CrossRef]
47. Kops, G.J.; Dansen, T.B.; Polderman, P.E.; Saarloos, I.; Wirtz, K.W.; Coffer, P.J.; Huang, T.T.; Bos, J.L.; Medema, R.H.; Burgering, B.M. Forkhead transcription factor FOXO3a protects quiescent cells from oxidative stress. *Nature* **2002**, *419*, 316–321. [CrossRef]

nutrients

MDPI

Article

The Bifidogenic Effect of 2′Fucosyllactose Is Driven by Age-Specific *Bifidobacterium* Species, Demonstrating Age as an Important Factor for Gut Microbiome Targeted Precision Medicine

Jenni Firrman [1], Stef Deyaert [2], Karley K. Mahalak [1], LinShu Liu [1], Aurélien Baudot [2], Marie Joossens [3], Jonas Poppe [2], Simon J. S. Cameron [4] and Pieter Van den Abbeele [2,*]

[1] United States Department of Agriculture, Agricultural Research Service, Eastern Regional Research Center, Dairy and Functional Foods Research Unit, 600 East Mermaid Lane, Wyndmoor, PA 19462, USA; Jenni.Firrman@usda.gov (J.F.)

[2] Cryptobiotix, Technologiepark-Zwijnaarde 82, 9052 Gent, Belgium

[3] Laboratory of Microbiology, Department of Biochemistry and Microbiology (WE10), Ghent University, 9000 Ghent, Belgium

[4] School of Biological Sciences and Institute for Global Food Security, Queen's University Belfast, 19 Chlorine Gardens, Belfast BT9 5DL, Northern Ireland, UK

* Correspondence: pieter.vandenabbeele@cryptobiotix.com (P.V.d.A.)

Abstract: Background: The human gut microbiota develops in concordance with its host over a lifetime, resulting in age-related shifts in community structure and metabolic function. Little is known about whether these changes impact the community's response to microbiome-targeted therapeutics. Providing critical information on this subject, faecal microbiomes of subjects from six age groups, spanning from infancy to 70-year-old adults (n = six per age group) were harvested. The responses of these divergent communities to treatment with the human milk oligosaccharide 2′-fucosyllactose (2′FL), fructo-oligosaccharides (FOS), and lactose was investigated using the *Ex vivo* SIFR® technology that employs bioreactor fermentation and is validated to be predictive of clinical findings. Additionally, it was evaluated whether combining faecal microbiomes of a given age group into a single pooled microbiome produced similar results as the individual microbiomes. Results: First, marked age-dependent changes in community structure were identified. *Bifidobacterium* levels strongly declined as age increased, and *Bifidobacterium* species composition was age-dependent: *B. longum*, *B. catenulatum/pseudocatenulatum*, and *B. adolescentis* were most prevalent for breastfed infants, toddlers/children, and adults, respectively. Metabolomic analyses (LA-REIMS) demonstrated that these age-dependent differences particularly impacted treatment effects of 2′FL (more than FOS/lactose). Further analysis revealed that while 2′FL enhanced production of short-chain fatty acids (SCFAs) and exerted potent bifidogenic effects, regardless of age, the specific *Bifidobacterium* species enhanced by 2′FL, as well as subsequent cross-feeding interactions, were highly age-dependent. Furthermore, single-pooled microbiomes produced results that were indicative of the average treatment response for each age group. Nevertheless, pooled microbiomes had an artificially high diversity, thus overestimating treatment responses (especially for infants), did not recapitulate interindividual variation, and disallowed for the correlative analysis required to unravel mechanistic actions. Conclusions: Age is an important factor in shaping the gut microbiome, with the dominant taxa and their metabolites changing over a lifetime. This divergence affects the response of the microbiota to therapeutics, demonstrated in this study using 2′FL. These results evidence the importance of screening across multiple age groups separately to provide granularity of how therapeutics impact the microbiome and, consequently, human health.

Keywords: 2′-fucosyllactose; *Bifidobacterium*; prebiotic; systemic intestinal fermentation research (SIFR®), gut microbiota; precision medicine; senescence; LA-REIMS; metagenomics

1. Background

There is a well-established link between the gut microbiota, nutrition, and human health [1]. This association is used advantageously by developers of prebiotics, probiotics, or therapeutics that target the gut microbiome to maintain or restore human health, or potentially prevent or ameliorate disease symptoms [2]. However, understanding and predicting the benefits of delivered therapeutics is often complicated by the individualistic nature of the gut microbiota, which uniquely coevolves with its host in response to a number of factors, i.e., the environment, genetic background, diet, and medication usage [3–5]. As these factors change for the host over the course of a lifetime so does the gut microbiota, and although the gut microbes themselves do not age, there is a documented age-related shift in this community's structure and function that occurs [6–8].

Beginning after birth, the infant gut microbiome has low diversity that increases with age, and a high prevalence of *Bifidobacterium* [9]. By 3 years of age, the gut microbiota is estimated to share 40–60% similarly with an adult, showing that the community evolves towards an adult-like state during the first years of life [10–12]. As a person ages, there are again specific changes that occur such as decreases in abundance of *Bifidobacterium* and *Faecalibacterium prausnitzii*, in contrast to increased levels of *Escherichia coli* and Bacteroidota as reported for elderly adults [9–12]. Functionally, for adults, it has been previously reported that levels of short-chain fatty acids (SCFAs) are reduced as age progresses [13]. Although it is well-documented that the gut microbiome consistently evolves in response to age-related environmental changes, there remains a lack of knowledge on how this impacts the community's response to microbial modifiers, such as prebiotics, probiotics, or other therapeutic administrations. Understanding the relationship between age, the gut microbiome, and its response to therapeutics becomes increasingly important when considering the application of precision medicine, which is personalized treatment tailored to an individual, because specific treatments may not remain effective, or produce desired effects to the same extent, as a person ages [14].

Exemplifying age-directed changes that occur to the gut microbiome is the genus *Bifidobacterium*, which is well-studied due to its known positive health benefits and is often used as a probiotic itself, or as the target of prebiotic administration [15,16]. This is a prominent taxa following birth, but upon reaching adulthood it is estimated that the gut microbiota contains only 0–18% *Bifidobacterium*, which is further reduced as aging progresses [17]. Additionally, the prominent species of *Bifidobacterium* present in the community is age-dependent; species *B. longum*, *B. infantis*, and *B. bifidum* that preferentially metabolize human milk oligosaccharides (HMOs) are more abundant in breastfed infants (BF infants) while *B. adolescentis*, which metabolizes other complex carbohydrates such as starch, is more abundant in adults [15,18]. Research has demonstrated that levels of *Bifidobacterium* within the gut microbiota positively corresponds with longevity and overall human health and negatively correlates with immunoscenescence, metabolic disorders, and other conditions such as IBS in elderly adults [17,19].

Although age is known to affect the abundance and dominant species of *Bifidobacterium* present in the community, there is minimal information available on how these age-related changes may influence the community's response to a prebiotic with bifidogenic properties, such as 2′-fucosyllactose. 2′FL is a soluble milk glycan undigested in the upper gastrointestinal tract that is fermented by the gut microbiota producing positive benefits to both the microbial community and human health [20]. Both *in vitro* and *in vivo* studies have reported that 2′FL produces a strong bifidogenic effect in infants and toddlers [21,22]. Due to these reported health benefits, 2′FL has gained interest as a potential prebiotic for all age groups, expanding its application beyond early life up to end of life [23,24].

To provide critical information on the relationship between age and the gut microbiota, filling in these identified gaps in knowledge, a comparative evaluation was performed using the *ex vivo* Systemic Intestinal Fermentation Research (SIFR®) technology. Gut microbial communities were cultured from subjects spanning 0–70 years of age divided into six distinct age groups: breastfed (BF) infants (0–0.3 y), toddlers (1–1.5 y), children (5–7 y), and three groups of adults (25–35 y, 35–50 y, and 50–70 y) [25]. Data generated from metagenomics, flow cytometry, metabolic quantification, and REIMS analysis were combined in order to provide a comprehensive understanding of how age affects the gut microbiome in terms of structure, function, and phenotype. To further expand on this topic, the influence of age on the community's response to therapeutic administration was tested using the well-known prebiotic 2′FL. The results of this study provided granularity on the changes to the gut microbiome that correspond with chronological age and how this may impact a therapeutic response. Of particular importance were the changes identified to species within *Bifidobacterium*, which were found to be highly age-dependent in terms of dominant species and community abundance. Together, the results demonstrate the importance of age when considering therapeutic administration and its role in the development of precision medicine.

2. Methods

Test products: Test products 2′FL, (Glycom, GlyCare™ 2FL 9000, DSM-Firmenich, Maastricht, The Netherlands), Fructooligosaccharide (FOS) from chicory root, (F8052, Sigma-Aldrich, St. Gallen, Switzerland), and lactose, (6868, Carl Roth, Karlsruhe, Germany) were purchased commercially. All tested products were used at a concentration of 5 g/L. Additionally included was an unsupplemented parallel control (no substrate control = NSC), in which the fecal microbiome was grown in the absence of additional test products [25,26].

Ex vivo experimental design: Feces were harvested from subjects living in Belgium that fell within one of the six following age categories at a 1:1 male to female ratio: BF infants (0–0.3 y), toddlers (1–1.5 y), children (5–7 y), adults (25–35 y), adults (35–50 y), adults (50–70 y). All adults had a BMI < 30 and were non-smokers, consumed less than three alcoholic beverages a day, were antibiotic free, prebiotic free, and probiotic free for at least three months, not pregnant or lactating, had no GI disorders including cancers, ulcers, and inflammatory bowel disease (IBD), and were not taking any anti-psychotics or anti-allergy drugs (Table S1). Fresh feces were collected according to a procedure approved by the Ethics Committee of the University Hospital Ghent (reference number BC-09977) that required a signed informed consent. For underage participants, the responsible adult provided consent. *Ex vivo* SIFR® experiments were performed as recently described using a bioreactor management device (Cryptobiotix, Ghent, Belgium) (Figure 1) [25]. Briefly, individual bioreactors containing 5 mLs of nutritional medium (M001, Cryptobiotix, Ghent, Belgium) were inoculated with freshly collected feces from a single donor. For pooled samples, an equal volume of each donor's sample within each age group were combined and used as the inoculum. Various test compounds were added, and bioreactors were sealed individually in an anaerobic environment, then incubated for 24 h at 37 °C with continuous agitation (140 rpm) (MaxQ 6000, Thermo Scientific, Merelbeke, Belgium) [27,28]. In an initial preliminary experiment, the effects of three known products with prebiotic qualities, lactose, FOS, and 2′FL were screened for activity using rapid evaporation ionization mass spectrometry (REIMS) to identify which substrate produced the largest change in phenotype based on significant features identified (Figure S1). Administration with 2′FL produced the most changes, specifically to lipids and lipid-like molecules, and was therefore selected for continued use in the experiment. Based on these results, 2′FL was selected to determine the impact of age on prebiotic potential, which was evaluated using a combination of in-depth analyses as described below. For DNA sequencing, a 1 mL volume of culture was centrifuged at 5000× g for 10 min, and the pellet was used for DNA extraction. The supernatant was separated and used for metabolomics and SCFA analysis. For flow cytometry, culture was harvested and used directly.

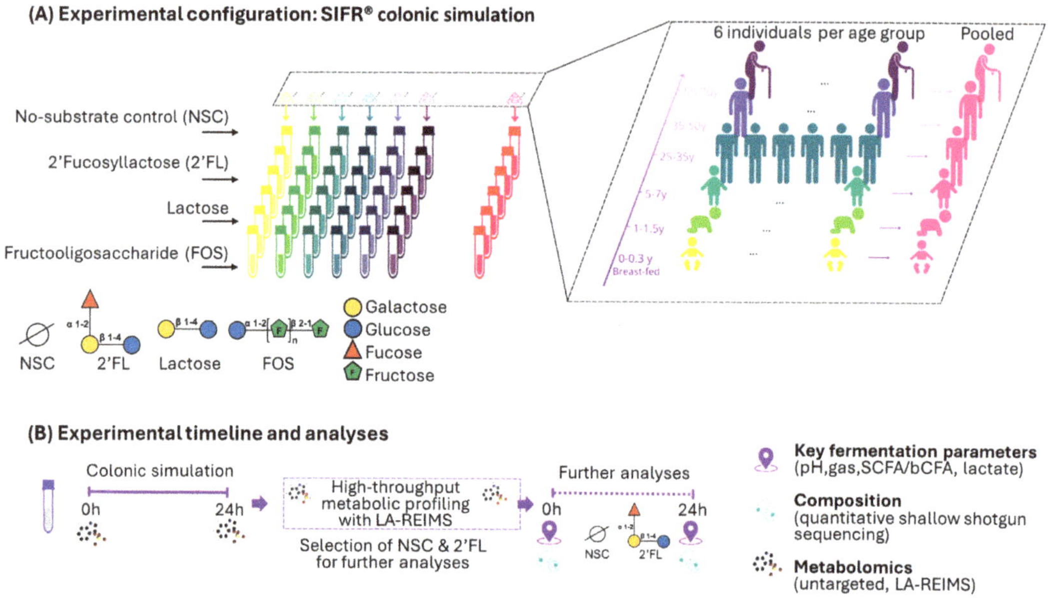

Figure 1. Schematic depicting the experimental design using the *Ex vivo* SIFR® technology to examine the impact of 2′FL (along with FOS and lactose) on the gut microbiota of six different age groups, ranging from BF infants over toddlers and children up to three adult groups (25–35, 35–50, 50–70) compared to an unsupplemented parallel control (NSC). For each age group, incubations were conducted for six individual microbiomes, along with an incubation with a single pooled sample of the six microbiomes. SIFR = Systemic Intestinal Fermentation Research; 2′FL = 2′Fucosyllactose; FOS = fructo-oligosaccharides; NSC = no substrate control; SCFA = short-chain fatty acids; bCFA = branched chain fatty acids, LA = lactate; LA-REIMS = Laser-assisted rapid evaporative ionization mass spectrometry.

DNA sequencing and analysis: DNA was extracted via the SPINeasy DNA Kit for Soil (MP Biomedicals, Eschwege, Germany), according to the manufacturer's instructions. Subsequently, DNA libraries were prepared using the Nextera XT DNA Library Preparation Kit (Illumina, San Diego, CA, USA) and IDT Unique Dual Indexes with total DNA input of 1 ng [26]. Genomic DNA was fragmented using Illumina Nextera XT fragmentation enzyme, and indexes were added to each sample followed by 12 cycles of PCR to construct libraries [29]. DNA libraries were purified using AMpure magnetic Beads (Beckman Coulter, Brea, CA, USA), eluted in QIAGEN EB buffer, quantified using a Qubit 4 fluorometer and a Qubit dsDNA HS Assay Kit, and sequenced on an Illumina Nextseq 2000 platform 2 × 150 bp. Unassembled sequencing reads were converted to relative abundances (%) using the CosmosID-HUB Microbiome Platform (CosmosID Inc., Germantown, MD, USA;

accessed on 16 February 2022). This platform was also used to calculate the Chao1, Shannon, and reciprocal Simpson diversity index.

Bioinformatical analysis and statistics: All univariate and multivariate analyses were performed using R (version 4.2.2; www.r-project.org; accessed on 13 May 2024). This software was used to make a series of violin plots and heat maps. While violin plots present the actual values, heat maps present log_2-transformed fold changes for the different treatments compared to the parallel control arm (NSC). For the principal component (PCA) analysis, the FactoMineR package was used [30]. Regularized Canonical Correlation Analysis (rCCA) was executed using the mixOmics package with the shrinkage method for estimation of penalization parameters (version 6.20.3) [31]. Significance of supplementation effects compared to parallel un-supplemented controls were assessed via repeated measures ANOVA analyses, with p-value correction according to Benjamini–Hochberg [32]. For the analysis of microbial composition, three measures were taken. First, the aforementioned statistical analysis was performed on log_{10}-transformed values. Second, a value of a given taxonomic group below the limit of detection (LOD) was considered equal to the overall LOD. Finally, a threshold was set to retain the 100 most abundant species in the analysis.

SCFA quantification and environmental parameters: SCFAs (acetate, propionate, butyrate, and valerate) and branched-chain fatty acids (bCFA; sum of isobutyrate, isocaproate, and isovalerate) were determined using a Trace 1300 chromato-graph (Thermo Fisher Scientific, Merelbeke, Belgium) equipped with a Stabilwax-DA capillary GC column, a flame ionization detector, and a split injector using nitrogen gas as the carrier, as previously described [25,29]. Environmental pH was measured using an electrode (Hannah Instruments Edge HI2002, Temse, Belgium) [25,26]. Gas was measured at the beginning and end of the experiment [29]. Lactate was quantified using an enzymatic method (EnzytecTM, R-Biopharm, Darmstadt, Germany). To determine total bacteria counts, samples were diluted in anaerobic phosphate-buffered saline (PBS), followed by cell staining with SYTO 16 at a final concentration of 1 μM, and counted via a BD FACS Verse flow cytometer (BD, Erembodegem, Belgium) [25,29]. Data were analyzed using FlowJo, version 10.8.1. Quantitative insights were obtained by correcting proportions (%; 16S rRNA gene profiling) with total counts (cells/mL; flow cytometry), resulting in estimated cells/mL of different taxa.

Rapid evaporation ionization mass spectrometry (REIMS) methodology: The analytical platform used was a modification of that previously reported [33] with a carbon dioxide laser (A.R.C., Nürnberg, Germany) used for sample heating and evaporation and an XYZ gantry robot (igus, Northampton, UK) used for automated movement of the laser focusing lens piece. The CO_2 focusing lens was moved to ≈2 mm above the sample pellet within the well of a 96-well plate (Greiner Bio-One, Frickenhausen, Germany). The pellet was produced through centrifugation of 200 μL of sample for 10 m at 4000× g in a refrigerated (4 °C) chamber and supernatant removed. Each plate was analyzed in a column-by-column pattern with sample heating occurring for approximately 5 s, followed by 10 s to allow washout of the evacuation tubing. The CO_2 laser was set at 2 W and 20 Hz pulsatile operation. The analyte-containing smoke produced through sample heating was aspirated through PTFE tubing with a 1.5 mm internal diameter. This was linked to the CO_2 focusing lens through a 3D resin-printed capture head that channels the Xevo G2-XS QToF (Waters, Wilmslow, UK) mass spectrometer's native vacuum for smoke evacuation. The PTFE tubing was linked to a stainless-steel T-piece that allowed mixing of the analyte-containing smoke with 2-propanol solvent containing leucine enkephalin at a concentration of 0.1 ng/μL introduced at a flow rate of 250 μL/m using an Acquity I-Class Plus binary solvent manager (Waters, Milford, MA, USA). The combined mixture entered the REIMS interface (Waters, Wilmslow, UK), where it was heated to approximately 700 °C via collision with a Kanthal ribbon surface to remove the 2-propanol solvent prior to entry into the ion guide of the mass spectrometer. Mass spectra were acquired over a 50 to 1200 m/z range at a scan rate of two scans per second in negative ion detection mode.

REIMS Statistical Analysis: Acquired mass spectra were imported into Abstract Model Builder software (Version 1.0.1966.0, Waters, Budapest, Hungary), where it underwent lockmass correction, background subtraction, and peak binning to 0.1 Da-width bins. Data was exported as a comma-separated value file and processed within the R environment (Version 4.2.1) in R Studio (Version 2023.03.0+386). Any features which had a significant ($p < 0.05$) correlation value of more than 0.9 through Spearman correlation against the leucine enkephalin signal at bin 554.25 were removed from further analysis. MetaboAnalyst 5.0 [34] was used for univariate (ANOVA) and multivariate (PCA) analysis after data was subjected to total ion count normalization, Log_{10} transformation, and Pareto scaling. GraphPad Prism (Version 9.5.1.733) and Microsoft Excel 365 were used for creation of summary figures. Significant REIMS features identified through analysis were tentatively identified against the Human Metabolome Database (downloaded 25 April 2022) using an in-house R script with an accuracy threshold of less than 10 ppm, and with no preferential adduct selection. Correlation between OTU and REIMS features was conducted in the R environment, as above, using Spearman correlation with a significant threshold of less than 0.05, after Bonferroni correction, and R threshold of less than −0.5 or more than 0.5.

3. Results

3.1. Age Drives Divergence in Community Structure

Shotgun sequencing revealed that each subject used for this study produced a unique gut microbiome and that the communities clustered together according to age group (Figure 2A). The largest difference was observed between the BF infant age group and all others, represented by large separation along PC1 (23.4%). Both the BF infant and toddler groups were significantly distinct from all other age groups, whereas children and older were more similar in composition (Table S2). Nevertheless, LefSe analysis identified core taxa that were significantly enriched in each of the six age groups tested, indicating that a core microbiome could be identified for each age group (Table S3).

The strongest age-dependent difference in microbiota composition was the decrease in *Bifidobacteriaceae* as age increased (Figure 2B). In four of six BF infants, the microbiota was almost completely comprised of *Bifidobacterium* species (Figure 2C), but levels of *Bifidobacterium* decreased to <40% of the community for subjects in the toddler group and were further reduced to <10% for children and adults (Figure 2B). Not only did the prevalence of *Bifidobacterium* decrease with age, but the species that dominated the communities were highly age-dependent (Figure 2C,D). For the BF infant group, the most dominant species were *B. longum* followed by *B. breve* and *B. bifidum*. This changed markedly by 1–1.5 years of age; for toddlers and to lesser extent also for children, *B. catenulatum* and *B. pseudocatenulatum* were most prevalent. Finally, for all three adult groups *B. adolescentis* was the dominant *Bifidobacterium* species.

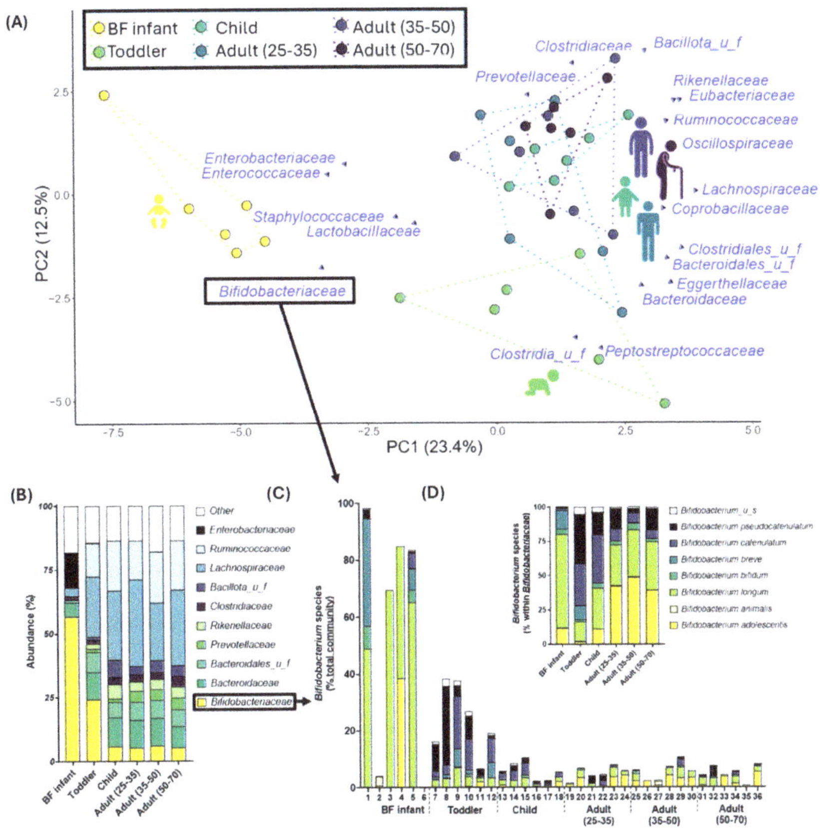

Figure 2. The gut microbiota was divergent across multiple age groups. (**A**) Principal Components Analysis (PCA) depicting the community structure for each test subject in relation to one another, with the 20 most dominant families being highlighted; (**B**) Abundance (%) of 10 most abundant families, averaged per age group (n = 6); (**C**) Absolute abundance of *Bifidobacterium* for each subject tested; (**D**) Relative abundance for each *Bifidobacterium* species (normalized compared to total *Bifidobacterium* levels), averaged per age group (n = 6).

3.2. Age-Related Differences in Community Structure Drove the Response to 2′FL Supplementation, Exemplified by Age-Dependent Bifidogenic Effect

2′FL elicited changes to the gut microbiome structure, with a significant increase in levels of Actinomycetota (synonym Actinobacteria) for all age groups (Figure 3A). The corresponding increase in cell density for 2′FL-treated communities compared to the no substrate control (NSC) indicated its use as carbon source able to support cellular growth (Figure 3A). At the family level, the increase in Actinomycetota was shown to be due to an increase in *Bifidobacteriaceae* for all age groups. This achieved statistical significance for the toddler and older age groups and corresponded with a decrease in families such as *Peptostreptococcaceae*, Clostridiales_u_f, and to a lesser extent *Clostridiaceae*, and *Oscillospiraceae* (Figure 3B). At the species level, more detailed insights were obtained. First, the response to 2′FL treatment was largely age-dependent (Figure 3C). Interestingly, the divergence between the NSC and 2′FL communities was driven by age-dependent *Bifidobacterium* species: *B. breve/longum* mostly increased for BF infants (positioning downwards), *B. catenulatum/pseudocatenulatum* mostly increased for toddlers/children (positioning to right bottom), and *B. adolescentis* mostly increased for adults. These results demonstrated that 2′FL exerted bifidogenic effects that were dependent on subject age. In other words, age was a determining factor in which *Bifidobacterium* were present in the community and, thus, directly influenced which *Bifidobacterium* species responded to 2′FL administration. Beyond *Bifidobacterium*, analysis at the species level also indicated that several commensal species were enhanced by 2′FL, particularly for the adult microbiota including, amongst others, *Phocaeicola dorei*, *Phocaeicola vulgatus*, *Anaerobutyricum hallii*, and *Mediterraneibacter faecis*. The statistical significance of specific findings are provided in Figures S2 and S3.

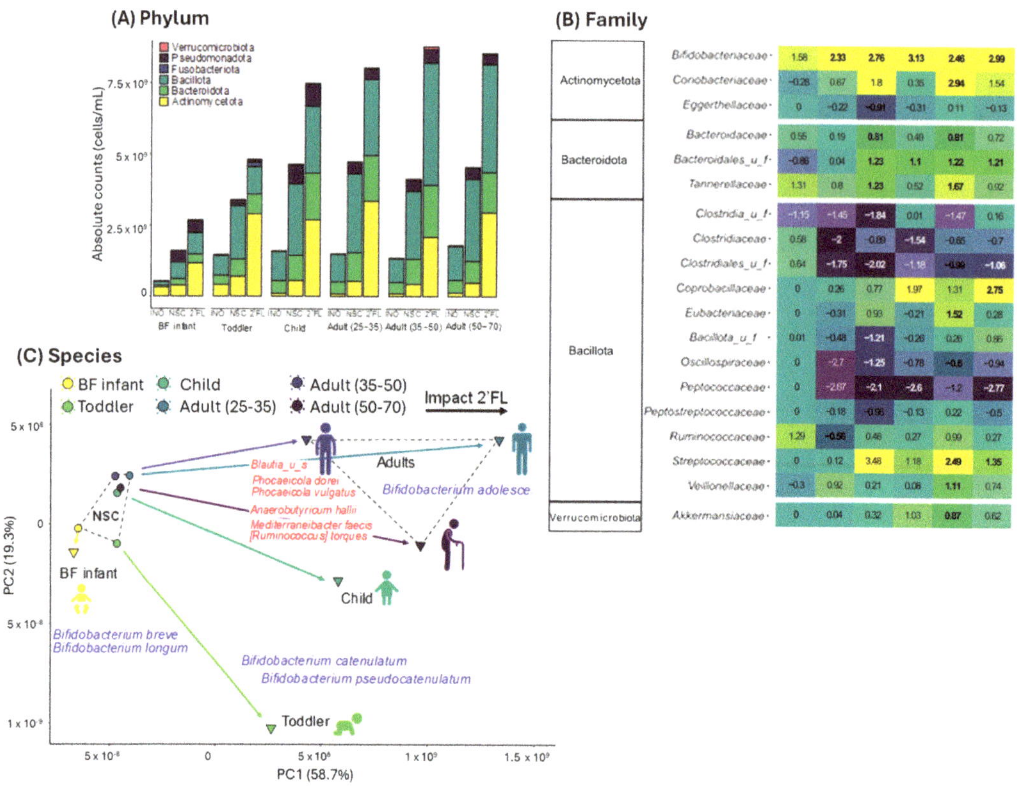

Figure 3. Treatment with 2′FL elicited structural changes to the gut microbiota, with an age-dependent effect on *Bifidobacterium* species. (**A**) Absolute levels at the phylum level for the original fecal sample at 0 h (INO) along with the untreated (NSC) and 2′FL treated communities at 24 h; (**B**) Heat map showing $\log_2$ fold change at the family level following 24 h of treatment with 2′FL. Significant differences are indicated by bold (FDR < 0.10); (**C**) PCA biplot based on centered values of microbial species (cells/mL). Bifidobacterium species are indicated in blue while other commensals are in red.

3.3. *Pooled Communities Only Provided Indicative Insights into the Response of the Gut Microbiota*

An additional research question was to assess the effect of combining microbiomes from multiple subjects to a single pooled microbiome. After creating a pooled sample per age group, this was treated with 2′FL and the results were compared to the findings of the six individual microbiomes to determine whether or not they would produce similar results. In terms of bacterial load determined by flow cytometry, the pooled communities grew to a density similar to the averaged communities for the BF infants and toddler groups (Figure 4A). However, for the child and older groups, the pooled communities were substantially lower in density than the averaged communities.

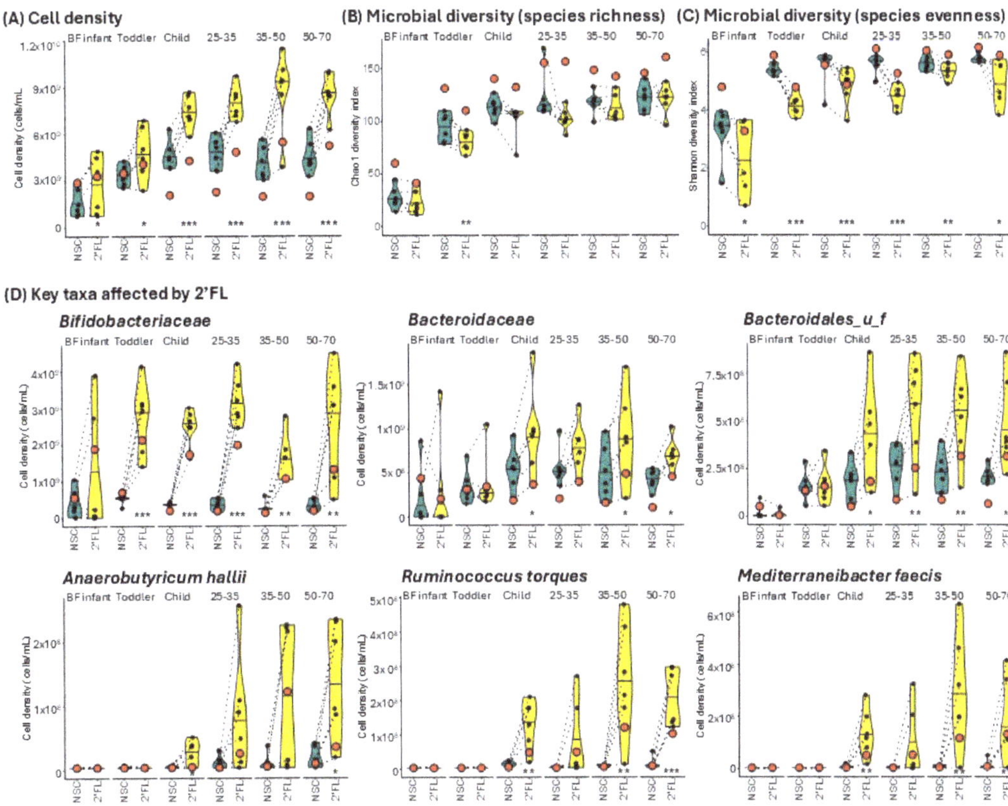

Figure 4. Pooled fecal communities provided indicative insights into the response of the gut microbiota to 2′FL treatment. (**A**) Cell density quantified by flow cytometry; Microbial diversity based on the (**B**) Chao1 diversity index; and (**C**) Shannon index; (**D**) Abundance of key microbial families and species affected by 2′FL treatment. Statistical significance was determined using repeated measures ANOVA with FDR correction. Adjusted p-values are indicated as follows: $p < 0.1$ *, $p < 0.05$ **, $p < 0.01$ ***. Pooled communities shown as a red dot. Headings 25–35, 35–50, and 50–70 are used to indicate the age groups Adults (25–35), Adults (35–50), and Adults (50–70), respectively.

In terms of microbial diversity, both species richness, determined by the Chao1 diversity index (Figure 4B), and community evenness, represented here using the Shannon's diversity index (Figure 4C), were artificially high for the pooled samples. When looking at taxa that were most affected by 2′FL, the results of the pooled sample provided only indicative insights (Figure 4D). With some exceptions, the direction of the response for the pooled microbiome was generally in line with the response across the six individual donors. However, the pooled sample did not recapitulate the interpersonal differences in treatment response. For instance, for BF infants, only two out of six subjects responded with a bifidogenic effect to 2′FL treatment. Based on the result of the pooled sample, such insight in responders and non-responders was not provided as the pooled sample only revealed a marked bifidogenic effect for BF infants (likely due to the presence of 2′FL-fermenting *Bifidobacterium* species of the two responders). Overall, results with the pooled microbiota sample were thus rather indicative.

3.4. 2′FL Treatment Altered Metabolic Output and Community Phenotype in a Manner Irrespective of Age, Which Was Poorly Recapitulated by Pooled Communities

To assess the effect of age on functional changes driven by the addition of 2′FL, metabolic output for each community was assessed through monitoring of the fermentation parameters- environmental pH and gas production, and quantification of short chain fatty acid (SCFA) and lactate production (Figure 5). 2′FL markedly decreased pH, most likely due to the increase in total SCFAs, and increased gas production, which achieved statistical significance for all age groups (Figure 5A–C). For toddlers and older, elevated total SCFAs was driven by increased acetate production, which is a known metabolic byproduct of *Bifidobacterium*, and propionate (Figure 5D,E) [35,36]. There were no statistically significant changes observed in butyrate, valerate, or branched SCFAS (BCFA) for any age group (Figure 5F–H). For infants this was due to a lack of production, but for toddlers and older this was due to large variability between subjects. In all age groups, following both the NSC and 2′FL treatment, the pooled communities aligned closely with a single donor in each age group, suggesting that the pooled community adopted characteristics of a single donor and was not representative of the average response (Figure S4). Together, the results demonstrated that pooled communities may have been able to fairly represent a community under control conditions, but they were unable to accurately portray a pattern of response to a stimulus, shown here using 2′FL as an example, and could be described as metabolic outliers.

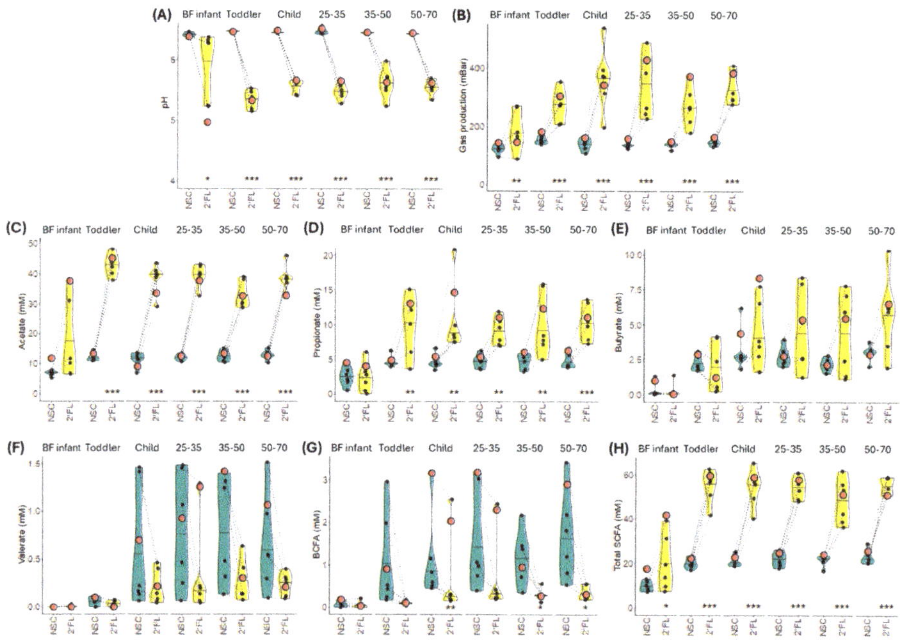

Figure 5. 2′FL treatment altered metabolic output and community phenotype in a manner irrespective of age, which was poorly recapitulated by pooled communities. Metabolic output in terms of (**A**) environmental pH, (**B**) gas production, (**C**) acetate, (**D**) propionate, (**E**) butyrate, (**F**) valerate, (**G**) BCFAs, and (**H**) total SCFAs. Statistical significance was determined using repeated measures ANOVA with FDR correction. Adjusted *p*-values are indicated as follows: $p < 0.1$ *, $p < 0.05$ **, $p < 0.01$ ***. Pooled communities are shown as a red dot. Headings 25–35, 35–50, and 50–70 are used to indicate the age groups Adults (25–35), Adults (35–50), and Adults (50–70), respectively.

3.5. Associations Between Structure and Metabolic Output Were Highly Age-Dependent

A correlation analysis was performed between metagenomic data and metabolic output in order to shed light on which taxa may be associated with production of the predominant SCFAs (Figure 6). Interestingly, for all age groups, *Bifidobacterium* species correlated positively to acetate production. Except for BF infants, *B. adolescentis* correlated positively with acetate, propionate, and butyrate, although to varying degrees. Looking at propionate and butyrate, which are not end products of 2′FL metabolism but were considered to have increased through cross-feeding interactions, the taxa correlated to these metabolites were highly age-dependent. Notably, for adults (25–35 y) and adults (35–50 y) there was a strong positive correlation between butyrate and *Anaerobutyricum hallii*. This correlation was also observed for adults (50–70 y), but to a lesser extent. This supported previous findings that metabolic byproducts released by *Bifidobacterium* in response to 2′FL administration are used by *A. hallii* to produce butyrate [37]. This observation was limited to the more mature microbial communities, as the child group had the same trend of increase for both of these taxa as well, but to a lesser extent. This indicated that age-specific cross feeding reactions were occurring.

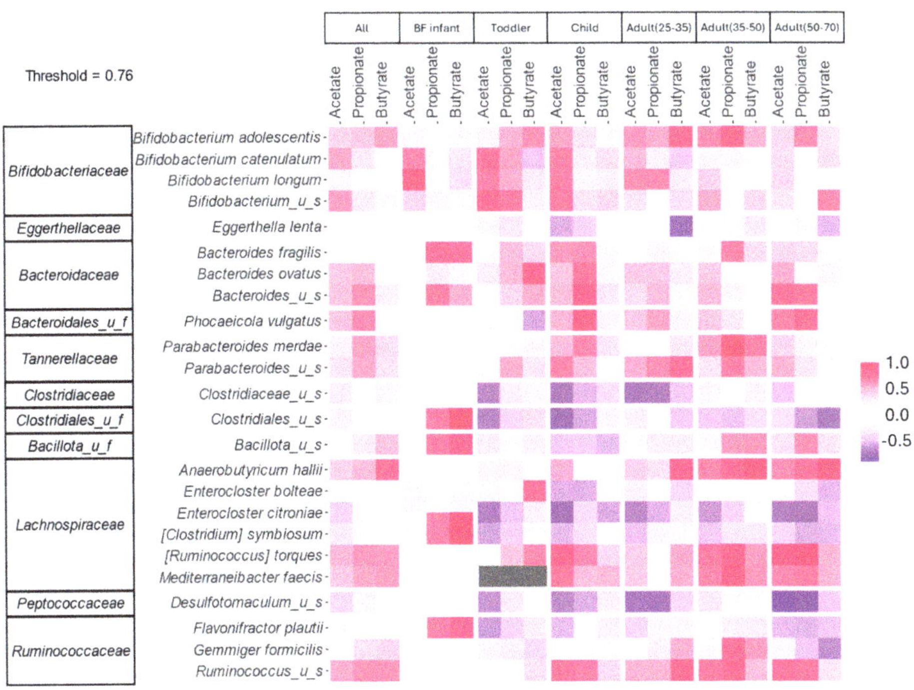

Figure 6. Correlation between structure and function for each age group. Taxa were limited to less than 20 for consideration. Only categories with a correlation > 0.5 or <−0.5 are depicted.

3.6. Age-Dependent Structure-Function Correlations Were Detected Using REIMS Regardless of 2′FL Administration

To delineate the structure-function relationship for communities of different age groups, a Spearman's correlation was conducted between taxonomic data and REIMS features. For this analysis, NSC and 2′FL treated communities within each age group were combined to increase statistical power. Both positive and negative correlations were identified, but there were more negative correlations observed for all age groups, with the largest number found within the BF infant group and smallest within the Adults

(35–50 y) group (Figure 7A). The number of correlations unique to a specific age group were calculated and displayed as a Venn diagram, which highlighted that there were a number of significant correlations that were age-dependent, and a number of correlations that were shared (Figure 7B). To provide further resolution, the chemical taxonomies for each correlating feature specific to an age group were identified at the superclass level and portrayed as heat maps presenting the absolute values and ratios (Figure 7C). Based on this data, lipids and lipid-like molecules were by far the most prevalent feature for all age groups, most likely due to their increase following 2′FL administration (Figure S1), but other chemical super classes that contributed to age-distinction were benzenoids, organic acid derivatives, organic oxygen compounds, organoheteroyclic compounds, and phenylpropanoids and polyketides. Together, this data demonstrated that the communities developed phenotypes unique to their respective age groups.

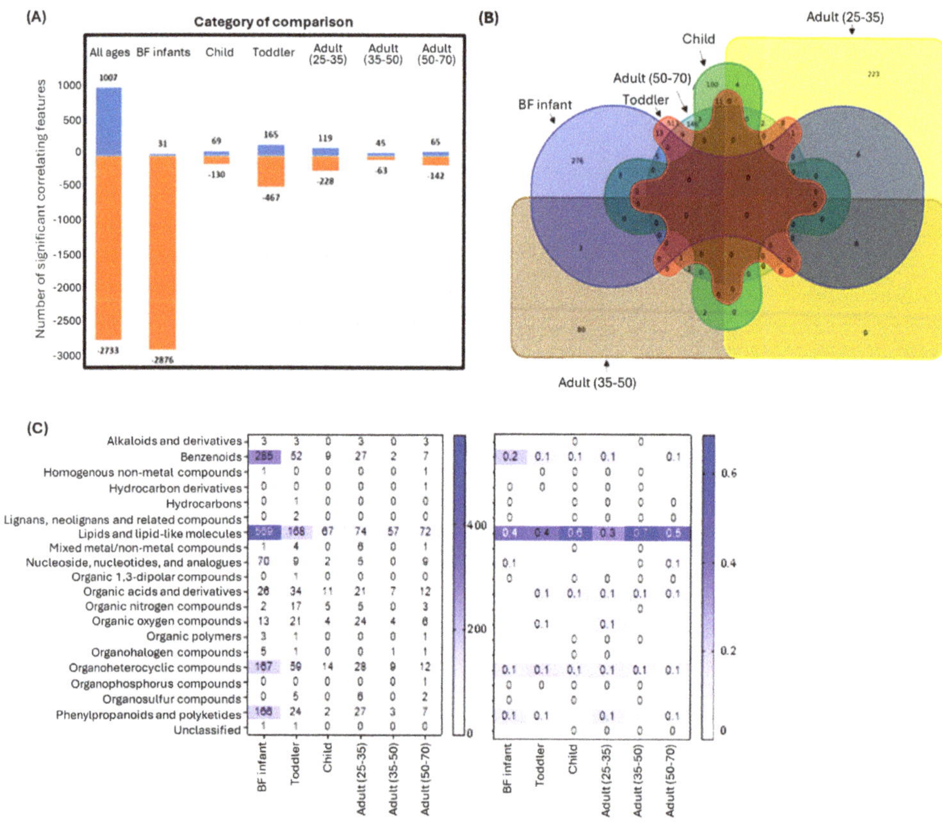

Figure 7. Spearman's correlations between taxonomic structure and REIMS features. Significant correlations were considered as $p < 0.05$ after Bonferroni correction and R value above 0.5 or below −0.5. (**A**) Bar plot depicting significant correlations observed with positive correlations in blue and negative correlations in orange; (**B**) Venn diagram depicting the number of unique correlations between OTU and REIMS features; (**C**) Heat maps showing chemical taxonomies of the different correlations at the superclass level. Left: absolute numbers. Right: proportional within each experimental class.

4. Discussion

It is well-recognized that the gut microbiome evolves in concert with its host over a lifetime, driven by changing conditions that alter the intestinal environment, i.e., diet, and/or epigenetic changes that occur due to cellular senescence [7,38–40]. Yet reports addressing age and the gut microbiota tend to highlight either early childhood, infants and BF infants, or elderly adults developing frailty. To provide much-needed clarification on how the gut microbiota is altered due to the aging process, in this study, comparative evaluation combining both metagenomics and metabolomics was performed on communities cultured from subjects spanning 0–70 years of age, divided into six distinct age groups, BF infants (0–0.3 y), toddlers (1–1.5 y), children (5–7 y), and adults belonging to three age ranges (25–35 y, 35–50 y, and 50–70 y). These communities were then treated with 2′FL to determine how the age-related changes to the gut microbiota translated to its ability to respond to therapeutic treatment. This was accomplished using an *Ex vivo* strategy (SIFR® technology), which has been previously validated and found to provide results that are predictive of clinical outcomes [24,25].

When looking simply at community structure, the largest shift related to age was observed between BF infants and all others, which was driven by the reduction in *Bifidobacteriaceae* corresponding with an increase in taxa associated with the mature gut microbiota, i.e., members of Bacillota and Bacteroidota (Figure 1A) [41]. Although distinct from the BF infant group, the toddler group remained mostly separate from the other groups, whereas the child and older age groups were structurally similar and more closely clustered together. These observations confirmed previous reports that the gut microbiota reaches maturity following the first few years of life and, therefore, the toddler group (1–1.5 y) represented a transitory community between infancy and maturity [9,10,40]. Once the mature community was established, here this refers to the child group (5–7 y), age-driven shifts were comparably more minimal. This pattern of progression was also observed when looking at community phenotype, profiled by combining metagenomic and REIMS data to identify correlating features between the community structure and function (Figure 6). In this analysis, the toddler group had the most age-specific correlations and the most shared correlations, pointing towards the toddler age group as transitionary between the BF infant and mature communities (child and older age groups). Although structurally the differences between the child and older groups were less apparent, phenotypically there were a number of structure-function correlations that changed with age even once the community was mature, providing further evidence towards the development of specific age-related features.

Exemplifying the changes to the gut microbiota that correspond with age, there was an identified successive switch in prevalent species of *Bifidobacterium* and their overall abundance in the communities, similar to what has been reported previously [42,43]. Here, the transition from BF infants to the child and older groups was marked by a stepped decrease in the abundance of *Bifidobacterium*, which was considered most likely due to the introduction of foods during weaning [40,44]. Levels of *Bifidobacterium* were further reduced between the toddler group and older groups, with the dominant species of *Bifidobacterium* converting from those able to utilize human milk components (*B. longum*, *B. bifidum*) in the BF infants to those preferentially metabolizing complex carbohydrates (*B. adolescentis*) in the adult groups [15,18]. It was considered likely that the changes to the gut microbiota structure corresponding with age were directly related to diet, as the types and amount of food consumed changes with age and is known to play a major role in shaping the gut microbiota [13,38]. The observed switch in *Bifidobacterium* supported this supposition, although it is not possible to know how much of an influence diet has on age-related changes to the gut microbiome from this data set.

The divergence in community structure between age groups was further realized upon treatment with the prebiotic 2′FL, an HMO with known prebiotic properties and a well-established bifidogenic effect [22,45,46]. Here, 2′FL was administered to provoke a measurable reaction that was used to identify how the age-related changes to the gut microbiome influenced the response of the communities to a stimulus. Here, the addition of 2′FL statistically increased levels of *Bifidobacteriaceae* for all age groups, except for the BF infants (Figure 2B,C). It was hypothesized that the increase in *Bifidobacteriaceae* for the infant group failed to reach significance due to large interpersonal differences that obscured the statistical results and because the communities within this age group were already predominantly *Bifidobacterium* (four of six subjects), and these subjects were already consuming HMOs in their diet.

Notably, the results here found that the species of *Bifidobacterium* that responded to 2′FL was highly age dependent and seemed to be a primary factor driving divergence of the age-specific communities. It was considered that this observation was most likely due to the changes in the species of *Bifidobacterium* present, and their abundance, that occurred with age, and not necessarily due to selection by 2′FL. For BF infants, *B. breve* was the most affected, which was logical as *B. breve* is typically associated with the infant gut and not the adult gut [42]. For toddlers and older, the species of *Bifidobacterium* that responded to the highest degrees were *B. catenulatum*, *pseudocatenulatum*, and *adolescentis*, although only the increase in *B. adolescentis* reached statistical significance for all of these age groups. It is impossible to know from this study whether or not these species were enhanced due to their direct metabolism of 2′FL or through cross-feeding interactions. There are strains of *B. pseudocatenulatum* and *catenulatum* able to metabolize fucosyllated HMOs to varying degrees [47–50]; yet *B. adolescentis* is primarily associated with metabolism of plant-based carbohydrates and considered unlikely to metabolize HMOs or other human-derived glycans, indicating that the increase to this taxon may be due to cross-feeding or other interactions [51,52].

Although the largest effect on community structure was the increase in *Bifidobacteriaceae*, treatment with 2′FL produced a number of other taxonomic shifts that drove the age-specific communities further away from one another when visualized by PCA (Figure 2B). It was considered that, similar to *B. adolescentis*, these were likely due to cross-feeding interactions as there have been previous reports of cross-feeding between *Bifidobacterium* and other butyrate producers such as *A. hallii* [19,53–56]. Expanding on this further, in this study, the taxa that were enhanced due to potential cross-feeding were age-dependent, a unique and important finding. This was apparent in the heat map showing the taxonomic changes that occurred following the addition of 2′FL (Figure 3B) but was also confirmed using correlative analysis (Figure 5A). Highlighting this finding was the identified correlation between *B. adolescentis*, *A. hallii*, and butyrate. This correlative network is similar to what has been previously proposed, that metabolic byproducts released by *Bifidobacterium* (for example, lactate) are used by *A. hallii* with the end production of butyrate, either directly or through a more complex interaction [55,57]. This correlation was only found in the adult age groups even though both *B. adolescentis* and *A. hallii* were also present in the child group, albeit at a lower abundance than the adults. Yet for the child group *B. adolescentis* and *A. hallii* were not correlated to butyrate levels. In this case, here, the identified correlation between *B. adolescentis*, *A. hallii*, and butyrate was age specific. This is quite important when considering a prebiotic treatment as it is difficult to elucidate exactly how the prebiotic will be metabolized and how this will influence the resident members of the community. Where administration of a prebiotic to selectively enhance levels of a specific taxa, or subset of taxa, could be categorized as a targeted therapeutic approach, the cross-feeding reactions that occur as a byproduct are not targeted and can be highly variable depending on community composition, and here this was shown to be dependent on age.

In terms of metabolic output, the observed increase in SCFAs following 2′FL administration in this study was expected and aligns with results from previously published reports [56,58]. The only difference in SCFA release observed here was between the BF infants, which did not have any statistical differences in SCFAs following 2′FL treatment, and all other communities, which had a large increase in levels of total SCFAs following 2′FL treatment (Figure 4B). In fact, it was notable that the toddler and older age groups produced very similar patterns of SCFA release under NSC conditions and responded to 2′FL treatment with a strong increase in acetate, which indicated that this response was not affected by the age of the subjects. In this case, the differences observed in community structure did not affect SCFA production. The increase in acetate was considered most likely due to the metabolism of 2′FL by *Bifidobacterium* itself, which releases acetate and lactate following metabolism of hexoses via the bifid shunt [59,60]. On the other hand, changes to levels of propionate and butyrate in response to 2′FL were highly variable between subjects. Since propionate and butyrate are not identified end products of 2′FL metabolism, it was assumed that any changes to their concentration were due to cross-feeding between community members, which was discussed in the paragraph above.

To provide a more dimensional view of metabolic function, SCFA quantification was complemented with REIMS analysis, which provided data on the full complement of metabolites released. When looking at the metabolic profiles determined by REIMS (Figure 4C), age-specific patterns were detectable when visualized by PCA under NSC conditions. This indicated that while the pattern of SCFA release was similar for toddlers and older, there were other metabolites produced that drove age-specific separation between these communities. Yet the addition of 2′FL caused these metabolic profiles to converge, with less distinct separation between age groups. This indicated that the metabolites produced by 2′FL metabolism were not all necessarily age-dependent. Together these results indicated that subject age affected the overall structure of the gut microbiota, which in turn affected which taxa were enhanced due to 2′FL administration, yet the metabolic fate of 2′FL itself was similar across the multiple age groups. This was considered logical as the metabolic breakdown of 2′FL would not necessarily differ among communities, but the taxa that perform the metabolism and those affected by the released byproducts would be dependent on community composition.

Although not the primary subject of this study, the relevance of data generated from pooling gut microbiome communities was evaluated as this is a common strategy employed for microbiome testing [61,62]. Pooling, or combining samples from multiple donors together to create a single inoculum (N = 1), is beneficial as it increases diversity of microbes tested without having to increase the number of individual replicates required. Contrary to previous findings that pooled communities produced results similar to those of single donors [63], the results here found that pooled communities did not effectively recapitulate the average response (Figures 3 and 4). While pooling did enrich the communities, which aligned with previous findings, here, pooling altered the structural changes that occurred due to 2′FL administration [63]. Furthermore, without the interindividual variation that occurs when comparing the response of the communities to treatment, statistical analysis was limited. Metabolically, the pooled communities seemed to take on the characteristics of a single subject (Figure 4), which was most apparent in the metabolic profiles determined using REIMS, where the pooled communities converged together following 2′FL treatment (Figure 4C). Together, this leads to the conclusion that pooled communities were not able to provide valuable information on the response to stimuli that may be variable among subjects.

5. Conclusions

In conclusion, the metagenomic results here indicated that subject age affected the community structure of the microbiome, and this translated into an age-dependent response of the communities to 2′FL treatment. In other words, the age of the subject was a driving factor in the community's response to 2′FL in terms of structure and which taxa were affected through cross-feeding interactions. In terms of community phenotype of metabolic profiles, there were age-specific distinctions that were detected. However, the metabolic fate of 2′FL was similar between the toddler and older age groups. The results confirmed age as a key determinant of the gut microbiome, which is an important finding because it demonstrates that age should be considered when studying therapeutic treatments, such as prebiotics/probiotics, or functional foods, or when considering an approach to modify the gut microbiome using precision medicine.

Supplementary Materials: The following supporting information can be downloaded at: https://www.mdpi.com/article/10.3390/nu17010151/s1, Table S1: Subject information; Figure S1: Selection of 2′FL; Table S2: Beta-diversity analysis indices: Table S3: Lefse analysis: Figure S2: Heatmap depicting structural changes directed by 2′FL; Figure S3: Age-dependent changes to *Bifidobacterium*; Figure S4: Functional PCA analysis.

Author Contributions: J.F., K.K.M., L.L., and P.V.d.A. designed the experiment. P.V.d.A., S.D., J.P., M.J., and A.B. performed the culturing experiment and functional analyses. S.J.S.C. performed REIMS analysis. J.F. and P.V.d.A. compiled the data and wrote the manuscript. J.F., K.K.M., L.L., P.V.d.A., S.D., J.P., M.J., A.B., and S.J.S.C. edited the manuscript. All authors have read and agreed to the published version of the manuscript.

Funding: This work was supported by the in-house Project 8072-41000-102-00D, "in vitro Human Intestinal Microbial Ecosystem: Effects of Diet".

Institutional Review Board Statement: Fresh feces were collected according to a procedure approved by the Ethics Committee of the University Hospital Ghent (reference number BC-09977; date 13 April 2021) that required a signed in-formed consent. For underage participants, the responsible adult provided consent.

Informed Consent Statement: Consent to participate was obtained from all subjects prior to collection of fecal samples.

Data Availability Statement: Data has been deposited in the NCBI SRA archives with Bioproject number PRJNA1177813.

Conflicts of Interest: The authors declare that the research was conducted in the absence of any commercial or financial relationships that could be construed as a potential conflict of interest.

References

1. Liu, Y.; Wang, J.; Wu, C. Modulation of Gut Microbiota and Immune System by Probiotics, Pre-biotics, and Post-biotics. *Front. Nutr.* **2021**, *8*, 634897. [CrossRef] [PubMed]
2. Holscher, H.D. Dietary fiber and prebiotics and the gastrointestinal microbiota. *Gut Microbes* **2017**, *8*, 172–184. [CrossRef] [PubMed]
3. Murga-Garrido, S.M.; Hong, Q.; Cross, T.W.L.; Hutchison, E.R.; Han, J.; Thomas, S.P.; Vivas, E.I.; Denu, J.; Ceschin, D.G.; Tang, Z.Z.; et al. Gut microbiome variation modulates the effects of dietary fiber on host metabolism. *Microbiome* **2021**, *9*, 117. [CrossRef]
4. Kok, C.R.; Rose, D.; Hutkins, R. Predicting Personalized Responses to Dietary Fiber Interventions: Opportunities for Modulation of the Gut Microbiome to Improve Health. *Annu. Rev. Food Sci. Technol.* **2022**, *14*, 157–182. [CrossRef]
5. Olsson, L.M.; Boulund, F.; Nilsson, S.; Khan, M.T.; Gummesson, A.; Fagerberg, L.; Engstrand, L.; Perkins, R.; Uhlen, M.; Bergström, G.; et al. Dynamics of the normal gut microbiota: A longitudinal one-year population study in Sweden. *Cell Host Microbe* **2022**, *30*, 726–739.e3. [CrossRef]
6. Buford, T.W. (Dis)Trust your gut: The gut microbiome in age-related inflammation, health, and disease. *Microbiome* **2017**, *5*, 80. [CrossRef] [PubMed]

7. O'Toole, P.W.; Jeffery, I.B. Gut microbiota and aging. *Science* **2015**, *350*, 1214–1215. [CrossRef]
8. Coman, V.; Vodnar, D.C. Gut microbiota and old age: Modulating factors and interventions for healthy longevity. *Exp. Gerontol.* **2020**, *141*, 111095. [CrossRef]
9. Yatsunenko, T.; Rey, F.E.; Manary, M.J.; Trehan, I.; Dominguez-Bello, M.G.; Contreras, M.; Magris, M.; Hidalgo, G.; Baldassano, R.N.; Anokhin, A.P.; et al. Human gut microbiome viewed across age and geography. *Nature* **2012**, *486*, 222–227. [CrossRef] [PubMed]
10. Jandhyala, S.M.; Talukdar, R.; Subramanyam, C.; Vuyyuru, H.; Sasikala, M.; Nageshwar Reddy, D. Role of the normal gut microbiota. *World J. Gastroenterol.* **2015**, *21*, 8787–8803. [CrossRef] [PubMed]
11. Mariat, D.; Firmesse, O.; Levenez, F.; Guimaraes, V.; Sokol, H.; Dore, J.; Corthier, G.; Furet, J.P. The Firmicutes/Bacteroidetes ratio of the human microbiota changes with age. *BMC Microbiol.* **2009**, *9*, 123. [CrossRef] [PubMed]
12. Dong, C.; Guan, Q.; Xu, W.; Zhang, X.; Jin, B.; Yu, S.; Xu, X.; Xia, Y. Disentangling the age-related manner in the associations between gut microbiome and women's health: A multi-cohort microbiome study. *Gut Microbes* **2023**, *15*, 2290320. [CrossRef] [PubMed]
13. Salazar, N.; Arboleya, S.; Fernandez-Navarro, T.; de Los Reyes-Gavilan, C.G.; Gonzalez, S.; Gueimonde, M. Age-Associated Changes in Gut Microbiota and Dietary Components Related with the Immune System in Adulthood and Old Age: A Cross-Sectional Study. *Nutrients* **2019**, *11*, 1765. [CrossRef] [PubMed]
14. Gao, X.; Zhao, J.; Chen, W.; Zhai, Q. Food and drug design for gut microbiota-directed regulation: Current experimental landscape and future innovation. *Pharmacol. Res.* **2023**, *194*, 106867. [CrossRef]
15. Hidalgo-Cantabrana, C.; Delgado, S.; Ruiz, L.; Ruas-Madiedo, P.; Sanchez, B.; Margolles, A. Bifidobacteria and Their Health-Promoting Effects. *Microbiol. Spectr.* **2017**, *5*, 73–98. [CrossRef] [PubMed]
16. Shi, S.; Zhang, Q.; Sang, Y.; Ge, S.; Wang, Q.; Wang, R.; He, J. Probiotic Bifidobacterium longum BB68S Improves Cognitive Functions in Healthy Older Adults: A Randomized, Double-Blind, Placebo-Controlled Trial. *Nutrients* **2022**, *15*, 51. [CrossRef]
17. O'Neill, I.; Schofield, Z.; Hall, L.J. Exploring the role of the microbiota member Bifidobacterium in modulating immune-linked diseases. *Emerg. Top. Life Sci.* **2017**, *1*, 333–349. [CrossRef] [PubMed]
18. Lu, J.; Zhang, L.; Zhang, H.; Chen, Y.; Zhao, J.; Chen, W.; Lu, W.; Li, M. Population-level variation in gut bifidobacterial composition and association with geography, age, ethnicity, and staple food. *NPJ Biofilms Microbiomes* **2023**, *9*, 98. [CrossRef] [PubMed]
19. Iribarren, C.; Tornblom, H.; Aziz, I.; Magnusson, M.K.; Sundin, J.; Vigsnaes, L.K.; Amundsen, I.D.; McConnell, B.; Seitzberg, D.; Ohman, L.; et al. Human milk oligosaccharide supplementation in irritable bowel syndrome patients: A parallel, randomized, double-blind, placebo-controlled study. *Neurogastroenterol. Motil.* **2020**, *32*, e13920. [CrossRef] [PubMed]
20. Castanys-Munoz, E.; Martin, M.J.; Prieto, P.A. 2′-fucosyllactose: An abundant, genetically determined soluble glycan present in human milk. *Nutr. Rev.* **2013**, *71*, 773–789. [CrossRef] [PubMed]
21. Van den Abbeele, P.; Sprenger, N.; Ghyselinck, J.; Marsaux, B.; Marzorati, M.; Rochat, F. A Comparison of the In Vitro Effects of 2′Fucosyllactose and Lactose on the Composition and Activity of Gut Microbiota from Infants and Toddlers. *Nutrients* **2021**, *13*, 726. [CrossRef] [PubMed]
22. Vandenplas, Y.; Berger, B.; Carnielli, V.P.; Ksiazyk, J.; Lagström, H.; Sanchez Luna, M.; Migacheva, N.; Mosselmans, J.-M.; Picaud, J.-C.; Possner, M.; et al. Human Milk Oligosaccharides: 2′-Fucosyllactose (2′-FL) and Lacto-N-Neotetraose (LNnT) in Infant Formula. *Nutrients* **2018**, *10*, 1161. [CrossRef] [PubMed]
23. Ryan, J.J.; Monteagudo-Mera, A.; Contractor, N.; Gibson, G.R. Impact of 2′-Fucosyllactose on Gut Microbiota Composition in Adults with Chronic Gastrointestinal Conditions: Batch Culture Fermentation Model and Pilot Clinical Trial Findings. *Nutrients* **2021**, *13*, 938. [CrossRef] [PubMed]
24. Jackson, P.P.; Wijeyesekera, A.; Williams, C.M.; Theis, S.; van Harsselaar, J.; Rastall, R.A. Inulin-type fructans and 2′fucosyllactose alter both microbial composition and appear to alleviate stress-induced mood state in a working population compared to placebo (maltodextrin): The EFFICAD Trial, a randomized, controlled trial. *Am. J. Clin. Nutr.* **2023**, *118*, 938–955. [CrossRef]
25. Van den Abbeele, P.; Deyaert, S.; Thabuis, C.; Perreau, C.; Bajic, D.; Wintergerst, E.; Joossens, M.; Firrman, J.; Walsh, D.; Baudot, A. Bridging preclinical and clinical gut microbiota research using the ex vivo SIFR((R)) technology. *Front. Microbiol.* **2023**, *14*, 1131662. [CrossRef] [PubMed]
26. Van den Abbeele, P.; Kunkler, C.N.; Poppe, J.; Rose, A.; van Hengel, I.A.J.; Baudot, A.; Warner, C.D. Serum-Derived Bovine Immunoglobulin Promotes Barrier Integrity and Lowers Inflammation for 24 Human Adults Ex Vivo. *Nutrients* **2024**, *16*, 1585. [CrossRef] [PubMed]
27. Van den Abbeele, P.; Deyaert, S.; Albers, R.; Baudot, A.; Mercenier, A. Carrot RG-I Reduces Interindividual Differences between 24 Adults through Consistent Effects on Gut Microbiota Composition and Function Ex Vivo. *Nutrients* **2023**, *15*, 2090. [CrossRef] [PubMed]
28. Van den Abbeele, P.; Detzel, C.; Rose, A.; Deyaert, S.; Baudot, A.; Warner, C. Serum-Derived Bovine Immunoglobulin Stimulates SCFA Production by Specific Microbes in the Ex Vivo SIFR((R)) Technology. *Microorganisms* **2023**, *11*, 659. [CrossRef] [PubMed]

29. Firrman, J.; Narrowe, A.; Liu, L.; Mahalak, K.; Lemons, J.; Van den Abbeele, P.; Baudot, A.; Deyaert, S.; Li, Y.; Yao, Y.; et al. Tomato seed extract promotes health of the gut microbiota and demonstrates a potential new way to valorize tomato waste. *PLoS ONE* **2024**, *19*, e0301381. [CrossRef] [PubMed]
30. Lê, S.; Josse, J.; Husson, F. FactoMineR: An R Package for Multivariate Analysis. *J. Stat. Softw.* **2008**, *25*, 1–18. [CrossRef]
31. Welham, Z.; Dejean, S.; Le Cao, K.A. Multivariate Analysis with the R Package mixOmics. *Methods Mol. Biol.* **2023**, *2426*, 333–359. [CrossRef] [PubMed]
32. Green, G.H.; Diggle, P.J. On the operational characteristics of the Benjamini and Hochberg False Discovery Rate procedure. *Stat. Appl. Genet. Mol. Biol.* **2007**, *6*, 27. [CrossRef] [PubMed]
33. Cameron, S.J.; Perdones-Montero, A.; Van Meulebroek, L.; Burke, A.; Alexander-Hardiman, K.; Simon, D.; Schaffer, R.; Balog, J.; Karancsi, T.; Rickards, T.; et al. Sample Preparation Free Mass Spectrometry Using Laser-Assisted Rapid Evaporative Ionization Mass Spectrometry: Applications to Microbiology, Metabolic Biofluid Phenotyping, and Food Authenticity. *J. Am. Soc. Mass Spectrom.* **2021**, *32*, 1393–1401. [CrossRef] [PubMed]
34. Xia, J.; Sinelnikov, I.V.; Han, B.; Wishart, D.S. MetaboAnalyst 3.0—Making Metabolomics More Meaningful. *Nucleic Acids Res.* **2015**, *43*, W251–W257. [CrossRef]
35. Riviere, A.; Selak, M.; Lantin, D.; Leroy, F.; De Vuyst, L. Bifidobacteria and Butyrate-Producing Colon Bacteria: Importance and Strategies for Their Stimulation in the Human Gut. *Front. Microbiol.* **2016**, *7*, 979. [CrossRef] [PubMed]
36. Pokusaeva, K.; Fitzgerald, G.F.; van Sinderen, D. Carbohydrate metabolism in Bifidobacteria. *Genes. Nutr.* **2011**, *6*, 285–306. [CrossRef]
37. Bunesova, V.; Lacroix, C.; Schwab, C. Mucin Cross-Feeding of Infant Bifidobacteria and Eubacterium hallii. *Microb. Ecol.* **2018**, *75*, 228–238. [CrossRef]
38. Claesson, M.J.; Jeffery, I.B.; Conde, S.; Power, S.E.; O'Connor, E.M.; Cusack, S.; Harris, H.M.; Coakley, M.; Lakshminarayanan, B.; O'Sullivan, O.; et al. Gut microbiota composition correlates with diet and health in the elderly. *Nature* **2012**, *488*, 178–184. [CrossRef] [PubMed]
39. Biagi, E.; Nylund, L.; Candela, M.; Ostan, R.; Bucci, L.; Pini, E.; Nikkila, J.; Monti, D.; Satokari, R.; Franceschi, C.; et al. Through ageing, and beyond: Gut microbiota and inflammatory status in seniors and centenarians. *PLoS ONE* **2010**, *5*, e10667. [CrossRef]
40. Ling, Z.; Liu, X.; Cheng, Y.; Yan, X.; Wu, S. Gut microbiota and aging. *Crit. Rev. Food Sci. Nutr.* **2022**, *62*, 3509–3534. [CrossRef] [PubMed]
41. Gomaa, E.Z. Human gut microbiota/microbiome in health and diseases: A review. *Antonie Leeuwenhoek* **2020**, *113*, 2019–2040. [CrossRef]
42. Avershina, E.; Storro, O.; Oien, T.; Johnsen, R.; Wilson, R.; Egeland, T.; Rudi, K. Bifidobacterial succession and correlation networks in a large unselected cohort of mothers and their children. *Appl. Environ. Microbiol.* **2013**, *79*, 497–507. [CrossRef]
43. Ladeira, R.; Tap, J.; Derrien, M. Exploring Bifidobacterium species community and functional variations with human gut microbiome structure and health beyond infancy. *Microbiome Res. Rep.* **2023**, *2*, 9. [CrossRef]
44. Plaza-Diaz, J.; Ruiz-Ojeda, F.J.; Morales, J.; Martin-Masot, R.; Climent, E.; Silva, A.; Martinez-Blanch, J.F.; Enrique, M.; Tortajada, M.; Ramon, D.; et al. Innova 2020: A Follow-Up Study of the Fecal Microbiota of Infants Using a Novel Infant Formula between 6 Months and 12 Months of Age. *Int. J. Mol. Sci.* **2023**, *24*, 7392. [CrossRef]
45. Bajic, D.; Wiens, F.; Wintergerst, E.; Deyaert, S.; Baudot, A.; Van den Abbeele, P. HMOs Exert Marked Bifidogenic Effects on Children's Gut Microbiota Ex Vivo, Due to Age-Related Bifidobacterium Species Composition. *Nutrients* **2023**, *15*, 1701. [CrossRef]
46. Li, H.; Lane, J.A.; Chen, J.; Lu, Z.; Wang, H.; Dhital, S.; Fu, X.; Huang, Q.; Liu, F.; Zhang, B. In vitro fermentation of human milk oligosaccharides by individual Bifidobacterium longum-dominant infant fecal inocula. *Carbohydr. Polym.* **2022**, *287*, 119322. [CrossRef]
47. Heiss, B.E.; Ehrlich, A.M.; Maldonado-Gomez, M.X.; Taft, D.H.; Larke, J.A.; Goodson, M.L.; Slupsky, C.M.; Tancredi, D.J.; Raybould, H.E.; Mills, D.A. Bifidobacterium catabolism of human milk oligosaccharides overrides endogenous competitive exclusion driving colonization and protection. *Gut Microbes* **2021**, *13*, 1986666. [CrossRef]
48. Shani, G.; Hoeflinger, J.L.; Heiss, B.E.; Masarweh, C.F.; Larke, J.A.; Jensen, N.M.; Wickramasinghe, S.; Davis, J.C.; Goonatilleke, E.; El-Hawiet, A.; et al. Fucosylated Human Milk Oligosaccharide Foraging within the Species Bifidobacterium pseudocatenulatum Is Driven by Glycosyl Hydrolase Content and Specificity. *Appl. Environ. Microbiol.* **2022**, *88*, e0170721. [CrossRef] [PubMed]
49. Larke, J.A.; Heiss, B.E.; Ehrlich, A.M.; Taft, D.H.; Raybould, H.E.; Mills, D.A.; Slupsky, C.M. Milk oligosaccharide-driven persistence of Bifidobacterium pseudocatenulatum modulates local and systemic microbial metabolites upon synbiotic treatment in conventionally colonized mice. *Microbiome* **2023**, *11*, 194. [CrossRef] [PubMed]
50. Liu, J.; Li, W.; Yao, C.; Yu, J.; Zhang, H. Comparative genomic analysis revealed genetic divergence between Bifidobacterium catenulatum subspecies present in infant versus adult guts. *BMC Microbiol.* **2022**, *22*, 158. [CrossRef] [PubMed]
51. Derrien, M.; Turroni, F.; Ventura, M.; van Sinderen, D. Insights into endogenous Bifidobacterium species in the human gut microbiota during adulthood. *Trends Microbiol.* **2022**, *30*, 940–947. [CrossRef] [PubMed]

52. Duranti, S.; Milani, C.; Lugli, G.A.; Mancabelli, L.; Turroni, F.; Ferrario, C.; Mangifesta, M.; Viappiani, A.; Sanchez, B.; Margolles, A.; et al. Evaluation of genetic diversity among strains of the human gut commensal Bifidobacterium adolescentis. *Sci. Rep.* **2016**, *6*, 23971. [CrossRef] [PubMed]
53. Luo, Y.; Xiao, Y.; Zhao, J.; Zhang, H.; Chen, W.; Zhai, Q. The role of mucin and oligosaccharides via cross-feeding activities by Bifidobacterium: A review. *Int. J. Biol. Macromol.* **2021**, *167*, 1329–1337. [CrossRef] [PubMed]
54. Zhao, S.; Lau, R.; Zhong, Y.; Chen, M.H. Lactate cross-feeding between Bifidobacterium species and Megasphaera indica contributes to butyrate formation in the human colonic environment. *Appl. Environ. Microbiol.* **2023**, *90*, e0101923. [CrossRef] [PubMed]
55. Belenguer, A.; Duncan, S.H.; Calder, A.G.; Holtrop, G.; Louis, P.; Lobley, G.E.; Flint, H.J. Two routes of metabolic cross-feeding between Bifidobacterium adolescentis and butyrate-producing anaerobes from the human gut. *Appl. Environ. Microbiol.* **2006**, *72*, 3593–3599. [CrossRef] [PubMed]
56. Elison, E.; Vigsnaes, L.K.; Rindom Krogsgaard, L.; Rasmussen, J.; Sorensen, N.; McConnell, B.; Hennet, T.; Sommer, M.O.; Bytzer, P. Oral supplementation of healthy adults with 2′-O-fucosyllactose and lacto-N-neotetraose is well tolerated and shifts the intestinal microbiota. *Br. J. Nutr.* **2016**, *116*, 1356–1368. [CrossRef]
57. Duncan, S.H.; Louis, P.; Flint, H.J. Lactate-utilizing bacteria, isolated from human feces, that produce butyrate as a major fermentation product. *Appl. Environ. Microbiol.* **2004**, *70*, 5810–5817. [CrossRef]
58. Suligoj, T.; Vigsnaes, L.K.; Abbeele, P.V.D.; Apostolou, A.; Karalis, K.; Savva, G.M.; McConnell, B.; Juge, N. Effects of Human Milk Oligosaccharides on the Adult Gut Microbiota and Barrier Function. *Nutrients* **2020**, *12*, 2808. [CrossRef] [PubMed]
59. Bunesova, V.; Lacroix, C.; Schwab, C. Fucosyllactose and L-fucose utilization of infant Bifidobacterium longum and Bifidobacterium kashiwanohense. *BMC Microbiol.* **2016**, *16*, 248. [CrossRef] [PubMed]
60. Fushinobu, S. Unique sugar metabolic pathways of bifidobacteria. *Biosci. Biotechnol. Biochem.* **2010**, *74*, 2374–2384. [CrossRef] [PubMed]
61. Strain, R.; Tran, T.T.T.; Mills, S.; Stanton, C.; Ross, R.P. A pilot study of dietary fibres on pathogen growth in an ex vivo colonic model reveals their potential ability to limit vancomycin-resistant Enterococcus expansion. *Microbiome Res. Rep.* **2023**, *2*, 22. [CrossRef] [PubMed]
62. Maurer Sost, M.; Stevens, Y.; Salden, B.; Troost, F.; Masclee, A.; Venema, K. Citrus Extract High in Flavonoids Beneficially Alters Intestinal Metabolic Responses in Subjects with Features of Metabolic Syndrome. *Foods* **2023**, *12*, 3413. [CrossRef] [PubMed]
63. Aguirre, M.; Ramiro-Garcia, J.; Koenen, M.E.; Venema, K. To pool or not to pool? Impact of the use of individual and pooled fecal samples for in vitro fermentation studies. *J. Microbiol. Methods* **2014**, *107*, 1–7. [CrossRef] [PubMed]

nutrients

MDPI

Article

Lactobacillus helveticus Induces Two Types of Dendritic Cell Activation and Effectively Suppresses Onset of the Common Cold: A Randomized, Double-Blind, Placebo-Controlled Trial

Hiroka Wada [1,*], Takashi Mawatari [1], Yasuo Saito [1], Naoki Azuma [1] and Yoshitaka Iwama [2]

1 R&D Laboratory, Ezaki Glico Co., Ltd., 4-6-5 Utajima, Nishiyodogawa-ku, Osaka 555-8502, Japan; takashi.mawatari@glico.com (T.M.); yasuo.saito@glico.com (Y.S.); naoki.azuma@glico.com (N.A.)
2 Nihonbashi Cardiology Clinic, Kyodo Bldg. #201, 13-4 Nihonbashi Kodenmacho, Chuo-ku, Tokyo 103-0001, Japan; yiwama@well-sleep.jp
* Correspondence: hiroka.wada@glico.com; Tel.: +81-50-1741-2971

Abstract: Background/Objectives: *Lactobacillus helveticus* GCL1815 is a lactic acid bacterium thought to activate dendritic cells. This randomized, placebo-controlled, double-blind study aimed to evaluate the effects of *L. helveticus* GCL1815 on human dendritic cells and the onset of the common cold. Methods: Two hundred participants were divided into two groups and took capsules containing either six billion *L. helveticus* GCL1815 cells or placebo for 8 weeks. Results: In the GCL1815 group, the cumulative incidence days of symptoms such as feverishness, fatigue, tiredness, runny nose, nasal congestion, and phlegm were significantly lower than in the placebo group. Moreover, the change in the expression of HLA-DR on plasmacytoid dendritic cells was significantly higher in the GCL1815 group than in the placebo group at 4 and 8 weeks of intake. The expression of CD86 on plasmacytoid dendritic cells was significantly increased in the GCL1815 group at 4 and 8 weeks compared with before intake. Additionally, the expression of HLA-DR on type 1 conventional dendritic cells was significantly higher in the GCL1815 group than in the placebo group at 8 weeks of intake. The expression of CD86 on type 1 conventional dendritic cells significantly decreased in the placebo group but remained statistically the same in the GCL1815 group after intake compared with before. Conclusions: These results suggest that GCL1815 intake may enhance the response to viruses by activating two types of dendritic cells, thereby preventing the onset of systemic and local common colds in healthy adults.

Keywords: lactic acid bacteria; *Lactobacillus*; *Lactobacillus helveticus* GCL1815; postbiotics; dendritic cell; humans; symptom; common cold

1. Introduction

Infectious diseases are high-risk diseases, with potentially severe outcomes in individuals with a compromised immune system [1]. For example, it is estimated that approximately 3–5 million people worldwide become severely ill with influenza each year [2]. Infectious diseases also lead to substantial economic losses worldwide due to treatment costs and work absences. In the United States, the direct medical cost of treating influenza is reported to be approximately USD 10.4 billion per year [3], and the economic cost of other upper respiratory tract infections is estimated to be USD 40 billion per year, with more than 315 million days of work and school absences per year [4]. For infectious diseases such as influenza, treatment with antiviral drugs is possible [5].

The common cold, one of the most frequent infections, is defined as a mild upper respiratory tract infection that resolves spontaneously. It is reported that children get a cold 7–10 times a year, while adults do so 2–5 times a year [6]. The main cause of the common cold is a viral infection, but more than 200 different viruses are known to cause common colds, including rhinoviruses and adenoviruses [7]. Because common cold symptoms are similar even when caused by different viruses, it is difficult to identify the causative virus based on symptoms alone, and thus it is difficult to tailor the treatment to the virus. Therefore, methods to prevent or reduce the onset of the common cold by modulating the host's immune function, such as by promoting viral infection defense, are desirable. One useful approach includes the intake of foods and beverages [8] such as green tea, herbs, and mushrooms. Foods containing lactic acid bacteria and bifidobacteria are also among these, and the results of clinical trials have suggested that these bacteria regulate immune function and help prevent the common cold [9,10]. For example, the combined intake of the strains *Lactobacillus gasseri* PA 16/8, *Bifidobacterium longum* SP 07/3, and *B. bifidum* MF 20/5 reduced the duration of common cold symptoms [11], and intake of the *Lacticaseibacillus paracasei* strain Shirota reduced the proportion of medical students with colds before taking exams [12]. In addition to their effect on the common cold, these strains have also been reported to increase $CD8^+$ T cells or activate natural killer (NK) cells, which play an important role in suppressing the onset of colds [11,13].

Meanwhile, dendritic cells (DCs), which are antigen-presenting cells found in almost all tissues of the body, also play an important role in suppressing onset of the common cold by regulating both innate immunity, which is the immediate response to invading foreign substances, and adaptive immunity, which is a specific response to foreign substances. DCs are divided into conventional DCs (cDCs) and plasmacytoid DCs (pDCs), which play central roles in the immune response against viral infections. cDCs are further classified into type 1 cDCs (cDC1s) and type 2 cDCs (cDC2s), which induce exceptional activation of $CD4^+$ T cells and $CD8^+$ T cells through antigen presentation [14]. pDCs are known to produce a large amount of type I interferon (IFN) when they recognize pathogens such as viruses and bacteria [15], directly or indirectly promoting viral replication inhibition as well as $CD8^+$ T-cell activation [16].

Lactic acid bacteria are also attracting attention as a means to induce the activation of DCs. For example, *Lacticaseibacillus rhamnosus* GG is reported to activate cDCs and induce IL-12 production *in vitro* [17] and to reduce the number of upper respiratory tract infections in children [18], while the *Lactococcus lactis* strain Plasma is reported to stimulate pDCs via Toll-like receptor 9 [19] and to reduce the cumulative number of influenza and cold-like symptoms in adults [20]. However, not all lactic acid bacteria activate DCs [21], and the immune-modulating functions activated by DCs are known to be strain-specific. Therefore, DCs are considered an important indicator for selecting lactic acid bacteria that can suppress onset of the common cold.

Lactobacillus helveticus GCL1815 (hereafter, GCL1815) is thought to activate cDCs [22]. It is reported that cross-presentation and induction of type 1 helper T cell differentiation by cDCs are promoted by type I IFN [16,23] and that cDC function may be reinforced by pDC activation. Because pDCs are also highly responsive to viruses, the present study focused on not only cDCs but also pDCs as key immune indicators in the fight against viral infection. The effects of lactic acid bacteria intake on both human pDCs and cDCs are largely unknown, and the effect of GCL1815, which is expected to have DC-activating capacity, on the onset of the common cold has not been investigated. Therefore, this study investigated the effects of GCL1815 intake on common cold symptoms and immune cells, with the aim of verifying whether GCL1815 can suppress the onset of the common cold in healthy adults.

2. Materials and Methods

2.1. Participants

Participants were healthy Japanese adults aged 20 to <65 years at the time of consent who fulfilled the inclusion criteria, did not meet the exclusion criteria, and were deemed eligible to participate by the principal investigator. The aim and other details of the study as well as the secondary use of surplus samples were explained to them, and they provided written consent to participate in the study. The inclusion criteria required that participants were fully informed about the purpose and content of the study, had the capacity to provide consent, voluntarily agreed to participate after fully understanding the study's purpose and content, and provided written consent to take part in the study. The exclusion criteria were (1) history of diabetes, renal or hepatic disease, or other serious illnesses, including thyroid disease, adrenal gland disease, psychiatric disease, autoimmune disease, or other metabolic diseases; (2) inability to abstain from foods containing lactic acid bacteria, bifidobacteria, oligosaccharides, or other bacteria during the study period; (3) regular consumption of foods that can affect immunity; (4) regular alcohol consumption, averaging around 20 g of pure alcohol per day; (5) inability to abstain from alcohol 2 days before each test; (6) presence of food allergies; (7) history of gastrointestinal diseases or gastrointestinal surgery; (8) pregnant, breastfeeding, or planning to become pregnant during the study period; (9) history of drug or alcohol dependence; (10) participation or intent to participate in other studies involving the use of other foods, medicines, or cosmetics; (11) regular use of medicines that may affect immunity or the inability to stop taking them during the study period; (12) hay fever, atopic dermatitis, allergic rhinitis, bronchial asthma, or chronic bronchitis; (13) oral problems involving bleeding or intent to undergo dental or oral treatment; (14) regular engagement in strenuous exercise; (15) intent to travel abroad during the study period; (16) having taken antibiotics within 1 month of the screening test; (17) smoking; (18) having collected or donated more than 400 mL of blood components within 3 months prior to the date of consent; (19) work schedule involving both day and night shifts, working late at night, or fully remote work or blue-collar work; (20) diagnosis of dry mouth; (21) absence of any cold symptoms within the last year; (22) body mass index of <18.5 or >30.0; and (23) determined to be inappropriate as a research participant by the principal investigator.

2.2. Test Foods

Capsules containing six billion heat-sterilized GCL1815 cells (test food) and capsules without GCL1815 (control food) were prepared as test food. The inactive ingredients of the test food were starch, calcium stearate, and silicon dioxide and thus the test food did not contain any allergenic substances.

2.3. Study Design

The study had a randomized, double-blind, placebo-controlled, parallel-group design. The participants were randomly assigned to two groups (1:1) using computer-generated randomization in blocks of four, with stratification by age, gender, salivary secretory immunoglobulin A (sIgA) levels, expression levels of surface markers on pDCs, and background survey results at screening. The allocation manager assigned participants to either the GCL1815 intake group or the placebo food intake group. The final target sample size was set at 200 based on previous studies reporting reductions in colds with lactic acid bacteria [20,24]. Participants took capsules containing either GCL1815 or placebo once daily for 8 weeks from January 2023 to March 2023. During the study period, both the participants and the observers were blinded to their group allocation. Double-blinding was ensured by labelling the test food with identification numbers only. The primary endpoint was the daily questionnaire on common cold symptoms. Secondary endpoints were expression levels of surface markers on pDCs and cDCs, NK cell cytotoxic activity, and salivary sIgA levels. Other endpoints were the Profile of Mood States 2nd edition (POMS-2) and safety assessment. Blood and saliva samples were collected from the 80 participants who took part in immunological assessments before intake and again at 4 and 8 weeks during the intake period. Surplus blood samples from the immunological assessments were stored at −80 °C and used for additional analysis. Blood samples from the remaining 120 participants were collected before and after the intake period for safety assessment. Additionally, serum cytokine levels were measured for participants with immunological assessments. Samples from participants with immunological assessments whose peripheral blood mononuclear cell (PBMC) counts exceeded the number of cells in the analysis criteria were also measured to determine the expression of surface markers on $CD4^+$ T cells, $CD8^+$ T cells, B cells, and NK cells. The number of analyzed samples was 40 before intake, 39 at 4 weeks, and 33 at 8 weeks of intake. The study was pre-registered in the University Hospital Medical Information Network Clinical Trials Registry (UMIN-CTR) (UMIN000049616, UMIN000053740) and was conducted at the Nihonbashi Cardiology Clinic (Tokyo, Japan) from January to March 2023. This article adheres to the Consolidated Standards of Reporting Trials (CONSORT) 2010 guidelines.

2.4. Questionnaire Analysis

Participants recorded daily symptoms of feverishness, chills, fatigue, low appetite, tiredness, joint discomfort, nasal congestion, runny nose, muscle pain, heavy headedness, throat discomfort, sneezing, cough, and phlegm. Participants rated symptoms as (1) normal, (2) slight, (3) mild, (4) moderate, or (5) severe. Days with mild, moderate, or severe symptoms were counted as symptomatic days, and the cumulative number of days with symptoms was calculated. Additionally, 'moderate' and 'severe' symptoms were grouped together as serious cases, and 'mild' symptoms were taken as mild cases. The numbers of mild and serious symptoms in each of the 14 categories were totaled to assess the proportion of serious symptoms among all symptoms.

The POMS-2 was administered before intake and at 4 and 8 weeks of intake to examine mood states. It consists of 65 questions with responses on a five-point Likert scale, and assess seven states: anger-hostility, confusion-bewilderment, depression-dejection, fatigue-inertia, tension-anxiety, vigor-activity, and friendliness.

2.5. Flow Cytometric Analysis

PBMCs were obtained from blood samples using centrifugation. For pDC labelling, PBMCs were stained with anti-CD123 FITC (BioLegend, San Diego, CA, USA), anti-CD304 APC (BioLegend), anti-CD86 PE (eBioscience, Santa Clara, CA, USA), and anti-HLA-DR PerCP-CyTM5.5 (BD Biosciences, Franklin Lakes, NJ, USA). For cDC labelling, $CD3^+$ $CD14^+$ $CD16^+$ cells were eliminated from PBMCs using anti-CD3 (BD Biosciences), anti-CD14 (BioLegend), and anti-CD16 (BioLegend), and the remaining fractions were stained with anti-CD11c FITC (BD Biosciences), anti-CD141 APC (BD Biosciences), anti-CD86 PE (eBioscience), and anti-HLA-DR PE (BD Biosciences). cDC1s and cDC2s were classified based on the presence or absence of CD141 expression. Cells were washed with stain buffer, fixed in paraformaldehyde, and measured using a flow cytometer (BD AccuriTM C6; BD Biosciences). Expression levels of HLA-DR and CD86, indicators of pDC and cDC activation, were measured using mean fluorescence intensity. Sample data with fewer than 50,000 PBMC events were treated as missing values. In the additional analysis, Pacific Blue™ anti-human CD3 antibody (BioLegend), Brilliant Violet 650™ anti-human CD4 antibody (BioLegend), APC/Fire™ 750™ anti-human CD8 antibody (BioLegend), Alexa

Fluor® 700 anti-human CD16 antibody (BioLegend), Brilliant Violet 605™ anti-human CD20 antibody (BioLegend), FITC anti-human CD56 (NCAM) antibody (BioLegend), and PE anti-human CD69 antibody (BioLegend) were used to label $CD4^+$ T cells, $CD8^+$ T cells, B cells, and NK cells by staining. Expression levels of CD69, an indicator of the activation of these cells, were measured using mean fluorescence intensity. Cells were then washed with fluorescence-activated cell sorting buffer and measured using a CytoFLEX S (Beckman Coulter, Brea, CA, USA).

2.6. Chromium 51 Release Assay

A chromium 51 (51Cr) release assay was performed to measure the cytotoxic activity of NK cells. K562 cells were labelled with 51Cr (PerkinElmer Japan, Yokohama, Japan), added to PBMCs, and incubated for 4 h at 37 °C and 5% CO_2. The released 51Cr was measured using a Wizard2 Automatic Gamma Counter (PerkinElmer, Waltham, MA, USA). NK cell cytotoxic activity was expressed as a percentage of cytotoxicity.

2.7. Measurement in Saliva

Saliva was collected by having participants hold a Salivet-attached sponge in their mouth for 2 min. The weight of their saliva was measured at the time of collection. The sIgA concentration in saliva was determined using the YK280 Human s-IgA ELISA kit (Yanaihara Institute Inc., Shizuoka, Japan). The sIgA secretion rate was calculated from the saliva weight and sIgA concentration.

2.8. Measurement of Cytokine Concentrations

A sandwich enzyme-linked immunosorbent assay was performed to measure the cytokine concentrations in serum supernatants. The aliquoted serum was assayed for cytokines, using the Luminex Discovery Assay (R&D Systems, Minneapolis, MN, USA), S-PLEX Human IFN-α2a (Mesoscale, Rockville, MD, USA), S-PLEX Human IFN-β (Mesoscale), S-PLEX Proinflammatory Panel 1 (Mesoscale), U-PLEX Biomarker Group 1 (Mesoscale), V-PLEX Cytokine Panel 1 Human Kit (Mesoscale), and MESO QuickPlex SQ 120MM (Mesoscale), following the instructions provided with each respective kit. The following parameters were measured: IFN-α, IFN-β, IFN-γ, IL-1, IL-2, IL-4, IL-6, IL-8, IL-10, IL-12, IL-15, IL-17, IL-18, IL-27, a proliferation-inducing ligand, B-cell activating factor, and tumor necrosis factor (TNF)-α1. Samples with values below the detection limit were treated as missing values.

2.9. Safety Assessment

The safety of the test food was assessed by testing blood and urine samples obtained from the participants before intake and at 8 weeks of intake. The following parameters were measured: blood pressure, pulse rate, body weight, body mass index, red blood cell count, white blood cell count, hemoglobin, hematocrit, mean corpuscular volume, mean corpuscular hemoglobin volume, mean corpuscular hemoglobin concentration, platelet count, leucogram, total protein, albumin, aspartate aminotransferase, alanine aminotransferase, lactate dehydrogenase, total bilirubin, alkaline phosphatase, gamma-glutamyl transferase, urea nitrogen, creatinine, uric acid, Na, Cl, K, Ca, total cholesterol, low density lipoprotein cholesterol, high-density lipoprotein cholesterol, triglycerides, glucose, glycated hemoglobin, urine protein qualitative data, urine glucose qualitative data, urine urobilinogen qualitative data, urine bilirubin qualitative data, urine pH, urine specific gravity, urine ketones, and urine occult blood reaction. Qualitative items were quantified as follows: '−' as 0, '+−' as 1, '+' as 2, '++' as 3, and '+++' as 4 for urine protein, urine glucose, urine bilirubin, urine ketones, and urine occult blood reaction. For urine urobilinogen, '+−'

was scored as 0, '+' as 1, and '++' as 2. In addition, medical consultations were conducted before intake and at 4 and 8 weeks of intake.

2.10. Statistical Analysis

The cumulative incidence days with symptoms based on the daily questionnaire was assessed using the chi-squared test. For immunological parameters, participants' characteristics and safety parameters, means, standard deviation, and standard errors were calculated using IBM® SPSS® Statistics 27 (IBM Corp., Armonk, NY, USA). Means, standard deviations, and standard errors were presented to the nearest significant figure, with the final digit rounded accordingly. Comparisons between the GCL1815 and placebo groups for each item were assessed with an unpaired *t*-test (two-tailed). Differences between pre-intake and 4 weeks and between pre-intake and 8 weeks of intake were each assessed using a paired *t*-test. For qualitative items, Wilcoxon's rank sum test was used for comparisons between the GCL1815 and the placebo groups. Missing data were treated as missing values, and no alternative values were used. The level of significance for all analyses was set at 5% (two-tailed test).

3. Results

3.1. Participant Characteristics

Of the 420 healthy adults who underwent screening, 200 were deemed eligible, and 100 each were enrolled in the GCL1815 and placebo groups. During the study period, five participants withdrew due to either an illness unrelated to the study, which prevented continuation, or deviation from the protocol. After the study period, three participants were excluded from the efficacy analysis due to high-frequency consumption of prohibited foods, and two of those had undergone immunological assessment. As a result, there were 96 participants in the GCL1815 group and 96 in the placebo group (Figure 1). The full analysis set for safety analysis contained all 200 participants, while the per-protocol set for efficacy analysis contained 192 participants. No differences at baseline were observed in the participants' characteristics between the GCL1815 group and the placebo group in the efficacy analysis (Table 1).

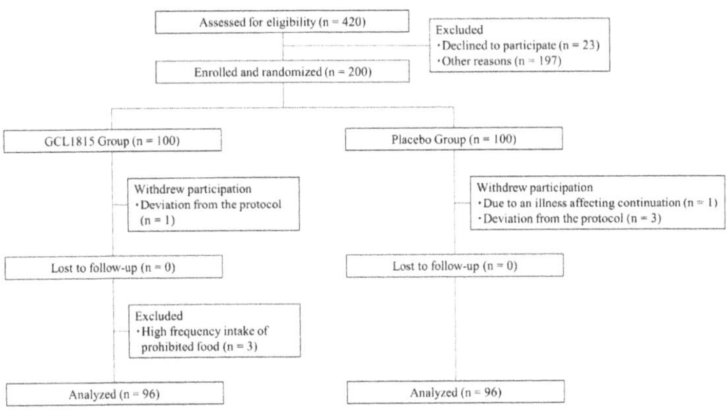

Figure 1. Flow chart of study participation. GCL1815 group, *Lactobacillus helveticus* GCL1815 group.

Table 1. Participant characteristics by group (per-protocol set).

	GCL1815		Placebo		p
	Mean	SE	Mean	SE	
Number of participants (Male: Female)	96 (44:52)		96 (42:54)		-
Age (years)	44.8	1.0	44.5	0.9	0.801
Body weight (kg)	61.3	1.0	60.7	0.9	0.646
Body mass index	22.3	0.3	22.2	0.2	0.675
Systolic blood pressure (mmHg)	129.3	1.5	126.0	1.5	0.120
Diastolic blood pressure (mmHg)	84.7	1.4	82.1	1.2	0.154
Pulse rate (bpm)	75.7	1.0	76.9	1.0	0.414

Data represent the baseline means, with the SE shown for each group and the results of unpaired t-tests. GCL1815, *Lactobacillus helveticus* GCL1815 group; Placebo, placebo group; SE, standard error.

3.2. Common Cold Symptoms and Other Sensory Effects

The effect of GCL1815 on clinical symptoms was evaluated based on the daily questionnaires on common cold symptoms. The cumulative incidence days of common cold-like symptoms was 938 days in the GCL1815 group, which was significantly less than the 1116 days in the placebo group (Table 2). Furthermore, when assessed by symptom, the GCL1815 group showed significantly fewer cumulative incidence days of feverishness, fatigue, tiredness, runny nose, nasal congestion, and phlegm compared with the placebo group (Table 3). The cumulative incidence days of chills was significantly less in the placebo group than in the GCL1815 group. There was no significant difference in the cumulative incidence days of low appetite, joint discomfort, muscle pain, heavy headedness, throat discomfort, sneezing, and cough. The cumulative incidence of mild and serious cases (moderate + severe) was calculated to confirm the palliative effect on severe illness, and the proportion of serious symptoms was assessed. In the GCL1815 group, the proportion of serious symptoms was significantly lower compared with the placebo group (Table 4). These results suggest that GCL1815 intake might have improved common cold symptoms. Furthermore, the results of the POMS-2, which was conducted to assess quality of life, showed a trend toward lower anger-hostility in the GCL1815 group compared with the placebo group at 4 weeks of intake (p = 0.088) (Supplementary Material, Figure S1). There were no significant differences between the GCL1815 group and placebo group in other indicators on the POMS-2 at either 4 weeks or 8 weeks of intake.

Table 2. Cumulative incidence days with common cold-like symptoms during the study period.

	Symptom (+)	Symptom (−)	p
GCL1815	938	4438	<0.001
Placebo	1116	4260	

Lactobacillus helveticus GCL1815 group: n = 5376 (96 healthy adults × 56 d); placebo group: n = 5376 (96 healthy adults × 56 d). Data represent the cumulative incidence days and the χ^2 test results.

Table 3. Cumulative incidence days with individual cold-like symptoms during the study period.

		Symptom (+)	Symptom (−)	p
Feverishness	GCL1815	17	5359	0.009
	Placebo	36	5340	
Chills	GCL1815	95	5281	<0.001
	Placebo	51	5325	

Table 3. *Cont.*

		Symptom (+)	Symptom (−)	p
Fatigue	GCL1815 Placebo	140 267	5236 5109	<0.001
Low appetite	GCL1815 Placebo	25 28	5351 5348	0.680
Tiredness	GCL1815 Placebo	312 539	5064 4837	<0.001
Joint discomfort	GCL1815 Placebo	72 73	5304 5303	0.933
Muscle pain	GCL1815 Placebo	94 116	5282 5260	0.125
Heavy headedness	GCL1815 Placebo	163 150	5213 5226	0.456
Sneezing	GCL1815 Placebo	211 197	5165 5179	0.480
Runny nose	GCL1815 Placebo	360 428	5016 4948	0.012
Nasal congestion	GCL1815 Placebo	140 253	5236 5123	<0.001
Throat discomfort	GCL1815 Placebo	185 161	5191 5215	0.190
Cough	GCL1815 Placebo	117 114	5259 5262	0.842
Phlegm	GCL1815 Placebo	62 156	5314 5220	<0.001

Lactobacillus helveticus GCL1815 group: n = 5376 (96 healthy adults × 56 d); placebo group: n = 5376 (96 volunteers × 56 d). Data represent the cumulative incidence numbers and the χ^2 test results.

Table 4. Cumulative incidence numbers of common cold-like symptoms during the study period, categorized by severity.

	Serious (Moderate + Severe)	Mild	p
GCL1815 Placebo	337 560	1656 2009	<0.001

Lactobacillus helveticus GCL1815 group: n = 1993; and placebo group: n = 2569. Data represent the cumulative incidence numbers categorized into two groups, including serious (moderate + severe), and mild, and the χ^2 test results.

3.3. Effect on Immune Cells and sIgA

Expression levels of surface markers on DCs, NK cell cytotoxic activity, and salivary sIgA levels were measured to assess the effects of GCL1815 intake on immune function. Figures 2A and 3A show the expression of HLA-DR and CD86 on DCs as measured, and Figures 2B and 3B show the change from before intake of the test food. The change in the expression levels of HLA-DR on pDCs from baseline was significantly higher in the GCL1815 group at both 4 and 8 weeks of intake compared with the placebo group (Figure 2B(i)). Meanwhile, the expression levels of HLA-DR on pDCs significantly decreased at 4 weeks of intake in the placebo group but not in the GCL1815 group (Figure 2A(i)). In addition, the expression levels of CD86 on pDCs increased significantly in the GCL1815 group at both 4 and 8 weeks of intake compared with before intake (Figure 2A(ii)). In contrast, the placebo group did not show any significant post-intake changes (Figure 2A(ii)).

The GCL1815 group showed significantly higher levels in the expression of HLA-DR on cDC1s compared with the placebo group, and a significant increase was noted at 8 weeks of intake (Figure 3A(i)). Meanwhile, the change in the expression levels of HLA-DR on cDC1s tended to be higher in the GCL1815 group compared with the placebo group at 8 weeks of intake ($p = 0.074$) (Figure 3B(i)). In addition, the placebo group showed a significant decrease in the expression levels of CD86 on cDC1s after intake, whereas there was no significant decrease in the GCL1815 group (Figure 3A(ii)).

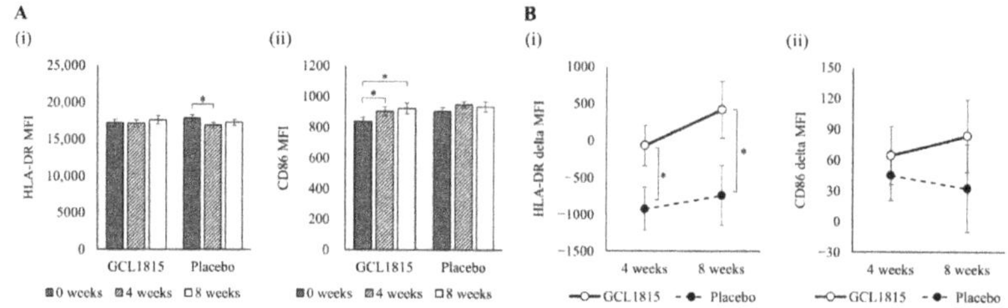

Figure 2. Expression levels of HLA-DR and CD86 on pDCs. Data are means, with the standard errors represented by vertical bars for each group. (**A**) Expression levels of (**i**) HLA-DR and (**ii**) CD86 on pDCs. (**B**) Change in the expression levels of (**i**) HLA-DR and (**ii**) CD86 on pDCs from before intake. The GCL1815 group and the placebo group consisted of 37 and 40 healthy adults, respectively, at 8 weeks. Comparisons of pre- and post-intake within each group were performed using paired *t*-tests, and comparisons between the two groups were performed using unpaired *t*-tests. GCL1815, *Lactobacillus helveticus* GCL1815 group; Placebo, placebo group; MFI, mean fluorescence intensity. * $p < 0.05$.

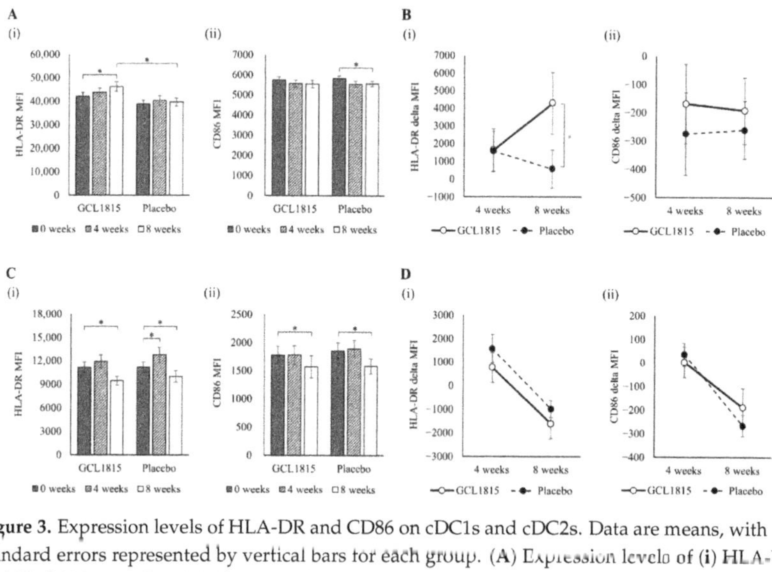

Figure 3. Expression levels of HLA-DR and CD86 on cDC1s and cDC2s. Data are means, with the standard errors represented by vertical bars for each group. (**A**) Expression levels of (**i**) HLA-DR and (**ii**) CD86 on cDC1s. (**B**) Change in the expression levels of (**i**) HLA-DR and (**ii**) CD86 on cDC1s from before intake. (**C**) Expression levels of (**i**) HLA-DR and (**ii**) CD86 on cDC2s. (**D**) Change in the expression levels of (**i**) HLA-DR and (**ii**) CD86 on cDC2s from before intake. The GCL1815 group and the placebo group consisted of 37 and 40 healthy adults, respectively, at 8 weeks. Comparisons of pre- and post-intake within each group were performed using paired *t*-tests, and comparisons between the two groups were performed using unpaired *t*-tests. GCL1815, *Lactobacillus helveticus* GCL1815 group; Placebo, placebo group; MFI, mean fluorescence intensity. * $p < 0.05$, # $p < 0.1$.

There were no significant differences between the GCL1815 group and placebo group in the expression of either HLA-DR or CD86 on cDC2s (Figure 3C,D). In contrast, both the placebo and GCL1815 groups showed a significant decrease in the expression levels of HLA-DR and CD86 on cDC2s at 8 weeks of intake (Figure 3C). The expression levels of HLA-DR on cDC2s significantly increased at 4 weeks of intake in the placebo group (Figure 3C(i)). However, the changes in the expression levels of both CD86 and HLA-DR on cDC2s were similar in both the GCL1815 group and placebo group (Figure 3D). NK cell cytotoxic activity, salivary sIgA concentration, and salivary sIgA secretion rate did not differ significantly between the GCL1815 group and placebo group at either 4 or 8 weeks of intake (Table 5). Additionally, no significant differences in the expression of CD69 on $CD4^+$ T cells, $CD8^+$ T cells, NK cells, or B cells were observed between the GCL1815 and placebo groups (Supplementary Material, Table S1).

Table 5. Changes in NK cell cytotoxic activity and salivary sIgA.

		At 4 Weeks			At 8 Weeks		
	Group	Mean	SE	p	Mean	SE	p
NK cell cytotoxic activity (%)	GCL1815 Placebo	2.0 4.1	2.2 1.4	0.427	2.9 4.0	1.7 1.8	0.664
sIgA secretion rate (μg/min)	GCL1815 Placebo	−3.1 8.3	6.4 5.5	0.179	−3.2 −3.7	10.7 8.0	0.965
sIgA concentration (μg/mL)	GCL1815 Placebo	−11.8 11.3	9.2 8.0	0.060	−9.7 −1.3	11.9 8.3	0.559

Data represent the mean changes from baseline, with the SE shown for each group and the results of unpaired t-tests. NK, natural killer; sIgA, secretory immunoglobulin A; SE, standard error.

3.4. Effect of GCL1815 Intake on Cytokines

The effect of GCL1815 intake on cytokine concentrations in serum was investigated. The results for representative cytokines related to pDCs and cDC1s [25] are shown in Table 6. The change in IL-12p40 concentration tended to be higher in the GCL1815 group compared with the placebo group at 8 weeks of intake (Table 6). There were no significant differences between the GCL1815 and placebo groups for other items after intake (Table 6, Supplementary Material, Table S1).

Table 6. Changes in cytokine concentrations.

	Group	At 4 Weeks			At 8 Weeks		
		Mean	SE	p	Mean	SE	p
IFN-α2A (fg/mL)	GCL1815 Placebo	20.4 11.1	3.1 5.7	0.155	11.1 8.6	4.6 9.0	0.809
IFN-β (fg/mL)	GCL1815 Placebo	−46.8 −56.6	10.5 8.4	0.470	−16.5 −33.2	18.2 12.4	0.451
IFN-γ (fg/mL)	GCL1815 Placebo	−18.8 −137.1	188.1 118.0	0.596	89.1 195.9	330.4 412.2	0.840
IL-6 (fg/mL)	GCL1815 Placebo	−182.5 −97.8	166.5 143.3	0.701	−86.3 23.2	240.6 217.8	0.737
IL-12p40 (pg/mL)	GCL1815 Placebo	−5.1 −11.4	2.6 3.5	0.156	−3.6 −12.7	3.5 3.8	0.080
IL-12p70 (fg/mL)	GCL1815 Placebo	2.4 38.9	18.4 15.9	0.139	4.3 34.3	46.4 14.1	0.538
TNF-α (fg/mL)	GCL1815 Placebo	−51.7 −77.4	14.5 18.5	0.279	−36.0 −64.6	18.4 20.3	0.301

Data represent the mean changes from baseline, with the SE shown for each group and the results of unpaired t-tests. SE, standard error; IFN, interferon; IL, interleukin; TNF, tumor necrosis factor.

3.5. Safety Assessment

During the study period, there were 37 adverse events in 23 of the 200 participants, but none was serious. All adverse events were judged to be not causally related to the study food by the principal investigator. Therefore, no adverse effects were reported. After intake, significant fluctuations were observed in albumin and Cl between GCL1815 and placebo groups (Supplementary Material, Table S2). However, these changes were minor physiological variations, and the study food was judged to be safe by the principal investigator.

4. Discussion

In this study, the effects of intake of heat-sterilized GCL1815 for 8 weeks on common cold symptoms and DCs in healthy adults were evaluated. Intake of GCL1815 led to the activation of pDCs and cDC1s as well as reduced incidence days of feverishness, fatigue, tiredness, runny nose, nasal congestion, and phlegm. These findings suggest that GCL1815 may promote viral infection responses by activating two types of DCs, thereby suppressing systemic and local common cold incidence in healthy adults.

The common cold is known to cause a wide range of symptoms throughout the body, including runny nose, nasal congestion, sneezing, coughing, fatigue, sore throat, and fever. In addition, symptoms of the common cold change over time, starting with early signs such as fever, fatigue, and sneezing, followed by symptoms such as runny nose, nasal congestion, and cough [7]. As a result, the common cold, with its variety of symptoms and different times of onset, has been reported to cause an average of 8.7 h of lost working time and reduced labor productivity [26]. Given that universal suppression of common cold symptoms is considered important for maintaining worker productivity, 14 of these symptoms were investigated in adults in the present study. GCL1815 showed efficacy in reducing the cumulative incidence days with common cold symptoms (Table 2), particularly runny nose, congestion, and phlegm as local symptoms, as well as feverishness, fatigue, and tiredness (Table 3). The suppressive effect of GCL1815 on the onset of the common colds was not concentrated on specific symptoms but rather extended from early symptoms such as fatigue to late symptoms such as runny nose, suggesting that GCL1815 effectively reduced the number of days with common cold symptoms. It has been reported that *Lacticaseibacillus rhamnosus* CRL1505 has a number of immunomodulatory effects, including activating DCs derived from intestinal Peyer's patches *in vitro*; increasing the number of $CD4^{+}IFN\text{-}\gamma^{+}$ T cells in the small intestine, which subsequently migrate to the respiratory tract to induce local IFN-γ production *in vivo* [27]; and reducing the number of respiratory symptoms in children [28]. In the present study, GCL1815 suppressed a wide range of symptoms, possibly by stimulating the activation of immune cells, starting with DCs in the small intestine, with some of these cells migrating to the upper respiratory tract and inducing the activation of immune cells in local lymph nodes and other sites. Although there were fewer overall incidence days of symptoms with GCL1815 intake (Table 2), there were significantly fewer cumulative incidence days of chills in the placebo group compared with the GCL1815 group. However, this was considered to be an incidental occurrence.

In addition to mild symptoms, GCL1815 might also alleviate more severe symptoms (Table 4). Because more severe infections can lead to complications such as otitis media, sinusitis, bronchiolitis, and pneumonia, the reduction in more severe symptoms is considered important, even for mild infections such as the common cold. In this study, each symptom was rated on a five-point scale, with mild or more severe symptoms being considered symptomatic. Furthermore, among those rated as symptomatic, when serious symptoms (moderate + severe) were analyzed separately from mild symptoms, intake of GCL1815 significantly reduced the proportion of serious symptoms compared with intake of placebo (Table 4). For infants and the elderly, who are at high risk of complications from the common cold, GCL1815 is expected to be useful as a countermeasure against severe colds.

pDCs and cDC1s were thought to play a central role in the suppression of the common cold by GCL1815 (Figures 2 and 3). Considering that common colds are caused primarily by viral infections [7], a DC-driven protective immune response against viruses is important in suppressing the onset of the common cold. pDCs produce large amounts of type I IFN early in the viral response, which promotes apoptosis of virus-infected cells and inhibits viral replication, thereby enhancing resistance to infection [16]. It is also known that pDCs have the ability to present antigens to $CD4^+$ T cells and $CD8^+$ T cells [29]. It has been recently reported that intake of lactic acid bacteria leads to suppression of colds and pDC activation [24]. Given that GCL1815 also led to pDC activation, it may also induce a high antiviral infection immune response via pDCs. However, because pDCs have been reported to have different reactivity to different viruses as well as a lower antigen-presenting capacity compared with cDCs [29,30], inducing activation of both pDCs and cDCs was considered important as a measure against viral infection. The intake of GCL1815 induced cDC1 activation; however, to our knowledge, the activation of these two types of DCs has not been reported in clinical trials of other lactic acid bacteria. cDC1s induce mainly cytotoxic T lymphocytes and type 1 helper T cell differentiation, whereas cDC2s induce mainly differentiation of type 2 and type 17 helper T cells [31]. In a clinical trial involving the *Lacticaseibacillus paracasei* strain Shirota, there was no activation of cDC1s, whereas significant activation of cDC2s was observed [32]. Although GCL1815 was suggested to induce cDC activation *in vitro* [22], cDC1s and cDC2s were not classified in that study. Thus, it was unclear whether GCL1815 induces activation of one or both. In the present study, GCL1815 was found to specifically induce cDC1 activation, suggesting that GCL1815 enhances the induction of cytotoxic T lymphocytes via antigen presentation to $CD8^+$ T cells by cDC1s, ultimately promoting the elimination of virus-infected cells.

The activation of pDCs and cDC1s by GCL1815 was suggested to promote the production of IL-12 (Table 6). cDC1s are well known to induce type 1 helper T cell differentiation and promote the activation of NK cells and macrophages via IL-12. Furthermore, IL-12 is also known to be produced by pDCs [33] and to enhance the cytotoxic activity of $CD8^+$ T cells [34]. The enhancement of IL-12 production via cDC1s by lactic acid bacteria has been confirmed *in vivo* using *Lacticaseibacillus rhamnosus* CRL1505. Namely, *L. rhamnosus* CRL1505 induced the expression of $CD11c^+CD103^+$ DCs and $CD11c^+CD11b^{high}$ DCs, and increased IL-12 production from $CD11c^+CD103^+$ DCs [27,35]. GCL1815 was also found to promote the production of IL-12 by DCs *in vitro* [22]. In the present study, IL-12 levels tended to be higher compared with the control. Thus, IL-12 production might be promoted through GCL1815-induced activation of pDCs and cDC1s, which may promote cytotoxic activity in NK cells and $CD8^+$ T cells. In this study, there were no significant differences in the expression of cell surface markers on NK cells or $CD8^+$ T cells between the GCL1815 and control, although their expression was higher in the GCL1815 group after intake. For instance, a clinical trial with a larger sample size than this study reported a significant increase in $CD8^+$ T cells along with a reduction in cold episodes [11]. Because the sample size in this study was insufficient, there may have been variability between samples, which might be one of the reasons why significant differences in the expression of surface markers on these cells could not be confirmed.

GCL1815-induced activation of pDCs is thought to further enhance the aforementioned cDC1 function. pDCs are important for cDC function. As reported *in vivo*, when pDCs were absent, cDCs did not produce IL-12 [36]. As reported *in vitro*, bacterial stimulation caused pDCs to mature, thereby promoting cDC activation [37]. It was also reported that pDCs might induce cDC1 migration to the site of infection early in viral infection [38]. It is considered that pDCs activated by GCL1815 reinforce the ability of cDC1s to uptake and present viral antigens, and that the combined action of pDCs and cDC1s promote an immune response to viral infection, thereby suppressing the onset of the common cold.

The study had several limitations. Regarding DC activation, the change in the expression of surface markers on pDCs from baseline was significantly higher in the GCL1815 group compared with the placebo group after intake. In contrast, despite considerable variability, the change in the expression of surface markers on cDC1s showed a tendency to be higher in the GCL1815 group compared with the placebo group after intake. Meanwhile, a significant increase in the expression of surface markers on cDC1s was observed after GCL1815 intake compared with before, and the expression of surface markers on cDC1s was significantly higher in the GCL1815 group compared with the placebo group after intake, suggesting that GCL1815 can induce cDC1 activation. In addition, the expression of surface markers on cDC2s decreased in both the placebo group and GCL1815 group after intake compared with before, but the change from baseline was similar between the two groups. Therefore, although the cause of the decrease in the expression of surface markers on cDC2s after intake of GCL1815 was not clear, it was not considered to be the result of GCL1815 intake. Furthermore, symptoms were recorded based on the participants' self-recognition. Thus, for a more objective assessment of cold prevention, it will be necessary in future studies to conduct tests that include measurements of body temperature and to obtain a medical diagnosis. Further investigation into the effect of GCL1815 in suppressing the onset of the common cold via DC activation is expected.

5. Conclusions

This study verified that intake of GCL1815 reduces the incidence of common cold symptoms and activates immune cells. Intake of GCL1815 for 8 weeks significantly induced activation of both pDCs and cDC1s and significantly reduced the cumulative incidence days of common cold symptoms in adults aged 20 to <65 years. These results suggest the possibility that continuous intake of GCL1815 may provide a preventive effect against the onset of the common cold in healthy adults. It is expected that GCL1815 will help to maintain daily physical condition by promoting two types of DC activation, which in turn will improve labor productivity in workers, reduce the severity of colds in the elderly, and reduce school absenteeism in children, thereby benefiting the lives of people of all ages.

Supplementary Materials: The following supporting information can be downloaded at: https://www.mdpi.com/article/10.3390/nu17010101/s1, Figure S1: T-scores of Profile of Mood States 2nd edition, Table S1: Changes in expression levels of surface markers on immune cells and cytokine concentrations, Table S2: Safety assessment.

Author Contributions: Conceptualization, H.W. and T.M.; Methodology, H.W. and T.M.; Validation, H.W.; Investigation, H.W. and T.M.; Writing-original draft preparation, H.W.; Writing-review and editing, H.W., Y.S., N.A. and Y.I.; Formal Analysis, H.W.; Visualization, H.W.; Supervision, Y.I. All authors have read and agreed to the published version of the manuscript.

Funding: This study received no external funding.

Institutional Review Board Statement: This study was conducted according to the guidelines laid down in the Declaration of Helsinki and all procedures involving patients were approved by the Clinical Research Ethics Committee of Kobuna Orthopedics Clinic (approval date: 8 September 2022; approval number: MK-2209-01). The secondary use of surplus samples was approved by the Clinical Research Ethics Committee of Ezaki Glico Co., Ltd. (approval date: 8 September 2023; approval number: 2023-27).

Informed Consent Statement: Informed consent was obtained from all subjects involved in the study.

Data Availability Statement: Datasets generated during the current study and/or analyzed during the current study are available from the responsible author upon reasonable request.

Acknowledgments: The authors would like to thank the staff of the R&D Laboratory, Ezaki Glico Co., Ltd., for preparing the test samples for the clinical trial.

Conflicts of Interest: H.W., T.M., Y.S., and N.A. are employees of Ezaki Glico Co., Ltd. Y.I. reports no conflict of interest in this work.

References

1. Falsey, A.R.; Walsh, E.E. Respiratory syncytial virus infection in elderly adults. *Drugs Aging* **2005**, *22*, 577–587. [CrossRef] [PubMed]
2. World Health Organization. Global Influenza Strategy 2019 to 2030. Available online: https://www.who.int/publications/i/item/9789241515320 (accessed on 18 September 2024).
3. Molinari, N.A.M.; Ortega-Sanchez, I.R.; Messonnier, M.L.; Thompson, W.W.; Wortley, P.M.; Weintraub, E.; Bridges, C.B. The annual impact of seasonal influenza in the US: Measuring disease burden and costs. *Vaccine* **2007**, *25*, 5086–5096. [CrossRef] [PubMed]
4. Fendrick, A.M.; Monto, A.S.; Nightengale, B.; Sarnes, M. The economic burden of non-influenza-related viral respiratory tract infection in the United States. *Arch. Intern. Med.* **2003**, *163*, 487–494. [CrossRef] [PubMed]
5. Adamson, C.S.; Chibale, K.; Goss, R.J.M.; Jaspars, M.; Newman, D.J.; Dorrington, R.A. Antiviral drug discovery: Preparing for the next pandemic. *Chem. Soc. Rev.* **2021**, *50*, 3647–3655. [CrossRef] [PubMed]
6. Monto, A.S. Epidemiology of viral respiratory infections. *Am. J. Med.* **2002**, *112*, 4–12. [CrossRef]
7. Mammas, I.N.; Drysdale, S.B.; Rath, B.; Theordoridou, M.; Papaioannou, G.; Papatheodoropoulou, A.; Koutsounaki, E.; Koutsaftiki, C.; Kozanidou, E.; Achtsidis, V.; et al. Update on current views and advances on RSV infection (Review). *Int. J. Mol. Med.* **2020**, *46*, 509–520. [CrossRef]
8. Wu, D.; Lewis, E.D.; Pae, M.; Meydani, S.N. Nutritional modulation of immune function: Analysis of evidence, mechanisms, and clinical relevance. *Front. Immunol.* **2019**, *9*, 3160. [CrossRef]
9. Berggren, A.; Ahrén, I.L.; Larsson, N.; Önning, G. Randomised, double-blind and placebo-controlled study using new probiotic lactobacilli for strengthening the body immune defence against viral infections. *Eur. J. Nutr.* **2011**, *50*, 203–210. [CrossRef]
10. Tavares-Silva, E.; Caris, A.V.; Santos, S.A.; Ravacci, G.R.; Thomatieli-Santos, R.V. Effect of multi-strain probiotic supplementation on URTI symptoms and cytokine production by monocytes after a marathon race: A randomized, double-blind, placebo study. *Nutrients* **2021**, *13*, 1478. [CrossRef]
11. de Vrese, M.; Winkler, P.; Rautenberg, P.; Harder, T.; Noah, C.; Laue, C.; Ott, S.; Hampe, J.; Schreiber, S.; Heller, K.; et al. Effect of *Lactobacillus gasseri* PA 16/8, *Bifidobacterium longum* SP 07/3, *B. bifidum* MF 20/5 on common cold episodes: A double blind, randomized, controlled trial. *Clin. Nutr.* **2005**, *24*, 481–491. [CrossRef]
12. Kato-Kataoka, A.; Nishida, K.; Takada, M.; Suda, K.; Kawai, M.; Shimizu, K.; Kushiro, A.; Hoshi, R.; Watanabe, O.; Igarashi, T.; et al. Fermented milk containing *Lactobacillus casei* strain Shirota prevents the onset of physical symptoms in medical students under academic examination stress. *Benef. Microbes* **2016**, *7*, 153–156. [CrossRef] [PubMed]
13. Nagao, F.; Nakayama, M.; Muto, T.; Okumura, K. Effects of a fermented milk drink containing *Lactobacillus casei* strain Shirota on the immune system in healthy human subjects. *Biosci. Biotechnol. Biochem.* **2000**, *64*, 2706–2708. [CrossRef] [PubMed]
14. Murphy, T.L.; Grajales-Reyes, G.E.; Wu, X.; Tussiwand, R.; Briseño, C.G.; Iwata, A.; Kretzer, N.M.; Durai, V.; Murphy, K.M. Transcriptional control of dendritic cell development. *Annu. Rev. Immunol.* **2016**, *34*, 93–119. [CrossRef] [PubMed]
15. Siegal, F.P.; Kadowaki, N.; Shodell, M.; Fitzgerald-Bocarsly, P.A.; Shah, K.; Ho, S.; Antonenko, S.; Liu, Y.J. The nature of the principal type 1 interferon-producing cells in human blood. *Science* **1999**, *284*, 1835–1837. [CrossRef]
16. Trinchieri, G. Type I interferon: Friend or foe? *J. Exp. Med.* **2010**, *207*, 2053–2063. [CrossRef]
17. Cai, S.; Kandasamy, M.; Rahmat, J.N.; Tham, S.M.; Bay, B.H.; Lee, Y.K.; Mahendran, R. *Lactobacillus rhamnosus* GG activation of dendritic cells and neutrophils depends on the dose and time of exposure. *J. Immunol. Res.* **2016**, *2016*, 7402760. [CrossRef]
18. Hatakka, K.; Savilahti, E.; Pönkä, A.; Meurman, J.H.; Poussa, T.; Näse, L.; Saxelin, M.; Korpela, R. Effect of long term consumption of probiotic milk on infections in children attending day care centres: Double blind, randomised trial. *BMJ* **2001**, *322*, 1327. [CrossRef]
19. Jounai, K.; Ikado, K.; Sugimura, T.; Ano, Y.; Braun, J.; Fujiwara, D. Spherical lactic acid bacteria activate plasmacytoid dendritic cells immunomodulatory function via TLR9-dependent crosstalk with myeloid dendritic cells. *PLoS ONE* **2012**, *7*, e32588. [CrossRef]
20. Sugimura, T.; Takahashi, H.; Jounai, K.; Ohshio, K.; Kanayama, M.; Tazumi, K.; Tanihata, Y.; Miura, Y.; Fujiwara, D.; Yamamoto, N. Effects of oral intake of plasmacytoid dendritic cells-stimulative lactic acid bacterial strain on pathogenesis of influenza-like illness and immunological response to influenza virus. *Br. J. Nutr.* **2015**, *114*, 727–733. [CrossRef]

21. Christensen, H.R.; Frøkiær, H.; Pestka, J.J. Lactobacilli differentially modulate expression of cytokines and maturation surface markers in murine dendritic cells. *J. Immunol.* **2002**, *168*, 171–178. [CrossRef]
22. Tsuruno, K.; Mawatari, T.; Tanaka-Azuma, Y.; Yamatsu, A.; Tanabe, S. Screening of novel lactic acid bacteria with high induction of IgA production, dendritic cell activation, and IL-12 production. *Biosci. Biotechnol. Biochem.* **2024**. [CrossRef] [PubMed]
23. Diamond, M.S.; Kinder, M.; Matsushita, H.; Mashayekhi, M.; Dunn, G.P.; Archambault, J.M.; Lee, H.; Arthur, C.D.; White, J.M.; Kalinke, U.; et al. Type I interferon is selectively required by dendritic cells for immune rejection of tumors. *J. Exp. Med.* **2011**, *208*, 1989–2003. [CrossRef]
24. Sugimura, T.; Jounai, K.; Ohshio, K.; Tanaka, T.; Suwa, M.; Fujiwara, D. Immunomodulatory effect of *Lactococcus lactis* JCM5805 on human plasmacytoid dendritic cells. *Clin. Immunol.* **2013**, *149*, 509–518. [CrossRef]
25. Schlitzer, A.; Zhang, W.; Song, M.; Ma, X. Recent advances in understanding dendritic cell development, classification, and phenotype. *F1000Research* **2018**, *7*, 1558. [CrossRef]
26. Bramley, T.J.; Lerner, D.; Sarnes, M. Productivity losses related to the common cold. *J. Occup. Environ. Med.* **2002**, *44*, 822–829. [CrossRef]
27. Kitazawa, H.; Villena, J. Modulation of respiratory TLR3-anti-viral response by probiotic microorganisms: Lessons learned from *Lactobacillus rhamnosus* CRL1505. *Front. Immunol.* **2014**, *5*, 201. [CrossRef]
28. Villena, J.C.; Salva, M.S.; Núñez, M.S.; Corzo, J.; Tolaba, R.; Faedda, J.; Font, G.M.; Alvarez, G.S. Probiotics for everyone! The novel immunobiotic *Lactobacillus rhamnosus* CRL1505 and the beginning of social probiotic programs in Argentina. *Int. J. Biotechnol. Wellness Ind.* **2012**, *1*, 189–198.
29. Villadangos, J.A.; Young, L. Antigen-presentation properties of plasmacytoid dendritic cells. *Immunity* **2008**, *29*, 352–361. [CrossRef]
30. Dalod, M.; Hamilton, T.; Salomon, R.; Salazar-Mather, T.P.; Henry, S.C.; Hamilton, J.D.; Biron, C.A. Dendritic cell responses to early murine cytomegalovirus infection: Subset functional specialization and differential regulation by interferon α/β. *J. Exp. Med.* **2003**, *197*, 885–898. [CrossRef]
31. Kumar, S.; Jeong, Y.; Ashraf, M.U.; Bae, Y.-S. Dendritic cell-mediated Th2 immunity and immune disorders. *Int. J. Mol. Sci.* **2019**, *20*, 2159. [CrossRef]
32. Naito, T.; Morikawa, M.; Yamamoto-Fujimura, M.; Iwata, A.; Maki, A.; Kato-Nagaoka, N.; Oana, K.; Kiyoshima-Shibata, J.; Matsuura, Y.; Kaji, R.; et al. Diverse impact of a probiotic strain, *Lacticaseibacillus paracasei* Shirota, on peripheral mononuclear phagocytic cells in healthy Japanese office workers: A randomized, double-blind, controlled trial. *Biosci. Microbiota Food Health* **2023**, *42*, 65–72. [CrossRef] [PubMed]
33. Matsui, T.; Connolly, J.E.; Michnevitz, M.; Chaussabel, D.; Yu, C.-I.; Glaser, C.; Tindle, S.; Pypaert, M.; Freitas, H.; Piqueras, B.; et al. CD2 distinguishes two subsets of human plasmacytoid dendritic cells with distinct phenotype and functions. *J. Immunol.* **2009**, *182*, 6815–6823. [CrossRef] [PubMed]
34. Mehrotra, P.T.; Wu, D.; Crim, J.A.; Mostowski, H.S.; Siegel, J.P. Effects of IL-12 on the generation of cytotoxic activity in human $CD8^+$ T lymphocytes. *J. Immunol.* **1993**, *151*, 2444–2452. [CrossRef] [PubMed]
35. Villena, J.; Chiba, E.; Tomosada, Y.; Salva, S.; Marranzino, G.; Kitazawa, H.; Alvarez, S. Orally administered *Lactobacillus rhamnosus* modulates the respiratory immune response triggered by the viral pathogen-associated molecular pattern poly(I:C). *BMC Immunol.* **2012**, *13*, 53. [CrossRef]
36. Kuwajima, S.; Sato, T.; Ishida, K.; Tada, H.; Tezuka, H.; Ohteki, T. Interleukin 15-dependent crosstalk between conventional and plasmacytoid dendritic cells is essential for CpG-induced immune activation. *Nat. Immunol.* **2006**, *7*, 740–746. [CrossRef]
37. Piccioli, D.; Sammicheli, C.; Tavarini, S.; Nuti, S.; Frigimelica, E.; Manetti, A.G.O.; Nuccitelli, A.; Aprea, S.; Valentini, S.; Borgogni, E.; et al. Human plasmacytoid dendritic cells are unresponsive to bacterial stimulation and require a novel type of cooperation with myeloid dendritic cells for maturation. *Blood* **2009**, *113*, 4232–4239. [CrossRef]
38. Brewitz, A.; Eickhoff, S.; Dähling, S.; Quast, T.; Bedoui, S.; Kroczek, R.A.; Kurts, C.; Garbi, N.; Barchet, W.; Iannacone, M.; et al. $CD8^+$ T cells orchestrate pDC-XCR1+ dendritic cell spatial and functional cooperativity to optimize priming. *Immunity* **2017**, *46*, 205–219. [CrossRef]

nutrients

MDPI

Article

Lactobacillus delbrueckii subsp. *lactis* CKDB001 Ameliorates Metabolic Complications in High-Fat Diet-Induced Obese Mice

Hyunsoo Jang [1,†], Hyunchae Joung [1,2,†], Jaeryang Chu [2], Minseo Cho [1], Yeon-Woo Kim [1], Kyung Hwan Kim [2], Chang Hun Shin [3], Jisu Lee [1,*] and Jung-Heun Ha [1,4,*]

1 Department of Food Science and Nutrition, Dankook University, Cheonan 31116, Republic of Korea
2 Microbiome Research Laboratory, Chong Kun Dang Bio (CKDBiO) Research Institute, Ansan 15604, Republic of Korea
3 Chong Kun Dang Bio (CKDBiO) Research Institute, Ansan 15604, Republic of Korea
4 Research Center for Industrialization of Natural Neutralization, Dankook University, Yongin 16890, Republic of Korea
* Correspondence: js72220247@dankook.ac.kr (J.L.); ha@dankook.ac.kr (J.-H.H.); Tel.: +82-41-550-6243 (J.L.); +82-41-550-3479 (J.-H.H.)
† These authors contributed equally to this work.

Abstract: Background/Objectives: Functional probiotics, particularly *Lactobacillus delbrueckii* subsp. *lactis* CKDB001, have shown potential as a therapeutic option for metabolic dysfunction-associated steatotic liver disease (MASLD). However, their effects have not been confirmed in in vivo systems. Here, we investigated the effects of *L. delbrueckii* subsp. *lactis* CKDB001 on insulin resistance, dyslipidemia, MASLD, and lipid metabolism in a murine model of high-fat diet (HFD)-induced obesity. Methods: The mice were divided into four groups (n = 12 per group)—normal chow diet (NCD), high fat diet (HFD), HFD with *L. delbrueckii* subsp. *lactis* CKDB001 (LL), and HFD with resmetirom (positive control (PC), a thyroid receptor β agonist). The experimental animals were fed NCD or HFD for 12 weeks, followed by an additional 12-week oral treatment with LL or resmetirom. Results: LL supplementation reduced body weight, insulin levels, and HOMA-IR compared with those in the HFD group, indicating improved insulin sensitivity. Additionally, LL reduced serum triglyceride (TG) levels without affecting total cholesterol (TC) levels. HFD consumption increased liver weight and hepatic TG and TC levels, indicating ectopic fat accumulation; however, LL supplementation reversed these changes, indicating a liver-specific effect on cholesterol metabolism. Furthermore, LL administration attenuated NAFLD activity scores, reduced hepatic fibrosis, improved liver function markers (aspartate aminotransferase), and enhanced Adenosine monophosphate-activated protein kinase (AMPK) phosphorylation. However, LL did not considerably affect the expression of genes related to lipid metabolism. In epididymal adipose tissue, LL treatment reduced leptin levels but had no effect on adiponectin; additionally, histological analysis showed an increase in adipocyte size, potentially linked to enhanced energy metabolism. Conclusions: Collectively, these findings suggest that LL could be a promising therapeutic candidate for improving insulin sensitivity, reducing hepatic lipid accumulation, and mitigating MASLD.

Keywords: MASLD; probiotics; *Lactobacillus delbrueckii* subsp. *lactis* CKDB001

1. Introduction

Obesity, a condition characterized by the accumulation of excess white adipose tissue (WAT), resulting in a body mass index (BMI) ≥ 30 kg/m^2, has become a global epidemic with major implications for public health [1]. Over the past few decades, the prevalence of obesity has considerably increased, driven by factors such as sedentary lifestyles [2] and the widespread adoption of Western dietary patterns [3], particularly high-fat diets (HFDs). According to the World Health Organization (WHO), the number of individuals with obesity has nearly tripled since 1975, with current estimates suggesting that approximately 1.3 billion adults worldwide are overweight, and more than 600 million of them are obese [4]. Obesity is not only an issue of excess weight but also a major risk factor for several chronic diseases. Excessive body fat accumulation increases the risk of developing various complications, including cardiovascular diseases (CVD) [5], type 2 diabetes (T2D) [6], hypertension [7], and cancer [8,9]. To address these worsening health outcomes, analyzing their underlying mechanisms and developing effective preventive strategies to mitigate the impact of obesity on overall physiological homeostasis is crucial.

One such remarkable impact is the negative effect of obesity on hepatic homeostasis. Obesity is a major risk factor for the development of non-alcoholic fatty liver disease (NAFLD), a condition characterized by excessive fat accumulation in the liver [10]. NAFLD occurs when ectopic fat builds up in the liver without the influence of alcohol consumption and may progress to more severe pathologic conditions such as hepatitis, fibrosis, and cirrhosis [11]. Recently, NAFLD was renamed as metabolic-associated fatty liver disease (MASLD) to emphasize the strong connection to metabolic abnormalities beyond just fat accumulation independent of alcohol consumption [12]. MASLD is estimated to affect approximately 30% of the global adult population, and the 15% increase in MASLD prevalence between 1991 and 2019 corresponds with the rise in obesity and obesity-related diseases [13,14]. The condition elevates the risk of developing hepatomegaly, excessive ectopic WAT accumulation in the liver, insulin resistance, dyslipidemia, and reduced lipid metabolism [15–17].

Currently, lifestyle changes involving dietary regulation and exercise are the primary preventive and therapeutic options for mitigating the MASLD caused by obesity. Although various therapeutic drugs have been released in the clinical market—such as pioglitazone, which improves insulin sensitivity through PPARγ activation [18,19]; GLP-1 receptor agonists such as liraglutide, which aid in weight loss by modulating appetite [20,21]; and SGLT2 inhibitors such as empagliflozin, which can lower blood glucose [22,23]—these medications are often associated with several side effects. For instance, pioglitazone can cause weight gain, fluid retention, and increased risk of heart failure [18,19]; liraglutide may cause nausea and vomiting; and empagliflozin may increase the risk of urinary tract infections and dehydration [21]. Given the challenges in developing effective pharmaceutical treatments, it is necessary to explore natural materials with beneficial effects and few side effects. However, medications alone cannot serve as preventive measures against obesity-induced MASLD; therefore, preventive approaches such as consuming functional nutraceuticals and probiotics are necessary.

Probiotics are defined by the Food and Agriculture Organization and WHO as "live microorganisms that, when administered in adequate amounts, confer a health benefit on the host" [24]. Healthy gut microbiota are essential for proper metabolic functions and homeostasis, playing a crucial role in the catabolism and anabolism of energy derived from diet [25,26]. Accordingly, the use of probiotics to selectively regulate the gut microbiota has emerged as a potential treatment strategy for managing obesity. Probiotics reduce WAT mass and positively regulate metabolic homeostasis [27]. For instance, studies on murine models of obesity induced by an HFD have demonstrated that probiotic treatment can alter bile acid composition and kinetics, thereby ameliorating insulin resistance [28]. Additionally, probiotic treatment has been found to alleviate dysbiosis caused by a high-fat diet by reducing total cholesterol (TC), triglycerides (TG), and LDL-C levels, as well as mitigating dyslipidemia [29]. While numerous studies have documented the effects of probiotics on obesity and related disorders, research on using probiotics to specifically modulate obesity and its associated metabolic complications remains at an early stage.

Among probiotics, the genus *Lactobacillus*, comprising Gram-positive, thermophilic bacteria, is particularly noteworthy for its economic importance in industrial applications. *Lactobacillus* species are notable for their ability to inhibit the growth of competing microorganisms by depleting available carbon sources and rapidly fermenting organic acids as metabolites [30]. Studies have shown that certain *Lactobacillus* strains are health-promoting and exhibit low levels of antibiotic resistance; thus, they are widely used as probiotic treatments in animal models of obesity. Among the 42 species within *Lactobacillus*, *L. delbrueckii* subsp. *lactis* is particularly important for the commercial production of fermented products such as yogurt and cheese [31]. Previous studies have demonstrated that *L. delbrueckii* subsp. *lactis* can reduce fasting blood glucose levels, inhibit the growth of pathogenic bacteria, and ameliorate ulcerative colitis [32–34]. Furthermore, we recently demonstrated the safety and effectiveness of *L. delbrueckii* subsp. *lactis* CKDB001 as a probiotic and potential therapeutic candidate for MASLD [35]. *L. delbrueckii* subsp. *lactis* CKDB001 reduces lipid accumulation in hepatic cells by promoting the expression of genes involved in fatty acid oxidation and suppressing that of those involved in fatty acid uptake [36]. Given its crucial role in reducing lipid accumulation in vitro, we aimed to evaluate the impact of *L. delbrueckii* subsp. *lactis* CKDB001 in vivo, which remains largely unexplored. Specifically, we examined the influence of *L. delbrueckii* subsp. *lactis* CKDB001 on insulin resistance, dyslipidemia, MASLD, and lipid metabolism in an HFD-induced obese murine experimental model.

2. Materials and Methods

2.1. Preparation for Probiotic Powder

Lactobacillus delbrueckii subsp. *lactis* CKDB001 (*L. lactis* CKDB001, KCTC 14149BP) was isolated from fermented milk. The *L. lactis* CKDB001 was inoculated into a flask containing de Man, Rogosa, and Sharpe (MRS) broth (BD/Difco, Franklin Lakes, NJ, USA) and incubated under facultative anaerobic conditions at 37 °C for 24 h. Stock solutions were prepared by mixing the cultured MRS broth with an equal volume of a 20% glycerol solution and then stored at −80 °C until use.

The seed culture was grown in a flask with MRS broth at 37 °C for 24 h. The cultured broth was subsequently inoculated into an optimized medium in a mini jar fermenter (Bio Control & Science, MARADO-05D-PS, Xiamen, Fujian, China). Fermentation was conducted at a constant pH of 5.5 to 6.0, maintained automatically by adding NaOH solution (25% *w*/*v*), with agitation at 120 rpm at 37 °C for 16 to 18 h. At the end of fermentation, cells were harvested by centrifugation at 6000 rpm for 10 min (Hanil, Supra R12, Daejeon, Republic of Korea). The resulting cell concentrate (40×) was lyophilized following the manufacturer's instructions (Cooling & Heating System, Lab-Mast 10, Seoul, Republic of Korea). After lyophilization, the colony-forming units (CFU) per gram of probiotic powder were determined using a serial dilution method. For daily use, *L. lactis* CKDB001 was suspended in phosphate-buffered saline (PBS, Bioneer, Daejeon, Republic of Korea) and adjusted to a concentration of 1.0×10^9 CFU per mouse.

2.2. Animal Experiments and Dietary Interventions

Four-week-old male C57BL/6J mice were purchased from DooYeol Biotech (Seoul, Republic of Korea) and housed under controlled conditions with a temperature of 20 ± 2 °C, humidity of 55 ± 5%, and an alternating 12 h light/dark cycle. After a 1-week acclimation period, the mice were divided into the following four groups (n = 12 per group): NCD (normal chow diet, based on the AIN-93G formulation; 10% of energy from fat), HFD (60% of energy from fat; Research Diets Inc., New Brunswick, NJ, USA), LL (HFD with *L. delbrueckii* subsp. *lactis* CKDB001), and PC (positive control, HFD with resmetirom). The experimental animals were fed either an NCD or HFD for 12 weeks. All the HFD-fed groups were provided with drinking water containing fructose at a concentration of 12.5%. After feeding an NCD or HFD to each group for 12 weeks, *L. delbrueckii* subsp. *lactis* CKDB001 or resmetirom was additionally administered orally for another 12 weeks. The

LL group mice received *L. delbrueckii* subsp. *lactis* CKDB001 in PBS containing probiotic strains at 1.0×10^9 CFU/g once daily for 12 weeks. The PC group was treated with resmetirom (MedChemExpress, Beytelsbach, Germany) at a dosage of 3 mg/kg (Figure 1). The resmetirom dose was selected based on previous studies [37–39]. The NCD and HFD groups were administered the same amount of PBS instead of the treatments. Throughout the experiment, water and food were provided ad libitum. After a 12 h fasting period, the mice were sacrificed via thoracotomy after CO_2 narcosis. Whole blood samples were collected via cardiac puncture and centrifuged at 3000× *g* and 4 °C for 20 min to obtain the serum. The liver, epididymal adipose tissue (EAT), subcutaneous adipose tissue (SAT), and mesenteric adipose tissue (MAT) were immediately weighed and stored at −80 °C until further analysis. All murine experimental procedures were approved by the Institutional Animal Care and Use Committee of Dankook University (No. DKU 2023-22-085).

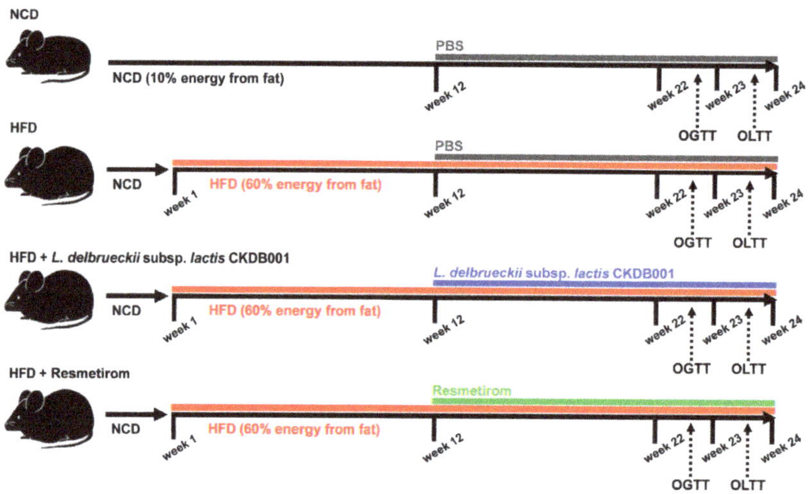

Figure 1. Overview of experimental design. Four-week-old male C57BL/6J mice (n = 12 per group) were subjected to the following dietary interventions for 24 weeks: normal chow diet (NCD), high-fat diet (HFD), HFD with *L. delbrueckii* subsp. *lactis* CKDB001 (LL), and HFD with resmetirom (positive control). Abbreviation: HFD, High-fat diet; LL, *L. delbrueckii* subsp. *lactis* CKDB001; NCD, normal chow diet; OGTT, Oral glucose tolerance test; OLTT, Oral lipid tolerance test; PBS, Phosphate buffered saline.

2.3. Oral Glucose Tolerance Test (OGTT) and Oral Lipid Tolerance Test (OLTT)

Following 22 weeks of dietary intervention, an OGTT was conducted on the mice after a 12 h fast. Briefly, a glucose solution (MB Cell, Seoul, Republic of Korea) was orally administered at a dose of 1 g/kg, and blood samples were collected from the tail vein 30, 60, 90, 120, and 240 min after glucose administration. Thereafter, blood glucose levels were measured using an Accu-Chek instant blood glucose meter (Accu-Chek, Seoul, Republic of Korea).

An OLTT was conducted on the mice after 12 h of fasting following 23 weeks of dietary intervention. Briefly, the mice were orally administered olive oil (Sigma-Aldrich, St. Louis, MO, USA) at a dose of 5 mL/kg, after which blood samples were collected from the tail vein 30, 60, 90, 120, and 240 min post-administration. Blood lipid levels were analyzed using Barogen triglyceride test strips and a Barogen lipid meter (Handok, Anseong, Republic of Korea) [40].

2.4. Analysis of Metabolic Parameters in the Serum

Hepatic function was evaluated by quantifying the serum levels of alanine aminotransferase (ALT) and aspartate aminotransferase (AST) using commercial kits (ALT assay, AST assay kit; Embiel, Gunpo, Republic of Korea). Additionally, the serum levels of triglycerides (TGs; Asan, Hwaseong, Republic of Korea), TC (Asan), HDL-C (Asan), and glucose (Crystal Chem, Downers Grove, IL, USA) were measured using commercial kits following established protocols. Low-density lipoprotein cholesterol (LDL-C) [41,42] and cardiac risk factor (CRF) calculations [6] were performed based on prior research.

2.5. Histopathological Evaluation of the Liver and EAT

Liver and EAT samples were fixed using 10% formalin and embedded in paraffin. Thereafter, sections were prepared for analysis using hematoxylin and eosin (H&E) and sirius red staining. Fatty liver classification followed the non-alcoholic steatohepatitis (NASH) clinical research network scoring system for NAFLD, with grades ranging from 0 to 3 based on the extent of steatosis [43]. Inflammation was graded from 0 to 3 based on foci per field. The NAFLD activity score (NAS) was calculated based on Kleiner's criteria, which consider steatosis, lobular inflammation, and ballooning. Patients were grouped into the following NAS categories for statistical analysis: NAS 0–2 (probable no NASH), NAS 3–4 (borderline), and NAS 5–8 (probable NASH) [44]. In the EAT, macrophage infiltration and adipocyte size were quantified using ImageJ software (imagej.net, NIH, Bethesda, MD, USA). The scoring criteria for each classification are shown in Table 1.

Table 1. Scoring system for histopathological assessment.

Item	Score	Extent
NAS	0	<5%
	1	5–33%
	2	34–66%
	3	>66%
Fibrosis	0	None
	1	Perisinusoidal or periportal
	1a	Mild, zone 3, perisinusoidal
	1b	Moderate, zone 3, perisinusoidal
	1c	Portal/periportal
	2	Perisinusoidal and portal/periportal
	3	Bridging fibrosis
	4	Cirrhosis
Macrophage infiltration	0	None
	1	Minimal (<10%)
	2	Mild (10–25%)
	3	Moderate (26–50%)
	4	Marked (>51%)

Abbreviation: NAS, non-alcoholic fatty liver disease activity score.

2.6. Quantification of Hepatic Lipid Levels

Hepatic lipids were extracted using a slightly modified version of the Bligh and Dyer method [45]. To quantify TG and TC in the liver, approximately 0.1 g of liver was homogenized in a chloroform (1:2, v/v) solution, followed by centrifugation at 805× g for 15 min. Next, the lower phase was carefully collected using a Pasteur pipette, and 1 mL n-hexane (3:2, v/v) was added to solubilize the lipids. The concentrations of TG and TC were measured using commercial kits (Embiel), and the results are expressed as mg per g of tissue weight.

2.7. Enzyme-Linked Immunosorbent Assay (ELISA)

An ELISA was used to quantify the serum levels of insulin (Mercodia, Uppsala, Sweden) and adipokine (leptin and adiponectin) in the EAT. EAT was treated using radioimmunoprecipitation assay (RIPA) buffer (ATTO, Tokyo, Japan) containing protease and phosphatase inhibitors (Thermo Fisher Scientific, Waltham, MA, USA). Thereafter, the lysates were analyzed using commercial ELISA kits (R&D Systems, Minneapolis, MN, USA). ELISA procedures were conducted according to the manufacturer's instructions. The homeostatic model assessment of insulin resistance (HOMA-IR) was performed using the following established formula: (HOMA-IR = serum insulin (μg/L) × serum glucose (mg/dL)/405 [5].

2.8. Quantitative Reverse Transcription-Polymerase Chain Reaction (qRT-PCR)

For mRNA analysis of the liver and EAT, total RNA was extracted using the NucleoZoL reagent (Macherey-Nagel, GmbH & Co. KG, Duren, Germany) as described previously [46]. Subsequently, 2 μg mRNA was used to synthesize cDNA using an iScriptTM cDNA synthesis kit (Bio-Rad Laboratories, Hercules, CA, USA). Afterward, the cDNA was combined with iQTM SYBR Green Supermix (Bio-Rad Laboratories), and qRT-PCR was performed using a CFX96 Real-Time PCR Detection System (Bio-Rad Laboratories). The relative expression of each gene was determined using the 2ΔΔCT method, with mouse Gapdh serving as the reference gene. The primers used in the qRT-PCR targeted the expression of lipolytic and adipogenic enzymes. The primers used are listed in Table 2 and previous studies [47].

Table 2. qRT-PCR primer sequences (5′ to 3′).

Transcript	Forward	Reverse
Acox1	CAGGAAGAGCAAGGAAGTGG	CCTTTCTGGCTGATCCCATA
Cpt1α	CTCCGCCTGAGCCATGAAG	CACCAGTGATGATGCCATTCT
Pparα	GTACGGTGTGTATGAAGCCATCTT	GCCGTACGCGATCAGCAT
Atgl	TGTGGCCTCATTCCTCCTAC	TCGTGGATGTTGGTGGAGCT
Hsl	GCTGGGCTGTCAAGCACTGT	GTAACTGGGTAGGCTGCCAT
Mgl	CGGACTTCCAAGTTTTTGTCAGA	GCAGCCACTAGGATGGAGATG
Acc	TGGACAGACTGATCGCAGAGAAAG	TGGAGAGCCCCACACACA
Fas	GGAGGTGGTGATAGCCGGTAT	TGGGTAATCCATAGAGCCCAG
Scd1	TTCTTGCGATACACTCTGGTGC	CGGGATTGAATGTTCTTGTCGT
Dgat1	GAGTCTATCACTCCAGTGGG	GGCGGCACCACAGGTTGACA
Pgc1α	CCCAGGCAGTAGATCCTCTTCAA	CCTTTCGTGCTCATAGGCTTCATA
Srebp1	GCAGCCACCATCTAGCCTG	CAGCAGTGAGTCTGCCTTGAT
Il-1β	GTCACAAGAAACCATGGCACAT	GCCCATCAGAGGCAAGGA
Il-6	CTGCAAGAGACTTCCATCCAGTT	AGGGAAGGCCGTGGTTGT
Tnf- α	GGCTGCCCCGACTACGT	ACTTTCTCCTGGTATGAGATAGCAAAT
Hmg-coa	GGCCCAGTGGTGCGTCTTCC	TGGTCCCACCACCCACGGTT
Ldlr	ACTCATGCAGCAGGAACC	GTCATTTTCACAGTCTAC
Gapdh	CATGGCCTTCCGTGTTCCTA	GCGGCACGTCAGATCCA

Abbreviation: *Acox1*, Peroxisomal acyl-coenzyme A oxidase 1; *Cpt1α*, Carnitine palmitoyl transferase I alpha; *Pparα*, Peroxisome proliferator-activated receptor alpha; *Atgl*, Adipose triglyceride lipase; *Hsl*, Hormone-sensitive lipase; *Mgl*, Monoacylglycerol lipase; *Acc*, Acetyl-CoA carboxylase; *Fas*, Fatty acid synthase; *Scd1*, Stearoyl-CoA 9-desaturase; *Dgat1*, Diacylglycerol O-acyltransferase; *Pgc1α*, Peroxisome proliferator-activated receptor gamma coactivator 1 alpha; *Srebp1c*, Sterol regulatory element-binding protein-1c; *Il*, Interleukin; *Tnf-α*, Tumor necrosis factor alpha; *Hmg-coa*, 3-Hydroxy-3-Methylglutaryl-Coenzyme A; *Ldlr*, Low-Density Lipoprotein Receptor; *Gapdh*, Glyceraldehyde-3-phosphate dehydrogenase.

2.9. Western Blot Analysis

Western blot analysis was conducted based on previous research [48]. Briefly, liver tissue proteins were isolated using a Branson 450 Digital Sonifier Homogenizer (Branson, Danbury, CT, USA) in ice-cold RIPA lysis buffer (ATTO) containing protease and phosphatase inhibitors (Thermo Fisher Scientific). Next, equal amounts of protein (30 μg) were separated using 10% sodium dodecyl sulfate-polyacrylamide gel electrophoresis and transferred onto polyvinylidene difluoride membranes (Bio-Rad Laboratories). After blocking with 5% skim milk (Difco; BD Biosciences, Franklin Lakes, NJ, USA), the membranes were incubated with primary antibodies against phospho-AMP-activated protein kinase

(p-AMPK [#2531]; Cell Signaling Technology, Danvers, MA, USA), total-AMP-activated protein kinase (t-AMPK [#2532]; Cell Signaling Technology), and glyceraldehyde-3-phosphate dehydrogenase (GAPDH [#sc-365062]; Santa Cruz, Dallas, TX, USA) overnight at 4 °C. Subsequently, the membranes were washed and exposed to secondary antibodies for 1 h at room temperature. After secondary antibody treatment, a chemiluminescent substrate solution (Thermo Fisher Scientific) was used for visualization using an Azure Biosystems Imaging System (Azure Biosystems, Dublin, CA, USA). Blot intensity was quantitatively analyzed using ImageJ Software (v.1.8; National Institutes of Health, Bethesda, MD, USA) (Table 3).

Table 3. Antibodies used for Western blot analysis.

Type	Antibody	Dilution Factor	Corporation	Catalog Number
Primary	*p*-AMPK	1:1000	Cell Signaling	2531
	t-AMPK	1:1000	Cell Signaling	2532
	GAPDH	1:2000	Santa Cruz	365,062
Secondary	Anti-rabbit IgG	1:3000	Cell Signaling	7074
	Anti-mouse IgG	1:1000	Cell Signaling	7076

Abbreviation: *p*-AMPK, Phospho-AMP-activated protein kinase; t-AMPK, Total-AMP-activated protein kinase; GAPDH, Glyceraldehyde-3-phosphate dehydrogenase; Anti-rabbit IgG, Peroxidase antibody to rabbit Immunoglobulin G produced in goat; Anti-mouse, Peroxidase antibody to mouse Immunoglobulin G produced in goat.

2.10. Statistical Analysis

The results are reported as means with their corresponding standard deviations (SDs). All figures were generated using GraphPad Prism 5 (GraphPad Software, Inc., San Diego, CA, USA). Statistical analysis was conducted using a one-way ANOVA followed by Tukey's post hoc test, for comparing the NCD and HFD groups. Additionally, comparisons were made among the HFD, LL, and PC groups. The analysis was performed using XLAST 2012 statistical software (Addinsoft Inc., Paris, France). Statistical significance was set at $p < 0.05$ [49].

3. Results

3.1. Effects of LL on Body Weight (BW) and Food Efficiency

Experimental C57BL/6J mice were fed either an NCD or HFD for a total of 24 weeks. After 12 weeks of designated dietary feeding, the mice were orally administered PBS, *L. lactis* CKDB001, or resmetirom to evaluate the effects of *L. lactis* CKDB001 in response to HFD consumption. Changes in BW over the 24-week dietary intervention period are shown in Figure 2A. In the HFD, BW noticeably increased by 4 weeks after dietary intervention. In contrast, BW decreased significantly in the LL group compared with that in the HFD. PC showed a significant reduction in BW compared with that in the HFD group from week 12 onward. Consequently, final BW was higher in the HFD than in the NCD group, whereas it was 0.92- and 0.89-fold lower in the LL and PC groups, respectively, although these differences were not statistically significant (Figure 2B). However, there were no significant differences in daily food intake and energy intake between the groups. According to the food efficiency ratio (FER) assessment, the NCD group had the lowest FER, whereas the HFD group had the highest FER. However, the LL and PC groups had remarkably lower FERs compared with that of the HFD group (Figure 2E).

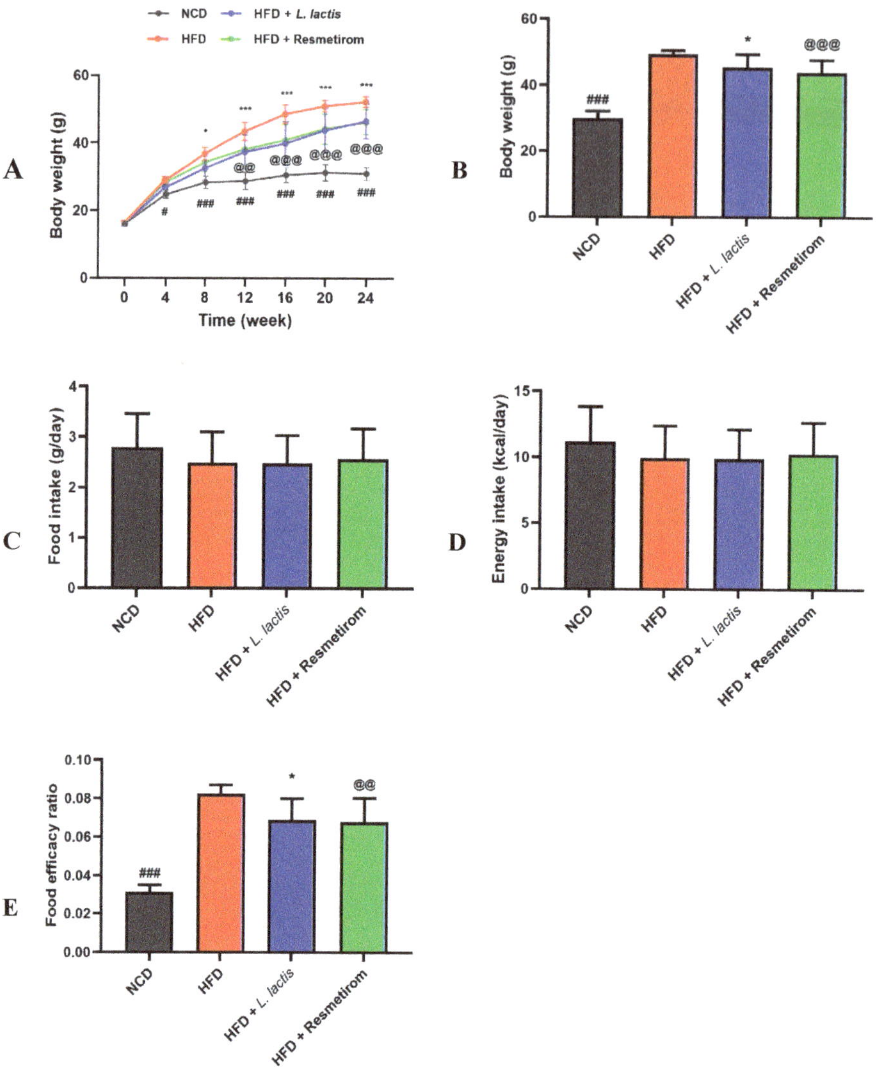

Figure 2. Effects of *L. delbrueckii* subsp. *lactis* CKDB001 on the body weight, final body weight, daily feed intake, energy intake, and food efficiency ratio of mice. The mice were subjected to the following dietary interventions for 24 weeks: normal chow diet (NCD), high-fat diet (HFD), HFD with *L. delbrueckii* subsp. *lactis* CKDB001 (LL), and HFD with resmetirom (positive control). (**A**) Weekly body weight over 24 weeks induced by HFD; (**B**) final body weight; (**C**) daily food intake; (**D**) energy intake; (**E**) food efficiency ratio. Values are presented as mean ± standard deviation (SD), and organ weights are expressed as a percentage of body weight (% of BW). # $p < 0.05$, ### $p < 0.0001$ between NCD and HFD; * $p < 0.05$, *** $p < 0.001$ between HFD and LL; @@ $p < 0.01$, @@@ $p < 0.001$ between HFD and PC.

3.2. Effect of LL on Liver and WAT Weights

In metabolic complications, increased liver weight and excessive adipose tissue accumulation are associated with several health risks, including inflammation, insulin resistance, and dyslipidemia [50]. To assess changes in the weight of central metabolic organs, the weights of the liver and WATs (EAT, SAT, and MAT) were measured and presented in Figure 3 as a percentage of BW. In the HFD group, liver weight was significantly higher than that in the NCD group. However, LL and PC treatment resulted in significantly lower liver weights [0.75- ($p < 0.01$) and 0.63-fold ($p < 0.001$), respectively, compared with that in the HFD group (Figure 3A). In the HFD group, the relative weight of EAT was higher than that of the NCD group. Notably, EAT weight in the LL and PC groups was 1.29- and 1.22-fold higher, respectively, than that in the HFD group ($p < 0.05$; Figure 3B). Furthermore, the weights of SAT, MAT, and total WATs in the HFD group were significantly higher than those in the NCD group ($p < 0.0001$), but they did not significantly differ between the HFD and LL or PC groups (Figure 3C–E). These results suggest that LL consumption could prevent HFD-induced hepatomegaly, but do not markedly affect overall fat weight gain.

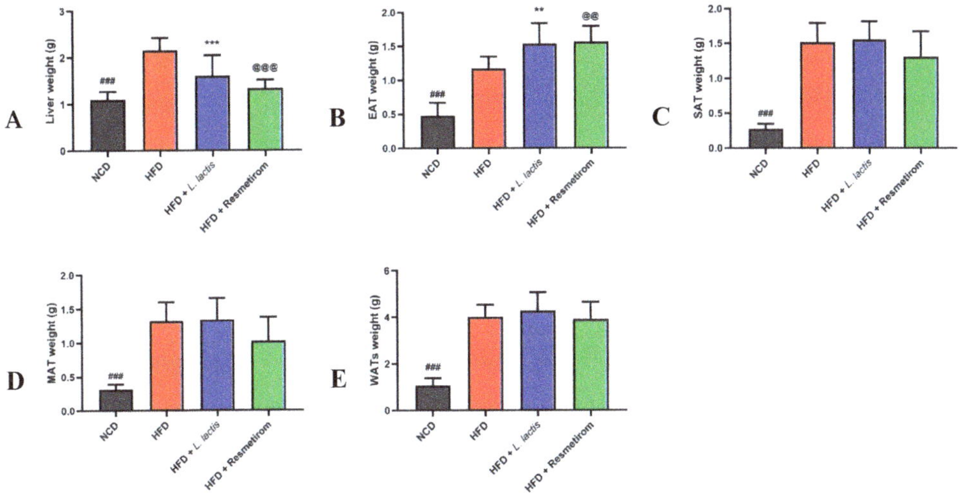

Figure 3. Effects of *L. delbrueckii* subsp. *lactis* CKDB001 on mouse organ weights. The mice were subjected to the following dietary interventions for 24 weeks: normal chow diet (NCD), high-fat diet (HFD), HFD with *L. delbrueckii* subsp. *lactis* CKDB001 (LL), and HFD with resmetirom (positive control). (**A**) Liver, (**B**) EAT, (**C**) SAT, (**D**) MAT, and (**E**) WATs weights. Values are presented as mean ± standard deviation (SD). ### $p < 0.001$ between NCD and HFD; ** $p < 0.01$, *** $p < 0.001$ between HFD and LL; @@ $p < 0.01$, @@@ $p < 0.001$ between HFD and PC. Abbreviation: EAT, epididymal adipose tissue; SAT, subcutaneous adipose tissue; MAT, mesenteric adipose tissue; WAT, white adipose tissue.

3.3. LL Maintains Intact Insulin Sensitivity in HFD-Induced Mice

To assess the impact of LL supplementation on insulin resistance, we conducted OGTTs. The results showed significantly higher glucose levels in the HFD group compared with those in the NCD group, but those in the HFD, LL, and PC groups did not significantly differ (Figure 4A,B). Similarly, the serum glucose levels in the HFD group were significantly higher than those in the NCD group ($p < 0.05$). The serum glucose levels in the LL and PC groups were 0.94- and 0.88-fold lower, respectively, relative to those in the HFD group, but these differences were not significant (Figure 4C). Additionally, the HFD group displayed 10.96-fold higher serum insulin levels than those in the NCD group ($p < 0.001$). However, the insulin levels in the LL and PC groups were 0.64- and 0.60-fold lower than those in the HFD group, respectively ($p < 0.05$; Figure 4D). Consequently, the HOMA-IR calculated from glucose and insulin levels was significantly lower in the NCD group compared with that in the HFD group. Similarly, both LL and PC groups also showed significantly lower levels ($p < 0.05$; Figure 4E). Accordingly, while LL consumption may show potential for improving insulin sensitivity against HFD-induced metabolic syndrome by regulating pancreatic insulin secretion, the current results did not reveal statistically significant differences in serum glucose levels.

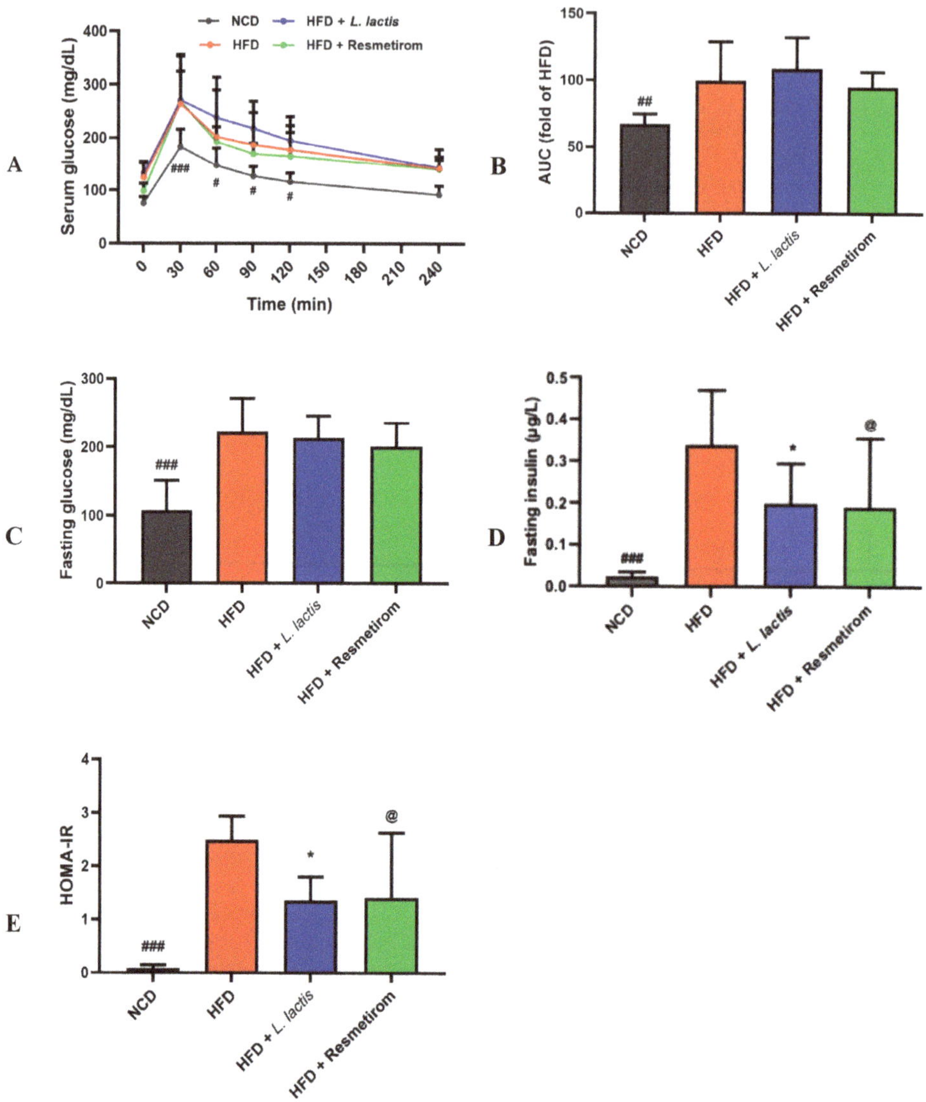

Figure 4. Effects of *L. delbrueckii* subsp. *lactis* CKDB001 on serum glucose levels of mice. The mice were subjected to the following dietary interventions for 24 weeks: normal chow diet (NCD), high-fat diet (HFD), HFD with *L. delbrueckii* subsp. *lactis* CKDB001 (LL), and HFD with resmetirom (positive control). (**A**) Serum glucose; (**B**) AUC of OGTT; (**C**) fasting glucose; (**D**) fasting insulin; (**E**) HOMA-IR. Values are presented as mean ± standard deviation (SD). # $p < 0.05$, ## $p < 0.01$, ### $p < 0.001$ between NCD and HFD; * $p < 0.05$ between HFD and LL; @ $p < 0.05$ between HFD and PC. Abbreviation: AUC, area under the curve; OGTT, oral glucose tolerance test; HOMA-IR, homeostasis model assessment-estimated insulin resistance.

3.4. LL Attenuates CVD Risk Markers in HFD-Induced Mice

To determine whether LL prevents hyperlipidemia induced by an HFD, we conducted OLTTs. The results showed that blood lipid levels were significantly higher in the HFD group compared with those in the NCD group. Although the LL group showed 0.90-fold lower blood lipid levels than those in the HFD group, the difference did not reach statistical significance (Figure 5A,B). Additionally, Cmax was 0.80- and 0.95-fold lower in the NCD and LL groups, respectively, than in the HFD group, but these differences were also not significant. However, the PC group exhibited a 1.39-fold higher Cmax than that of the HFD group (Figure 5C). The Tmax was similar across all groups, with no notable differences (Figure 5D).

Furthermore, to evaluate the effects of LL on lipid reduction and CVD risk factors in diet-induced dyslipidemia, we conducted lipid panel assessments and analyzed CRFs through biochemical serum analysis. Serum TG and TC levels in the HFD group were 1.61- and 2.18-fold higher than those in the NCD group (Figure 5E,F). Notably, serum TG levels were 0.59- and 0.57-fold lower in the LL and PC groups, respectively, compared with those in the HFD group ($p < 0.001$; Figure 5E). However, while serum TC levels were 0.72-fold lower in the PC group ($p < 0.001$), LL did not reduce TC levels (Figure 5F).

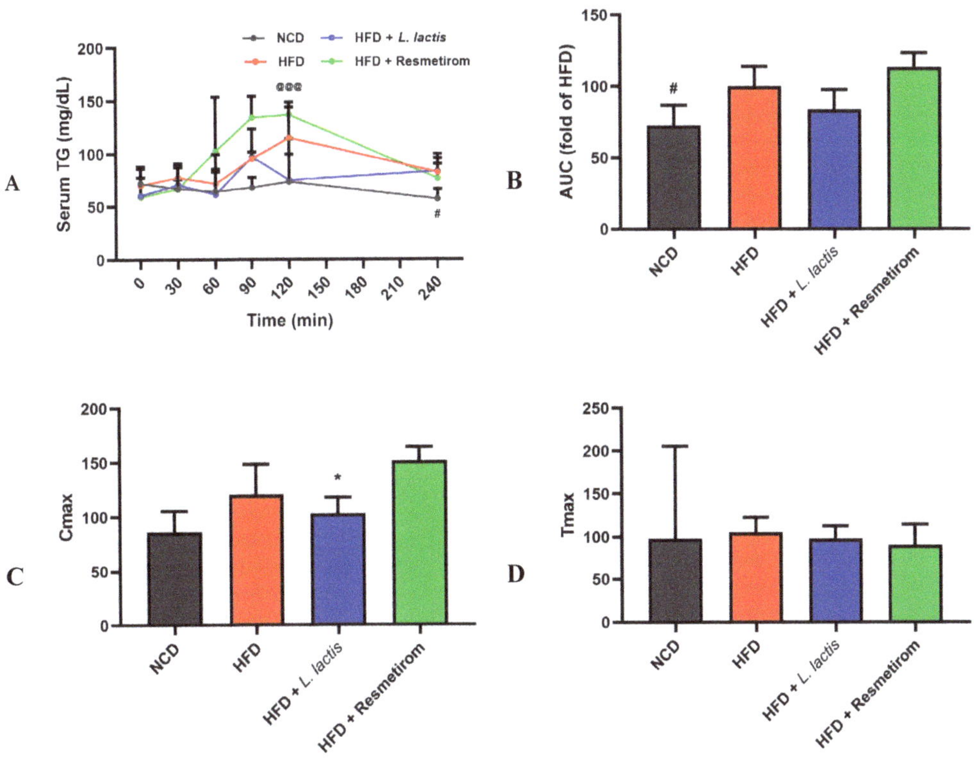

Figure 5. *Cont.*

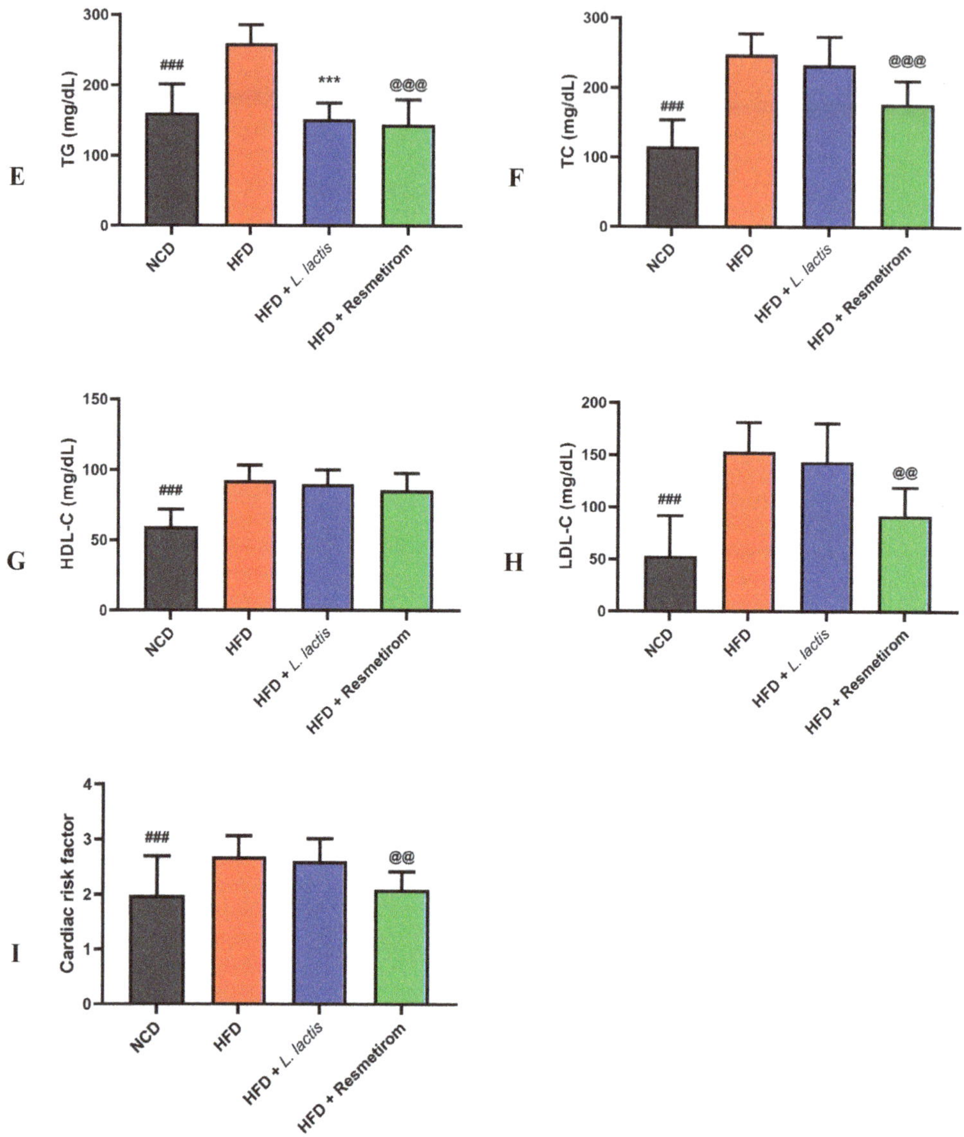

Figure 5. Effects of *L. delbrueckii* subsp. *lactis* CKDB001 on serum TC, TG, HDL-c, LDL-c, and CRF in mice. The mice were subjected to the following dietary interventions for 24 weeks: normal chow diet (NCD), high-fat diet (HFD), HFD with *L. delbrueckii* subsp. *lactis* CKDB001 (LL), and HFD with resmetirom (positive control). (**A**) Serum TG; (**B**) AUC of OLTT; (**C**) Cmax; (**D**) Tmax; (**E**) TG; (**F**) serum TC; (**G**) serum HDL-cholesterol; (**H**) serum LDL-cholesterol; (**I**) cardiac risk factor. Values are presented as mean ± standard deviation (SD). # $p < 0.05$, ### $p < 0.001$ between NCD and HFD; * $p < 0.05$, *** $p < 0.001$ between HFD and LL; @@ $p < 0.01$, @@@ $p < 0.001$ between HFD and PC. Abbreviation: TG, triglyceride; AUC, area under the curve; OLTT, oral lipid tolerance test; TC, total cholesterol; HDL, high-density lipoprotein; LDL, low-density lipoprotein.

Serum HDL-C levels were significantly higher in the HFD group compared with those in the NCD group ($p < 0.001$), but they did not significantly differ between the HFD, LL, and PC groups (Figure 5G). LDL-C levels were significantly higher in the HFD than in the NCD group ($p < 0.001$). LL did not significantly lower LDL-C levels relative to those in the HFD group, but those in the PC group were 0.60-fold lower (Figure 5H). Similarly to the LDL-C results, CRF levels were higher in the HFD than in the NCD group, significantly contributing to dyslipidemia ($p < 0.05$; Figure 5I). While LL tended to decrease CRF levels, significance was not reached; however, the PC group exhibited significantly lower levels.

In summary, our findings indicate that LL supplementation may improve catabolic lipid metabolism or enhance the clearance of TG from the bloodstream, potentially reducing the risk of associated metabolic disorders. However, LL did not significantly reduce TC or LDL-C levels. Therefore, while LL may have potential lipid-lowering effects and contribute to cardiovascular homeostasis, further research under different pathologic experimental conditions is necessary to confirm these findings.

3.5. LL Ameliorates Hepatic Lipid Accumulation and Function in HFD-Induced Mice

To determine whether systemic metabolic disorders induced by HFD intake cause pathological stress in hepatocytes, we measured hepatic lipid levels, histological characteristics, and liver enzyme activities. Hepatic TG and TC levels were 2.61- ($p < 0.001$) and 1.41-fold ($p < 0.05$) higher in the HFD group, respectively, relative to those in the NCD group (Figure 6A,B). In the PC group, TG and TC levels were 0.49- and 0.72-fold lower, respectively ($p < 0.001$). In the LL group, TG and TC levels were 0.92- and 0.76-fold lower, respectively, but only the decrease in TG levels was statistically significant (Figure 6A,B).

Histological evaluation of the liver using H&E staining revealed severe vacuolation in the HFD group, which was characterized by micro- and macrovascular steatosis due to ectopic WAT deposition in hepatocytes. Contrastingly, visual inspection showed reduced steatosis and fibrosis in the LL and PC groups compared with those in the HFD group (Figure 6C,D). Quantification of NAS and fibrosis from hepatic histological analysis showed significantly higher levels in the HFD than in the NCD group. In the LL group, NAS and fibrosis showed a decreasing trend compared with that in the HFD group, but the differences were not significant (Figure 6E,F). However, the PC group showed significantly lower NAS and fibrosis than those in the HFD group (Figure 6E,F).

A

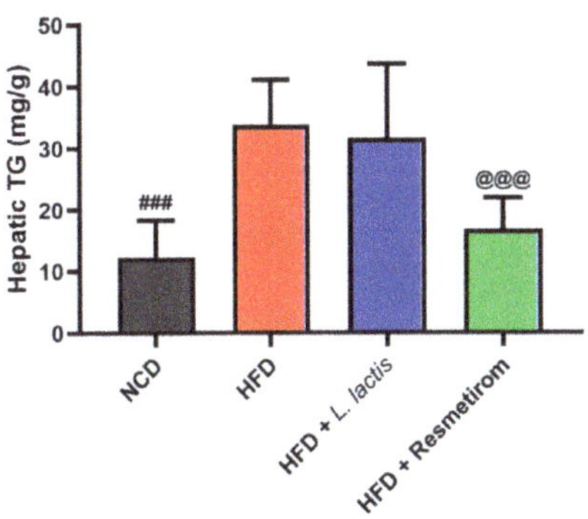

B

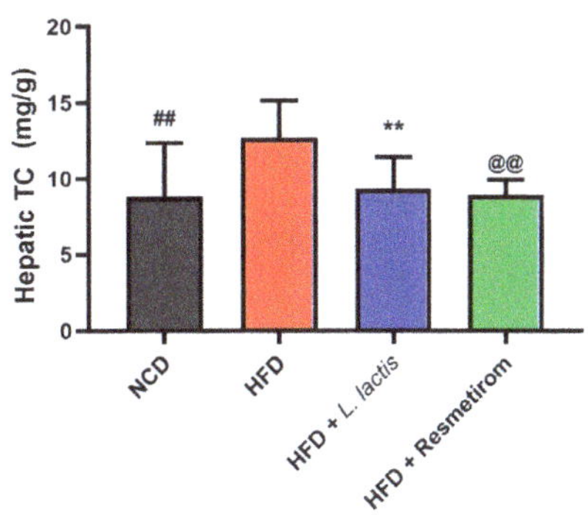

Figure 6. *Cont.*

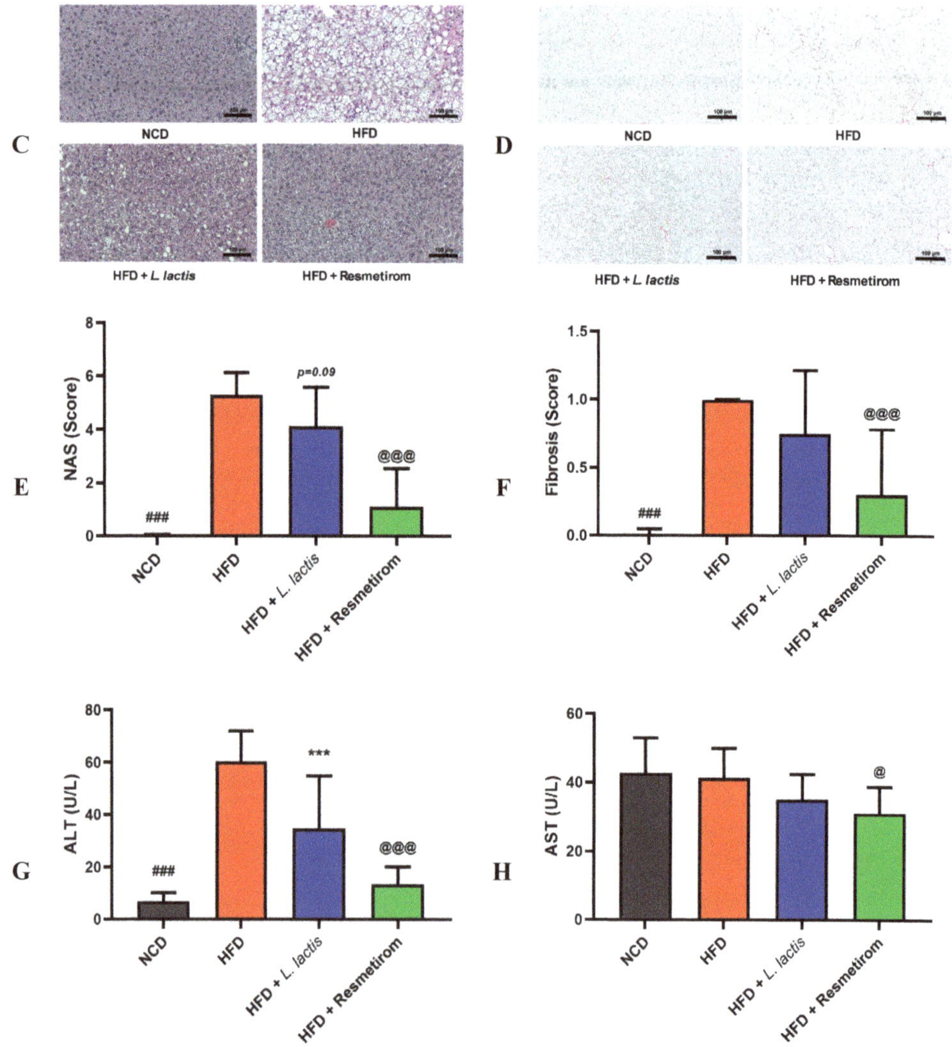

Figure 6. Effects of *L. delbrueckii* subsp. *lactis* CKDB001 on serum hepatic TG, hepatic TC, histology, NAS, fibrosis, ALT, and AST levels of mice. The mice were subjected to the following dietary interventions for 24 weeks: normal chow diet (NCD), high-fat diet (HFD), HFD with *L. delbrueckii* subsp. *lactis* CKDB001 (LL), and HFD with resmetirom (positive control). (**A**) Hepatic TG; (**B**) hepatic TC. (**C**) H&E and (**D**) sirius red staining images of the liver. (**E**) NAS; (**F**) hepatic fibrosis; (**G**) serum ALT; (**H**) serum AST. Values are presented as mean ± standard deviation (SD). ## $p < 0.01$, ### $p < 0.001$ between NCD and HFD; ** $p < 0.01$, *** $p < 0.001$ between HFD and LL; @ $p < 0.05$, @@ $p < 0.01$, @@@ $p < 0.001$ between HFD and PC. Abbreviations: TG; triglyceride, TC; total cholesterol, H&E; hematoxylin and eosin, NAS; NAFLD activity score, ALT; alanine aminotransferase, AST; aspartate aminotransferase.

Furthermore, serum ALT and AST activities were examined to evaluate the effects of LL on liver enzymatic function. The ALT levels were significantly higher in the HFD than in the NCD group ($p < 0.001$; Figure 6G). However, the LL and PC groups exhibited significantly lower ALT levels (0.57- and 0.22-fold, respectively) than those in the HFD group (Figure 6G). AST levels did not significantly differ between the dietary intervention groups, except for the PC group (Figure 6H). Therefore, systemic metabolic disorders induced by HFD intake resulted in hepatic lipid accumulation, increased liver injury markers, and worsened histological characteristics. Hepatic pathology caused by HFD consumption was mitigated by LL and PC interventions, as evidenced by reductions in hepatic TG and TC levels, improved histological features, and decreased ALT levels.

3.6. LL Modulates AMPK and Lipid Metabolism-Related Gene Expression in the Liver

The HFD-induced metabolic disturbances in energy and lipid metabolism in the liver may lead to various pathological progressions [51]. However, LL treatment significantly mitigated HFD-induced metabolic disturbances; therefore, we logically postulated that LL treatment would also alter energy and lipid metabolism beneficially. Therefore, the expression levels of energy and lipid metabolism-related biomarkers in the liver were measured following HFD intake. The *p*-AMPK levels in the liver were 4.50-fold lower in the HFD than in the NCD group ($p < 0.05$; Figure 7A,B). Notably, LL and PC treatments resulted in 7.47- ($p < 0.001$) and 5.79-fold ($p < 0.05$) higher *p*-AMPK levels, respectively, compared with those in the HFD group (Figure 7A,B). Additionally, the expression levels of genes involved in fatty acid β-oxidation were measured to determine the effects of LL on lipid metabolism. Anabolic gene expression related to de novo ectopic adipogenesis, including *Acox1*, *Cpt1α*, *Pparα*, *Pgc1α*, *Acc*, *Fas*, *Srebp1c*, *Scd1*, and *Dgat1*, was measured by qRT-PCR. The HFD groups exhibited significantly lower expressions of adipogenic genes, such as *Acox1*, *Cpt1α*, *Pgc1α*, *Acc*, *Scd1*, and *Dgat1*, reaching levels as low as 51.5%, 38.3%, 38.0%, 63.0%, 54.5%, and 59.3%, respectively, compared to those in the NCD group (Figure 7C–K). Interestingly, among the anabolic gene expressions, hepatic *Scd1* expression in the LL group was significantly decreased compared to the HFD group (Figure 7J). Furthermore, hepatic *Srebp1c* expression in the LL group (~54%) was significantly lower than in the HFD group, which was elevated by HFD consumption compared to the NCD, *Il-6*, *Tnf-α*, *Hmgcoa reductase*, and *Ldlr* in the liver were analyzed by qRT-PCR (Figure 7J,P,Q,S). However, LL did not significantly alter lipolysis, cytokine, or cholesterol regulatory gene expressions. These results suggest that LL treatment significantly improves *p*-AMPK levels and influences gene expression associated not with catabolic, but with anabolic responses in lipid metabolism, including lipid synthesis. Our findings imply potential therapeutic benefits in managing HFD-induced metabolic disturbances in the liver.

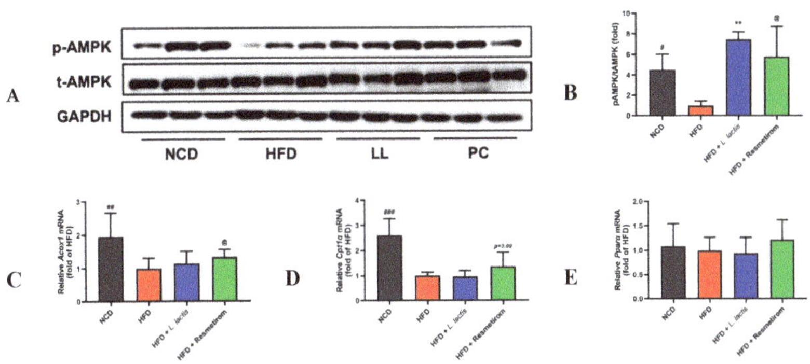

Figure 7. *Cont.*

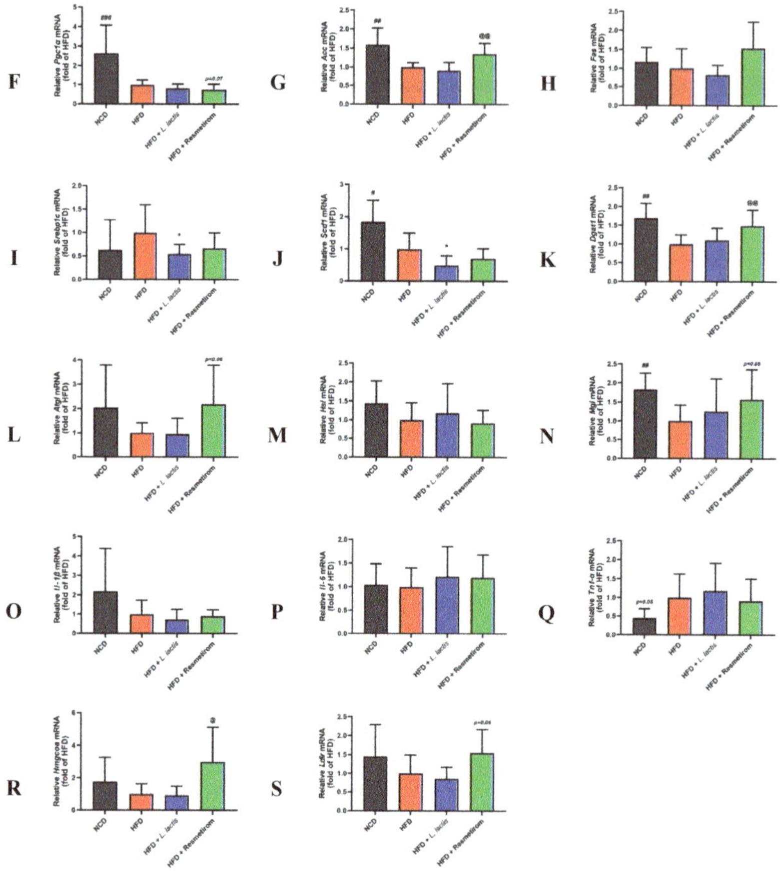

Figure 7. Effects of *L. delbrueckii* subsp. *lactis* CKDB001 on hepatic AMPK activity and mRNA levels associated with mouse lipid metabolism. The mice were subjected to the following dietary interventions for 24 weeks: normal chow diet (NCD), high-fat diet (HFD), HFD with *L. delbrueckii* subsp. *lactis* CKDB001 (LL), and HFD with resmetirom (positive control). (**A**) Representative Western blot images. (**B**) *p*-AMPK levels; relative gene expression of (**C**) *Acox1*; (**D**) *Cpt1α*; (**E**) *Pparα*; (**F**) *Pgc1α*; (**G**) *Acc*; (**H**) *Fas*; (**I**) *Srebp1c*; (**J**) *Scd1*; (**K**) *Dgat1*; (**L**) *Atgl*; (**M**) *Hsl*; (**N**) *Mgl*; (**O**) *Il-1β*; (**P**) *Il-6*; (**Q**) *Tnf-α*; (**R**) *Hmg-coa reductase*; (**S**) *Ldlr*. Values are presented as mean ± standard deviation (SD). # $p < 0.05$, ## $p < 0.01$, ### $p < 0.001$ between NCD and HFD; * $p < 0.05$, ** $p < 0.01$ between HFD and LL; @ $p < 0.05$, @@ $p < 0.01$ between HFD and PC. Abbreviation: *p*-AMPK, phospho-AMP-activated protein kinase; *Acox1*, Peroxisomal acyl-coenzyme A oxidase 1; *Cpt1α*, Carnitine palmitoyl transferase I; *Pparα*, Peroxisome proliferator-activated receptor alpha; *Pgc1α*, Peroxisome proliferator-activated receptor gamma coactivator 1 alpha; *Acc*, Acetyl-CoA carboxylase; *Fas*, fatty acid synthase; *Srebp1c*, Sterol regulatory element-binding protein-1c; *Scd1*, Stearoyl-CoA 9-desaturase; *Dgat1*, Diacylglycerol O-acyltransferase 1; *Atgl*, Adipose triglyceride lipase; *Hsl*, hormone-sensitive lipase; *Mgl*, Monoacylglycerol lipase; *Il*, Interleukin; *Tnf-α*, tumor necrosis factor alpha; *Hmg-coa*, Hydroxymethylglutaryl-CoA reductase; *Ldlr*, low-density lipoprotein receptor.

3.7. LL Inhibits Lipid Accumulation and Modulates Leptin and Adiponectin Levels in HFD-Induced Mice

Epididymal adipose tissue (EAT) is a crucial endocrine organ that regulates energy metabolism and immune responses. Excessive EAT accumulation due to an HFD is closely linked to various metabolic complications [52]. Histological analysis of EAT revealed that adipocyte size in the HFD group was significantly higher (1.69-fold) than that in the NCD group, while LL and PC treatment led to significantly higher adipocyte sizes (1.25- and 1.23-fold, respectively) compared with those in the HFD group (Figure 8A,B). However, macrophage infiltration among the groups did not significantly differ (Figure 8C). Additionally, the effect of LL on the expression of leptin and adiponectin, hormones involved in energy balance and metabolic regulation, was examined in the lysates of EAT. Although no significant differences were observed in leptin and adiponectin levels between the NCD and HFD groups, leptin expression was 0.84-fold lower in the LL than in the HFD group ($p < 0.05$, Figure 8D,E). Collectively, these findings indicate that LL treatment further induced the increased adipocyte size in EAT caused by an HFD. Despite no significant differences in macrophage infiltration or adiponectin levels, LL treatment notably reduced leptin expression, suggesting potential benefits in managing HFD-induced metabolic disturbances in EAT.

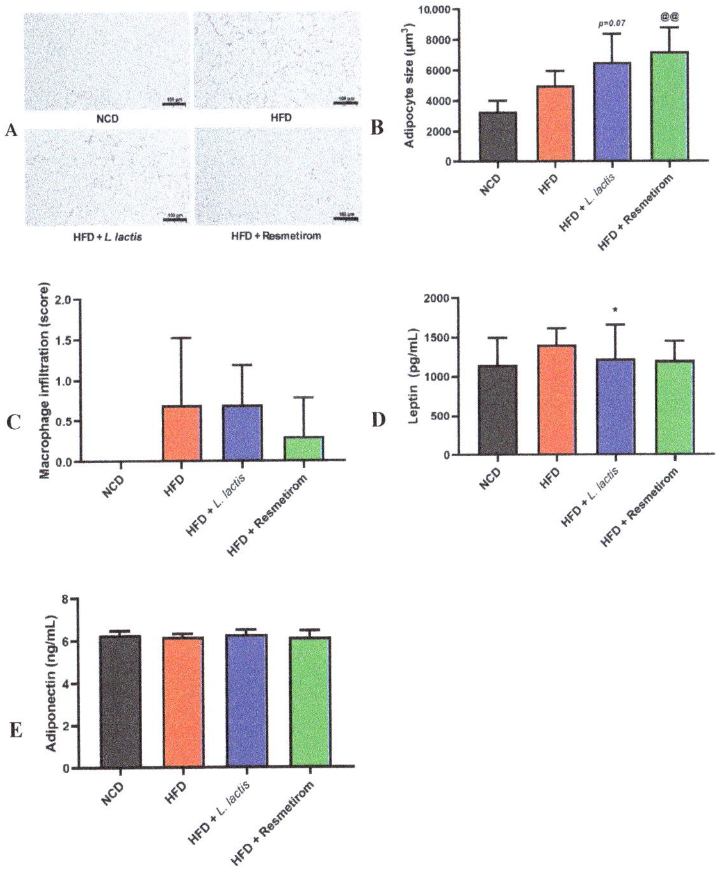

Figure 8. Effects of *L. delbrueckii* subsp. *lactis* CKDB001 on mouse lipid metabolism. The mice were subjected to the following dietary interventions for 24 weeks: normal chow diet (NCD), high-fat diet (HFD), HFD with *L. delbrueckii* subsp. *lactis* CKDB001 (LL), and HFD with resmetirom (positive control). (**A**) H&E staining image of EAT. (**B**) Adipocyte size in EAT. (**C**) Macrophage infiltration; (**D**) Leptin; (**E**) Adiponectin. Values are presented as mean ± standard deviation (SD). * $p < 0.05$ between HFD and LL; @@ $p < 0.01$ between HFD and PC. Abbreviation: H&E staining image of EAT; EAT, epididymal adipose tissue.

4. Discussion

Probiotics have emerged as a promising therapeutic approach for patients with MASLD, formerly known as NAFLD. Probiotics play a crucial role in restoring gut microbiota balance by increasing the abundance of beneficial bacteria and reducing that of harmful bacteria in the gut [53]. The gut microbiota, consisting of trillions of microorganisms in the gastrointestinal tract, are essential for maintaining host health and homeostasis, with compositional changes playing a major role in various diseases [54,55]. Recent studies have highlighted the involvement of the gut microbiota in liver homeostasis, particularly via regulation of the gut–liver axis [56]. The liver and gut communicate primarily via two pathways—the hepatic portal vein and bile acids (BAs) [57]. The hepatic portal vein carries most of the blood from the intestines to the liver, while BAs transport metabolites from the liver to the intestines [58]. Owing to the intertwined physiological relationship between the gut and liver, alterations in the gut microbiome by probiotics have gained attention as a potential therapeutic approach for liver diseases, including MASLD [59].

Additionally, probiotics have demonstrated positive effects on metabolic parameters associated with MASLD, such as improved insulin sensitivity [60,61] and lipid metabolism [62,63]. These metabolic improvements are essential for preventing or managing MASLD, as the condition is closely linked to metabolic dysfunction. Some studies have suggested that probiotics may serve as an alternative to antibiotics in MASLD treatment [64]. For instance, certain probiotic strains, such as *Lactococcus lactis*, have shown promise in mitigating MASLD by reducing lipid accumulation and improving liver health [65,66]. Previous research demonstrated that *L. delbrueckii* subsp. *lactis* CKDB001 reduces lipid accumulation and improves the lipid profiles of hepatic cells [35]. Moreover, Lee et al. found that *L. delbrueckii* subsp. *lactis* CKDB001 alleviated the Western diet-induced NAFLD by improving the liver-to-BW ratio, reducing steatosis, and lowering inflammation grade and NAS in the liver [36]. However, despite these promising results, the precise mechanisms through which *L. delbrueckii* subsp. *lactis* CKDB001 affects lipid metabolism remain unclear. Furthermore, issues such as low bioavailability and limited clinical data still hinder the use of *L. delbrueckii* subsp. *lactis* CKDB001 in the treatment of patients with MASLD [67,68].

A high dietary fat intake facilitates excessive caloric accumulation, elevating the risk of obesity by promoting WAT deposition [69]. Diets high in saturated fat, such as HFDs, are major contributors to obesity due to their high energy density. Obesity, in turn, is associated with an increased risk of metabolic disorders, including dyslipidemia, insulin resistance, and CVD [70]. Several studies have established obesity models in experimental mice using HFDs, which induce ectopic fat accumulation in the liver and BW gain [71]. Furthermore, HFD consumption ultimately leads to metabolic diseases such as hepatic steatosis, hypertension, and insulin resistance [72]. Previous research has demonstrated that HFDs, particularly those comprising 60% fat, are linked to obesity, hepatomegaly, and compromised liver function [73]. The existing studies primarily focused on reducing calorically dense fat intake to manage obesity while exploring nutraceuticals that may prevent obesity and its metabolic complications. Contrastingly, the present study aimed to investigate the impact of *L. delbrueckii* subsp. *lactis* CKDB001 on insulin resistance, dyslipidemia, MASLD, and lipid metabolism in an HFD-induced obese mouse model.

We investigated the effects of *L. delbrueckii* subsp. *lactis* CKDB001 on obesity and assessed its protective effects against the progression of metabolic disorders associated with obesity. BW is commonly used as a primary indicator of obesity [74], and our findings demonstrated that HFD-fed mice showed significant weight gain compared with those on an NCD. However, LL supplementation resulted in a notable reduction in BW. Additionally, LL supplementation reduced food efficiency, meaning that despite increased food intake, weight gain was less, indicating effective weight management. HFD-induced obesity and overweight are closely linked to peripheral insulin resistance and hyperinsulinemia, both of which contribute to metabolic disorders [75]. In the present study, HFD intake markedly elevated fasting blood glucose levels along with serum insulin levels compared with those in the NCD group. Notably, LL administration reduced the serum insulin levels in HFD-fed mice. These findings suggest that LL reduced HOMA-IR levels, a widely used indicator for assessing β-cell function and insulin resistance under steady-state conditions [76]. Elevated HOMA-IR values are associated with reduced insulin sensitivity, indicating insulin resistance [77]. The observed reduction in HOMA-IR levels suggests that LL treatment may effectively prevent or mitigate insulin resistance induced by HFD. However, no significant changes in blood glucose levels were observed with LL treatment, possibly due to the short dietary intervention period of this study. Previous studies have shown reduced blood glucose levels with longer HFD feeding periods, such as over 30 weeks [78]. Therefore, future studies should consider longer intervention durations to fully understand the effects of LL on glucose homeostasis.

Insulin resistance plays a key role in the development of dyslipidemia, even in individuals with normal glucose tolerance [79]. Dyslipidemia associated with insulin resistance is typically characterized by elevated TG and LDL-C levels, along with reduced HDL-C levels, commonly referred to as the "atherogenic lipid triad", which considerably increases the risk of CVD [79,80]. To evaluate the effects of LL on dyslipidemia, serum TG and TC levels were analyzed. HFD feeding led to higher TG and TC levels than those in the NCD group, but LL treatment reduced TG levels without significantly affecting TC levels. Consistent with these findings, other studies have also reported that *L. lactis* treatment reduces serum TG levels [81]. The reduction in TG levels is possibly due to the ability of LL to modulate the gut microbiota, which inhibits the growth of harmful bacteria while promoting beneficial bacteria, thereby improving gut health and reducing serum TG levels. Nevertheless, future studies are necessary to examine changes in the distribution of gut microbiota to better understand the interaction between LL, gut microbiota, and lipid metabolism. Although LL supplementation tended to reduce TC, LDL-C, and CRF levels, this reduction was not statistically significant relative to that in the HFD group. HFD feeding also led to increased HDL-C levels, which may be linked to elevated free cholesterol (FC) levels [82]. Rosales et al. recently suggested that high plasma concentrations of HDL-C, combined with elevated FC content, may facilitate the net transfer of FC into tissues, potentially leading to an atherogenic process [78]. Since FC movement between lipid surfaces is reversible, increased HDL-FC bioavailability could result in the deposition of excess FC in cells in vivo [83]. Future studies should focus on how FC levels are modulated by LL treatment.

MASLD is diagnosed when more than 5% of the liver has ectopic fat [84]. The pathogenesis of MASLD is often explained by the "two-hit hypothesis" [85]. The first hit involves the accumulation of lipids in hepatocytes, primarily TG, leading to steatosis. The second hit encompasses various factors that promote injury, inflammation, and fibrosis [86]. Persistent ectopic fat accumulation in the liver may lead to hepatic inflammation, contributing to metabolic dysfunction-associated steatohepatitis (MASH) development [57]. The progression from simple steatosis to MASH aligns with the second hit in the hypothesis. Prolonged MASLD or MASH, accompanied by inflammatory responses, may progress to liver fibrosis, cirrhosis, or hepatocellular carcinoma [87]. Preventing ectopic fat accumulation in the liver is crucial for effectively managing and treating MASLD, as it addresses the initial hit in disease progression [88]. In the present study, HFD consumption led to increased liver weight and hepatic TG and TC levels, indicating ectopic fat accumulation and the successful establishment of a MASLD model. LL consumption resulted in reduced liver weight and hepatic TC levels, suggesting a liver-specific effect on cholesterol metabolism. The lipid-lowering effect of LL treatment may be due to enhanced excretion of cholesterol, inhibition of hepatic cholesterol synthesis, or improved clearance of cholesterol from the bloodstream. These effects could help mitigate fatty liver disease and protect against liver cell lipotoxicity, potentially targeting both the first and second hits in MASLD pathogenesis. LL supplementation also attenuated NASs, hepatic fibrosis, and liver function indices such as AST. The decrease in hepatic TC levels may correlate with the reduction in NASs and fibrosis [89].

Moreover, HFD intake reduced AMPK phosphorylation in the liver, whereas LL treatment enhanced AMPK phosphorylation. AMPK plays a crucial role in regulating energy metabolism, acting as a cellular energy sensor and master regulator of metabolic homeostasis. AMPK activation promotes energy-producing pathways, such as fatty acid oxidation and glucose uptake, while inhibiting energy-consuming processes, such as fatty acid and protein synthesis [90–92]. The beneficial effects of AMPK activation, including improved insulin sensitivity [93–95], enhanced mitochondrial function [96], and reduced lipid accumulation [97–99] in the liver, contribute to improved liver function and reduced risk of MASLD. Experimental studies have demonstrated that both genetic and pharmacological activation of AMPK ameliorates fatty liver disease [100,101]. Accordingly, enhancing AMPK activity is considered a promising therapeutic approach for treating MASLD.

In the current study, LL intake protected against the HFD-induced reduction in hepatic AMPK phosphorylation, resulting in associated benefits in hepatic lipid metabolism. LL may have acted as an AMPK agonist, contributing to the reduction in ectopic fat accumulation in the liver. The observed reduction in liver weight and hepatic TC levels following LL consumption suggests that LL enhanced AMPK activity, potentially leading to increased fatty acid oxidation and decreased lipogenesis. The AMPK-induced effect played a crucial role in alleviating ectopic fat accumulation in the liver, thus counteracting MASLD development [102,103]. Notably, LL supplementation enhanced AMPK phosphorylation along with hepatic gene expressions related to de novo adipogenesis, such as Scd1 and Srebp1c. These findings suggest that the beneficial effects of LL on liver metabolism are primarily mediated through post-translational modifications and the suppressive transcriptional regulation of adipogenic gene expressions. Therefore, the beneficial effects of LL on liver metabolism may occur mainly via AMPK activation and subsequent post-translational modifications and changes in transcriptional expression.

MASLD primarily involves ectopic fat accumulation in the liver, but fat deposition in other tissues, such as EAT, also plays a crucial role in the progression of the disease [104]. EAT is metabolically sensitive and secretes adipokines such as leptin and adiponectin, which regulate metabolic homeostasis [105]. Under conditions of obesity and MASLD, adipokine secretion becomes imbalanced, promoting systemic inflammation and insulin resistance [106]. In the current study, LL treatment reduced leptin levels in EAT without significantly affecting adiponectin levels, consistent with previous findings [107]. The reduction in leptin levels is particularly relevant, as elevated leptin levels are linked to leptin resistance, a condition commonly observed in obesity and MASLD, which further exacerbates systemic inflammation and insulin resistance. A reduction in leptin levels may indicate improved leptin sensitivity, which could reduce inflammation and insulin resistance [108], thereby restoring metabolic balance and supporting beneficial outcomes in insulin sensitivity and lipid metabolism [109]. These findings are consistent with the broad effects of LL observed in the current study, including reduced BW, improved insulin sensitivity, and decreased serum TG levels.

Interestingly, histological analysis revealed that HFD intake increased adipocyte size, and notably, LL treatment also increased adipocyte size, potentially due to enhanced glucose uptake and mitochondrial function. The increase in adipocyte size following LL treatment suggests that LL supplementation induced hypertrophy in a metabolically healthier manner by promoting mitochondrial biogenesis and energy utilization, rather than simply increasing fat storage.

This study demonstrates the therapeutic potential of *L. delbrueckii* subsp. *lactis* CKDB001 (LL) in addressing metabolic dysfunctions associated with MASLD, including reductions in BW, improvements in insulin sensitivity, decreases in serum TG levels, and enhancements in AMPK phosphorylation in the liver. The comprehensive experimental design, utilizing a well-established HFD-induced murine model and detailed physiological and biochemical analyses, provides valuable insights into the role of *L. delbrueckii* subsp. *lactis* CKDB001 in lipid metabolism and gut microbiota modulation. However, the precise mechanisms underlying these effects remain unclear, and the short intervention duration may have limited observations of long-term outcomes. Challenges in translating findings to clinical applications are noted due to low bioavailability and limited human data. Additionally, while liver-specific effects were emphasized, further investigation into extrahepatic outcomes and direct evidence of gut microbiota interactions is needed to fully understand the therapeutic potential of *L. delbrueckii* subsp. *lactis* CKDB001.

5. Conclusions

In conclusion, LL supplementation ameliorated the HFD-induced metabolic dysregulation associated with MASLD, i.e., reduced hepatomegaly, decreased NASs and fibrosis, and enhanced AMPK phosphorylation in the liver. LL supplementation also modulated leptin levels, suggesting its potential role in regulating energy metabolism. These findings collectively highlight the potential of LL as a therapeutic candidate for ameliorating HFD-induced MASLD. However, several important areas require further investigation to fully understand the efficacy of LL as a potential probiotic supplement. Future studies should focus on assessing the bioavailability of LL in clinical settings and explore methods to enhance stability or absorption in the body. Additionally, as the present study lacks a detailed understanding of how LL affects specific bacterial strains and gut composition during gut microbiota modulation, a comprehensive investigation of gut microbiota changes is required.

Author Contributions: Conceptualization, H.J. (Hyunsoo Jang), H.J. (Hyunchae Joung), J.C., K.H.K., C.H.S., and J.-H.H.; methodology, H.J. (Hyunsoo Jang), H.J. (Hyunchae Joung)., M.C., Y.-W.K., and J.L.; software, H.J. (Hyunsoo Jang), H.J. (Hyunchae Joung), M.C., Y.-W.K., J.L., and J.-H.H.; validation, H.J. (Hyunsoo Jang), H.J. (Hyunchae Joung), J.L, and J.-H.H.; formal analysis, H.J. (Hyunsoo Jang), H.J. (Hyunchae Joung), and J.L.; investigation, K.H.K., C.H.S., and J.-H.H.; resources, K.H.K. and C.H.S.; data curation, H.J. (Hyunsoo Jang), H.J. (Hyunchae Joung), J.L., and J.-H.H.; writing—original draft preparation, H.J. (Hyunsoo Jang), H.J. (Hyunchae Joung), J.C., M.C., Y.-W.K., K.H.K., C.H.S., J.L., and J.-H.H.; writing—review and editing, H.J. (Hyunsoo Jang), H.J. (Hyunchae Joung), J.C., M.C., Y.-W.K., K.H.K., C.H.S., J.L., and J.-H.H.; visualization, H.J. (Hyunsoo Jang), H.J. (Hyunchae Joung) and J.L.; supervision, K.H.K. and J.-H.H.; project administration, K.H.K. and J.-H.H.; funding acquisition, K.H.K. All authors have read and agreed to the published version of the manuscript.

Funding: This research was funded by the National Research Foundation of Korea (NRF) grants funded by the Korea government (MSIT) (RS-2023-00227274).

Institutional Review Board Statement: All murine experimental procedures were approved by the Institutional Animal Care and Use Committee of Dankook University (No. DKU 2023-22-085) on 20 January 2023.

Informed Consent Statement: Not applicable.

Data Availability Statement: The datasets used in this study are available from the corresponding author upon reasonable request.

Conflicts of Interest: The authors affiliated with CKDBiO disclose that *Lactobacillus delbrueckii* subsp. *lactis* CKDB001 (KCTC14149BP, KR10-2128098) is patented by CKDBiO. Additionally, authors affiliated with Dankook University contributed to scientific research on this strain at the university. The funders participated in the design of the study, the collection, analyses, and interpretation of data, as well as the writing of the manuscript. However, the authors affiliated with Dankook University maintained full independence throughout the research process. No other conflicts of interest relevant to this article have been declared.

Abbreviations

Acc	Acetyl-Coa Carboxylase
Acox1	Peroxisomal Acyl-Coenzyme A Oxidase 1
ALT	Alanine Aminotransferase
AMPK	Adenosine Monophosphate-Activated Protein Kinase
AST	Aspartate Aminotransferase
AUC	Area Under the Curve
Atgl	Adipose Triglyceride Lipase

BAs	Bile Acids
BMI	Body Mass Index
BW	Body Weight
CFU	Colony-Forming Units
Cmax	Maximum Plasma Concentration
Cpt1α	Carnitine Palmitoyl Transferase I Alpha
CRF	Cardiac Risk Factor
CVD	Cardiovascular Disease
Dgat1	Diacylglycerol O-Acyltransferase 1
EAT	Epididymal Adipose Tissue
ELISA	Enzyme-Linked Immunosorbent Assay
Fas	Fatty Acid Synthase
FC	Free Cholesterol
FER	Food Efficiency Ratio
Gapdh	Glyceraldehyde-3-Phosphate Dehydrogenase
H&E	Hematoxylin and Eosin
HDL-C	High-Density Lipoprotein Cholesterol
HFD	High Fat Diet
Hmg-coa	3-Hydroxy-3-Methylglutaryl-Coenzyme A
HOMA-IR	Homeostasis Model Assessment of Insulin Resistance
Hsl	Hormone-Sensitive Lipase
Il-1β	Interleukin 1 Beta
Il-6	Interleukin 6
Ldlr	Low-Density Lipoprotein Receptor
LDL-C	Low-Density Lipoprotein Cholesterol
LL	Lactobacillus delbrueckii subsp. lactis CKDB001
MASLD	Metabolic-Associated Steatotic Liver Disease
MASH	Metabolic Dysfunction-Associated Steatohepatitis
MAT	Mesenteric Adipose Tissue
Mgl	Monoacylglycerol Lipase
NAFLD	Non-Alcoholic Fatty Liver Disease
NAS	Non-Alcoholic Fatty Liver Disease Activity Score
NASH	Non-Alcoholic Steatohepatitis
NCD	Normal Chow Diet
OGTT	Oral Glucose Tolerance Test
OLTT	Oral Lipid Tolerance Test
PBS	Phosphate-Buffered Saline
PC	Positive Control
Pgc1α	Peroxisome Proliferator-Activated Receptor Gamma Coactivator 1 Alpha
PPAR-GAMMA	Peroxisome Proliferator-Activated Receptor Gamma
Pparα	Peroxisome Proliferator-Activated Receptor Alpha
QRT-PCR	Quantitative Reverse Transcription-Polymerase Chain Reaction
RIPA	Radioimmunoprecipitation Assay
SAT	Subcutaneous Adipose Tissue
Scd1	Stearoyl-CoA 9-Desaturase
SDS	Standard Deviations
Srebp1c	Sterol Regulatory Element-Binding Protein 1c
T2D	Type 2 Diabetes
TC	Total Cholesterol
TG	Triglycerides
TMAX	Time to Reach Maximum Plasma Concentration
Tnf-α	Tumor Necrosis Factor Alpha
T-AMPK	Total-AMP-Activated Protein Kinase
WAT	White Adipose Tissue
WHO	World Health Organization

References

1. Lin, X.; Li, H. Obesity: Epidemiology, Pathophysiology, and Therapeutics. *Front. Endocrinol.* **2021**, *12*, 706978. [CrossRef] [PubMed]
2. Church, T.S.; Thomas, D.M.; Tudor-Locke, C.; Katzmarzyk, P.T.; Earnest, C.P.; Rodarte, R.Q.; Martin, C.K.; Blair, S.N.; Bouchard, C. Trends over 5 Decades in U.S. Occupation-Related Physical Activity and Their Associations with Obesity. *PLoS ONE* **2011**, *6*, e19657. [CrossRef] [PubMed]
3. Clemente-Suárez, V.J.; Beltrán-Velasco, A.I.; Redondo-Flórez, L.; Martín-Rodríguez, A.; Tornero-Aguilera, J.F. Global Impacts of Western Diet and Its Effects on Metabolism and Health: A Narrative Review. *Nutrients* **2023**, *15*, 2749. [CrossRef] [PubMed]
4. Galicia-Garcia, U.; Benito-Vicente, A.; Jebari, S.; Larrea-Sebal, A.; Siddiqi, H.; Uribe, K.B.; Ostolaza, H.; Martín, C. Pathophysiology of Type 2 Diabetes Mellitus. *Int. J. Mol. Sci.* **2020**, *21*, 6275. [CrossRef]
5. Zheng, J.; Lee, J.; Byun, J.; Yu, D.; Ha, J.H. Partial Replacement of High-Fat Diet with n-3 PUFAs Enhanced Beef Tallow Attenuates Dyslipidemia and Endoplasmic Reticulum Stress in Tunicamycin-Injected Rats. *Front. Nutr.* **2023**, *10*, 1155436. [CrossRef]
6. Lee, J.; Lee, J.K.; Lee, J.J.; Park, S.; Jung, S.; Lee, H.J.; Ha, J.H. Partial Replacement of High-Fat Diet with Beef Tallow Attenuates Dyslipidemia and Endoplasmic Reticulum Stress in db/db Mice. *J. Med. Food* **2022**, *25*, 660–674. [CrossRef]
7. Carter, J.L.; Abdullah, N.; Bragg, F.; Murad, N.A.A.; Taylor, H.; Fong, C.S.; Lacey, B.; Sherliker, P.; Karpe, F.; Jamal, R.; et al. Body Composition and Risk Factors for Cardiovascular Disease in Global Multi-Ethnic Populations. *Int. J. Obes.* **2023**, *47*, 855–864. [CrossRef]
8. Tan, P.Y.; Teng, K.T. Role of Dietary Fat on Obesity-Related Postmenopausal Breast Cancer: Insights from Mouse Models and Methodological Considerations. *Breast Cancer* **2021**, *28*, 556–571. [CrossRef] [PubMed]
9. Kim, W.G.; Cheng, S.Y. Mechanisms Linking Obesity and Thyroid Cancer Development and Progression in Mouse Models. *Horm. Cancer* **2018**, *9*, 108–116. [CrossRef]
10. Machado, M.V.; Cortez-Pinto, H. Non-Alcoholic Fatty Liver Disease: What the Clinician Needs to Know. *World. J. Gastroenterol.* **2014**, *20*, 12956–12980. [CrossRef]
11. Fabbrini, E.; Sullivan, S.; Klein, S. Obesity and Nonalcoholic Fatty Liver Disease: Biochemical, Metabolic, and Clinical Implications. *Hepatology* **2010**, *51*, 679–689. [CrossRef] [PubMed]
12. Staufer, K.; Stauber, R.E. Steatotic Liver Disease: Metabolic Dysfunction, Alcohol, or Both? *Biomedicines* **2023**, *11*, 2108. [CrossRef] [PubMed]
13. Huh, Y.; Cho, Y.J.; Nam, G.E. Recent Epidemiology and Risk Factors of Nonalcoholic Fatty Liver Disease. *J. Obes. Metab. Syndr.* **2022**, *31*, 17–27. [CrossRef]
14. Le, M.H.; Yeo, Y.-H.; Li, X.; Li, J.; Zou, B.; Wu, Y.; Ye, Q.; Huang, D.Q.; Zhao, C.; Nguyen, M.H.; et al. 2019 Global NAFLD Prevalence: A Systematic Review and Meta-analysis. *Clin. Gastroenterol. Hepatol.* **2022**, *20*, 2809–2817. [CrossRef] [PubMed]
15. Sandireddy, R.; Sakthivel, S.; Gupta, P.; Behari, J.; Tripathi, M.; Singh, B.K. Systemic Impacts of Metabolic Dysfunction-Associated Steatotic Liver Disease (MASLD) and Metabolic Dysfunction-Associated Steatohepatitis (MASH) on Heart, Muscle, and Kidney Related Diseases. *Front. Cell Dev. Biol.* **2024**, *12*, 1433857. [CrossRef]
16. Petito-da-Silva, T.I.; Souza-Mello, V.; Barbosa-da-Silva, S. Empaglifozin Mitigates NAFLD in High-Fat-Fed Mice by Alleviating Insulin Resistance, Lipogenesis and ER stress. *Mol. Cell. Endocrinol.* **2019**, *498*, 110539. [CrossRef]
17. Gaggini, M.; Morelli, M.; Buzzigoli, E.; DeFronzo, R.A.; Bugianesi, E.; Gastaldelli, A. Non-Alcoholic Fatty Liver Disease (NAFLD) and Its Connection with Insulin Resistance, Dyslipidemia, Atherosclerosis and Coronary Heart Disease. *Nutrients* **2013**, *5*, 1544–1560. [CrossRef]
18. Shah, P.; Mudaliar, S. Pioglitazone: Side Effect and Safety Profile. *Expert. Opin. Drug. Saf.* **2010**, *9*, 347–354. [CrossRef]
19. Pioglitazone. Available online: https://www.drugs.com/mtm/pioglitazone.html (accessed on 9 October 2024).
20. Armstrong, M.J.; Gaunt, P.; Aithal, G.P.; Barton, D.; Hull, D.; Parker, R.; Hazlehurst, J.M.; Guo, K.; Aldersley, M.K.; Newsome, P.N.; et al. Liraglutide Safety and Efficacy in Patients with Non-alcoholic Steatohepatitis (LEAN): A Multicentre, Double-Blind, Randomised, Placebo-Controlled Phase 2 Study. *Lancet* **2016**, *387*, 679–690. [CrossRef]
21. Liraglutide. Available online: https://www.drugs.com/mtm/liraglutide.html (accessed on 9 October 2024).
22. Radlinger, B.; Ress, C.; Folie, S.; Salzmann, K.; Lechuga, A.; Weiss, B.; Salvenmoser, W.; Graber, M.; Hirsch, J.; Kaser, S.; et al. Empagliflozin Protects Mice against Diet-Induced Obesity, Insulin Resistance and Hepatic Steatosis. *Diabetologia* **2023**, *66*, 754–767. [CrossRef]
23. Empagliflozin (Monograph). Available online: https://www.drugs.com/monograph/empagliflozin.html (accessed on 9 October 2024).
24. Hotel, A.C.P.; Cordoba, A. Health and Nutritional Properties of Probiotics in Food Including Powder Milk with Live Lactic Acid Bacteria. *Prevention* **2001**, *5*, 1–10.
25. Belizário, J.E.; Faintuch, J.; Garay-Malpartida, M. Gut Microbiome Dysbiosis and Immunometabolism: New Frontiers for Treatment of Metabolic Diseases. *Mediat. Inflamm.* **2018**, *2018*, 2037838. [CrossRef] [PubMed]
26. Vajro, P.; Paolella, G.; Fasano, A. Microbiota and Gut-liver Axis: Their Influences on Obesity and Obesity-Related Liver Disease. *J. Pediatr. Gastroenterol. Nutr.* **2013**, *56*, 461–468. [CrossRef] [PubMed]
27. Gérard, P. Gut Microbiota and Obesity. *Cell. Mol. Life. Sci.* **2016**, *73*, 147–162. [CrossRef]
28. Cai, H.; Zhang, J.; Liu, C.; Le, T.N.; Lu, Y.; Feng, F.; Zhao, M. High-Fat Diet-Induced Decreased Circulating Bile Acids Contribute to Obesity Associated with Gut Microbiota in Mice. *Foods* **2024**, *13*, 699. [CrossRef]

29. Madjd, A.; Taylor, M.A.; Mousavi, N.; Delavari, A.; Malekzadeh, R.; Macdonald, I.A.; Farshchi, H.R. Comparison of the Effect of Daily Consumption of Probiotic Compared with Low-Fat Conventional Yogurt on Weight Loss in Healthy Obese Women Following an Energy-restricted Diet: A Randomized Controlled Trial. *Am. J. Clin. Nutr.* **2016**, *103*, 323–329. [CrossRef]
30. Savijoki, K.; Nyman, T.A.; Kainulainen, V.; Miettinen, I.; Siljamäki, P.; Fallarero, A.; Sandholm, J.; Satokari, R.; Varmanen, P. Growth Mode and Carbon Source Impact the Surfaceome Dynamics of *Lactobacillus rhamnosus* GG. *Front. Microbiol.* **2019**, *10*, 1272. [CrossRef]
31. Rizzello, C.G.; Angelis, M.D. Lactic Acid Bacteria -Lactobacillus spp.: Lactobacillus delbrueckii Group. In *Encyclopedia of Dairy Sciences*, 2nd ed.; John, W.F., Ed.; Academic Press: Cambridge, MA, USA, 2011; Volume 3, pp. 119–124. ISBN 978-0-1237-4407-4.
32. Hallajzadeh, J.; Eslami, R.D.; Tanomand, A. Effect of *Lactobacillus delbrueckii* Subsp. *lactis* PTCC1057 on Serum Glucose, Fetuin-A, and Sestrin 3 Levels in Streptozotocin-Induced Diabetic Mice. *Probiotics Antimicrob. Proteins* **2021**, *13*, 383–389.
33. De Jesus, L.C.L.; Drumond, M.M.; Aburjaile, F.F.; Sousa, T.D.J.; Coelho-Rocha, N.D.; Profeta, R.; Brenig, B.; Mancha-Agresti, P.; Azevedo, V. Probiogenomics of *Lactobacillus delbrueckii* subsp. *lactis* CIDCA 133: In Silico, In Vitro, and In Vivo Approaches. *Microorganisms* **2021**, *9*, 829.
34. Chen, C.L.; Hsu, P.Y.; Pan, T.M. Therapeutic Effects of Lactobacillus paracasei subsp. *paracasei* NTU 101 Powder on Dextran Sulfate Sodium-Induced Colitis in Mice. *J. Food Drug Anal.* **2019**, *27*, 83–92.
35. Joung, H.; Chu, J.; Kwon, Y.J.; Kim, K.H.; Shin, C.H.; Ha, J.H. Assessment of the safety and hepatic lipid-lowering effects of *Lactobacillus delbrueckii* subsp. *lactis CKDB001*. *Appl. Biol. Chem.* **2024**, *67*, 101. [CrossRef]
36. Lee, N.Y.; Yoon, S.J.; Han, D.H.; Gupta, H.; Youn, G.S.; Shin, M.J.; Ham, Y.L.; Kwak, M.J.; Kim, M.J.; Suk, K.T.; et al. *Lactobacillus* and *Pediococcus* Ameliorate Progression of Non-Alcoholic Fatty Liver Disease through Modulation of the Gut Microbiome. *Gut Microbes* **2020**, *11*, 882–899. [CrossRef] [PubMed]
37. Kannt, A.; Wohlfart, P.; Madsen, A.N.; Veidal, S.S.; Feigh, M.; Schmoll, D. Activation of Thyroid Hormone Receptor-β Improved Disease Activity and Metabolism Independent of Body Weight in a Mouse Model of Non-Alcoholic Steatohepatitis and Fibrosis. *Br. J. Pharmacol.* **2021**, *178*, 2412–2423. [CrossRef] [PubMed]
38. Wang, X.; Wang, L.; Geng, L.; Tanaka, N.; Ye, B. Resmetirom Ameliorates NASH-Model Mice by Suppressing STAT3 and NF-κB Signaling Pathways in an RGS5-Dependent Manner. *Int. J. Mol. Sci.* **2023**, *24*, 5843. [CrossRef]
39. Kelly, M.J.; Pietranico-Cole, S.; Larigan, J.D.; Haynes, N.E.; Reynolds, C.H.; Scott, N.; Vermeulen, J.; Dvorozniak, M.; Conde-Knape, K.; Tilley, J.; et al. Discovery of 2-[3,5-Dichloro-4-(5-isopropyl-6-oxo-1,6-dihydropyridazin-3-yloxy)phenyl]-3,5-dioxo-2,3,4,5-tetrahydro [1,2,4]triazine-6-carbonitrile (MGL-3196), a Highly Selective Thyroid Hormone Receptor β Agonist in Clinical Trials for the Treatment of Dyslipidemia. *J. Med. Chem.* **2014**, *57*, 3912–3923.
40. Park, S.; Lee, J.J.; Lee, J.; Lee, J.K.; Byun, J.; Kim, I.; Ha, J.H. Lowering n-6/ n-3 Ratio as an Important Dietary Intervention to Prevent LPS-Inducible Dyslipidemia and Hepatic Abnormalities in ob/ob Mice. *Int. J. Mol. Sci.* **2022**, *23*, 6384. [CrossRef]
41. Son, H.K.; Kim, B.H.; Lee, J.; Park, S.; Oh, C.B.; Jung, S.; Lee, J.K.; Ha, J. Partial Replacement of Dietary Fat with Krill Oil or Coconut Oil Alleviates Dyslipidemia by Partly Modulating Lipid Metabolism in Lipopolysaccharide-Injected Rats on a High-Fat Diet. *Int. J. Environ. Res. Public Health* **2022**, *19*, 843. [CrossRef]
42. Friedewald, W.T.; Levy, R.I.; Fredrickson, D.S. Estimation of the Concentration of Low-Density Lipoprotein Cholesterol in Plasma, without Use of the Preparative Ultracentrifuge. *Clin. Chem.* **1972**, *18*, 499–502. [CrossRef]
43. Liang, W.; Menke, A.L.; Driessen, A.; Koek, G.H.; Lindeman, J.H.; Stoop, R.; Havekes, L.M.; Kleemann, R.; van den Hoek, A.M. Establishment of a General NAFLD Scoring System for Rodent Models and Comparison to Human Liver Pathology. *PLoS ONE* **2014**, *9*, e115922. [CrossRef]
44. Kleiner, D.E.; Brunt, E.M.; Van Natta, M.; Behling, C.; Contos, M.J.; Cummings, O.W.; Ferrell, L.D.; Liu, Y.-C.; Torbenson, M.S.; Unalp-Arida, A.; et al. Design and Validation of a Histological Scoring System for Nonalcoholic Fatty Liver Disease. *Hepatology* **2005**, *41*, 1313–1321. [CrossRef]
45. Bligh, E.G.; Dyer, W.J. A Rapid Method of Total Lipid Extraction and Purification. *Can. J. Biochem. Physiol.* **1959**, *37*, 911–917. [CrossRef] [PubMed]
46. Ha, J.H.; Doguer, C.; Wang, X.; Flores, S.R.; Collins, J.F. High-Iron Consumption Impairs Growth and Causes Copper-Deficiency Anemia in Weanling Sprague-Dawley Rats. *PLoS ONE* **2016**, *11*, e0161033. [CrossRef]
47. Jeong, S.; Bae, S.; Shin, E.C.; Lee, J.H.; Ha, J.H. Ellagic Acid Prevents Particulate Matter-Induced Pulmonary Inflammation and Hyperactivity in Mice: A Pilot Study. *Int. J. Environ. Res. Public Health* **2023**, *20*, 4523. [CrossRef]
48. Jeong, S.; Shin, E.C.; Lee, J.H.; Ha, J.H. Particulate Matter Elevates Ocular Inflammation and Endoplasmic Reticulum Stress in Human Retinal Pigmented Epithelium Cells. *Int. J. Environ. Res. Public Health* **2023**, *20*, 4766. [CrossRef] [PubMed]
49. Lee, J.; Jang, H.; Kang, D.; Kim, I.; Ha, J.-H. Physicochemical Properties of Yanggaeng with Added Tempeh Powder. *Prev. Nutr. Food. Sci.* **2023**, *28*, 514–519.
50. Qureshi, K.; Abrams, G.A. Metabolic Liver Disease of Obesity and Role of Adipose Tissue in the Pathogenesis of Nonalcoholic Fatty Liver Disease. *World J. Gastroenterol.* **2007**, *13*, 3540–3553. [CrossRef] [PubMed]
51. Mashek, D.G. Hepatic Lipid Droplets: A Balancing Act Between Energy Storage and Metabolic Dysfunction in NAFLD. *Mol. Metab.* **2021**, *50*, 101115. [CrossRef]
52. Franczyk, M.P.; He, M.; Yoshino, J. Removal of Epididymal Visceral Adipose Tissue Prevents Obesity-Induced Multi-organ Insulin Resistance in Male Mice. *J. Endocr. Soc.* **2021**, *5*, bvab024. [CrossRef]

53. Azad, M.A.K.; Sarker, M.; Li, T.; Yin, J. Probiotic Species in the Modulation of Gut Microbiota: An Overview. *Biomed Res. Int.* **2018**, *2018*, 9478630. [CrossRef]
54. Zhou, D.; Fan, J.G. Microbial Metabolites in Non-Alcoholic Fatty Liver Disease. *World J. Gastroenterol.* **2019**, *25*, 2019–2028. [CrossRef]
55. Lindheim, L.; Bashir, M.; Münzker, J.; Trummer, C.; Zachhuber, V.; Leber, B.; Horvath, A.; Pieber, T.R.; Gorkiewicz, G.; Stadlbauer, V.; et al. Alterations in Gut Microbiome Composition and Barrier Function Are Associated with Reproductive and Metabolic Defects in Women with Polycystic Ovary Syndrome (PCOS): A Pilot Study. *PLoS ONE* **2017**, *12*, e0168390. [CrossRef] [PubMed]
56. Milosevic, I.; Vujovic, A.; Barac, A.; Djelic, M.; Korac, M.; Radovanovic Spurnic, A.; Gmizic, I.; Stevanovic, O.; Djordjevic, V.; Lekic, N.; et al. Gut-Liver Axis, Gut Microbiota, and Its Modulation in the Management of Liver Diseases: A Review of the Literature. *Int. J. Mol. Sci.* **2019**, *20*, 395. [CrossRef] [PubMed]
57. Tripathi, A.; Debelius, J.; Brenner, D.A.; Karin, M.; Loomba, R.; Schnabl, B.; Knight, R. The gut-liver axis and the intersection with the microbiome. *Nat. Rev. Gastroenterol. Hepatol.* **2018**, *15*, 397–411. [CrossRef] [PubMed]
58. Chiang, J.Y.L.; Ferrell, J.M. Bile Acid Metabolism in Liver Pathobiology. *Gene Expr.* **2018**, *18*, 71–87. [CrossRef] [PubMed]
59. Ni, Y.; Ni, L.; Zhuge, F.; Fu, Z. The Gut Microbiota and Its Metabolites, Novel Targets for Treating and Preventing Non-Alcoholic Fatty Liver Disease. *Mol. Nutr. Food Res.* **2020**, *64*, e2000375. [CrossRef] [PubMed]
60. Zeng, Z.; Yuan, Q.; Yu, R.; Zhang, J.; Ma, H.; Chen, S. Ameliorative Effects of Probiotic Lactobacillus paracasei NL41 on Insulin Sensitivity, Oxidative Stress, and Beta-Cell Function in a Type 2 Diabetes Mellitus Rat Model. *Mol. Nutr. Food Res.* **2019**, *63*, e1900457. [CrossRef]
61. Rajkumar, H.; Kumar, M.; Das, N.; Kumar, S.N.; Challa, H.R.; Nagpal, R. Effect of Probiotic *Lactobacillus salivarius* UBL S22 and Prebiotic Fructo-oligosaccharide on Serum Lipids, Inflammatory Markers, Insulin Sensitivity, and Gut Bacteria in Healthy Young Volunteers: A Randomized Controlled Single-Blind Pilot Study. *J. Cardiovasc. Pharmacol. Ther.* **2015**, *20*, 289–298. [CrossRef]
62. Li, H.; Liu, F.; Lu, J.; Shi, J.; Guan, J.; Yan, F.; Li, B.; Huo, G. Probiotic Mixture of Lactobacillus plantarum Strains Improves Lipid Metabolism and Gut Microbiota Structure in High Fat Diet-Fed Mice. *Front. Microbiol.* **2020**, *11*, 512. [CrossRef]
63. Yoo, S.R.; Kim, Y.J.; Park, D.Y.; Jung, U.J.; Jeon, S.M.; Ahn, Y.T.; Huh, C.S.; McGregor, R.; Choi, M.S. Probiotics *L. Plantarum* and *L. Curvatus* in Combination Alter Hepatic Lipid Metabolism and Suppress Diet-Induced Obesity. *Obesity* **2013**, *21*, 2571–2578. [CrossRef]
64. Zhang, F.; Lo, E.K.K.; Chen, J.; Wang, K.; Felicianna; Ismaiah, M.J.; Leung, H.K.M.; Zhao, D.; Lee, J.C.; El-Nezami, H. Probiotic Mixture Ameliorates a Diet-Induced MASLD/MASH Murine Model Through the Regulation of Hepatic Lipid Metabolism and the Gut Microbiome. *J. Agric. Food Chem.* **2024**, *72*, 8536–8549. [CrossRef]
65. Yu, J.S.; Youn, G.S.; Choi, J.; Kim, C.H.; Kim, B.Y.; Yang, S.J.; Lee, J.H.; Park, T.S.; Kim, B.K.; Kim, Y.B.; et al. *Lactobacillus lactis* and *Pediococcus pentosaceus*-Driven Reprogramming of Gut Microbiome and Metabolome Ameliorates the Progression of Non-alcoholic Fatty Liver Disease. *Clin. Transl. Med.* **2021**, *11*, e634. [CrossRef] [PubMed]
66. Yu, J.S.; Youn, G.S.; Choi, J.; Kim, C.H.; Kim, B.Y.; Yang, S.J.; Lee, J.H.; Park, T.S.; Kim, B.K.; Kim, Y.B.; et al. Gut-Microbial and-Metabolomic Signatures in the Prevention of Non-Alcoholic Fatty Liver Disease by *Lactobacillus lactis* and *Pediococcus pentosaceus*. *Res. Sq.* **2020**, preprint. [CrossRef]
67. Samedi, L.; Charles, A.L. Viability of 4 Probiotic Bacteria Microencapsulated with Arrowroot Starch in the Simulated Gastrointestinal Tract (GIT) and Yoghurt. *Foods* **2019**, *8*, 175. [CrossRef]
68. Merenstein, D.; Pot, B.; Leyer, G.; Ouwehand, A.C.; Preidis, G.A.; Elkins, C.A.; Hill, C.; Lewis, Z.T.; Shane, A.L.; Zmora, N.; et al. Emerging issues in probiotic safety. *Gut Microbes* **2023**, *15*, 2185034. [CrossRef]
69. Demaria, T.M.; Crepaldi, L.D.; Costa-Bartuli, E.; Branco, J.R.; Zancan, P.; Sola-Penna, M. Once A Week Consumption of Western Diet Over Twelve Weeks Promotes Sustained Insulin Resistance and Non-Alcoholic Fat Liver Disease in C57BL/6J Mice. *Sci. Rep.* **2023**, *13*, 3058. [CrossRef]
70. Chiu, S.; Williams, P.T.; Krauss, R.M. Effects of A Very High Saturated Fat Diet on LDL Particles in Adults with Atherogenic Dyslipidemia: A Randomized Controlled Trial. *PLoS ONE* **2017**, *12*, e0170664. [CrossRef]
71. Snel, M.; Jonker, J.T.; Schoones, J.; Lamb, H.; de Roos, A.; Pijl, H.; Smit, J.W.; Meinders, A.E.; Jazet, I.M. Ectopic Fat and Insulin Resistance: Pathophysiology and Effect of Diet and Lifestyle Interventions. *Int. J. Endocrinol.* **2012**, *2012*, 983814. [CrossRef] [PubMed]
72. Longato, L.; Tong, M.; Wands, J.R.; de la Monte, S.M. High Fat Diet Induced Hepatic Steatosis and Insulin Resistance: Role of Dysregulated Ceramide Metabolism. *Hepatol. Res.* **2012**, *42*, 412–427. [CrossRef]
73. Kim, M.; Pichiah, P.B.T.; Kim, D.E.; Cha, Y.S. Black Adzuki Bean (*Vigna angularis*) Extract Exerts Phenotypic Effects on White Adipose Tissue and Reverses Liver Steatosis in Diet-Induced Obese Mice. *J. Food Biochem.* **2016**, *41*, e12333. [CrossRef]
74. Ghesmaty Sangachin, M.; Cavuoto, L.A.; Wang, Y. Use of Various Obesity Measurement and Classification Methods in Occupational Safety and Health Research: A Systematic Review of the Literature. *BMC Obes.* **2018**, *5*, 28. [CrossRef]
75. Lackey, D.E.; Lazaro, R.G.; Li, P.; Johnson, A.; Hernandez-Carretero, A.; Weber, N.; Vorobyova, I.; Tsukomoto, H.; Osborn, O. The Role of Dietary Fat in Obesity-Induced Insulin Resistance. *Am. J. Physiol. Endocrinol. Metab.* **2016**, *311*, E989–E997. [CrossRef] [PubMed]
76. Boyko, E.J.; Magliano, D.; Shaw, J.E. Insulin Sensitivity and Insulin Secretion Determined by Homeostasis Model Assessment and Risk of Diabetes in a Multiethnic Cohort of Women: The Women's Health Initiative Observational Study. *Diabetes Care* **2007**, *30*, 1747–1752. [CrossRef] [PubMed]

77. Petrelli, A.; Cugnata, F.; Carnovale, D.; Bosi, E.; Libman, I.M.; Piemonti, L.; Cuthbertson, D.; Sosenko, J.M. HOMA-IR and the Matsuda Index as Predictors of Progression to Type 1 Diabetes in Autoantibody-Positive Relatives. *Diabetologia* **2024**, *67*, 290–300. [CrossRef]
78. Kim, D.Y.; Park, J.Y.; Gee, H.Y. Lactobacillus plantarum Ameliorates NASH-Related Inflammation by Upregulating L-Arginine Production. *Exp. Mol. Med.* **2023**, *55*, 2332–2345. [CrossRef] [PubMed]
79. Steinberger, J.; Daniels, S.R.; American Heart Association Atherosclerosis, Hypertension, and Obesity in the Young Committee (Council on Cardiovascular Disease in the Young); American Heart Association Diabetes Committee (Council on Nutrition, Physical Activity, and Metabolism). Obesity, Insulin Resistance, Diabetes, and Cardiovascular Risk in Children: An American Heart Association scientific statement from the Atherosclerosis, Hypertension, and Obesity in the Young Committee (Council on Cardiovascular Disease in the Young) and the Diabetes Committee (Council on Nutrition, Physical Activity, and Metabolism). *Circulation* **2003**, *107*, 1448–1453.
80. Klop, B.; Elte, J.W.; Cabezas, M.C. Dyslipidemia in Obesity: Mechanisms and Potential Targets. *Nutrients* **2013**, *5*, 1218–1240. [CrossRef]
81. Hong, Y.; Song, G.; Feng, X.; Niu, J.; Wang, L.; Yang, C.; Luo, X.; Zhou, S.; Ma, W. The Probiotic Kluyveromyces *lactis* JSA 18 Alleviates Obesity and Hyperlipidemia in High-Fat Diet C57BL/6J Mice. *Foods* **2024**, *13*, 1124. [CrossRef] [PubMed]
82. Shinohata, R.; Shibakura, M.; Arao, Y.; Watanabe, S.; Hirohata, S.; Usui, S. A High-Fat/High-Cholesterol Diet, but Not High-Cholesterol Alone, Increases Free Cholesterol and ApoE-Rich HDL Serum Levels in Rats and Upregulates Hepatic ABCA1 Expression. *Biochimie* **2022**, *197*, 49–58. [CrossRef]
83. Rosales, C.; Gillard, B.K.; Xu, B.; Gotto, A.M., Jr.; Pownall, H.J. Revisiting Reverse Cholesterol Transport in the Context of High-Density Lipoprotein Free Cholesterol Bioavailability. *Methodist Debakey Cardiovasc. J.* **2019**, *15*, 47–54. [CrossRef]
84. Chan, W.K.; Chuah, K.H.; Rajaram, R.B.; Lim, L.L.; Ratnasingam, J.; Vethakkan, S.R. Metabolic Dysfunction-Associated Steatotic Liver Disease (MASLD): A State-of-the-Art Review. *J. Obes. Metab. Syndr.* **2023**, *32*, 197–213. [CrossRef]
85. Tilg, H.; Moschen, A.R. Evolution of Inflammation in Nonalcoholic Fatty Liver Disease: The Multiple Parallel Hits Hypothesis. *Hepatology* **2010**, *52*, 1836–1846. [CrossRef] [PubMed]
86. Day, C.P.; James, O.F. Steatohepatitis: A Tale of Two "Hits"? *Gastroenterology* **1998**, *114*, 842–845. [CrossRef]
87. Younossi, Z.; Anstee, Q.M.; Marietti, M.; Hardy, T.; Henry, L.; Eslam, M.; George, J.; Bugianesi, E. Global burden of NAFLD and NASH: Trends, Predictions, Risk Factors and Prevention. *Nat. Rev. Gastroenterol. Hepatol.* **2018**, *15*, 11–20. [CrossRef] [PubMed]
88. Elshaer, A.; Chascsa, D.M.H.; Lizaola-Mayo, B.C. Exploring Varied Treatment Strategies for Metabolic Dysfunction-Associated Steatotic Liver Disease (MASLD). *Life* **2024**, *17*, 844. [CrossRef] [PubMed]
89. Kim, S.Y.; Mun, S.; Yu, J.H.; Jin, Y.J.; Suh, Y.J.; Cho, S.H.; Lee, J.W. Association between small dense LDL levels and hepatic fibrosis in patients with nonalcoholic fatty liver disease. *Medicine* **2022**, *101*, e30527.
90. Garcia, D.; Shaw, R.J. AMPK: Mechanisms of Cellular Energy Sensing and Restoration of Metabolic Balance. *Mol. Cell* **2017**, *66*, 789–800. [CrossRef]
91. Cui, Y.; Chen, J.; Zhang, Z.; Shi, H.; Sun, W.; Yi, Q. The Role of AMPK in Macrophage Metabolism, Function and Polarisation. *J. Transl. Med.* **2023**, *21*, 892. [CrossRef]
92. Gupta, R.; Kasturi, P.; Bracher, A.; Loew, C.; Zheng, M.; Villella, A.; Garza, D.; Hartl, F.U.; Raychaudhuri, S. Firefly Luciferase Mutants as Sensors of Proteome Stress. *Nat. Methods* **2011**, *8*, 879–884. [CrossRef]
93. Xiao, Z.; Chu, Y.; Qin, W. IGFBP5 Modulates Lipid Metabolism and Insulin Sensitivity through Activating AMPK Pathway in Non-Alcoholic Fatty Liver Disease. *Life Sci.* **2020**, *256*, 117997. [CrossRef]
94. Zachariah Tom, R.; Garcia-Roves, P.M.; Sjögren, R.J.; Jiang, L.Q.; Holmström, M.H.; Deshmukh, A.S.; Vieira, E.; Chibalin, A.V.; Björnholm, M.; Zierath, J.R. Effects of AMPK Activation on Insulin Sensitivity and Metabolism in Leptin-Deficient ob/ob Mice. *Diabetes* **2014**, *63*, 1560–1571. [CrossRef]
95. Chularojmontri, L.; Nanna, U.; Tingpej, P.; Hansakul, P.; Jansom, C.; Wattanapitayakul, S.; Naowaboot, J. *Raphanus sativus* L. var. *caudatus* Extract Alleviates Impairment of Lipid and Glucose Homeostasis in Liver of High-Fat Diet-Induced Obesity and Insulin Resistance in Mice. *Prev. Nutr. Food Sci.* **2022**, *27*, 399–406. [PubMed]
96. Zhang, J.; Zhang, W.; Yang, L.; Zhao, W.; Liu, Z.; Wang, E.; Wang, J. Phytochemical Gallic Acid Alleviates Nonalcoholic Fatty Liver Disease via AMPK-ACC-PPARa Axis through Dual Regulation of Lipid Metabolism and Mitochondrial Function. *Phytomedicine* **2023**, *109*, 154589. [CrossRef] [PubMed]
97. Tu, Z.; Moss-Pierce, T.; Ford, P.; Jiang, T.A. Rosemary (*Rosmarinus officinalis* L.) Extract Regulates Glucose and Lipid Metabolism by Activating AMPK and PPAR Pathways in HepG2 Cells. *J. Agric. Food Chem.* **2013**, *61*, 2803–2810. [CrossRef] [PubMed]
98. Yao, H.; Tao, X.; Xu, L.; Qi, Y.; Yin, L.; Han, X.; Xu, Y.; Zheng, L.; Peng, J. Dioscin Alleviates Non-Alcoholic Fatty Liver Disease through Adjusting Lipid Metabolism via SIRT1/AMPK Signaling Pathway. *Pharmacol. Res.* **2018**, *131*, 51–60. [CrossRef] [PubMed]
99. Yu, P.; Xu, X.; Zhang, J.; Xia, X.; Xu, F.; Weng, J.; Lai, X.; Shen, Y. Liraglutide Attenuates Nonalcoholic Fatty Liver Disease through Adjusting Lipid Metabolism via SHP1/AMPK Signaling Pathway. *Int. J. Endocrinol.* **2019**, *2019*, 1567095. [CrossRef] [PubMed]
100. Esquejo, R.M.; Salatto, C.T.; Delmore, J.; Albuquerque, B.; Reyes, A.; Shi, Y.; Moccia, R.; Cokorinos, E.; Peloquin, M.; Monetti, M.; et al. Activation of Liver AMPK with PF-06409577 Corrects NAFLD and Lowers Cholesterol in Rodent and Primate Preclinical Models. *EBioMedicine* **2018**, *31*, 122–132. [CrossRef]

101. Garcia, D.; Hellberg, K.; Chaix, A.; Wallace, M.; Herzig, S.; Badur, M.G.; Lin, T.; Shokhirev, M.N.; Pinto, A.F.M.; Ross, D.S.; et al. Genetic Liver-Specific AMPK Activation Protects against Diet-Induced Obesity and NAFLD. *Cell Rep.* **2019**, *26*, 192–208.e6. [CrossRef]
102. Li, D.; Liu, F.; Wang, X.; Li, X. Apple Polyphenol Extract Alleviates High-Fat-Diet-Induced Hepatic Steatosis in Male C57BL/6 Mice by Targeting LKB1/AMPK Pathway. *J. Agric. Food Chem.* **2019**, *67*, 12208–12218. [CrossRef]
103. Smith, B.K.; Marcinko, K.; Desjardins, E.M.; Lally, J.S.; Ford, R.J.; Steinberg, G.R. Treatment of Nonalcoholic Fatty Liver Disease: Role of AMPK. *Am. J. Physiol. Endocrinol. Metab.* **2016**, *311*, E730–E740. [CrossRef]
104. Mulder, P.; Morrison, M.C.; Wielinga, P.Y.; van Duyvenvoorde, W.; Kooistra, T.; Kleemann, R. Surgical Removal of Inflamed Epididymal White Adipose Tissue Attenuates the Development of Non-alcoholic Steatohepatitis in Obesity. *Int. J. Obes.* **2016**, *40*, 675–684. [CrossRef]
105. Clemente-Suárez, V.J.; Redondo-Flórez, L.; Beltrán-Velasco, A.I.; Martín-Rodríguez, A.; Martínez-Guardado, I.; Navarro-Jiménez, E.; Laborde-Cárdenas, C.C.; Tornero-Aguilera, J.F. The Role of Adipokines in Health and Disease. *Biomedicines* **2023**, *11*, 1290. [CrossRef] [PubMed]
106. Feijóo-Bandín, S.; Aragón-Herrera, A.; Moraña-Fernández, S.; Anido-Varela, L.; Tarazón, E.; Roselló-Lletí, E.; Portolés, M.; Moscoso, I.; Gualillo, O.; González-Juanatey, J.R.; et al. Adipokines and Inflammation: Focus on Cardiovascular Diseases. *Int. J. Mol. Sci.* **2020**, *21*, 7711. [CrossRef] [PubMed]
107. Gan, X.T.; Ettinger, G.; Huang, C.X.; Burton, J.P.; Haist, J.V.; Rajapurohitam, V.; Sidaway, J.E.; Martin, G.; Gloor, G.B.; Swann, J.R.; et al. Probiotic Administration Attenuates Myocardial Hypertrophy and Heart Failure after Myocardial Infarction in the Rat. *Circ. Heart Fail.* **2014**, *7*, 491–499. [CrossRef] [PubMed]
108. Muskiet, F.A.J.; Carrera-Bastos, P.; Pruimboom, L.; Lucia, A.; Furman, D. Obesity and Leptin Resistance in the Regulation of the Type I Interferon Early Response and the Increased Risk for Severe COVID-19. *Nutrients* **2022**, *14*, 1388. [CrossRef]
109. Pereira, S.; Cline, D.L.; Glavas, M.M.; Covey, S.D.; Kieffer, T.J. Tissue-Specific Effects of Leptin on Glucose and Lipid Metabolism. *Endocr. Rev.* **2021**, *42*, 1–28. [CrossRef]

nutrients

MDPI

Article

Limosilactobacillus fermentum MG5368 and *Lactiplantibacillus plantarum* MG989 Regulates Skin Health in UVB-Induced HaCaT Cells and Hairless Mice Model

Jeong-Yong Park [1,†], Ji Yeon Lee [1,†], Seonghwa Hong [2], Huijin Heo [2], Hana Lee [2], Yong Gyeong Kim [1], Byoung-Kook Kim [1], Soo-Im Choi [1,*] and Junsoo Lee [2,*]

1 Mediogen, Co., Ltd., Biovalley 1-ro, Jecheon-si 27159, Republic of Korea; pjy@mediogen.co.kr (J.-Y.P.); ljy@mediogen.co.kr (J.Y.L.); kyk@mediogen.co.kr (Y.G.K.); kbk@mediogen.co.kr (B.-K.K.)
2 Department of Food Science and Biotechnology, Chungbuk National University, Cheongju-si 28644, Republic of Korea; tjd3465@naver.com (S.H.); pltreasure11@gmail.com (H.H.); dlgksk0514@naver.com (H.L.)
* Correspondence: csi@mediogen.co.kr (S.-I.C.); junsoo@cbnu.ac.kr (J.L.)
† These authors contributed equally to this work.

Abstract: Background: Photoaging, induced by chronic ultraviolet B (UVB) exposure, results in the degradation of extracellular matrix (ECM) components, leading to skin roughness, wrinkle formation, and reduced elasticity. Recent studies have explored probiotics as potential inhibitors of extrinsic aging, primarily through mechanisms that protect the skin barrier and reduce collagen breakdown. Methods: This study investigates the anti-photoaging effects of *Limosilactobacillus fermentum* MG5368 (*L. fermentum* MG5368) and *Lactiplantibacillus plantarum* MG989 (*L. plantarum* MG989) in UVB-exposed keratinocytes and an SKH-1 hairless mice model. Results: Both strains demonstrated significant efficacy in preserving collagen through the inhibition of activating protein-1 (AP-1) and reducing the expression of matrix metalloproteinase (MMP)-1 and MMP-3. Additionally, both strains restored COL1A1 protein expressions, thereby enhancing collagen synthesis and ECM stability. Enhanced skin elasticity was observed, attributed to restored levels of hyaluronic acid and hyaluronan synthase 2 (HAS2) protein expressions. Conclusions: These findings suggest that *L. fermentum* MG5368 and *L. plantarum* MG989 may serve as promising probiotic-based agents for anti-photoaging applications.

Keywords: ultraviolet B; wrinkle; collagen; *Limosilactobacillus fermentum*; *Lactiplantibacillus plantarum*

1. Introduction

As the largest organ of the human body, the skin constitutes approximately 16% of total body mass and functions as the first line of defense against external environmental factors [1]. The skin consists of two main layers, the epidermis and the dermis, with the epidermis being the outermost layer and acting as a barrier against environmental stressors such as ultraviolet (UV) exposure [2]. Epidermal keratinocytes migrate outward to form keratinocytes, forming the main barrier of the epidermal layer [3]. Skin aging involves a progressive decline in both structural integrity and physiological function, generally categorized into intrinsic aging, associated with natural biological processes, and extrinsic aging, driven by environmental factors such as pollution and UV exposure [4]. Among the types of UV radiation, UVB has particularly pronounced effects on skin health, contributing to dryness, hyperpigmentation, and wrinkle formation through its rapid interaction with cellular processes [5]. The most characteristic change in aged skin is a decline in both the quantity and structural alteration of collagen, primarily due to accelerated degradation processes and reduced biosynthesis [6]. Recently, some natural extracts have been used as dietary ingredients to prevent photoaging, but they have been reported to have high prices and side effects. [7]. Therefore, there is considerable interest in identifying cost-effective and safe materials to mitigate skin damage and photoaging caused by UV exposure.

In general, probiotics are beneficial bacteria that eliminate harmful microorganisms and benefit the health of the host [8]. Probiotics maintain the natural balance of gut bacteria and modulate immune responses [9]. Probiotics maintain the natural balance of gut bacteria and modulate immune responses [10]. Probiotics have been extensively studied for their gut health benefits, but recent studies have also shown that they have the potential to address antioxidant, anti-inflammatory, and immune properties [11,12]. In particular, probiotics such as *Limosilactobacillus fermentum* (*L. fermentum*) and *Lactiplantibacillus plantarum* (*L. plantarum*) have been reported to have high antioxidant potential [13]. Substances with antioxidant properties have a high potential for improving skin health caused by photoaging [14]. Therefore, this study investigated the protective effects and potential mechanisms of *L. fermentum* and *L. plantarum* strains against UVB-exposed keratinocytes and SKH-1 hairless mice.

2. Materials and Methods

2.1. Preparation of Bacterial Samples

The eight bacterial strains (*L. fermentum* MG5368, MG4294, MG5159, MG4538, MG5091, *L. plantarum* MG989, MG5530, and MG5023) were isolated from healthy infant feces or breast milk (Table 1). These strains were inoculated in Man Rogosa Sharpe broth (Difco, Sparks, MD, USA) and cultured at 37 °C for 18 h. The strains were centrifuged at 1500× *g* for 10 min, and the cell-free supernatant (CFS) was collected and filtered with a 0.22 µm polytetrafluoroethylene membrane filter (ADVANTEC, Tokyo, Japan). The prepared CFS was used for the in vitro study [15]. For the in vivo test, the harvested *L. fermentum* MG5368 and *L. plantarum* MG989 pellets were freeze-dried. The powdered strains were harvested, mixed with maltodextrin for dilution at a final concentration of 1×10^{11} CFU/g, and stored at 4 °C until further use.

Table 1. The origin and accession number of bacterial strains used in this study.

Spp.	Strain	Origin	NCBI Accession No.
Limosilactobacillus fermentum	MG5368	Food	ON631268.1
	MG4294	Human	MW404502.1
	MG5159	Food	MN435579.1
	MG4538	Human	MN368558.1
	MG5091	Food	OP102518.1
Lactiplantibacillus plantarum	MG989	Human	MN061270.1
	MG5530	Food	ON668221.1
	MG5023	Food	OP102478.1

2.2. In Vitro Test

2.2.1. Cell Culture

The HaCaT keratinocytes (provided by the School of Cosmetic Science and Beauty Biotechnology, Semyung University, Jecheon, Republic of Korea) and HT-29 cells (Korea Cell Line Bank, Seoul, Republic of Korea) were cultured as described in previous reports [16].

2.2.2. Ultraviolet B (UVB) Exposure and Cell Viability

The HaCaT keratinocytes were seeded in a 96-well plate (1×10^4 cell/well) and incubated at 37 °C for 24 h. Then, CFS of probiotics samples, 3% in serum-free DMEM (*v*/*v*), were pre-treated for 24 h. The cells were then irradiated with UVB (20 mJ/cm^2) using a UVB lamp (Sankyo Denki Lamps, GL20SE, Marine, Kanagawa, Japan). The intensity was monitored using a UV light meter (LT Lutron, UV-340A, Taipei, Taiwan). After exposure, cells were treated with probiotics samples for an additional 24 h [17]. Following treatment, 3-(4,5-dimethylthiazol-2-yl)-2,5-diphenyltetrazolium bromide (MTT) was added to each well, and cells were incubated for 2 h [18]. After incubation, the formazan was dissolved in dimethyl sulfoxide. The absorbance was measured at 550 nm using a microplate reader (BioTek, Winooski, VT, USA).

2.3. *In Vivo Test*

2.3.1. Animal Experiment and UVB Exposure

The 5-week-old SKH-1 female hairless mice (OrientBio Co., Ltd., Seongnam, Republic of Korea) were housed in the following environment (22 ± 2 °C, 50 ± 10% humidity, and less than 60 dB with a 12 h photoperiod and free access to food and water). The experimental animals were divided into four groups so that the average body weight and standard deviation of each group were uniform (n = 8): (1) normal group (no UVB exposure), (2) UVB exposure group, (3) i.p. *L. fermentum* MG5368 (1×10^9 CFU/day) with UVB exposure group, and (4) i.p. *L. plantarum* MG989 (1×10^9 CFU/day) with UVB exposure group. Each probiotic strain was orally administered for 12 weeks with UVB exposure. The animals were exposed to UVB 3 times per week for 12 weeks, and total irradiation was 7.56 J/cm^2 using a UV Crosslinking Chamber (UVP CL-1000, Upland, CA, USA). The UVB irradiation started with 1 Minimal Erythema Dose (MED; 0.06 J/cm^2) during the first week and increased by 1 MED every week until the 4 weeks. UVB exposure was maintained at 4 MED from 4 to 12 weeks shown in Figure 1. [19]. The UVB intensity was monitored by a UV light meter (VLX-3W radiometer, UVITEC, Milton, Cambridge, UK). There were no deaths by the end of the experiment. At the end of the animal experiment, all mice were anesthetized with 3% isoflurane, and skin wrinkle and elasticity were assessed with no exclusions.

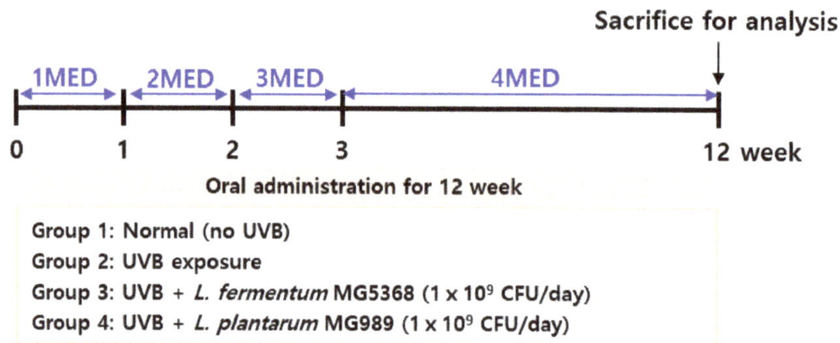

Figure 1. Animal experimental procedure of UVB-exposed SKH-1 hairless mice. The dorsal skin of the SKH-1 mice was exposed to UVB at 1 minimal erythema dose (MED) was 60 mJ/cm^2.

2.3.2. Evaluation of Skin Wrinkle and Skin Elasticity

The dorsal skin exposed to UVB was imaged using a 3D imaging system equipped with a high-resolution sensor (Primos^{CR}, Canfield, OH, USA) [20]. The mean of wrinkle depth, maximum of wrinkle depth, and skin roughness (Rz) were analyzed by Primos 5.0 software (Canfield, OH, USA). The dorsal skin elasticity was measured by a Cutometer (Courage and Khazaka, Kőln, Germany) [21]. The measuring mode was used with a constant negative pressure of 450 mbar consecutively three times of suction for two seconds each. The parameters of R2 (gross elasticity), R5 (net elasticity), and R7 (biological elasticity) were analyzed.

2.3.3. Analysis of Histopathology and Collagen Content

The dorsal skin was biopsied, fixed with 10% paraformaldehyde, and embedded in paraffin block. The slides were made by sectioning into 3 µm thick and subjected to a hydration process. The slides of skin dorsal tissues were stained with hematoxylin and eosin (H&E) solution to measure skin thickness. The collagen production was stained with Biebrich Scarlet-acid Fuchsin solution for 5 min, washed, and stained with phosphotungtic/phosphomolybdic acid for 5 min [22]. All stained tissue was pictured using an optical microscope (Olympus, Tokyo, Japan). The thickness of the skin and the production of collagen were analyzed by the ImageJ program (https://imagej.net/ij/, The National Institutes of Health, Bethesda, MD, USA).

2.4. Enzyme-Linked Immunosorbent Assay (ELISA)

In keratinocytes, matrix metalloproteinase (MMP)-1, MMP-3 (Merck & Co. Inc., Whitehouse Station, NJ, USA), and collagen content (Sircol Soluble Collagen Assay Kit, Biocolor, Belfast, UK) production were measured by according to the manufacturer's instructions. Hyaluronic acid (HA) contents in keratinocytes and dorsal skin were evaluated by using an HA ELISA assay kit (R&D systems, Minneapolis, MN, USA) according to the manufacturer's instructions.

2.5. Western Blotting

Western blot antibodies were obtained from Cell Signaling Technology (Beverly, MA, USA) and Santa Cruz Biotechnology (Dallas, TX, USA). The HaCaT keratinocytes and dorsal skin were lysed with a Pro-Prep protein extraction solution (iNtRON, Seongnam-si, Republic of Korea). Proteins were separated using SDS-PAGE and transferred onto an NC membrane (Cytiva, Marlborough, MA, USA). The membranes were blocked with 5% bovine serum albumin (BSA; fatty acid-free, purity ≥98%) for 1 h at room temperature and subsequently incubated 24 h at 4 °C with primary antibodies at dilutions of 1:500. After primary antibody incubation, the blots were incubated with secondary antibodies diluted 1:1000 for 1 h. Chemiluminescence was detected using ECLTM (ThermoFisher, Waltham, MA, USA). Specific protein bands were quantified using ATTO CS Analyzer 4 software (ATTO, Tokyo, Japan).

2.6. Statistical Analysis

GraphPad Prism 10 (GraphPad Software Inc., Boston, MA, USA) was used for all statistical analyses. All data are reported as the mean ± standard error of mean (SEM) for at least three replicates. Parametric data were analyzed by one-way analysis of variance (ANOVA) followed by Dunnett's multiple comparison test.

3. Results

3.1. Cell Protective Effects of CFS from Bacterial Strains in UVB-Exposed HaCaT Keratinocytes Including MMPs, HA, and Collagen Production

To determine the appropriate concentration of CFS, cell viability was assessed without UVB irradiation. To establish the UVB intensity, cell viability was measured following exposure to 10, 20, and 30 mJ/cm^2. With a cell viability of 74.7% observed at 20 mJ/cm^2, this intensity was chosen for subsequent experiments (Figure S1). The protective effect of CFS on UVB-exposed HaCaT keratinocytes was evaluated, and the results showed that CFS of *L. fermentum* MG5368, MG4294, and MG4538 and *L. plantarum* MG989 did not exhibit a significant recovery in cell viability (Figure 2A). The evaluation of MMP-1 and MMP-3 production in the four strains revealed that CFS of *L. fermentum* MG5368 and *L. plantarum* MG989 were significantly regulated in UVB-exposed HaCaT keratinocytes (Figure 2B,C). Additionally, *L. fermentum* MG5368 and *L. plantarum* MG989 significantly restored the collagen production levels that were reduced by UVB irradiation in HaCaT keratinocytes (Figure S2). The HA production was significantly increased in UVB-exposed HaCaT keratinocytes treated with CFS of the four strains (Figure 2D).

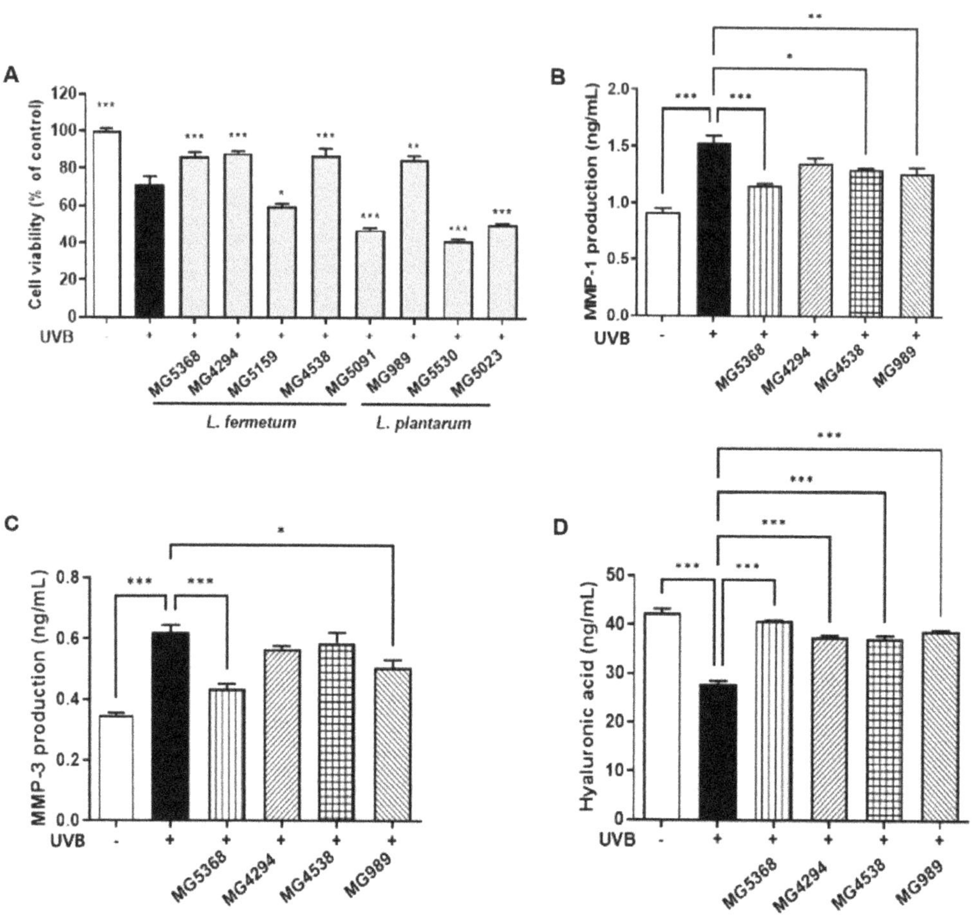

Figure 2. Effect on (**A**) cell viability, (**B**) MMP-3, (**C**) MMP-1, and (**D**) hyaluronic acid production of CFS in UVB-exposed HaCaT keratinocytes. The cells were pre-treated with CFS (3%) for 24 h and then exposed to UVB (20 mJ/cm^2), followed by additional treatment with CFS (3%) for 24 h. Values are expressed as the mean ± SEM (n = 3). * $p < 0.05$, ** $p < 0.01$, and *** $p < 0.001$, significant difference compared to UVB-exposed group. White bar, no-exposed group; black bar, UVB-exposed group.

3.2. CFS of L. fermentum MG5368 and L. plantarum MG989 Regulates the AP-1/Smad Signaling Pathway in UVB-Exposed HaCaT Keratinocytes

In HaCaT keratinocytes, the activator protein (AP)-1 signaling pathway, including phosphorylation of c-Fos and c-Jun protein expression, stimulated by UVB exposure was significantly reversed by CFS of *L. fermentum* MG5368 and *L. plantarum* MG989 (Figure 3A). CFS of *L. fermentum* MG5368 and *L. plantarum* MG989 also strongly increased phosphorylation of Smad 2/3, collagen type I, alpha 1 (COL1A1), and hyaluronan synthase (HAS) 2 protein expression in UVB-exposed HaCaT keratinocytes (Figure 3B).

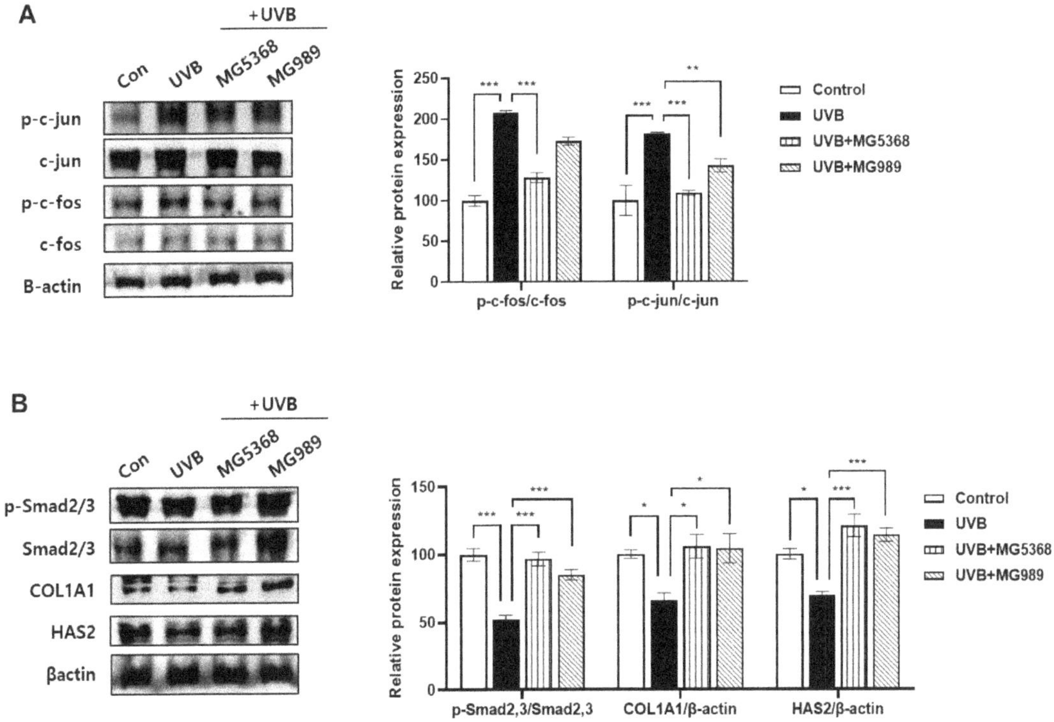

Figure 3. Effect of CFS on (**A**) AP-1 (p-c-fos, c-fos, p-c-jun, and c-jun) and (**B**) p-Smad 2/3, Smad 2/3, COL1A1, and HAS2 in UVB-exposed HaCaT keratinocytes. The cells were pre-treated with CFS (3%) for 24 h and then exposed to UVB (20 mJ/cm^2), followed by additional treatment with CFS (3%) for 24 h. The representative blotting images and relative expression were evaluated by Western blotting. The β-actin was used as a loading control. Values are expressed as the mean ± SEM (n = 3). * $p < 0.05$, ** $p < 0.01$, and *** $p < 0.001$, significant difference compared to the UVB-exposed group.

3.3. Oral Administration of L. fermentum MG5368 and L. plantarum MG989 Decreases Wrinkle and Elasticity in the Dorsal Skin of the UVB-Exposed SKH-1 Hairless Mice

Wrinkle formation was similar prior to UVB exposure; however, after 12 weeks of UVB exposure, wrinkles developed in the dorsal skin of SKH-1 hairless mice. Oral administration of *L. fermentum* MG5368 and *L. plantarum* MG989 significantly reduced wrinkle formation induced by UVB exposure at 12 weeks (Figure 4A). The mean and maximum wrinkle depth and skin roughness in UVB-exposed SKH-1 hairless mice were improved by the intake of *L. fermentum* MG5368 and *L. plantarum* MG989 (Figure 4B–D). The R2, R5, and R7, which indicate skin elasticity parameters, showed a decrease following UVB exposure; however, oral administration of *L. fermentum* MG5368 and *L. plantarum* MG989 significantly increased these parameters (Figure 4E).

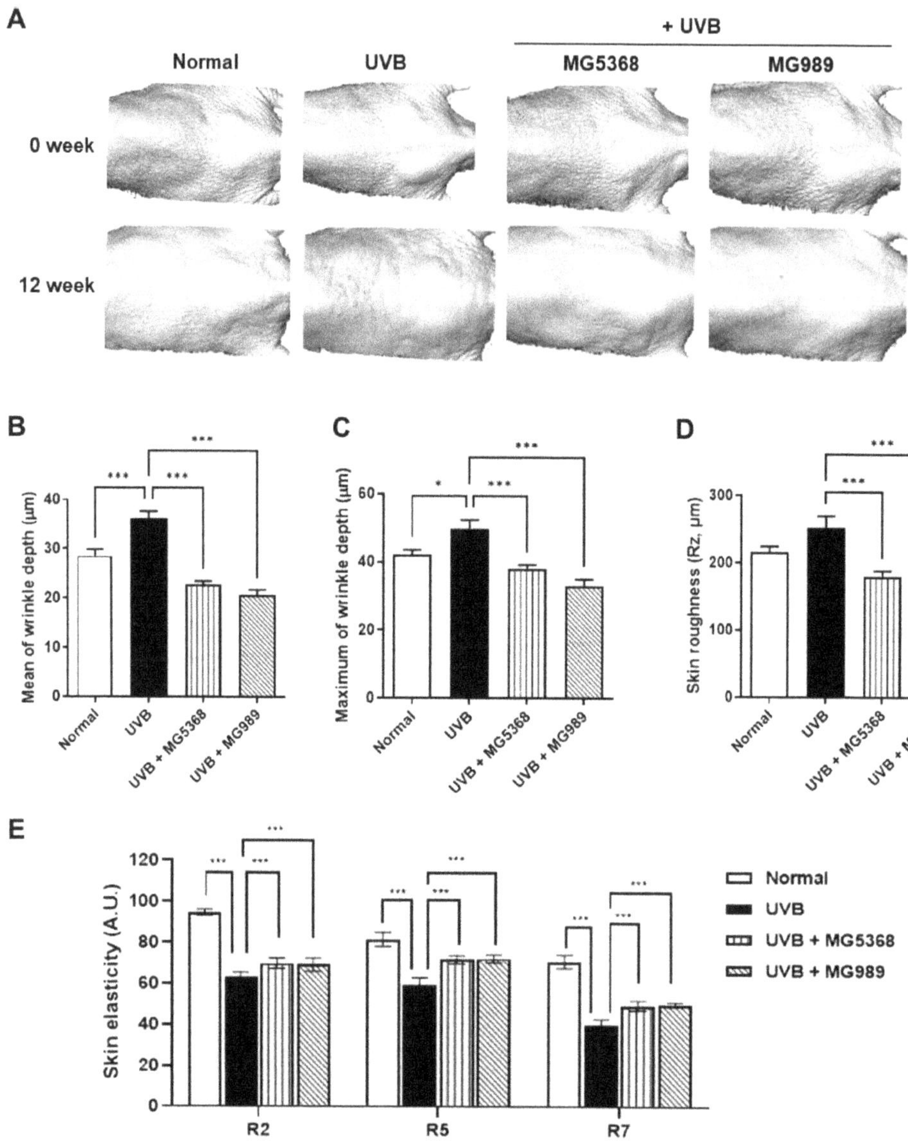

Figure 4. Effect of *L. fermentum* MG5368 and *L. plantarum* MG989 on wrinkle formation, roughness, and elasticity in UVB-exposed SKH-1 hairless mice. HR-1 hairless mice were orally administrated with *L. fermentum* MG5368 and *L. plantarum* MG989 (1×10^9 CFU/day) and were irradiated with UVB for 12 weeks. (**A**) Representative photographs of the mouse dorsal skin. (**B**) Mean of wrinkle depth, (**C**) maximum of wrinkle depth, (**D**) skin roughness (Rz), and (**E**) skin elasticity (A.U.) were analyzed. Values are expressed as the mean ± SEM ($n = 8$). * $p < 0.05$, and *** $p < 0.001$, significant difference compared to UVB-exposed group.

3.4. Oral Administration of L. fermentum MG5368 and L. plantarum MG989 Reduces Epidermis Thickness, Collagen, and HA in the Dorsal Skin of the UVB-Exposed SKH-1 Hairless Mice

Histological changes visualized by H&E and MT staining and HA levels in dorsal skin are shown in Figure 5. After UVB exposure to the dorsal skin of SKH-1 hairless mice, epidermis thickness was significantly increased, while oral administration of *L. fermentum* MG5368 significantly reduced epidermis thickness via H&E staining. MT staining revealed collagen fiber deposition and organization, which were quantified to measure collagen density. The collagen density was reduced by UVB exposure; however, the administration of *L. fermentum* MG5368 and *L. plantarum* MG989 significantly restored these levels to those observed in the normal group. Additionally, the administration of *L. fermentum* MG5368 and *L.s plantarum* MG989 significantly increased HA levels that had been reduced by UVB exposure.

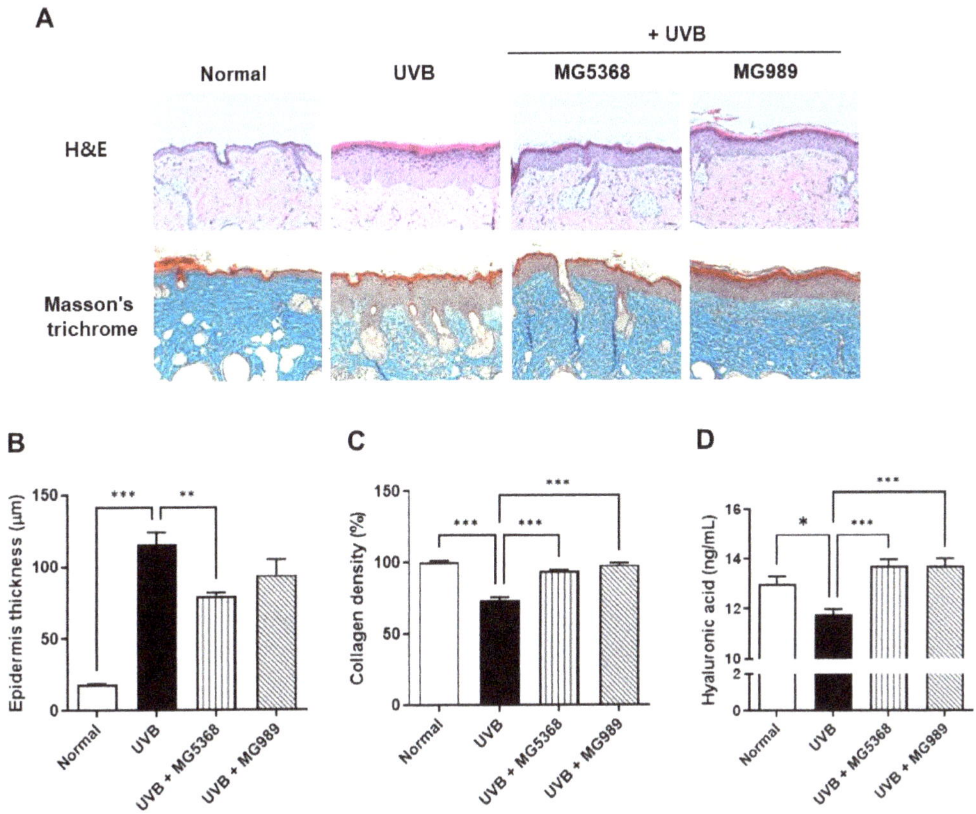

Figure 5. Histological observation and hyaluronic acid (HA) contents on SKH-1 hairless mice dorsal skin orally administrated with *L. fermentum* MG5368 and *L. plantarum* MG989 (1×10^9 CFU/day) and were exposed with UVB for 12 weeks. (**A**) Representative images of H&E and Masson's trichrome (MT) staining of the mouse dorsal skin. (**B**) Epidermis thickness by H&E stain, (**C**) collagen density by Masson's trichrome stain, and (**D**) HA analyzed by ELISA. Values are expressed as the mean ± SEM ($n = 8$). * $p < 0.05$, ** $p < 0.01$, and *** $p < 0.001$, significant difference compared to UVB-exposed group.

3.5. Oral Administration of L. fermentum MG5368 and L. plantarum MG989 Regulated AP-1/Smad Signaling Pathway in the Dorsal Skin of the UVB-Exposed SKH-1 Hairless Mice

In UVB-exposed dorsal skin of mice, phosphorylation of c-fos and c-jun, including in the AP-1 signaling pathway, was significantly reduced by the administration of *L. fermentum* MG5368 and *L. plantarum* MG989 (Figure 6A). Additionally, administration of *L. fermentum* MG5368 and *L. plantarum* MG989 significantly increased the phosphorylation of Smad 2/3 and the expression of COL1A1 and HAS2 proteins, which were reduced by UVB exposure (Figure 6B).

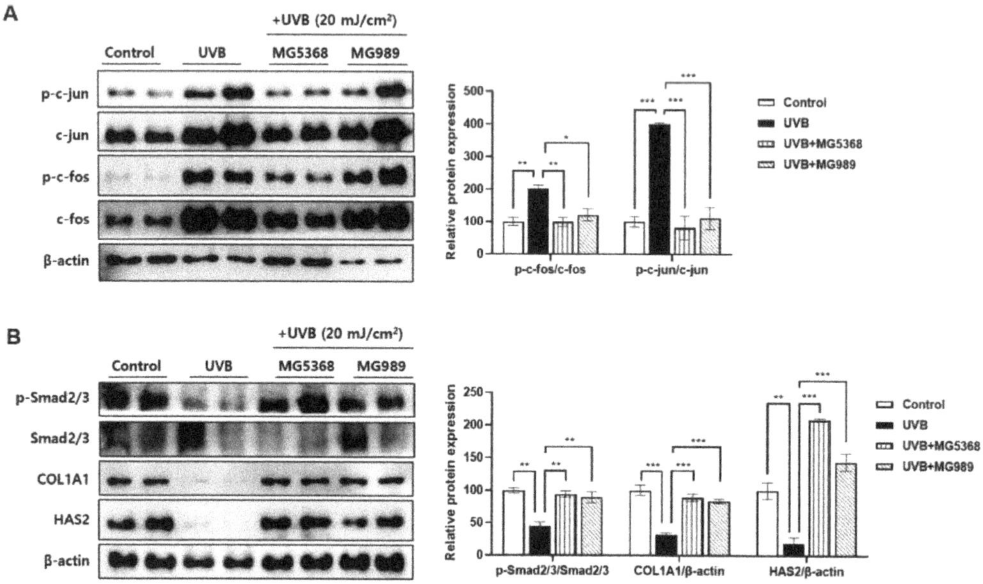

Figure 6. Effects of *L. fermentum* MG5368 and *L. plantarum* MG989 on the AP-1/Smad pathway in UVB-exposed SKH-1 hairless mice. HR-1 hairless mice were orally administrated with *L. fermentum* MG5368 and *L. plantarum* MG989 (1×10^9 CFU/day) and were irradiated with UVB for 12 weeks. The representative blotting images and relative expression of (**A**) AP-1 (p-c-fos, c-fos, p-c-jun, and c-jun) and (**B**) p-Smad 2/3, Smad 2/3, COL1A1, and HAS2 were evaluated by Western blotting. The β-actin was used as a loading control. Values are expressed as the mean ± SEM (n = 8). * $p < 0.05$, ** $p < 0.01$, and *** $p < 0.001$, significant difference compared to UVB-exposed group.

4. Discussion

One of the strategies to prevent photoaging is to use natural substances that can inhibit collagen breakdown. Recently, probiotics, rather than synthetic substances, have been studied extensively as alternatives with skin-preventing effects against extrinsic aging [1]. The *Lactobacillus* genus is commonly found and may be beneficial to the skin [23]. Probiotics attached to the gut can influence the microbial community, and probiotic metabolites, including lipoteichoic acid, lactic acid, and acetic acid, improve the skin barrier [8]. *L. plantarum* HY7714 maintained skin moisture and prevented wrinkles in vitro, in vivo, and in clinical trials [24,25]. Our previous study demonstrated that *Lactobacillus fermentum* MG5368 exhibited photoprotective effects against UVB exposure in human dermal fibroblasts, while *Lactobacillus plantarum* MG989 showed significant radical-scavenging activity and anti-inflammatory effects in RAW264.7 cells stimulated with LPS [8,26]. Nevertheless, the molecular mechanisms of photoprotective effects from *L. fermentum* MG5368 and *L. plantarum* MG989 remain unclear. Therefore, in this study, we investigated the photoprotective mechanism of *L. fermentum* MG5368 and *L. plantarum* MG989 in keratinocytes and in vivo.

One of the mechanisms for preventing skin aging is to maintain the skin barrier components [7]. Recent studies have shown that extracellular matrix (ECM) degradation is a major factor in wrinkle formation, specifically inducing ECM structural changes and dehydration [27]. Chronic UVB exposure induces collagen degradation, which leads to skin roughness, wrinkles, and loss of elasticity [28,29]. *L. fermentum* MG5368 and *L. plantarum* MG989 significantly restored collagen in keratinocytes and in vivo models against UVB. In addition, *L. fermentum* MG5368 and *L. plantarum* MG989 restored the average and maximum wrinkle depth, skin roughness, and elasticity parameters R2, R5, and R7 to normal levels.

The thickening of the epidermis and dermis is a primary defensive response to UV exposure, with prolonged UV exposure leading to an increase in the thickness of both the epidermal and dermal layers [30]. In our study, *L. fermentum* MG5368 and *L. plantarum* MG989 restored epidermis thickness in a UVB-exposed in vivo model. These findings indicate that the two strains improved wrinkle-related parameters by enhancing collagen production, a key component of the skin barrier.

Complex signaling induced by UV exposure leads to an increase in the expression of MMPs, which in turn promotes the degradation of proteins that constitute the ECM [31]. In the various types of MMP enzymes, UV exposure increases the expression of MMP-1 and MMP-3 in the dermal fibroblast and keratinocytes [32,33]. MMP-1 is a key enzyme in the collagen degradation process, cleaving collagen into two fragments and initiating collagen breakdown [34]. MMP-3, also known as stromelysin-1, degrades various types of ECM and activates MMP enzymes [33]. AP-1, composed of subunits of c-fos and c-jun, is activated by UVB and acts as a transcription factor that activates MMPs [7]. UVB exposure also damages the Smad 2/3 signaling pathway, resulting in decreased collagen synthesis [30]. Phosphorylation of Smad 2 and Smad 3 prompts their translocation from the cytoplasm to the nucleus and induces gene expression for collagen and collagen receptors, including COL1A1, thereby regulating collagen synthesis [35,36]. In our study, we investigated the effects on collagen production and degradation. *L. fermentum* MG5368 and *L. plantarum* MG989 were identified to have a molecular mechanism to reduce MMP-1 and MMP-3 by inhibiting AP-1 in UVB-exposed keratinocytes. In addition, these strains were identified to upregulate COL1A1 in UVB-exposed keratinocytes and in vivo models, thereby regulating the expression of factors involved in both collagen production and degradation.

An additional approach to prevent skin aging involves enhancing factors that maintain skin hydration levels [7]. HA is a crucial component of the ECM, essential for maintaining skin hydration and elasticity [37]. Exposure to UVB accelerates the breakdown of HA, leading to decreased moisture levels and reduced elasticity in the skin [38]. HAS2 is one of the primary enzymes that induces HA production, and it has a major role in epidermal cells [39]. In our study, *L. fermentum* MG5368 and *L. plantarum* MG989 significantly restored HA expression by upregulating HAS2 in UVB-exposed epidermal keratinocytes, with levels returning to normal in the in vivo models.

In this study, we confirmed the protective and anti-aging effects of *L. fermentum* MG5368 and *L. plantarum* MG989 against UVB-exposed skin damage. These strains contributed to collagen maintenance by inhibiting the expression of MMP-1 and MMP-3 and reducing collagen degradation by inhibiting the AP-1 pathway while promoting COL1A1 expression to maintain the ECM component and strengthen the skin barrier. Additionally, these strains positively affected skin elasticity by influencing skin moisture by restoring HA and HAS2 expression. Therefore, this study suggests that *L. fermentum* MG5368 and *L. plantarum* MG989 have the potential to be utilized as probiotic-based skin aging prevention agents, and further clinical trials and safety are needed to verify. However, further clinical trials are needed to validate the efficacy and safety of these strains.

5. Conclusions

In conclusion, this study demonstrates the potential of *L. fermentum* MG5368 and *L. plantarum* MG989 as effective probiotics for preventing UVB-induced skin aging. These strains exhibit significant protective effects on skin health by promoting collagen preservation and reducing ECM degradation. Specifically, *L. fermentum* MG5368 and *L. plantarum* MG989 effectively inhibited MMP-1 and MMP-3 expression by downregulating AP-1 activation, thereby mitigating collagen breakdown in UVB-exposed keratinocytes and in vivo models. Furthermore, these strains enhanced COL1A1 expression by regulating the Smad 2/3 pathway, promoting collagen synthesis and maintaining skin elasticity while inhibiting wrinkle formation. Additionally, they restored HA and HAS2 levels, which are essential for skin hydration and further supporting elasticity. These findings suggest that *L. fer-*

mentum MG5368 and *L. plantarum* MG989 hold promise as effective alternatives for skin aging prevention.

Supplementary Materials: The following supporting information can be downloaded at https://www.mdpi.com/article/10.3390/nu16234083/s1, Figure S1: The cell viability according to UVB exposure in HaCaT keratinocytes. Figure S2: Effect on collagen content of CFS in UVB-exposed HaCaT keratinocytes.

Author Contributions: Conceptualization, S.-I.C. and J.L.; methodology, J.-Y.P., J.Y.L. and S.-I.C.; formal analysis, J.Y.L., S.H. and H.H.; investigation, J.-Y.P., S.H., H.H. and H.L.; resources, B.-K.K.; data curation, J.Y.L., H.H. and H.L.; writing—original draft preparation, J.-Y.P. and J.Y.L.; writing—review and editing, S.H., H.H., H.L., Y.G.K., B.-K.K., S.-I.C. and J.L.; visualization, J.Y.L., S.H. and H.H.; supervision, B.-K.K. and J.L.; project administration, S.-I.C. and J.L.; funding acquisition, J.Y.L. and J.L. All authors have read and agreed to the published version of the manuscript.

Funding: This research was supported by the "Regional Innovation Strategy (RIS)" through the National Research Foundation of Korea (NRF), funded by the Ministry of Education (MOE), grant number 2021RIS-001.

Institutional Review Board Statement: The animal study protocol was approved by the Institutional Review Board of Seoul National University Bundang Hospital (BA-2307-371-003-02; approval date, 6 July 2023).

Informed Consent Statement: Not applicable.

Data Availability Statement: The datasets generated during and/or analyzed during the current study are available from the corresponding author upon reasonable request.

Conflicts of Interest: Authors Jeong-Yong Park, Ji Yeon Lee, Yong Gyeong Kim, Byoung-Kook Kim and Soo-Im Choi were employed by the company Mediogen, Co., Ltd. The remaining authors declare that the research was conducted in the absence of any commercial or financial relationships that could be construed as a potential conflict of interest.

References

1. Lee, J.Y.; Park, J.-Y.; Kim, Y.; Kang, C.-H. Protective effect of Bifidobacterium animalis subs. lactis MG741 as probiotics against UVB-exposed fibroblasts and hairless mice. *Microorganisms* **2022**, *10*, 2343. [CrossRef] [PubMed]
2. D'Orazio, J.; Jarrett, S.; Amaro-Ortiz, A.; Scott, T. UV radiation and the skin. *Int. J. Mol. Sci.* **2013**, *14*, 12222–12248. [CrossRef] [PubMed]
3. Proksch, E.; Brandner, J.M.; Jensen, J.M. The skin: An indispensable barrier. *Exp. Dermatol.* **2008**, *17*, 1063–1072. [CrossRef]
4. Park, J.-Y.; Lee, J.Y.; Kim, Y.; Kang, C.-H. *Latilactobacillus sakei* Wikim0066 protects skin through MMP regulation on UVB-irradiated in vitro and in vivo model. *Nutrients* **2023**, *15*, 726. [CrossRef]
5. Ichihashi, M.; Ando, H.; Yoshida, M.; Niki, Y.; Matsui, M. Photoaging of the skin. *Anti-Aging Med.* **2009**, *6*, 46–59. [CrossRef]
6. Quan, T.; Fisher, G.J. Role of age-associated alterations of the dermal extracellular matrix microenvironment in human skin aging: A mini-review. *Gerontology* **2015**, *61*, 427–434. [CrossRef]
7. Han, H.-S.; Shin, J.-S.; Myung, D.-B.; Ahn, H.S.; Lee, S.H.; Kim, H.J.; Lee, K.-T. *Hydrangea serrata* (Thunb.) Ser. extract attenuate UVB-induced photoaging through MAPK/AP-1 inactivation in human skin fibroblasts and hairless mice. *Nutrients* **2019**, *11*, 533. [CrossRef] [PubMed]
8. Park, J.-Y.; Lee, J.Y.; Kim, Y.; Kang, C.-H. Lactic acid bacteria improve the photoprotective effect via MAPK/AP-1/MMP signaling pathway on skin fibroblasts. *Microorganisms* **2022**, *10*, 2481. [CrossRef]
9. Yu, Y.; Dunaway, S.; Champer, J.; Kim, J.; Alikhan, A. Changing our microbiome: Probiotics in dermatology. *Br. J. Dermatol.* **2020**, *182*, 39–46. [CrossRef]
10. Jwo, J.Y.; Chang, Y.T.; Huang, Y.C. Effects of probiotics supplementation on skin photoaging and skin barrier function: A systematic review and meta-analysis. *Photodermatol. Photoimmunol. Photomed.* **2023**, *39*, 122–131. [CrossRef]
11. Morshedi, M.; Hashemi, R.; Moazzen, S.; Sahebkar, A.; Hosseinifard, E.-S. Immunomodulatory and anti-inflammatory effects of probiotics in multiple sclerosis: A systematic review. *J. Neuroinflammation* **2019**, *16*, 231. [CrossRef] [PubMed]
12. Kim, K.-T.; Kim, J.-W.; Kim, S.-I.; Kim, S.; Nguyen, T.H.; Kang, C.-H. Antioxidant and anti-inflammatory effect and probiotic properties of lactic acid bacteria isolated from canine and feline feces. *Microorganisms* **2021**, *9*, 1971. [CrossRef] [PubMed]
13. Mishra, V.; Shah, C.; Mokashe, N.; Chavan, R.; Yadav, H.; Prajapati, J. Probiotics as potential antioxidants: A systematic review. *J. Agric. Food Chem.* **2015**, *63*, 3615–3626. [CrossRef] [PubMed]

14. Calvo, M.J.; Navarro, C.; Durán, P.; Galan-Freyle, N.J.; Parra Hernández, L.A.; Pacheco-Londoño, L.C.; Castelanich, D.; Bermúdez, V.; Chacin, M. Antioxidants in Photoaging: From Molecular Insights to Clinical Applications. *Int. J. Mol. Sci.* **2024**, *25*, 2403. [CrossRef]
15. Kim, S.; Lee, J.Y.; Jeong, Y.; Kang, C.-H. Antioxidant activity and probiotic properties of lactic acid bacteria. *Fermentation* **2022**, *8*, 29. [CrossRef]
16. Lee, J.Y.; Park, Y.; Jeong, Y.; Kang, H. Anti-Inflammatory Response in TNFα/IFNγ-Induced HaCaT Keratinocytes and Probiotic Properties of *Lacticaseibacillus rhamnosus* MG4644, *Lacticaseibacillus paracasei* MG4693, and *Lactococcus lactis* MG5474. *J. Microbiol. Biotechnol.* **2023**, *33*, 1039. [CrossRef]
17. Xu, X.; Ding, Z.; Pu, C.; Kong, C.; Chen, S.; Lu, W.; Zhang, J. The structural characterization and UV-protective properties of an exopolysaccharide from a Paenibacillus isolate. *Front. Pharmacol.* **2024**, *15*, 1434136. [CrossRef]
18. Lee, J.Y.; Kim, Y.; Kim, J.-I.; Lee, H.-Y.; Moon, G.-S.; Kang, C.-H. Improvements in human keratinocytes and antimicrobial effect mediated by cell-free supernatants derived from probiotics. *Fermentation* **2022**, *8*, 332. [CrossRef]
19. Kim, J.-O.; An, G.; Choi, J.-H. Protective effect of mixture of *Acanthopanax sessiliflorum* and *Chaenomeles sinensis* against ultraviolet B-induced photodamage in human fibroblast and hairless mouse. *Food Sci. Biotechnol.* **2024**, *33*, 1715–1725. [CrossRef]
20. Carlos da Silva, G.; Barbosa, M.B.; Júnior, F.B.C.; Moreira, P.L.; Werka, R.; Martin, A.A. Detection of skin wrinkles and quantification of roughness using a novel image processing technique from a dermatoscope device. *Ski. Res. Technol.* **2023**, *29*, e13335. [CrossRef]
21. Kim, Y.J.; Lee, J.O.; Kim, S.Y.; Lee, J.M.; Lee, E.; Na, J.; Yoo, K.H.; Park, S.J.; Kim, B.J. Effect of A. polygama APEE (*Actinidia polygama* ethanol extract) or APWE (*Actinidia polygama* water extract) on wrinkle formation in UVB-irradiated hairless mice. *J. Cosmet. Dermatol.* **2023**, *22*, 311–319. [CrossRef] [PubMed]
22. Arnal-Forné, M.; Molina-García, T.; Ortega, M.; Marcos-Garcés, V.; Molina, P.; Ferrández-Izquierdo, A.; Sepulveda, P.; Bodí, V.; Ríos-Navarro, C.; Ruiz-Saurí, A. Changes in human skin composition due to intrinsic aging: A histologic and morphometric study. *Histochem. Cell Biol.* **2024**, *162*, 259–271. [CrossRef]
23. Lolou, V.; Panayiotidis, M.I. Functional role of probiotics and prebiotics on skin health and disease. *Fermentation* **2019**, *5*, 41. [CrossRef]
24. Ra, J.; Lee, D.E.; Kim, S.H.; Jeong, J.-W.; Ku, H.K.; Kim, T.-Y.; Choi, I.-D.; Jeung, W.; Sim, J.-H.; Ahn, Y.-T. Effect of oral administration of *Lactobacillus plantarum* HY7714 on epidermal hydration in ultraviolet B-irradiated hairless mice. *J. Microbiol. Biotechnol.* **2014**, *24*, 1736–1743. [CrossRef]
25. Lee, D.E.; Huh, C.-S.; Ra, J.; Choi, I.-D.; Jeong, J.-W.; Kim, S.-H.; Ryu, J.H.; Seo, Y.K.; Koh, J.S.; Lee, J.-H. Clinical evidence of effects of *Lactobacillus plantarum* HY7714 on skin aging: A randomized, double blind, placebo-controlled study. *J. Microbiol. Biotechnol.* **2015**, *25*, 2160–2168. [CrossRef] [PubMed]
26. Kang, C.-H.; Kim, J.-S.; Park, H.M.; Kim, S.; Paek, N.-S. Antioxidant activity and short-chain fatty acid production of lactic acid bacteria isolated from Korean individuals and fermented foods. *3 Biotech* **2021**, *11*, 217. [CrossRef] [PubMed]
27. Sparavigna, A. Role of the extracellular matrix in skin aging and dedicated treatment-state of the art. *Plast. Aesthet. Res* **2020**, *7*, 14. [CrossRef]
28. Hachiya, A.; Sriwiriyanont, P.; Fujimura, T.; Ohuchi, A.; Kitahara, T.; Takema, Y.; Kitzmiller, W.J.; Visscher, M.O.; Tsuboi, R.; Boissy, R.E. Mechanistic effects of long-term ultraviolet B irradiation induce epidermal and dermal changes in human skin xenografts. *Am. J. Pathol.* **2009**, *174*, 401–413. [CrossRef]
29. Yuksel Egrilmez, M.; Kocturk, S.; Aktan, S.; Oktay, G.; Resmi, H.; Simsek Keskin, H.; Guner Akdogan, G.; Ozkan, S. Melatonin prevents UVB-induced skin photoaging by inhibiting oxidative damage and MMP expression through JNK/AP-1 signaling pathway in human dermal fibroblasts. *Life* **2022**, *12*, 950. [CrossRef]
30. Kim, J.-M.; Chung, K.-S.; Yoon, Y.-S.; Jang, S.-Y.; Heo, S.-W.; Park, G.; Jang, Y.-P.; Ahn, H.-S.; Shin, Y.-K.; Lee, S.-H. Dieckol isolated from *Eisenia bicyclis* ameliorates wrinkling and improves skin hydration via MAPK/AP-1 and TGF-β/Smad signaling pathways in UVB-irradiated hairless mice. *Mar. Drugs* **2022**, *20*, 779. [CrossRef]
31. Kim, M.-J.; Woo, S.W.; Kim, M.-S.; Park, J.-E.; Hwang, J.-K. Anti-photoaging effect of aaptamine in UVB-irradiated human dermal fibroblasts and epidermal keratinocytes. *J. Asian Nat. Prod. Res.* **2014**, *16*, 1139–1147. [CrossRef] [PubMed]
32. Quan, T.; Qin, Z.; Xia, W.; Shao, Y.; Voorhees, J.J.; Fisher, G.J. Matrix-degrading metalloproteinases in photoaging. *J. Investig. Dermatol. Symp. Proc.* **2009**, *14*, 20–24. [CrossRef] [PubMed]
33. Noh, E.-M.; Lee, G.; Lim, C.-H.; Kwon, K.B.; Kim, J.-M.; Song, H.-K.; Yang, H.J.; Kim, M.J.; Kim, M.-s.; Lee, Y.-R. Protective effects of Evodiae Fructus extract against ultraviolet-induced MMP-1 and MMP-3 expression in human dermal fibroblasts. *J. Herb. Med.* **2022**, *35*, 100586. [CrossRef]
34. Brennan, M.; Bhatti, H.; Nerusu, K.C.; Bhagavathula, N.; Kang, S.; Fisher, G.J.; Varani, J.; Voorhees, J.J. Matrix metalloproteinase-1 is the major collagenolytic enzyme responsible for collagen damage in UV-irradiated human skin. *Photochem. Photobiol.* **2003**, *78*, 43–48. [CrossRef]
35. Lee, J.-J.; Ng, S.-C.; Ni, Y.-T.; Liu, J.-S.; Chen, C.-J.; Padma, V.V.; Huang, C.-Y.; Kuo, W.-W. Protective effects of galangin against H2O2/UVB-induced dermal fibroblast collagen degradation via hsa-microRNA-4535-mediated TGFβ/Smad signaling. *Aging* **2021**, *13*, 25342. [CrossRef]
36. Devos, H.; Zoidakis, J.; Roubelakis, M.G.; Latosinska, A.; Vlahou, A. Reviewing the regulators of COL1A1. *Int. J. Mol. Sci.* **2023**, *24*, 10004. [CrossRef]

37. Papakonstantinou, E.; Roth, M.; Karakiulakis, G. Hyaluronic acid: A key molecule in skin aging. *Derm. Endocrinol.* **2012**, *4*, 253–258. [CrossRef]
38. Kang, M.C.; Yumnam, S.; Kim, S.Y. Oral intake of collagen peptide attenuates ultraviolet B irradiation-induced skin dehydration in vivo by regulating hyaluronic acid synthesis. *Int. J. Mol. Sci.* **2018**, *19*, 3551. [CrossRef]
39. Abe, M.; Masuda, M.; Mizukami, Y.; Inoue, S.; Mizutani, Y. Epidermal keratinocytes regulate hyaluronan metabolism via extracellularly secreted hyaluronidase 1 and hyaluronan synthase 3. *J. Biol. Chem.* **2024**, *300*, 107449. [CrossRef]

nutrients

MDPI

Article

Effect of Postbiotic *Bifidobacterium longum* CECT 7347 on Gastrointestinal Symptoms, Serum Biochemistry, and Intestinal Microbiota in Healthy Adults: A Randomised, Parallel, Double-Blind, Placebo-Controlled Pilot Study

Malwina Naghibi [1], Adria Pont-Beltran [2], Araceli Lamelas [2], Laura Llobregat [2], Juan F. Martinez-Blanch [2], Antonia Rojas [2], Beatriz Álvarez [2], Bricia López Plaza [3,4], Lucia Arcos Castellanos [3], Empar Chenoll [2], Vineetha Vijayakumar [1,*] and Richard Day [1]

[1] Medical Department, ADM Health & Wellness, London SE1 7NT, UK
[2] ADM Research and Development Center-Valencia, ADM Health & Wellness, Parc Científic Universitat de València, 46980 València, Spain
[3] Food, Nutrition and Health Platform, Hospital La Paz Institzonulute for Health Research (IdiPAZ), 28046 Madrid, Spain
[4] Medicine Department, Faculty of Medicine, Complutense University of Madrid, Plaza de Ramón y Cajal, s/n, 28040 Madrid, Spain
* Correspondence: vineetha.vijayakumar@adm.com

Abstract: Objectives: A randomised, double-blind, placebo-controlled pilot trial was conducted to assess the effect of heat-treated *Bifidobacterium longum* CECT 7347 (HT-ES1) in healthy adults with mild to moderate digestive symptoms. A total of 60 participants were recruited and received either HT-ES1 or an identical placebo for 8 weeks with a further follow-up at week 10. Methods: This study monitored changes in the total Gastrointestinal Symptom Rating Scale for IBS score (GSRS-IBS), Irritable Bowel Syndrome Symptom Severity Scale (IBS-SSS), IBS Quality of Life index (IBS-QoL), gut microbiome using 16S rRNA sequencing, and the Visceral Sensitivity Index, as well as a range of biochemical markers, anthropometric parameters, and adverse events. Results: While minimal changes were observed in gastrointestinal (GI) symptoms, the HT-ES1 group showed a significant decrease in total and non-HDL cholesterol compared to the placebo. The intervention group also exhibited a significant increase in the abundance of the genera *Faecalibacterium* and *Anaerobutyricum*, both of which were positively correlated with butyrate concentrations. Faecal calprotectin significantly increased over time in the placebo group but remained stable in the HT-ES1 group. Conclusions: Overall, these findings suggest that HT-ES1 may promote gut health by increasing butyrate-producing bacteria in the gut, maintaining normal levels of faecal calprotectin and reducing serum cholesterol.

Keywords: postbiotics; gut health; microbiome; SCFAs; butyrate; healthy population; inflammation; calprotectin; abundance; *Faecalibacterium*; *Anaerobutyricum*; *Phocaeicola*; *Anaerostripes*; *Blautia*

1. Introduction

In recent years, there have been many developments in the research of functional foods and non-pharmacological bioactives for digestive health. Much of this research has been conducted in the microbiome space, including prebiotics, probiotics, and—more recently—postbiotics. This increase in research may be in part driven by the high prevalence of mild gastrointestinal (GI) symptoms experienced by the general population [1]. GI symptoms in otherwise healthy adults can have important consequences on overall well-being and quality of life. In a 2018 study, out of a total of 71,812 Americans, 61% reported at least one GI symptom, including heartburn, abdominal pain, bloating, diarrhoea, or constipation over a one-week period [1].

The GI microbiota is the collection of all the bacteria, archaea, and eukarya inhabiting the GI tract, and evidence indicates that the composition of the intestinal microbiota in those who have GI symptoms may be altered compared to symptom-free individuals [2]. Furthermore, it is known that a number of digestive disorders are characterised by imbalances in the composition of the *Bifidobacterium* genus [3,4]. Probiotics are defined as live microorganisms that, when administered in adequate amounts, confer a health benefit to the host [5]. Probiotics, including those belonging to the *Lactobacillus* and *Bifidobacterium* genera, have been indicated as potential candidates for the management of GI disorders such as irritable bowel syndrome (IBS) [6,7]. The genus *Bifidobacterium* has been studied extensively, and there are numerous studies indicating its potential health benefits; these include protecting against pathogenic bacteria, modulating mucosal barrier function, regulating immune and inflammatory responses, and exerting beneficial effects against conditions ranging between coeliac disease, IBS, ulcerative colitis, immunoglobulin E-associated conditions, and atopic dermatitis [8–10].

One strain of interest in digestive health is the breast milk isolate *Bifidobacterium longum* CECT 7347 (ES1), which has been shown in several studies to have physiological effects that may be beneficial for digestive health. In a paediatric clinical trial, children with newly diagnosed coeliac disease experienced decreased peripheral lymphocytes and decreased levels of TNF-α following supplementation with ES1 [11]. Additionally, a pilot study in a non-coeliac gluten-sensitive population demonstrated that a combination of diet and ES1 supplementation improved intestinal and extra-intestinal symptoms [12]. Notably, the beneficial probiotic bacterial–host interactions have been shown to be mediated by extracellular probiotic compounds, including organic acids, antimicrobial compounds, enzymes, and components related to the cell envelope (lipoteichoic acids, exopolysaccharides, or peptidoglycan-derived molecules) [13]. These findings underscore the potential of ES1 to exert its effects in its viable probiotic form.

Thus, considering that ES1 demonstrates significant bioactivities as a probiotic, there is interest in exploring how these effects may persist in its heat-treated form, here referred to as a postbiotic [14]. The use of postbiotics has been indicated to have several advantages over the use of live probiotic cultures, including better stability, longer shelf-life, and the ability to be included in food matrices and survive extreme conditions of processing [15]. Additionally, in populations where there may be safety concerns over the use of live bacteria, postbiotics may be a preferential alternative as they have potential applications in medical and early life nutrition [16,17]. Notably, *B. longum* CECT 7347 has been shown to retain certain functionalities in its heat-treated postbiotic form (referred to hereafter as "HT-ES1"), such as reducing inflammation in intestinal cells in an in vivo model [18]. In a recent study in an IBS population, daily consumption of either live ES1 or HT-ES1 for a period of 12 weeks was associated with statistically significant and clinically meaningful improvements in IBS-SSS, IBS-QoL, abdominal pain severity, and anxiety scores compared to placebo [7].

Despite positive preliminary data on the potential of postbiotics to improve GI symptoms, to our knowledge, the effects of postbiotic supplementation on the gut microbiome of healthy populations without any formal diagnosis of a GI disorder are yet to be explored. Here, we aim to evaluate the ability of an HT-ES1 to modulate gut microbiome composition as well as assess its ability to influence mild GI symptoms, serum biochemistry, and intestinal inflammation in a healthy adult population.

2. Materials and Methods

2.1. Compliance with Ethical Standards

This study was conducted in compliance with the Declaration of Helsinki and National Ethical Guidelines for Biomedical and Health Research involving Human Participants, and the study protocol was approved by the Research Ethics Committee with Medical Products Hospital La Paz Institute for Health Research (10 November 2021, Ref: 57/458465.9/21; IdiPAZ). This study was registered with the USA National Library of Medicine clinical trials registry ClinicalTrials.gov (Identifier: NCT05367427) and run from the Clinical Nutrition and Dietetics Unit of the University Hospital La Paz, Madrid, Spain. Written informed consent was obtained from all participants before initiation of the study procedures. No formal patient and public involvement (PPI) activity was undertaken, so, as a result, participants were not involved in the trial design, the choice of outcomes, or the recruitment strategy for the trial.

2.2. Study Participants

A total of 154 healthy volunteers were screened for eligibility; of those, 60 participants (11 males and 49 females) aged 18–65 years who scored between 13 and 39 points on the GI Symptom Rating Scale for IBS (GSRS-IBS) were included (Figure 1). More detailed inclusion and exclusion criteria are presented in Supplementary Section S1. Of the 60 randomised participants, 53 completed the study (n = 27 in placebo and n = 26 in intervention group). A total of 7 participants dropped out due to a broken tibia (n = 1), cancer diagnosis (n = 2), GI issues and hives (n = 1), due to distance, relocation, or non-compliance (n = 3). Reasons for withdrawal were determined to be unrelated to the investigational product. Therefore, the final per-protocol analysis was conducted on 53 participants.

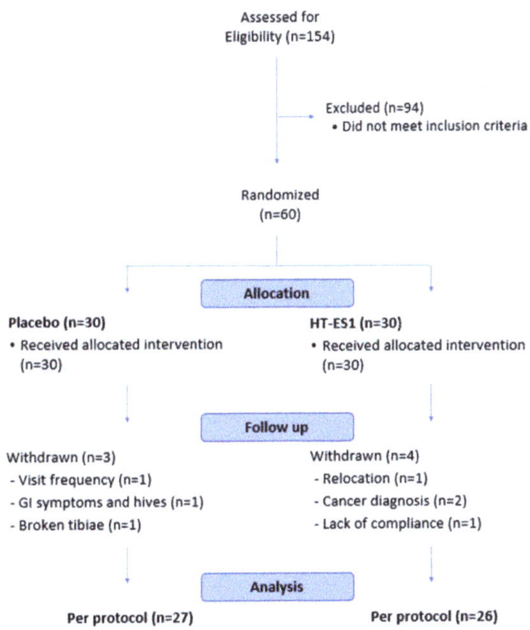

Figure 1. Consort flow diagram. n: number of subjects.

2.3. Study Design and Product

This is a single-centred, placebo-controlled, pilot study to explore the safety and efficacy of the postbiotic HT-ES1 in healthy adults with mild GI symptoms. This clinical trial was carried out between February and October 2022. Participants were randomised by the Biostatistics Unit of La Paz Hospital using a 1:1 allocation ratio between the intervention group (n = 30) and the placebo group (n = 30). Participants, investigators, and assessors collecting outcome data were blinded to the assigned intervention during the study.

The intervention group was instructed to take two capsules of postbiotic HT-ES1 daily, with breakfast (2.5×10^9 cells/day equivalent to 50 mg/day when prepared from a postbiotic batch at a concentration of 5×10^{10} cells/g), and the placebo group was given an identical placebo (Maltodextrin) for a period of 8 weeks. HT-ES1 was prepared through a proprietary method of heat treatment of the probiotic solution followed by a drying step to create a dry powder. Capsules were produced by Korott, Alcoi, Spain. The presentation and exterior characteristics of the active and placebo were visually identical. *Bifidobacterium longum* CECT 7347 is a strain deposited in the Spanish Culture Type Collection and patented by the Spanish National Research Council.

Clinical examination and sample collection were performed at baseline and after 4 and 8 weeks of intervention. A follow-up phone call was conducted 2 weeks after cessation of the intervention (week 10) (Figure 2).

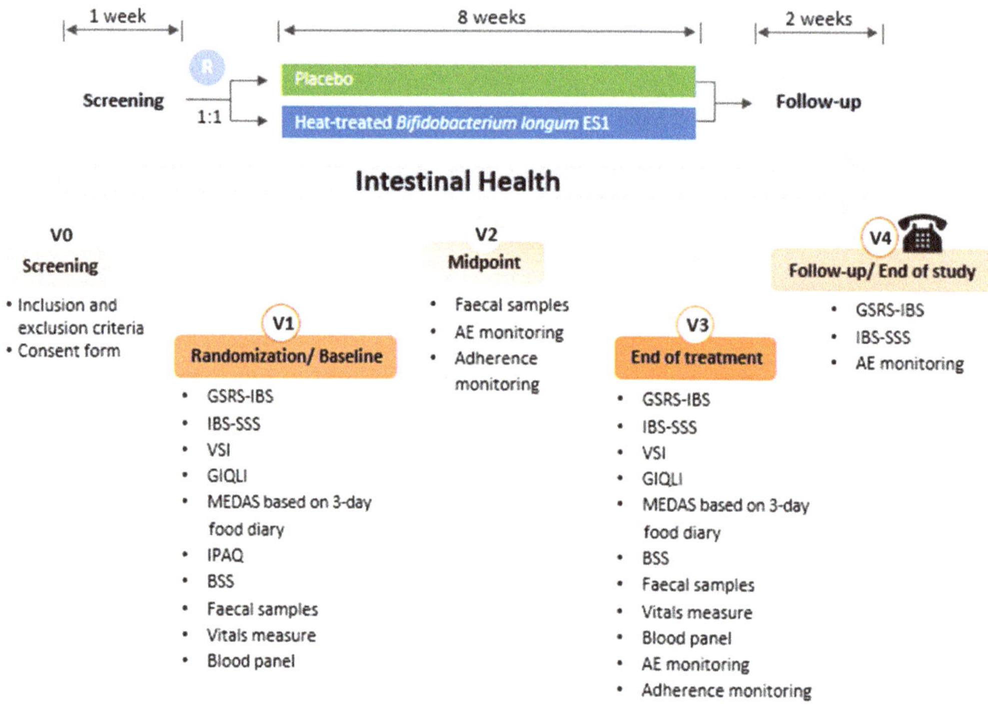

Figure 2. Study visit schedule. GSRS-IBS: GI Symptom Rating Scale for IBS; VSI: Visceral Sensitivity Index; IBS-SSS: Irritable Bowel Syndrome Symptom Severity Scale; GIQLI: Gastrointestinal Quality of Life Index; MEDAS: Mediterranean Diet Adherence Screener; IPAQ: International Physical Activity Questionnaire; BSS: Bristol Stool Scale; R: Randomisation.

2.4. Outcome Measures

2.4.1. Baseline and Safety Measures

The study cohort was assessed at the baseline for standard characteristics, including health habits (smoking, alcohol consumption), diet (the Mediterranean Diet Adherence Screener (MEDAS)), physical activity levels (the International Physical Activity Questionnaire (IPAQ)), and medical history. MEDAS score was also evaluated at week 8 to monitor any changes in dietary habits. Detailed methods of the assessment tools are described in the Supplementary Materials (Section S2).

Blood samples were collected at weeks 0 and 8 and analysed for full blood counts, urea and electrolytes, glucose, protein (Protein, Albumin, Prealbumin), and lipid metabolism markers (Triglycerides, HDL, LDL, non-HDL, and total cholesterol). Serum minerals (calcium, phosphorus, sodium, potassium, magnesium, chlorine) and vitamin (A, E, D, folic acid, vitamin B12) levels were also determined. Additionally, markers of inflammation (hsCRP, TNF-α, IL-4, IL-6, IL-10, and IL-12) were measured. Anthropometrics (weight, height, waist circumference, BMI) were evaluated, and bioelectrical impedance (BIA, INBODY S10) was used to assess body composition at weeks 0 and 8.

Safety variables collected at weeks 0 and 8 included blood pressure (systolic and diastolic), heart rate, and liver and kidney function (creatinine, glomerular filtration rate (GFR), alanine aminotransferase (ALT), and bilirubin).

2.4.2. GI Assessment Tools

The primary outcome measure is the change in the GSRS-IBS score. The GSRS-IBS is a validated questionnaire used to assess the severity and frequency of GI symptoms related to IBS, such as abdominal pain and discomfort, bloating and flatulence, stool urgency, frequency and form, as well as satiety after meals. The GSRS-IBS includes 13 questions, and each question is rated on a Likert scale of 6 points, where 0 represents no discomfort and 6 is severe discomfort. The GSRS-IBS questionnaire was collected at weeks 0, 8, and 10 as the primary outcome of this study. Symptom severity was then classified based on the total score: mild (0–19), moderate (20–39), or severe (40–78).

As secondary outcomes, patients also completed the Irritable Bowel Syndrome Symptom Severity Scale (IBS-SSS) questionnaire at weeks 0, 8, and 10. Additionally, at the beginning and end of the intervention (weeks 0 and 8), they completed the following: the GI Quality of Life Index (GIQLI) and the Visceral Sensitivity Index (VSI) questionnaires. The Bristol Stool Form Scale (BSS) was recorded daily for 7 days prior to study visit at weeks 0 and 8. Detailed methods for the assessment tools are described in the Supplementary Materials (Section S2).

2.4.3. Assessment of Faecal Samples

Microbiome Biochemistry

Faecal samples were collected at baseline, week 4, and week 8 using a faecal collection kit (FeelGut, Alderley edge, UK) and analysed by the ADM Research & Development Center Valencia, Spain. The concentrations of short-chain fatty acids (SCFAs) (butyric, acetic and propionic acid, and total SCFAs) in the samples were measured by high-performance liquid chromatography with refractive index detector (HPLC-RID) (Waters Corporation, Milford, MA, USA). SCFA concentration values were multiplied by 12, the dilution factor. Faecal samples were tested for calprotectin and lactoferrin using a commercially available kit (CALPRO, Abyntek Biopharma, Zamudio, Spain). The concentration of zonulin in stool was determined with an enzyme-linked immunosorbent assay (ELISA) kit (DRG Instruments GmbH, Marburg, Germany), following the manufacturer's instructions, in Hospital La Paz Institute for Health Research (IdiPAZ).

Microbiome Composition

Microbial DNA was extracted from stool using the QIAsymphony PowerFecal Pro DNA Kit (Qiagen, Hilden, Germany). The V3–V4 hypervariable region of the 16S rRNA gene was amplified from genomic DNA using primers 341F (CCTACGGGNGGCWGCAG) and 805R (GACTACHVGGG TATCTAATCC). 16S-based libraries were quantified by fluorimetry using the Quant-iT™ Picofreen™ dsDNA Assay Kit (Thermofisher, Waltham, MA, USA). Libraries were pooled before sequencing on the MiSeq platform (Illumina, San Diego, CA, USA) with a 300 cycles paired reads configuration. The size and quantity of the pool were assessed on the Bioanalyzer 2100 (Agilent, Santa Clara, CA, USA) and with the Library Quantification Kit for Illumina (Kapa Biosciences, Oslo, Norway), respectively. The PhiX Control library (v3) (Illumina) was combined with the amplicon library. Image analysis, base calling, and data quality assessment were performed on the MiSeq instrument (MiSeq Control Software (MCS v2.6.2.1)). Forward and reverse sequences were merged using the BBMerge package of BBMap V.38 software [19]. The amplification primers were trimmed to reduce the bias in the annotation step using Cutadapt v 1.8.1 [20].

A quality filter was applied to delete poor-quality sequences using the Reformat package of BBMap V.38 software. Sequences lower than 200 nts were removed from the analysis. Those bases in extreme positions that did not reach Q20 or a greater Phred score were removed. Sequences whose average quality did not surpass the Q20 threshold, as a mean quality of the whole sequence, were also deleted. The reads were processed using the DADA2 algorithm 'denoise-single' command [21]. Error rates were learned from a set of subsampled reads using 'learnErrors', and the sample inference algorithm was applied with the 'dada' function to generate the Amplicon Sequence Variants (ASVs). The chimeric ASVs were removed using the 'removeChimeraDenovo' function. The taxonomy of the ASVs was annotated against the NCBI 16S rRNA database version 2023 using blastn version 2.2.29+ [22]. The taxonomy of the ASVs that had been assigned with a lower percentage identity than 97% was reassigned using the NBAYES algorithm [23] from QIIME2 platform v2021.8 [24]. The NBAYES classifier was previously trained on V3-V4 regions of the 16S rRNA gene from the SILVA v.138 database [25]. ASVs identified to a bacteria kingdom and with at least 0.05% of relative frequency in at least 5 samples were kept for the statistical analysis. Sequence files and metadata for the microbiome analyses were deposited in NCBI SRA under BioProject PRJNA1164946.

2.4.4. Compliance and Adverse Event Reporting

Compliance was assessed by monitoring the number of capsules returned at each visit, and once the intervention period was over, the remaining containers were returned to the Principal Investigator. Concomitant medication and adverse events were also monitored.

2.5. Statistical Analysis

2.5.1. Statistical Analysis of Questionnaires and Physical and Biochemical Parameters

Normally distributed data were analysed using Student's *t*-tests, and non-parametric data were analysed using the Mann–Whitney U-test. Between-group changes from the baseline were analysed using an independent *t*-test. Within group analyses were conducted using paired sample *t*-tests. All tests were two-tailed with significance set at $p < 0.05$. Analyses were conducted on per-protocol (PP) populations using SPSS 21.0 at La Paz University Hospital's Biostatistics Section.

The Wilcoxon test was used to find differences in calprotectin, lactoferrin, and short-chain fatty acid concentrations between times on each group and between groups on each time.

2.5.2. Microbiome Data

Data were normalised using a rarefaction technique from Phyloseq R package v1.34 [26] to perform alpha diversity analysis. Shannon, Simpson, and Richness indexes were calculated using vegan R package v2.5-7 [27]. The Bray–Curtis dissimilarity matrix and permutational analysis of variance (PERMANOVA) analysis for beta diversity were performed using vegan R package v2.5-7 after normalisation by relative frequency for each sample. PERMANOVA was used to assess the differences in the microbiome composition among groups, times, and subjects and was also used to evaluate the influence of the MEDAS index on the microbiome.

Differential taxa abundance was analysed using the DESeq2 R package v.1.30.1 [28]. The normalisation was based on the 'Relative Log Expression' method. The 'EstimateSizeFactors' function was used to calculate the scaling factors using the median ratio between taxa abundances and the geometric mean. We used the 'PosCounts' method, which deals with taxa that have multiple zeros in most of the samples, as usually occurs in metagenomics. A taxon was considered differentially abundant with a Benjamani–Hochberg ("BH") multiple testing correction adjusted p-value < 0.05 and if it was present in at least 50% of the samples of one of the compared groups. Heatmaps were constructed using ComplexHeatmap R package v.2.11.1 [29]. For this analysis, only subjects with three samples obtained thought time were considered.

MaAslin2 R package v1.4 [30] was used to study correlations between microbial abundances and organic compounds. A linear model test was performed for each variable, with the variable as the fixed effect. The microbial taxa counts were normalised using the DESeq2 normalisation method, and the normalised counts were log-transformed. Only taxa present in more than 10% of the samples were considered.

The Wilcoxon test was used to find differences in alpha diversity metrics between times on each group and between groups on each time. It was also used to find differences in the intra-subject over-time changes between the groups on certain taxa abundances.

3. Results

3.1. Baseline Characteristics of Participants

The baseline characteristics of the enrolled subjects were comparable (Table S1A–C). The IPAQ showed no significant differences between groups at the baseline, with 73.3% of the population reporting moderate physical activity, 10% stating a predominantly sedentary lifestyle, and 16.7% of the cohort reporting high physical activity. Regarding dietary habits, the MEDAS index indicated that the placebo group followed a more Mediterranean-style diet compared to the HT-ES1 group at the baseline [placebo: 8.0 ± 1.2 vs. HT-ES1: 7.1 ± 1.4, $p = 0.007$]. However, it is important to note that the mean score for neither group reached the nine-point threshold, which has been previously established as the cut-off for a diet that meets the recommendations of the Mediterranean diet [31].

3.2. Biochemical Outcomes and Safety Parameters

The blood biochemical assessment over the study duration indicated that there was a significant between-group difference in the change in total cholesterol, [HT-ES1: −12.83 ± 46 vs. placebo: +8.04 ± 22.42 ($p = 0.01$)] and non-HDL cholesterol [HT-ES1: −0.85 ± 17.06 vs. placebo: +8.3 ± 19.32 ($p = 0.044$)] at the end of the intervention (Tables 1 and S2).

Table 1. Per-protocol analysis of changes in serum biochemistry and faecal parameters.

	HT-ES1 n = 26		Control n = 27		
	Week 0	Week 8	Week 0	Week 8	*p*-Value #
Serum Biochemistry					
Glucose (mg/dL)	92.85 ± 6.69	90.62 ± 7.27	91.7 ± 5.92	91.52 ± 8.34	ns
Cholesterol (mg/dL)	193 ± 29.18	180.17 ± 48.72	191.63 ± 28.79	199.67 ± 33.95	0.01
HDL (mg/dL)	57.88 ± 13.01	55.46 ± 13.4	64.44 ± 15.03	64.15 ± 14.69	ns
Non-HDL (mg/dL)	135 ± 26.51	134.15 ± 29.87	127.19 ± 30.45	135.48 ± 37.44 *	0.044
LDL (mg/dL)	118.32 ± 23.29	128.92 ± 31.05 **	110.3 ± 27.09	127.48 ± 37.43 ***	ns
Triglycerides (mg/dL)	84.12 ± 46.61	93.77 ± 64.44	86.07 ± 39.71	91.85 ± 51.69	ns
Total proteins (g/dL)	7.16 ± 0.33	7.06 ± 0.37	7.24 ± 0.62	7.07 ± 0.56 *	ns
Albumin (mg/dL)	4.58 ± 0.21	4.32 ± 0.31 ***	4.56 ± 0.32	4.35 ± 0.33 **	ns
Prealbumin (mg/dL)	24.51 ± 4.58	25.06 ± 4.55	25.86 ± 3.44	27.04 ± 4.26	ns
Ferritin (ng/mL)	77.38 ± 75.26	79.62 ± 66.93	51.04 ± 47.02	61.48 ± 43.53 ***	ns
Faecal parameters					
Zonulin (ng/mg)	177.38 ± 127.69	208.87 ± 137.89	185.69 ± 98.37	241.31 ± 222.74	ns

Change of HT-ES1 vs. placebo. Intragroup change from baseline: * $p < 0.05$, ** $p < 0.01$, *** $p < 0.001$. ns: non-significant.

Significant within-group changes were observed in LDL cholesterol, albumin, ferritin, vitamin D, vitamin E, fat mass, urate, bilirubin, and systolic blood pressure (SBP) in both groups, or specifically in either the placebo or probiotic group (Tables 1, S2 and S3). Of note, during the course of the study, three participants (two in HT-ES1 group and one in placebo) were given vitamin D supplements due to deficiencies.

Safety variables such as blood pressure (systolic and diastolic), heart rate, and kidney and liver function (creatinine, GFR, ALT, and bilirubin levels) were comparable between the groups throughout the intervention (Table S3).

3.3. Adverse Event

Overall, 27 participants (15 in HT-ES1, 12 in placebo) reported a total of 39 adverse events (AEs). Only two of the AEs were classified as related to the consumption of the investigational product (gastralgia and foul gases), and three others (nausea, bloating, and reflux) were deemed to be possibly related to the postbiotic. In the placebo group, three AEs (nausea, diarrhoea, foul gases) were suspected to be related to the study product. There were no SAEs related to the investigational product reported.

3.4. GI Assessment

No significant between-group differences were observed for the total GSRS-IBS, IBS-SSS, GIQLI, VSI, or BSS scores after 8 weeks of intervention (Table 2).

Table 2. Health questionnaire total scores.

Questionnaire	HT-ES1 (n = 26)	Placebo (n = 27)	*p*-Value #
	GSRS-IBS: Total Score		
Baseline (week 0)	27.08 ± 8.32	28.62 ± 9.25	ns
End of intervention (week 8)	26.48 ± 13.08	26.31 ± 14.53	ns
End of follow-up (week 10)	21.92 ± 14.1 *	22.35 ± 14.19 *	ns
	IBS-SSS: Total Score		
Baseline (week 0)	154.2 ± 72.58	187.88 ± 93	ns
End of intervention (week 8)	140.2 ± 78.14	166.92 ± 93.39	ns
End of follow-up (week 10)	143.4 ± 73.65	163.65 ± 80.41 *	ns
	GIQLI: Total Score		
Baseline (week 0)	99.32 ± 9.68	99.35 ± 14.69	ns
End of intervention (week 8)	101.68 ± 10.76	101.88 ± 15.28	ns
	VSI: Total Score		
Baseline (week 0)	54.96 ± 19.04	55.54 ± 19.49	ns
End of intervention (week 8)	60.64 ± 16.65	64.58 ± 15.62 *	ns
	Bowel movements/week		
Baseline (week 0)	10.52 ± 6.25	8.58 ± 3.68	ns
End of intervention (week 8)	10.48 ± 6.84	8.96 ± 3.8	ns
	Bowel movements/day		
Baseline (week 0)	1.5 ± 0.89	1.23 ± 0.53	ns
End of intervention (week 8)	1.5 ± 0.98	1.28 ± 0.54	ns

Change in HT-ES1 vs. placebo, ns: non-significant. Intragroup change from baseline: * $p < 0.05$.

Some outcomes exhibited a significant within-group decrease at the 10-week follow-up. The diarrhoea subscale of the GSRS showed a significant within-group decrease in both groups [HT-ES1 2.03 ± 0.65 vs. 1.49 ± 1.09 $p < 0.01$ and placebo 2.2 ± 0.91 vs. 1.52 ± 1.13 $p < 0.05$]. Additionally, a significant within-group reduction in the total GSRS-IBS score was observed at the follow-up in both groups [HT-ES1 27.08 ± 8.32 vs. 21.92 ± 14.1 $p < 0.05$ and placebo 28.62 ± 9.25 vs. 22.35 ± 14.19 $p < 0.05$] (Table S4). The placebo group also showed a significant within-group decrease in total IBS-SSS scores [187.88 ± 93 vs. 163.65 ± 80.41, $p < 0.05$]. However, despite being statistically significant, this change is not considered clinically meaningful, and baseline values, although not significantly different, reflected different severity categories between groups.

3.5. Faecal Health Biomarkers

3.5.1. Inflammation Markers

Calprotectin and lactoferrin were measured in faecal samples at the baseline, week 4, and week 8. There was no significant difference in the faecal calprotectin concentration between the intervention and placebo groups at the end of the study. However, in the placebo arm, a significant increase in faecal calprotectin levels between weeks 4 and 8 of the intervention period was observed [wk4: 26.84 ± 59.84 vs. wk8: 75.40 ± 95.04 $p = 0.039$] (Figure 3A). No within-group changes were observed in the HT-ES1 group. The lactoferrin concentration did not vary significantly over time in either group.

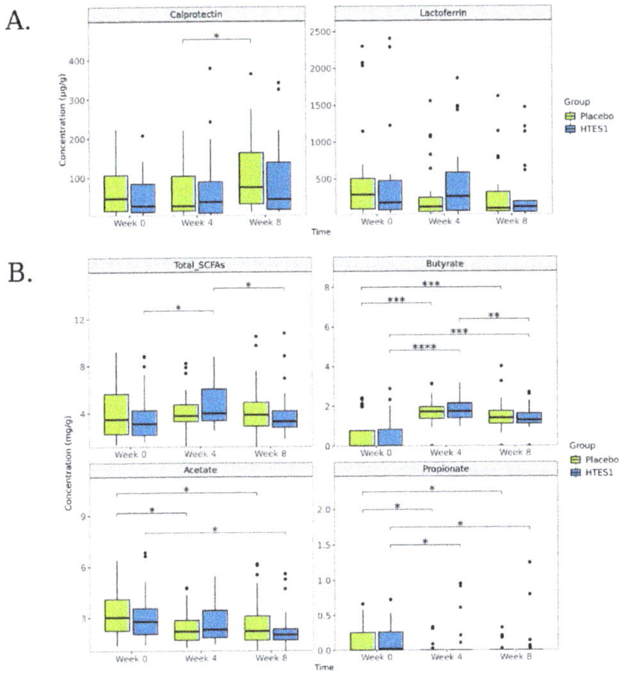

Figure 3. (**A**) Boxplots on calprotectin and lactoferrin concentrations and (**B**) organic compound concentrations in each group over time; weeks 0, 4, and 8. The Wilcox test was applied between times in each group and between groups on each time. * $p < 0.05$, ** $p < 0.01$, *** $p < 0.001$, **** $p < 0.0001$.

3.5.2. Short-Chain Fatty Acids

No significant differences in SCFAs were observed between groups at any time point (Figure 3B). A significant within-group change in total SCFA was observed in the HT-ES1 arm from week 0 to week 4 [3.09 ± 2.15 vs. 3.97 ± 1.77 ($p = 0.027$)], and there was a significant decrease from week 4 to 8 [3.97 ± 1.77 vs. 3.27 ± 2.07 ($p = 0.031$)]. In contrast, no significant changes in the total SCFA concentration were observed over time in the placebo group.

While analysing individual SCFAs, within-group changes were observed in both groups for butyric acid, propionic acid, and acetic acid (Figure 3B). A significant increase in the butyric acid concentration was noted in both groups over time [placebo: wk0: 0 ± 0.88 vs. wk4: 1.72 ± 0.64 ($p = 0.0002$) and vs. wk8: 1.41 ± 0.78 ($p = 0.0004$) and HT-ES1 group: wk0: 0 ± 0.88 vs. wk4: 1.74 ± 0.61 ($p = 0.000004$) and vs. wk8: 1.30 ± 0.56 ($p = 0.0002$)]. A significant decrease in the propionic and acetic acid concentration was observed in both groups over time: propionic acid [placebo: wk0: 0 ± 0.21 vs. wk4: 0 ± 0.08 ($p = 0.025$) and vs. wk8: 0 ± 0.09 ($p = 0.045$) and HT-ES1 group: wk0: 0.02 ± 0.21 vs. wk4: 0 ± 0.27 ($p = 0.05$) and vs. wk8: 0 ± 0.28 ($p = 0.037$)]; acetic acid [placebo: wk0: 3.02 ± 1.38 vs. wk8: 2.19 ± 1.49 ($p = 0.05$), and HT-ES1: wk0: 2.78 ± 1.42 vs. wk8: 1.97 ± 1.17 ($p = 0.011$)] (Figure 3B).

3.6. Microbiome Composition

3.6.1. Composition of Gut Microbiome

A total of 947 ASVs were taxonomically identified as bacteria and passed the prevalence filter. In total, 82.58% of these ASV were classified at the genus level. Overall, the study population had a microbiome mainly dominated by the genera *Phocaeicola* (10.31 ± 5.46%), *Faecalibacterium* (7.68 ± 3.52%), *Bacteroides* (6.49 ± 3.98%), *Blautia* (6.46 ± 3.55%), and *Bifidobacterium* (4.79 ± 4.33%) (Figure S1).

3.6.2. Diversity Analysis

No significant differences were observed in richness or alpha diversity, measured by the Shannon or Simpson indices, at either time point when comparing the HT-ES1 or placebo groups (Figure 4A). Additionally, we performed principal coordinate analysis (PCoA) using the Bray–Curtis distance to assess whether the overall gut microbiome composition differed between time points and groups. The analysis revealed no distinct clustering by either group or time (Figure 4B).

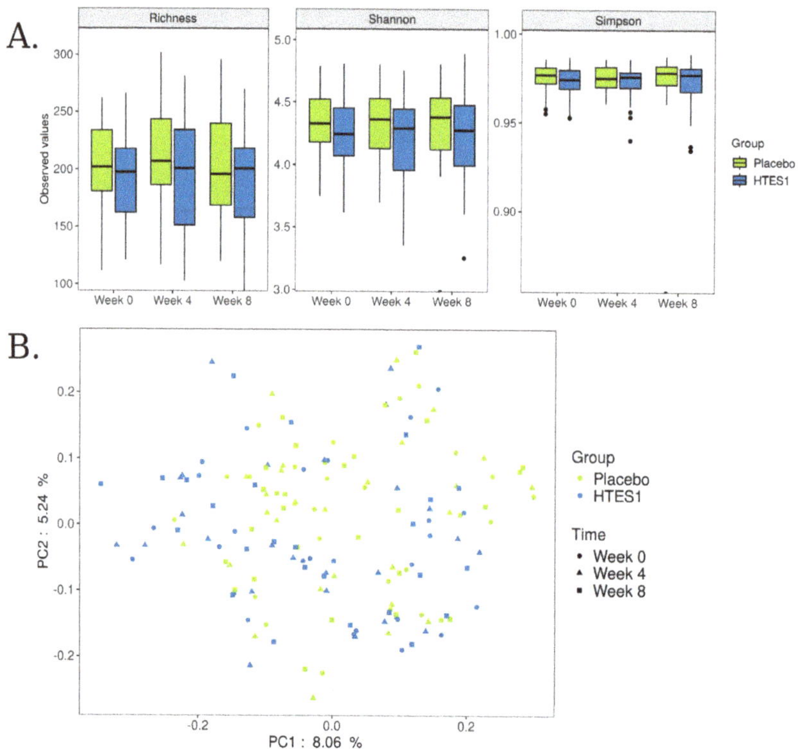

Figure 4. (**A**) Boxplots of Richness, Shannon, and Simpson indexes in placebo and HT-ES1 groups over weeks 0, 4, and 8. The Wilcoxon test was applied between times on each group and between groups on each time, with no significant results. (**B**) PCoA plot of beta diversity based on Bray–Curtis distance analysis in different groups and times.

3.6.3. Permutational Analysis of Variance

A PERMANOVA analysis using the Bray–Curtis distance method, and including the MEDAS index as a factor, showed that MEDAS had no significant influence on the microbiome variability [$R = 0.002$, ($p = 0.7$)] (Table S5A). Moreover, no significant correlation score was found between the MEDAS index and other organic compounds and clinical variables (Figure S2). The PERMANOVA analysis based on a simplified model indicated significant differences in microbiome profiles among groups [R = 0.0192, (p = 0.001)], time [R = 0.0084, (p = 0.001)], and subject [R = 0.8251, (p = 0.001)] (Table S5B).

3.6.4. Differential Abundance of Bacterial Taxonomic Features

Differential abundance analysis identified a number of bacterial taxa for which abundance significantly differed over time within the placebo or HT-ES1 group. The differences in abundance were primarily observed between week 0 and 4 (Figure 5). At the genus level (Figure 5A), within the placebo group, *Anaerotaenia* experienced a significant increase between week 4 vs. 8 and week 0 vs. 8, while no significant difference was observed in the HT-ES1 group. Additionally, *Haemophilus* was shown to significantly decrease in the placebo group at week 0 vs. 4 [adj. $p < 0.05$], which did not occur in the HT-ES1 group.

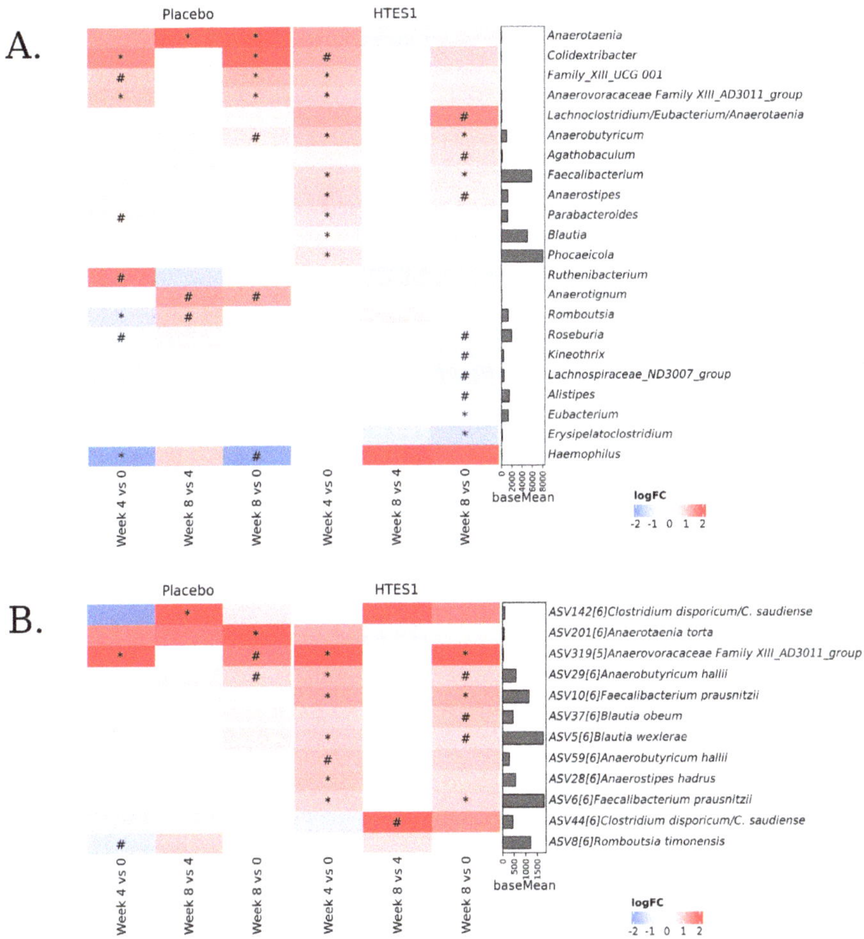

Figure 5. Differentially abundant taxa by DESeq2. Heatmaps showing the 'log fold change' (Log2FC) resulting from between time comparisons per group on (**A**) genera and (**B**) ASV abundances. Red indicates that the taxon is over-represented in the first group of the comparison, while blue indicates that the taxon is over-represented in the second group. # 0.05 < adj. $p < 0.1$, * adj. $p < 0.05$. In # and *, the presence of the taxon in at least 50% of samples of at least one of the compared groups. BaseMean bar plots show the mean abundances of each genus.

A significant increase in abundance, for butyrate-producing bacteria such as *Faecalibacterium, Anaerobutyricum, Phocaeicola, Anaerostripes*, and *Blautia*, at week 0 vs. 4 was observed only in the HT-ES1 group [adj. $p < 0.05$]. *Faecalibacterium* and *Anaerobutyricum* abundances were also significantly increased between week 0 and 8 [adj. $p < 0.05$] in the HT-ES1 group. Of note, *Anaerobutyricum* showed a non-significant increase in the placebo group. In the HT-ES1 arm, a significant decrease in *Eubacterium* and *Erysipelatclostridium* was observed at week 8 vs. 0.

The ASV annotated as *Faecalibacterium prausnitzii* (ASV10 and ASV6), *Anaerobutyricum hallii* (ASV29), *Anaerostripes hadrus* (ASV28), and *Blautia wexlerae* (ASV5) had a significant abundance increase at week 0 vs. 4 in the HT-ES1 group, which was not observed in the placebo group at the same time interval (Figure 5B). The abundance of *Faecalibacterium prausnitzii* remained significantly increased at week 0 vs. 8, while the abundance of *A. hallii*, *B. obeum* (ASV37), and *B. wexlerae* had a trending increase at week 0 vs. 8 (Figure 5B).

The genera identified as significantly abundant by DESeq2 were further analysed, examining the differences per subject during intervals of weeks 0–4 and 4–8. To evaluate specific abundance increases, the Wilcoxon test was performed comparing the placebo and HT-ES1 groups for each period. *Faecalibacterium, Phocaeicola*, and *Anaerobutyricum* were found to be significantly increased in the HT-ES1 group compared to the placebo group at weeks 0–4 (Figure 6A). In all cases, variations in the increments were shown only in the first period of study (weeks 0–4). When the same analysis was applied at the ASV level, *F. prausnitzii* and *A. hallii* were shown to have a significant abundance increment [$p < 0.05$] in the HT-ES1 vs. placebo group and, as in the case of the genus level, they remained stable at weeks 4–8 (Figure 6B).

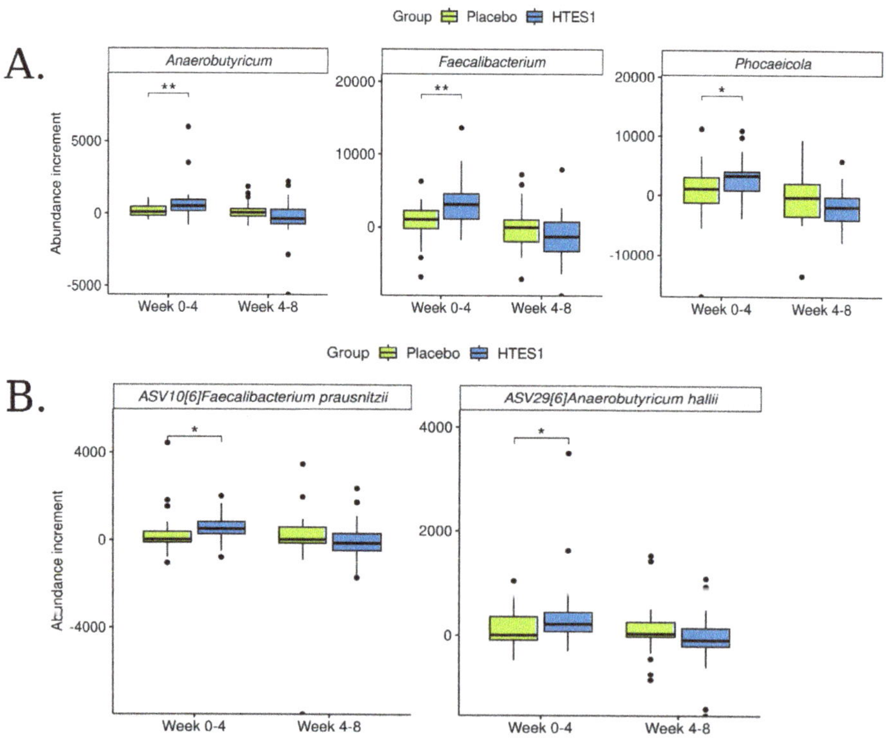

Figure 6. Boxplots on intra-subject differences between weeks 0–4 and weeks 4–8 times on each group of (**A**) genera and (**B**) ASV abundances normalised by DESeq2. Wilcox test was applied between groups on each period. * $p < 0.05$, ** $p < 0.01$.

3.6.5. Correlation Analysis

A linear mixed-effects model using the Maaslin2 tool was implemented to determine if correlations between genera and levels of SCFAs, butyric acid and acetic acid, and the clinical questionnaires existed. The genera *Agathobaculum*, *Faecalibacterium*, *Blautia*, *Anaerostripes*, *Phocaeicola*, and *Anaerobutyricum* positively correlated with butyric acid concentration, while *Haemophilus* abundance correlated with acetic acid content (Figure 7A). At the ASVs level, butyrate-producing species *F. prausnitzii*, *A. hallii*, *B. wexlerae*, *B. luti*, *A. hadrus*, and *Anaerovoracaceae* family XIII_AD3011_group had a positive correlation with butyric content [$p < 0.05$] (Figure S3). *Faecalibacterium* genus abundance positively correlated with the GIQLI, with higher scores indicating better gut health (Figure 7B).

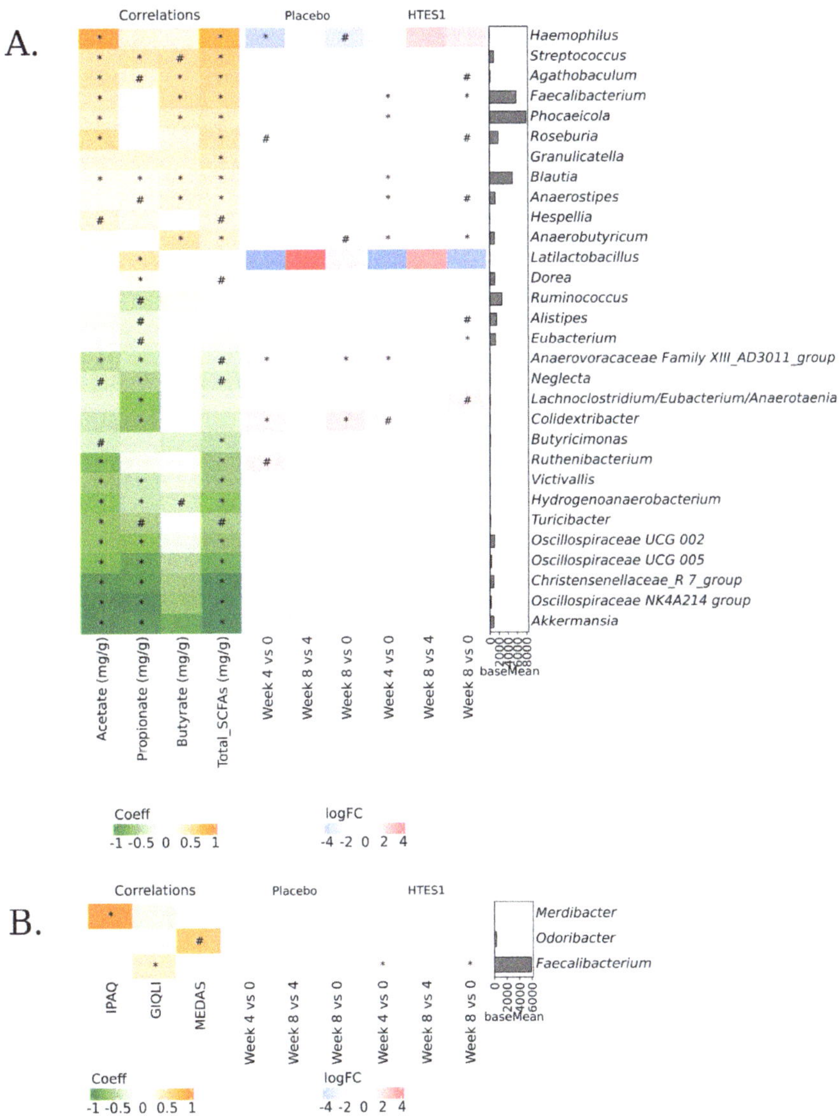

Figure 7. Correlations: heatmaps showing the Maaslin2 Coefficient (Coeff) of correlations between (**A**) organic compound concentrations and genera abundances and (**B**) questionnaires and genera

abundances. # $0.05 <$ adj. $p < 0.1$, * adj. $p < 0.05$. Orange colour means it is directly correlated, while green colour means inversely correlated. Red colour means that the taxon is over-represented in the first group of the comparison, while blue colour means that the taxon is over-represented in the second group. # $0.05 <$ adj. $p < 0.1$, * adj. $p < 0.05$. In # and *, the presence of the taxon occurs in at least 50% of samples of at least one of the compared groups. BaseMean bar plots show the mean abundances of each genus.

4. Discussion

This study investigated the potential of postbiotic HT-ES1 to modulate the intestinal microbiota, influence clinical presentation, and impact a range of commonly assessed haematological and biochemical parameters in healthy adults experiencing mild GI symptoms. Our results demonstrate that 8 weeks of HT-ES1 intake significantly reduced total and non-HDL cholesterol levels. The postbiotic notably increased butyrate-producing bacteria while maintaining stable calprotectin levels. However, HT-ES1 did not outperform the placebo when comparing scores from commonly used GI ratings tools in this population of healthy individuals with occasional digestive symptoms. The incidence of AEs in this study was low, with only two AEs attributed to HT-ES1 and three being potentially related. All AEs were considered mild and resolved quickly. There were no significant differences between groups in AEs reporting or in the safety parameters measured (vital signs, liver function, kidney function), adding to the safety profile of the postbiotic.

An increase in butyrate-producing bacteria is frequently considered to be desirable as butyrate acts as an energy source for colonocytes, plays an integral role in the maintenance of colonic health [32], and is therefore considered a reference indicator when screening for "next-generation probiotics" [33]. Additionally, butyrate has been shown to influence cell proliferation and differentiation, iron absorption, intestinal motility and barrier function, oxidative stress, immune regulation, and cholesterol synthesis [34]. In this study, butyric acid producers, belonging to the phylum Firmicutes: *Faecalibacterium*, *Anaerobutyricum*, *Phocaeicola*, *Anaerostripes*, and *Blautia*, showed a significant increase in the HT-ES1 group which was not observed in the placebo group. Furthermore, correlation analysis also revealed that the genera *Faecalibacterium*, *Anaerobutyricum*, *Phocaeicola*, *Anaerostripes*, and *Blautia* positively correlated with butyric acid concentrations. Species belonging to these genera have been associated with a variety of health benefits. The *Faecalibacterium* genus in particular has been identified as having promising health associations [35], while its reduced abundance has been associated with various conditions, including inflammatory bowel diseases (IBD), Alzheimer's disease, and post-acute COVID-19 syndrome (long COVID) [36–38]. Thus, finding ways to increase the abundance of this health-associated genus is highly desirable. Notably, the genus *Faecalibacterium* belongs to the *Oscillospiraceae* family, which also observed a significant within-group increase between weeks 0 and 4 and a trend increase between weeks 0 and 8 in the HT-ES1 group. Sequencing data and metabolic profiling suggest that members of the *Oscillospiraceae* family, such as *Oscillospira*, may have the ability to produce SCFAs such as butyrate [33]. *Anaerobutyricum*, a known butyrate producer [39] and species belonging to this genus (*A. halii*), has recently been termed a next-generation probiotic as a result of its associated bioactive properties [40]. The *Phocaeicola* genus, which belongs to the family *Bacteroidaceae* (phylum Bacteroidetes), has been indicated to play a critical role in gut health [41], contributing not only to the degradation of complex heteropolysaccharides but also vitamin synthesis [42]. In recent years, several studies have indicated that *Blautia* may play a role in the aetiology of certain inflammatory and neoplastic conditions; its abundance has been shown to be significantly reduced in patients with Crohn's disease and colorectal cancer [43]. This is in contrast to earlier studies that showed a higher abundance of *Blautia* in subjects with IBS and ulcerative colitis [43]. This may indicate that health effects may be exhibited by specific species or even strains rather than the whole genus, highlighting the importance of analysing the microbiome at the species level to obtain a holistic insight into the specific bioactivities associated with different bacterial species.

Considering this, we conducted ASV-level microbiome analysis, identifying an increased abundance of specific butyric acid-producing species: *Faecalibacterium prausnitzii, Anaerobutyricum hallii, Anaerostripes hadrus,* and *Blautia wexlerae* [44–47]. Notably, levels of butyrate increased from week 0 to 4 in both groups. In the HT-ES1 group, this increase can be attributed to the increase in butyrate producers *Faecalibacterium, Anaerobutyricum, Phocaeicola, Anaerostripes,* and *Blautia*, which were positively correlated with butyric acid concentrations. The non-significant increase in butyrate-producing *Anaerobutyricum*, genera observed in the placebo arm, offers an explanation for why butyrate production remained similar in both groups. An interesting observation in this study was that acetate production was decreased in both groups following treatment. Indigenous intestinal species from the genera *Faecalibacterium (F. prausnitzii), Anaerostipes, Eubacterium,* and *Roseburia* can utilise cross-feeding pathways, converting acetate and lactate to butyrate [10]. In fact, acetate is a major driver of butyrate production by members of the *Faecalibacterium* genus [48], and in in vitro assays, culture medium supplemented with acetate has been shown to increase the growth of *Faecalibacterium* [49–51].

Butyric acid-producing bacteria play important roles in maintaining gastrointestinal homeostasis. *B. wexlerae* has been linked to reducing inflammation associated with obesity-related complications, and thus methods to increase its levels offer potential microbiota-based strategies for supporting overall health [52]. Similarly, *F. prausnitzii* has been shown to inhibit NF-kB expression and IL-8 secretion in the context of colitis, reducing inflammation while in parallel preventing pathogen colonisation [36,53]. During our 8-week study, there were no significant changes in serum anti-inflammatory (IL-4, IL-10) or pro-inflammatory parameters (IL-6, IL-12, TNF-α). However, faecal calprotectin, which is a marker of inflammation in the intestine [54,55] and a surrogate marker of IBD [56], was increased in the placebo group but remained stable in the HT-ES1 group. While these findings suggest that HT-ES1 may have a stabilising effect on intestinal inflammation, only mild changes in symptoms were observed in this population. The validated assessment tools used to measure GI symptoms (IBS-SSS and GSRS-IBS) are designed to measure changes in individuals with a clinical diagnosis of IBS. Our previous publication involving IBS-D predominant individuals demonstrated a clinically meaningful improvement in GI symptoms following HT-ES1 intake [7].

Notably, a significant difference in the change in total cholesterol and non-HDL cholesterol in the HT-ES1 group in comparison to the placebo was observed. Preclinical and clinical studies have indicated that probiotic supplementation may have a beneficial effect on serum lipid profiles [57,58]. Meta-analysis of 32 randomised controlled trials (RCTs) involving 1971 patients demonstrated that probiotics may reduce total cholesterol (TC), and specific species such as *L. acidophilus* and *Bifidobacterium lactis* were shown to significantly reduce serum TC [59].

In the HT-ES1 group, a significant increase in vitamin D level from the baseline was observed. However, during data analysis, it was noted that three subjects were supplemented for their vitamin D deficiency over the duration of the intervention (two in the HT-ES1 and one in the placebo group). Furthermore, this clinical trial was carried out between February to October, and it is possible that seasonal variation in vitamin D occurred. To establish the role of HT-ES1 in vitamin D homeostasis, future studies should take into account the possibility of seasonal variation as well as supplementation. Indeed, a recent systematic review and meta-analysis of 308 studies with 7,947,359 participants found that 15.7%, 47.9%, and 76.6% of participants had serum 25-hydroxyvitamin D levels less than 12, 20, and 30 ng/mL, respectively [60], with normal ranges falling between 30 and 100 ng/mL. Interestingly, evidence indicated that combined supplementation of vitamin D and probiotics may have superior bioactivity in modulating the intestinal microbiome and metabolome [61–63]. Furthermore, probiotics have been shown to increase the intestinal absorption of vitamin D [62].

Although our study brings new insights into the effects of HT-ES1 on a generally healthy population with mild GI symptoms, we acknowledge that this clinical study had some limitations. Firstly, as this was a pilot study, no formal sample size calculation was performed. This might have led to the study population being underpowered, limiting the ability to detect differences between groups. Secondly, the population was selected from a healthy cohort with mild symptoms, which may have contributed to the absence of statistically significant changes in the primary outcome and the scores from the other GI assessment tools. Thirdly, because this was a feasibility study, some parameters such as supplement intake were not considered as exclusion criteria, and this may have affected some of the outcomes measured.

Despite its limitations, our study has several strengths. It is the first to evaluate the effects of HT-ES1 on a generally healthy population with mild GI symptoms. In addition to the previously published trial using HT-ES1, the results from this trial further contribute to the valuable safety data on postbiotics and specifically on HT-ES1. HT-ES1 demonstrated an interesting modulatory effect on the GI microbiome of this cohort, as evidenced by increased levels of beneficial butyrate-producing genera (*Faecalibacterium, Anaerobutyricum, Phocaeicola, Anaerostripes, and Blautia*) and species (*F. prausnitzii, A. hallii, A. hadrus*, and *B. wexlerae*) in the GI tract. This microbiome-modulatory effect is the first time such data have been published for this strain and represents one of the few published studies to date which show the microbiome-modulating effects of a postbiotic on a healthy adult population. Additionally, interesting effects were observed on cholesterol, vitamin D, and calprotectin levels.

Additional research will help to further define the potential of the postbiotic HT-ES1, especially examining the mechanisms behind HT-ES1′s microbiome modulation. The increase in *Faecalibacterium* and *Anaerobutyricum* from HT-ES1 supplementation may stem from cross-feeding interactions, where metabolites produced by *B. longum* (like lactate and acetate) support the growth of these butyrate-producing bacteria [64]. In vitro experiments and animal models indicate that *Bifidobacterium longum* has anti-inflammatory effects on intestinal cells [65], thereby creating a favourable environment for these beneficial microbes. Studies focusing on metabolite profiling could clarify the pathways through which HT-ES1 enhances the abundance of these butyrate-producing genera. Further larger and focused studies could provide valuable insights into HT-ES1′s impact on inflammation markers, cholesterol levels, and sustained microbiome changes, thereby contributing to the promotion of overall digestive and gut health.

5. Conclusions

The results of this randomised, double-blind, placebo-controlled pilot trial demonstrate that the consumption of HT-ES1 for 8 weeks increased the abundance of butyrate-producing bacteria, a key source of bacterial SCFAs essential for intestinal health. Furthermore, the calprotectin levels remained stable in the HT-ES1 group, while a significant increase was noted in the placebo group between week 4 and 8, suggesting a potential protective effect of the postbiotic against intestinal inflammation. Interestingly, a significant decrease in total cholesterol from baseline to week 8 was noted in the HT-ES1 group compared to placebo. Adverse event reporting demonstrated that the postbiotic was safe for use, as the observed AEs were consistent with expectations and aligned with those reported in published trials of similar products. Overall, these findings suggest that HT-ES1 is effective in promoting beneficial gut microbiota and maintaining intestinal health while demonstrating a favourable safety profile.

Supplementary Materials: The following supporting information can be downloaded at: https://www.mdpi.com/article/10.3390/nu16223952/s1, Figure S1: Relative abundances of the thirty most abundant genera of all the samples. Figure S2: Correlation plot showing Spearman's rank correlation coefficient between all clinical variables and organic compound concentrations; Figure S3: Correlations: Heatmaps showing the Maaslin2 Coefficient (Coeff) of correlations between organic compound concentrations and ASVs abundances. Label others includes the rest of the genera and the taxa that could not be annotated at genus level; Table S1: Baseline participant (A) characteristics, (B) habits, and (C) medical history. Table S2: Per-protocol participant characteristics over the intervention.

Table S3: Safety parameters over the intervention period. Table S4: Full questionnaire scores. Table S5: PERMANOVA analysis. (***) p-value < 0.001. (A) The time, group, the Group:Time interaction the subject and the MEDAS index were included in the model for testing. Only samples with MEDAS index available were included. R^2: partial R^2. F: pseudo-F statistic. (B) The time, group, the Group:Time interaction and the subject were included in the model for testing. R^2: partial R^2. F: pseudo-F statistic. Section S1: Inclusion and exclusion criteria; Section S2: Detailed methods of assessment tools.

Author Contributions: Study concept and design: A.R., B.L.P., M.N. and R.D.; data analysis: A.P.-B., A.L., B.Á. and E.C.; data sequencing: L.L. and J.F.M.-B.; drafting of the manuscript: A.P.-B., A.L. and V.V.; revision of the manuscript: all authors. Trial site investigators: L.A.C. All authors have read and agreed to the published version of the manuscript.

Funding: This study received funding from ADM and the Spanish Ministry of Economy and Competitiveness under the CDTI Project TOLERA IDI-20170876. The funder had the following involvement with the study: study design and writing and reviewing of the manuscript. M.N., A.P.-B., A.L., L.L., J.F.M.-B., A.R., B.Á., E.C., V.V., and R.D. are employed by ADM.

Institutional Review Board Statement: This study was conducted in compliance with the Declaration of Helsinki and National Ethical Guidelines for Biomedical and Health Research involving Human Participants and the study protocol was approved by the Research Ethics Committee with Medical Products Hospital La Paz Institute for Health Research (IdiPAZ), code: Ref: 57/458465.9/21, date: 10 November 2021.

Informed Consent Statement: Informed consent was obtained from all subjects involved in the study.

Data Availability Statement: The data that support the findings of this study are available from the corresponding author upon reasonable request.

Acknowledgments: The authors would like to thank the Hospital La Paz Institute for Health Research (IdiPAZ), Madrid, Spain, for their valuable contribution to conducting the clinical trial, which was essential to the success of this study. We also extend our gratitude to the trial participants, and the Spanish Ministry of Economy and Competitiveness for providing the necessary funding. Additionally, we acknowledge the administrative and technical support received throughout the project, with special thanks to Elisabet Navarro, Erinn Quinn, and Ana Matos Cardoso.

Conflicts of Interest: This study was partly funded by ADM. Authors M.N., A.P.-B., A.L., L.L., J.F.M.-B., A.R., B.Á., E.C., V.V., and R.D. were employed by ADM. The remaining authors declare that the research was conducted in the absence of any commercial or financial relationship that could be construed as a potential conflict of interest.

References

1. Almario, C.V.; Ballal, M.L.; Chey, W.D.; Nordstrom, C.; Khanna, D.; Spiegel, B.M.R. Burden of Gastrointestinal Symptoms in the United States: Results of a Nationally Representative Survey of Over 71,000 Americans. *Am. J. Gastroenterol.* **2018**, *113*, 1701. [CrossRef] [PubMed]
2. Wu, X.; Xia, Y.; He, F.; Zhu, C.; Ren, W. Intestinal Mycobiota in Health and Diseases: From a Disrupted Equilibrium to Clinical Opportunities. *Microbiome* **2021**, *9*, 60. [CrossRef]
3. Nouvenne, A.; Ticinesi, A.; Tana, C.; Prati, B.; Catania, P.; Miraglia, C.; De' Angelis, G.L.; Di Mario, F.; Meschi, T. Digestive Disorders and Intestinal Microbiota. *Acta Biomed.* **2018**, *89*, 47–51. [CrossRef]
4. Thursby, E.; Juge, N. Introduction to the Human Gut Microbiota. *Biochem. J.* **2017**, *474*, 1823. [CrossRef]
5. Hill, C.; Guarner, F.; Reid, G.; Gibson, G.R.; Merenstein, D.J.; Pot, B.; Morelli, L.; Canani, R.B.; Flint, H.J.; Salminen, S.; et al. The International Scientific Association for Probiotics and Prebiotics Consensus Statement on the Scope and Appropriate Use of the Term Probiotic. *Nat. Rev. Gastroenterol. Hepatol.* **2014**, *11*, 506–514. [CrossRef] [PubMed]
6. Ishaque, M.S.; Khosruzzaman, S.M.; Ahmed, D.S.; Sah, M.P. A Randomized Placebo-Controlled Clinical Trial of a Multi-Strain Probiotic Formulation (Bio-Kult®) in the Management of Diarrheapredominant Irritable Bowel Syndrome. *Med. Counc.* **2018**, *18*, 71. [CrossRef]
7. Srivastava, S.; Basak, U.; Naghibi, M.; Vijayakumar, V.; Parihar, R.; Patel, J.; Jadon, P.S.; Pandit, A.; Dargad, R.R.; Khanna, S.; et al. A Randomized Double-Blind, Placebo-Controlled Trial to Evaluate the Safety and Efficacy of Live Bifidobacterium Longum CECT 7347 (ES1) and Heat-Treated Bifidobacterium Longum CECT 7347 (HT-ES1) in Participants with Diarrhea-Predominant Irritable Bowel Syndrome. *Gut Microbes* **2024**, *16*, 2338322. [CrossRef]

8. Buffie, C.G.; Pamer, E.G. Microbiota-Mediated Colonization Resistance against Intestinal Pathogens. *Nat. Rev. Immunol.* **2013**, *13*, 790–801. [CrossRef]
9. Hidalgo-Cantabrana, C.; Delgado, S.; Ruiz, L.; Ruas-Madiedo, P.; Sánchez, B.; Margolles, A. Bifidobacteria and Their Health-Promoting Effects. *Microbiol. Spectr.* **2017**, *5*, 73–98. [CrossRef]
10. Quinn, E.M.; Slattery, H.; Walsh, D.; Joshi, L.; Hickey, R.M. Bifidobacterium Longum Subsp. Infantis ATCC 15697 and Goat Milk Oligosaccharides Show Synergism In Vitro as Anti-Infectives against Campylobacter Jejuni. *Foods* **2020**, *9*, 348. [CrossRef]
11. Olivares, M.; Castillejo, G.; Varea, V.; Sanz, Y. Double-Blind, Randomised, Placebo-Controlled Intervention Trial to Evaluate the Effects of Bifidobacterium Longum CECT 7347 in Children with Newly Diagnosed Coeliac Disease. *Br. J. Nutr.* **2014**, *112*, 30–40. [CrossRef] [PubMed]
12. Di Pierro, F.; Bergomas, F.; Marraccini, P.; Ingenito, M.R.; Ferrari, L.; Vigna, L. Pilot Study on Non-Celiac Gluten Sensitivity: Effects of Bifidobacterium Longum ES1 Co-Administered with a Gluten-Free Diet. *Minerva Gastroenterol. Dietol.* **2020**, *66*, 187–193. [CrossRef] [PubMed]
13. Indira, M.; Venkateswarulu, T.C.; Abraham Peele, K.; Nazneen Bobby, M.; Krupanidhi, S. Bioactive Molecules of Probiotic Bacteria and Their Mechanism of Action: A Review. *3 Biotech* **2019**, *9*, 306. [CrossRef] [PubMed]
14. Maria Carmen, C.; Seppo, S.; Vinderola, G. Postbiotics: Defining the Impact of Inactivated Microbes and Their Metabolites on Promotion of Health. In *The Human Microbiome in Early Life: Implications to Health and Disease*; Academic Press: New York, NY, USA, 2021. [CrossRef]
15. Nataraj, B.H.; Ali, S.A.; Behare, P.V.; Yadav, H. Postbiotics-Parabiotics: The New Horizons in Microbial Biotherapy and Functional Foods. *Microb. Cell Factories* **2020**, *19*, 168. [CrossRef]
16. Piqué, N.; Berlanga, M.; Miñana-Galbis, D. Health Benefits of Heat-Killed (Tyndallized) Probiotics: An Overview. *Int. J. Mol. Sci.* **2019**, *20*, 2534. [CrossRef]
17. Wegh, C.A.M.; Geerlings, S.Y.; Knol, J.; Roeselers, G.; Belzer, C. Postbiotics and Their Potential Applications in Early Life Nutrition and Beyond. *Int. J. Mol. Sci.* **2019**, *20*, 4673. [CrossRef]
18. Martorell, P.; Alvarez, B.; Llopis, S.; Navarro, V.; Ortiz, P.; Gonzalez, N.; Balaguer, F.; Rojas, A.; Chenoll, E.; Ramón, D.; et al. Heat-Treated Bifidobacterium Longum CECT-7347: A Whole-Cell Postbiotic with Antioxidant, Anti-Inflammatory, and Gut-Barrier Protection Properties. *Antioxidants* **2021**, *10*, 536. [CrossRef]
19. BBMap—Bushnell B. Available online: https://sourceforge.net/projects/bbmap/ (accessed on 8 December 2016).
20. Martin, M. Cutadapt Removes Adapter Sequences from High-Throughput Sequencing Reads. *EMBnet J.* **2011**, *17*, 10–12. [CrossRef]
21. Callahan, B.J.; McMurdie, P.J.; Rosen, M.J.; Han, A.W.; Johnson, A.J.A.; Holmes, S.P. DADA2: High-Resolution Sample Inference from Illumina Amplicon Data. *Nat. Methods* **2016**, *13*, 581–583. [CrossRef]
22. Altschul, S.F.; Gish, W.; Miller, W.; Myers, E.W.; Lipman, D.J. Basic Local Alignment Search Tool. *J. Mol. Biol.* **1990**, *215*. [CrossRef]
23. Bokulich, N.A.; Kaehler, B.D.; Rideout, J.R.; Dillon, M.; Bolyen, E.; Knight, R.; Huttley, G.A.; Gregory Caporaso, J. Optimizing Taxonomic Classification of Marker-Gene Amplicon Sequences with QIIME 2's Q2-Feature-Classifier Plugin. *Microbiome* **2018**, *6*, 90. [CrossRef] [PubMed]
24. Bolyen, E.; Rideout, J.R.; Dillon, M.R.; Bokulich, N.A.; Abnet, C.C.; Al-Ghalith, G.A.; Alexander, H.; Alm, E.J.; Arumugam, M.; Asnicar, F.; et al. Reproducible, Interactive, Scalable and Extensible Microbiome Data Science Using QIIME 2. *Nat. Biotechnol.* **2019**, *37*, 852–857. [CrossRef] [PubMed]
25. Quast, C.; Pruesse, E.; Yilmaz, P.; Gerken, J.; Schweer, T.; Yarza, P.; Peplies, J.; Glöckner, F.O. The SILVA Ribosomal RNA Gene Database Project: Improved Data Processing and Web-Based Tools. *Nucleic Acids Res.* **2012**, *41*, D590–D596. [CrossRef] [PubMed]
26. McMurdie, P.J.; Holmes, S. Phyloseq: An R Package for Reproducible Interactive Analysis and Graphics of Microbiome Census Data. *PLoS ONE* **2013**, *8*, e61217. [CrossRef]
27. Oksanen, J.; Blanchet, F.G.; Kindt, R.; Legendre, P.; Minchin, P.R.; O'Hara, R.B.; Simpson, G.L.; Solymos, P.; Stevens, M.H.H.; Wagner, H. Vegan: Community Ecology R Package, Version 2.3-5. Vegan: Community Ecology Package. R. Package Version 2.4-1. Available online: https://CRAN.R-project.org/package=vegan (accessed on 8 December 2016).
28. Love, M.I.; Huber, W.; Anders, S. Moderated Estimation of Fold Change and Dispersion for RNA-Seq Data with DESeq2. *Genome Biol.* **2014**, *15*, 550. [CrossRef]
29. Gu, Z.; Eils, R.; Schlesner, M. Complex Heatmaps Reveal Patterns and Correlations in Multidimensional Genomic Data. *Bioinformatics* **2016**, *32*, 2847–2849. [CrossRef]
30. Mallick, H.; Rahnavard, A.; McIver, L.J.; Ma, S.; Zhang, Y.; Nguyen, L.H.; Tickle, T.L.; Weingart, G.; Ren, B.; Schwager, E.H.; et al. Multivariable Association Discovery in Population-Scale Meta-Omics Studies. *PLoS Comput. Biol.* **2021**, *17*, e1009442. [CrossRef]
31. Schröder, H.; Fitó, M.; Estruch, R.; Martínez-González, M.A.; Corella, D.; Salas-Salvadó, J.; Lamuela-Raventós, R.; Ros, E.; Salaverría, I.; Fiol, M.; et al. A Short Screener Is Valid for Assessing Mediterranean Diet Adherence among Older Spanish Men and Women. *J. Nutr.* **2011**, *141*, 1140–1145. [CrossRef] [PubMed]
32. Martin-Gallausiaux, C.; Marinelli, L.; Blottière, H.M.; Larraufie, P.; Lapaque, N. SCFA: Mechanisms and Functional Importance in the Gut. *Proc. Nutr. Soc.* **2021**, *80*, 37–49. [CrossRef]
33. Yang, J.; Li, Y.; Wen, Z.; Liu, W.; Meng, L.; Huang, H. Oscillospira—A Candidate for the next-Generation Probiotics. *Gut Microbes* **2021**, *13*, 1987783. [CrossRef]

34. Canani, R.B.; Di Costanzo, M.; Leone, L.; Pedata, M.; Meli, R.; Calignano, A. Potential Beneficial Effects of Butyrate in Intestinal and Extraintestinal Diseases. *World J. Gastroenterol.* **2011**, *17*, 1519–1528. [CrossRef]
35. Martín, R.; Rios-Covian, D.; Huillet, E.; Auger, S.; Khazaal, S.; Bermúdez-Humarán, L.G.; Sokol, H.; Chatel, J.M.; Langella, P. Faecalibacterium: A Bacterial Genus with Promising Human Health Applications. *FEMS Microbiol. Rev.* **2023**, *47*, fuad039. [CrossRef] [PubMed]
36. Sokol, H.; Pigneur, B.; Watterlot, L.; Lakhdari, O.; Bermúdez-Humarán, L.G.; Gratadoux, J.J.; Blugeon, S.; Bridonneau, C.; Furet, J.P.; Corthier, G.; et al. Faecalibacterium Prausnitzii Is an Anti-Inflammatory Commensal Bacterium Identified by Gut Microbiota Analysis of Crohn Disease Patients. *Proc. Natl. Acad. Sci. USA* **2008**, *105*, 16731–16736. [CrossRef] [PubMed]
37. Ueda, A.; Shinkai, S.; Shiroma, H.; Taniguchi, Y.; Tsuchida, S.; Kariya, T.; Kawahara, T.; Kobayashi, Y.; Kohda, N.; Ushida, K.; et al. Identification of Faecalibacterium Prausnitzii Strains for Gut Microbiome-Based Intervention in Alzheimer's-Type Dementia. *Cell Rep. Med.* **2021**, *2*, 100398. [CrossRef]
38. Hazan, S.; Stollman, N.; Bozkurt, H.S.; Dave, S.; Papoutsis, A.J.; Daniels, J.; Barrows, B.D.; Quigley, E.M.M.; Borody, T.J. Lost Microbes of COVID-19: Bifidobacterium, Faecalibacterium Depletion and Decreased Microbiome Diversity Associated with SARS-CoV-2 Infection Severity. *BMJ Open Gastroenterol.* **2022**, *9*, e000871. [CrossRef] [PubMed]
39. Singh, V.; Lee, G.D.; Son, H.W.; Koh, H.; Kim, E.S.; Unno, T.; Shin, J.H. Butyrate Producers, "The Sentinel of Gut": Their Intestinal Significance with and beyond Butyrate, and Prospective Use as Microbial Therapeutics. *Front. Microbiol.* **2023**, *13*, 1103836. [CrossRef] [PubMed]
40. Kumari, M.; Singh, P.; Nataraj, B.H.; Kokkiligadda, A.; Naithani, H.; Azmal Ali, S.; Behare, P.V.; Nagpal, R. Fostering Next-Generation Probiotics in Human Gut by Targeted Dietary Modulation: An Emerging Perspective. *Food Res. Int.* **2021**, *150 Pt A*, 110716. [CrossRef]
41. Wu, X.; Park, S. Fecal Bacterial Community and Metagenome Function in Asians with Type 2 Diabetes, According to Enterotypes. *Biomedicines* **2022**, *10*, 2998. [CrossRef]
42. Zafar, H.; Saier, M.H. Gut Bacteroides Species in Health and Disease. *Gut Microbes* **2021**, *13*, 1848158. [CrossRef]
43. Liu, X.; Mao, B.; Gu, J.; Wu, J.; Cui, S.; Wang, G.; Zhao, J.; Zhang, H.; Chen, W. Blautia—A New Functional Genus with Potential Probiotic Properties? *Gut Microbes* **2021**, *13*, 1875796. [CrossRef]
44. Zhou, L.; Zhang, M.; Wang, Y.; Dorfman, R.G.; Liu, H.; Yu, T.; Chen, X.; Tang, D.; Xu, L.; Yin, Y.; et al. Faecalibacterium Prausnitzii Produces Butyrate to Maintain Th17/Treg Balance and to Ameliorate Colorectal Colitis by Inhibiting Histone Deacetylase 1. *Inflamm. Bowel Dis.* **2018**, *24*, 1926–1940. [CrossRef] [PubMed]
45. Shetty, S.A.; Zuffa, S.; Bui, T.P.N.; Aalvink, S.; Smidt, H.; De Vos, W.M. Reclassification of Eubacterium Hallii as Anaerobutyricum Hallii Gen. Nov., Comb. Nov., and Description of Anaerobutyricum Soehngenii Sp. Nov., a Butyrate and Propionate-Producing Bacterium from Infant Faeces. *Int. J. Syst. Evol. Microbiol.* **2018**, *68*, 3741–3746. [CrossRef] [PubMed]
46. Liu, D.; Xie, L.-S.; Lian, S.; Li, K.; Yang, Y.; Wang, W.-Z.; Hu, S.; Liu, S.-J.; Liu, C.; He, Z. Anaerostipes Hadrus, a Butyrate-Producing Bacterium Capable of Metabolizing 5-Fluorouracil. *mSphere* **2024**, *9*, e0081623. [CrossRef] [PubMed]
47. Yang, J.; Martínez, I.; Walter, J.; Keshavarzian, A.; Rose, D.J. In Vitro Characterization of the Impact of Selected Dietary Fibers on Fecal Microbiota Composition and Short Chain Fatty Acid Production. *Anaerobe* **2013**, *23*, 74–81. [CrossRef] [PubMed]
48. Miquel, S.; Martín, R.; Rossi, O.; Bermúdez-Humarán, L.G.; Chatel, J.M.; Sokol, H.; Thomas, M.; Wells, J.M.; Langella, P. Faecalibacterium Prausnitzii and Human Intestinal Health. *Curr. Opin. Microbiol.* **2013**, *16*, 255–261. [CrossRef]
49. Duncan, S.H.; Hold, G.L.; Harmsen, H.J.M.; Stewart, C.S.; Flint, H.J. Growth Requirements and Fermentation Products of Fusobacterium Prausnitzii, and a Proposal to Reclassify It as Faecalibacterium Prausnitzii Gen. Nov., Comb. Nov. *Int. J. Syst. Evol. Microbiol.* **2002**, *52*, 2141–2146. [CrossRef]
50. Lopez-Siles, M.; Khan, T.M.; Duncan, S.H.; Harmsen, H.J.M.; Garcia-Gil, L.J.; Flint, H.J. Cultured Representatives of Two Major Phylogroups of Human Colonic Faecalibacterium Prausnitzii Can Utilize Pectin, Uronic Acids, and Host-Derived Substrates for Growth. *Appl. Environ. Microbiol.* **2012**, *78*, 420–428. [CrossRef]
51. D'hoe, K.; Conterno, L.; Fava, F.; Falony, G.; Vieira-Silva, S.; Vermeiren, J.; Tuohy, K.; Raes, J. Prebiotic Wheat Bran Fractions Induce Specific Microbiota Changes. *Front. Microbiol.* **2018**, *9*, 31. [CrossRef]
52. Benítez-Páez, A.; Gómez del Pugar, E.M.; López-Almela, I.; Moya-Pérez, Á.; Codoñer-Franch, P.; Sanz, Y. Depletion of Blautia Species in the Microbiota of Obese Children Relates to Intestinal Inflammation and Metabolic Phenotype Worsening. *mSystems* **2020**, *5*, e00857-19. [CrossRef]
53. Benus, R.F.; Harmsen, H.J.; Welling, G.W.; Spanjersberg, R.; Zijlstra, J.G.; Degener, J.E.; Van Der Werf, T.S. Impact of Digestive and Oropharyngeal Decontamination on the Intestinal Microbiota in ICU Patients. *Intensive Care Med.* **2010**, *36*, 1394–1402. [CrossRef]
54. Rubio, M.G.; Amo-Mensah, K.; Gray, J.M.; Nguyen, V.Q.; Nakat, S.; Grider, D.; Love, K.; Boone, J.H.; Sorrentino, D. Fecal Lactoferrin Accurately Reflects Mucosal Inflammation in Inflammatory Bowel Disease. *World J. Gastrointest. Pathophysiol.* **2019**, *10*, 54–63. [CrossRef] [PubMed]
55. Walsham, N.E.; Sherwood, R.A. Fecal Calprotectin in Inflammatory Bowel Disease. *Clin. Exp. Gastroenterol.* **2016**, *9*, 21–29. [CrossRef] [PubMed]
56. Van Rheenen, P.F.; Van De Vijver, E.; Fidler, V. Faecal Calprotectin for Screening of Patients with Suspected Inflammatory Bowel Disease: Diagnostic Meta-Analysis. *BMJ* **2010**, *341*, c3369. [CrossRef] [PubMed]
57. Huang, Y.; Zheng, Y. The Probiotic Lactobacillus Acidophilus Reduces Cholesterol Absorption through the Down-Regulation of Niemann-Pick C1-like 1 in Caco-2 Cells. *Br. J. Nutr.* **2010**, *103*, 473–478. [CrossRef] [PubMed]

58. Lye, H.S.; Rahmat-Ali, G.R.; Liong, M.T. Mechanisms of Cholesterol Removal by Lactobacilli under Conditions That Mimic the Human Gastrointestinal Tract. *Int. Dairy J.* **2010**, *20*, 169–175. [CrossRef]
59. Wang, L.; Guo, M.-J.; Gao, Q.; Yang, J.-F.; Yang, L.; Pang, X.-L.; Jiang, X.-J. The Effects of Probiotics on Total Cholesterol: A Meta-Analysis of Randomized Controlled Trials. *Medicine* **2018**, *97*, e9679. [CrossRef]
60. Cui, A.; Zhang, T.; Xiao, P.; Fan, Z.; Wang, H.; Zhuang, Y. Global and Regional Prevalence of Vitamin D Deficiency in Population-Based Studies from 2000 to 2022: A Pooled Analysis of 7.9 Million Participants. *Front. Nutr.* **2023**, *10*, 1070808. [CrossRef]
61. Abboud, M.; Rizk, R.; AlAnouti, F.; Papandreou, D.; Haidar, S.; Mahboub, N. The Health Effects of Vitamin D and Probiotic Co-Supplementation: A Systematic Review of Randomized Controlled Trials. *Nutrients* **2020**, *13*, 111. [CrossRef]
62. Dargenio, V.N.; Castellaneta, S.; Panico, S.; Papagni, M.E.; Dargenio, C.; Schettini, F.; Francavilla, R.; Cristofori, F. Probiotics and Gastrointestinal Diseases. *Minerva Pediatr.* **2022**, *74*, 703–723. [CrossRef]
63. Shang, M.; Sun, J. Vitamin D/VDR, Probiotics, and Gastrointestinal Diseases. *Curr. Med. Chem.* **2017**, *24*, 876. [CrossRef]
64. Ríos-Covián, D.; Ruas-Madiedo, P.; Margolles, A.; Gueimonde, M.; de los Reyes-Gavilán, C.G.; Salazar, N. Intestinal Short Chain Fatty Acids and Their Link with Diet and Human Health. *Front. Microbiol.* **2016**, *7*, 185. [CrossRef]
65. Yao, S.; Zhao, Z.; Wang, W.; Liu, X. Bifidobacterium Longum: Protection against Inflammatory Bowel Disease. *J. Immunol. Res.* **2021**, *2021*, 8030297. [CrossRef]

nutrients

MDPI

Article

Akkermansia muciniphila for the Prevention of Type 2 Diabetes and Obesity: A Meta-Analysis of Animal Studies

Ethan Liu [1], Xiangming Ji [2] and Kequan Zhou [1,*]

1 Department of Nutrition and Food Science, Wayne State University, Detroit, MI 48202, USA; ethanliu0307@gmail.com
2 Department of Nutritional Sciences, The College of Health and Human Development, The Pennsylvania State University, University Park, PA 16802, USA
* Correspondence: kzhou@wayne.edu

Abstract: Background: More than half of the states in the U.S. report that over 30% of adults are obese. Obesity increases the risk of many chronic diseases, including type 2 diabetes, hypertension, and cardiovascular disease, and can even reduce one's lifespan. Similarly, the prevalence of type 2 diabetes follows a comparable trend. As a result, researchers are striving to find solutions to reduce obesity rates, with a particular focus on gut health, which has been previously linked to both obesity and type 2 diabetes. Recent studies suggest that *Akkermansia muciniphila* (Akk) may have a positive probiotic effect on preventing the onset of type 2 diabetes and obesity. Methods: We conducted a quantitative meta-analysis of 15 qualified animal studies investigating the effects of Akk administration as a probiotic. Results: The statistical analyses showed that Akk administration significantly reduced body weight gain by 10.4% and fasting blood glucose by 21.2%, while also significantly improving glucose tolerance by 22.1% and increasing blood insulin levels by 26.9%. However, our analysis revealed substantial heterogeneity between the control and experimental groups across all subgroups. Conclusions: Overall, Akk appears to be effective at reducing the onset of type 2 diabetes and diet-induced obesity. Long-term studies with larger sample sizes are needed to confirm these beneficial effects, as the current animal studies were of short duration (less than 20 weeks).

Keywords: probiotic; *Akkermansia*; obesity; type 2 diabetes; animals; meta-analysis

1. Introduction

The alarming surge in obesity and diabetes rates within the USA is reaching critical levels, with 41.9% and 14.7%, respectively among American adults [1,2]. In 2022, 43% of adults in the world were overweight and 16% were living with obesity [3]. Moreover, obesity stands as a significant precursor to diabetes, amplifying the urgency of this health crisis [3]. Both conditions demand sustained attention and comprehensive care, presenting formidable challenges to public health. Addressing this pressing issue necessitates the development of innovative, sustainable long-term strategies. There has been strong evidence suggesting that both obesity and diabetes have been strongly linked to gut microbiota, the vast community of microbes in our intestines [4]. Studies have shown that lean mice gained significant weight after transferring gut bacteria from obese mice, suggesting that gut microbiota play a key role in managing body weight [5,6]. Other studies in animals and humans demonstrate an inverse relationship between obesity and diversity of gut microbiota, specifically symbionts including genera Bifidobacteria, Lactobacillus, and Verrucomicrobiota (in which Akk belongs to) [7,8]. In addition, gut microbiota has been shown to alter low-grade inflammation and insulin resistance upon modification via dietary interventions [9]. In particular, a group of gut bacterial metabolites such as short-chain fatty acids (SCFAs) are believed play a role in mediating the effects of gut microbiota [10]. For instance, diabetes patients were found to have a reduced population of SCFAs-producing gut bacteria, suggesting a potential link of gut bacteria with impaired blood sugar control [4]. Common SCFAs include acetate, butyrate, and propionate, and their anti-obesity and anti-diabetes bioactivities have been widely studied. These findings also suggest that a potential strategy to manage obesity and type 2 diabetes is targeting gut microbiota.

Akk is a gram-negative gut bacterium belonging to the phylum Verrucomicrobia. It is one of the most abundant gut bacteria in humans, representing 3–5% of the microbial community. A. muciniphila was first isolated and identified in 2004 in purified mucin as an oval-shaped, strictly anaerobic bacterium. Akk has the ability to utilize mucus glycans as carbon sources to grow. As a mucin-degrading bacterium, Akk in turn stimulates the growth of the protective gut lining and enhances gut barrier functions [11,12]. Akk has recently gained increased research interest due to its potential benefits against obesity and metabolic syndrome. Research has found that Akk is more abundant in healthy subjects than in diabetic and obese patients. Further support comes from intervention studies that have also found an inverse correlation between Akk abundance and body weight, metabolic syndrome, and type 2 diabetes [13–16].

Despite the growing body of evidence suggesting that Akk is a promising probiotic, the exact mechanisms by which it exerts its beneficial impact on health have not been fully elucidated (Figure 1). Studies have shown that Akk promotes the gut production of short-chain fatty acids (SCFAs), improving insulin resistance and host metabolism—factors linked to obesity and diabetes [12–15]. Moreover, Akk has been shown to modify the gut microbiota by stimulating other beneficial gut bacteria such as Bifidobacteria, thereby promoting a healthier gut ecosystem [13].

There have been a growing number of studies investigating the beneficial role of Akk on obesity and diabetes [7]. Animal studies have been particularly encouraging. For instance, dietary Akk supplementation has been shown to reduce body weight gain, fasting blood glucose, and insulin resistance in mice fed with a high-fat diet [14,15]. Similar findings have been demonstrated in other studies, suggesting the protective role of Akk against obesity and diabetes, though the exact mechanisms are not clear. A recent human trial, while demonstrating improved insulin sensitivity and reduced cholesterol in overweight/obese participants, did not show significant changes in weight or body fat composition [16]. This discrepancy highlights the need for a more comprehensive analysis of Akk effects on obesity and diabetes. A previous review that compared the effects of Akk on various metabolic diseases found a positive association with the onset of type 2 diabetes following Akk supplementation. However, this association lacked strong evidence [17]. To address this, our meta-analysis aims to systematically evaluate the latest research and compare the effects of Akk administration in different animal studies. We will employ the most comprehensive subgroup analyses possible to provide a more definitive understanding of the impact of Akk.

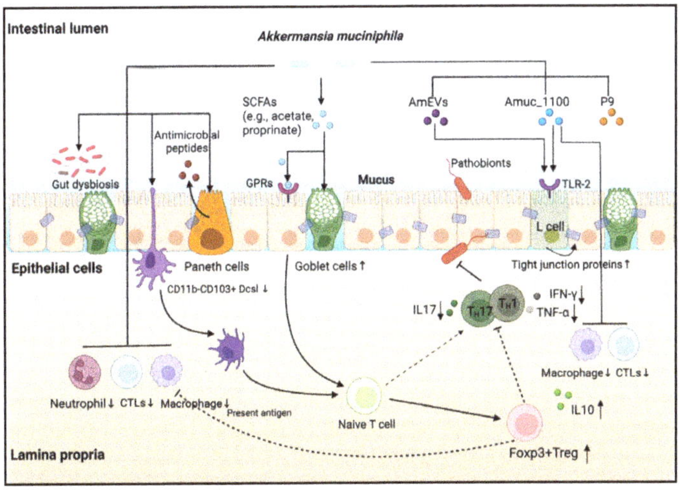

Figure 1. Various pathways and models associated with *A. muciniphila* [7].

2. Materials and Methods

2.1. Literature Search Strategy and Inclusion Criteria

This meta-analysis investigated the effect of Akk dietary intake on obesity and type 2 diabetes, focusing on animal studies that generated quantitative data. This study was conducted strictly following the guidelines of Preferred Reporting Items for Systematic Reviews and Meta-Analyses (PRISMA) [18]. The databases PubMed, EMBASE, Web of Science, and Cochrane Library were searched for animal trials on Akk to prevent obesity and type 2 diabetes.

Publications from the inception of the databases until February 2024 were collected. We employed a combination of terms from medical subject headings (MeSH) and keywords. The search strategy encompassed subject headings "Obesity" or "diabetes mellitus" or "metabolic syndromes" in conjunction with identifiers such as "animals" or "mice" or "rats." The search keywords included "probiotic(s)" and "*Akkermansia muciniphila*". All retrieved articles were systematically compiled using Endnote software (20th version). Additionally, we searched bibliographies to ensure inclusivity of relevant literature not initially captured by the database search.

Inclusion criteria: (1) randomized controlled trials in mice; (2) studies employing the Akk probiotic in experimental groups, with a placebo control group for comparison; (3) alternatively, studies utilizing a substrate containing Akk; and (4) studies reporting outcomes related to the risk and development of diabetes or obesity. Exclusion criteria: (1) duplicate studies; (2) studies that were non-blinded trials; (3) studies where the probiotics composition of the intervention was not specified. Article screening and data extraction were completed by 2 reviewers using Covidence software (https://www.covidence.org (accessed on 10 March 2024)), as recommended by the Cochrane Handbook for Systematic Reviews of Interventions and others [19].

2.2. Data Extraction and Quality Assessment

Two researchers independently selected the studies, resolving any disagreements through consultation with a third researcher. Data from the selected studies were extracted into a shared spreadsheet by one reviewer and validated by a second reviewer. The data extraction utilized a standardized form by an independent researcher. The primary outcome was the incidence or biomarkers of obesity or type 2 diabetes, along with any metabolic syndrome factors, upon administration of Akk in animal models. The secondary outcome included the incidence of adverse events or outlier outcomes. Additional extracted data encompassed demographics, indications for antibiotics, probiotic species and dosage, and duration of probiotic administration. Data were extracted as continuous variables [20].

The quality of the selected studies was assessed using the Cochrane Handbook for Systematic Reviews of Interventions [21]. Previously used study quality scales were adapted to evaluate study quality and possible bias risk [22,23]. The methodological assessment scale and its elements were informed by guidelines and publications from rigorous biomedical research such as the STAIR and RIGOR guidelines [24,25]. Taking into account the distinctive nature of the selected animal studies on Akk, the following parameters were considered for study quality assessment: presence or absence of exclusion statement, study pre-registration, inclusion of both sexes, aged and/or compromised animals, sample size, control of diet in the experimental group, clear description of infusion parameters (e.g., rate and/or duration, and dosage), and conflict of interest statements.

2.3. Statistical Analyses

Data analyses were performed using RStudio (version 4.3.3, Ann Arbor, MI, USA), with plots generated using the robumeta, metafor, and dplyr packages. Due to the variability in probiotic durations and infusion parameters, a random-effect meta-analysis model utilizing the Derismonian-Laird estimator was selected for all endpoints. The standardized mean differences (SMDs) were used for calculating effect sizes, with Hedge's G applied to correct for bias in studies with small sample sizes. Pooled relative risk (RR) and the 95% confidence interval (CI) were calculated using a random-effects model (DerSimonian-Laird method [26]) or a fixed-effects model (Mantel-Haenszel method [27]).

Meta-regression was conducted to evaluate heterogeneity, taking into account variables such as probiotic duration, infusion parameters (including temperature and rate volume), and methodological quality. Sensitivity and subgroup analyses were carried out in cases where unexpected or extreme outcomes were identified in the forest plots. Heterogeneity among the included studies was assessed using the Chi-squared (X^2) test and the I^2 statistic [28,29]. A $p < 0.1$ or $I^2 > 50\%$ indicated substantial heterogeneity, warranting the adoption of a random-effects model. In the absence of substantial heterogeneity, a fixed-effects model was applied. Publication bias was evaluated through funnel plots and further evaluated using the Begg and Egger tests [22,23].

3. Results

3.1. Eligible Studies

A comprehensive literature search was conducted in January 2024, yielding 1552 citations across four databases: PubMed (461), Cochrane Library (52), EMBASE (336), and Web of Science (703). After removing duplicates and conducting title and abstract screenings, 1030 studies were deemed potentially relevant for further evaluation. Of these, 952 of these studies were excluded due to irrelevance or methodological shortcomings. A full-text review of the remaining 78 studies led to the exclusion of 63 studies due to methodological issues (15 non-blinded, 14 non-randomized, 11 unknown probiotic composition) or irrelevant outcomes (seven reporting non-SCFA metabolites, four involving unrelated diseases, and two with missing outcome data). Ultimately, 15 studies met our inclusion criteria, encompassing a total of 586 animals and were selected for data analysis and extraction [30–44]. The search flow details are depicted in Figure 2.

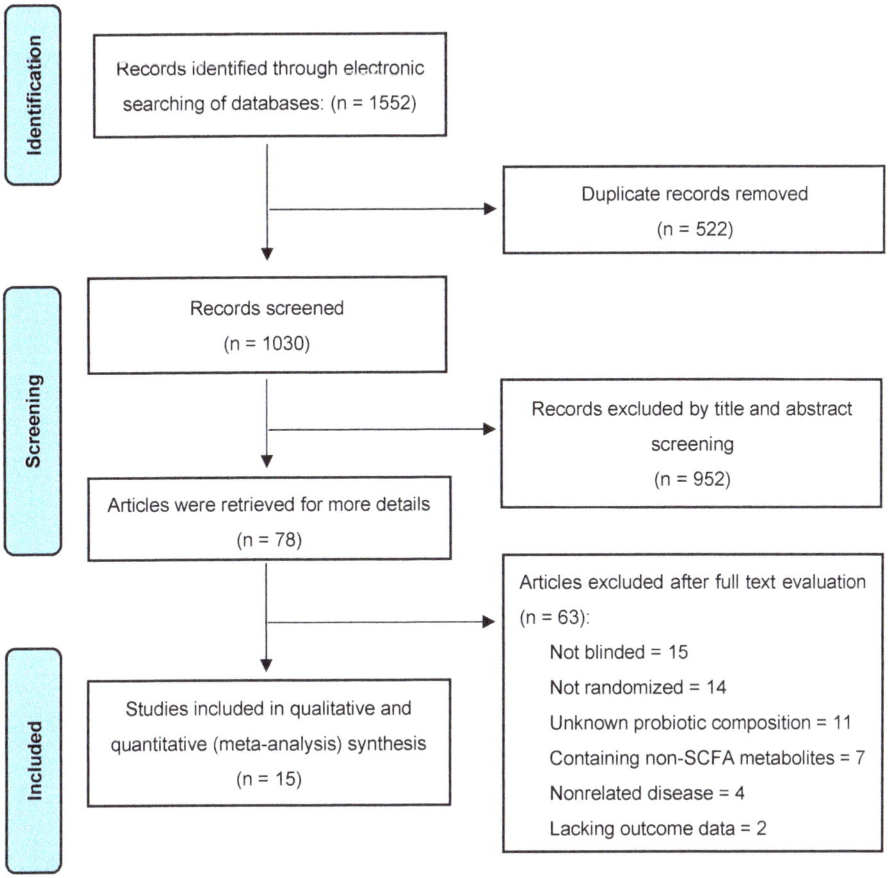

Figure 2. Selection of studies for the meta-analysis.

3.2. *Study Characteristics*

Table 1 summarizes the characteristics of the selected individual studies, such as animal models, sample size, and Akk treatment conditions (e.g., prior antibiotic use, single treatment or combination with other supplements, dosage, and duration). Regarding animal models used for Akk intervention, C57BL/6J was the most prevalent (73%), followed by db/db, NOD mice, and other less common models (27%). Notably, one study utilized a streptozotocin-induced diabetic model in Sprague–Dawley rats for oral Akk administration. Methodologically, 83% of the studies reported randomization, 60% mentioned exclusions, 47% disclosed conflicts of interest, 26% ensured complete blinding (during Akk administration and outcome assessment), and 11% included the mortality rate for both experimental and placebo groups (Table 1). None of the studies performed a priori group size calculations.

Table 1. Characteristics of the enrolled studies.

References	Risk of Bias	Setting	Sample Size (Treatment/Placebo Group)	Obesity/Type 2 Diabetes Definition	High-Fat Diet Composition %	Antibiotic(s)	Time from Antibiotic/HFD to Probiotic, d	Probiotic Species	Dosage per Day	Probiotic Duration	Experimental Period
Acharya et al. [30]	Low	C57BL/6J mice, female, 10-week-old	7/14	WHO	60%	Various	14	*A. muciniphila*	2×10^8 CFU	10 d	4 wk
Anhê et al. [31]	Low	C57BL/6 mice, male	18/18	WHO	65%	None	2	*A. muciniphila* (Cranberry extract)	1.5×10^{10} CFU	2 wk	8 wk
Chelakkot et al. [32]	Low	C57BL/6 mice, male, 6–8-week-old	12/12	Other definition	60%	None	14	*A. muciniphila*	4×10^{10} CFU	2 wk	12 wk
Chung et al. [33]	Low	C57BL/6 mice, male	24/24	WHO	58%	None	N/A	*A. muciniphila* (metaformin, tocotrienol)	2×10^{10} CFU, 8×10^{10} CFU	12 wk	14 wk
Everard et al. [34]	Low	C57BL/6 mice, male	10/10	WHO	60%	None	N/A	*A. muciniphila*	2×10^8 CFU	4 wk	14 wk
Hänninen et al. [35]	Medium	NOD/MrkTac mice, 7–8-week-old	16/21	WHO	N/A	None	N/A	*A. muciniphila*	1×10^{10} CFU	2 wk	18 wk
Okamura et al. [36]	Medium	7-week-old db/db mice	6/6	WHO	N/A	None	N/A	*A. muciniphila* (milk)	1×10^{10} CFU	8 wk	16 wk
Plovier et al. [37]	Medium	mice, male	6/6	WHO	HFD	None	N/A	*A. muciniphila*	2×10^8 CFU	2 wk	6 wk
Shin et al. [38]	Low	C57BL/6J mice	15/15	Other definition	HFD	None	N/A	*A. muciniphila* (metaformin)	1×10^{10} CFU	6 wk	6 wk
Song et al. [39]	Low	C57BL/6J mice	12/24	WHO	HFD	None	N/A	*A. muciniphila*	1×10^{10} CFU	4 wk	14 wk
Wang et al. [40]	Low	Villin Cre and Gko, adult male mice	10/10	WHO	N/A	None	N/A	*A. muciniphila*	5×10^{10} CFU	6 wk	12 wk
Wu et al. [41]	Medium	C57BL/6J	10/10	WHO	HFD	None	N/A	*A. muciniphila*	1×10^{10} CFU	2 wk	6 wk
Zhai et al. [42]	Low	C57BL/6 7-week-old male mice	10/30	WHO	N/A	None	N/A	*A. muciniphila*	2×10^{10} CFU	9 d	14 wk
Zhang, J et al. [43]	Low	C57BL/6J 8-week-old male mice	28/21	WHO	HFD	None	N/A	*A. muciniphila*	5×10^{10} CFU	15 wk	20 wk
Zhang, L et al. [44]	Medium	Sprague-Dawley rats	105/77	Other definition	66%	Streptozocin	3	*A. muciniphila*	1×10^{10} CFU	4 wk	8 wk

The experimental groups were predominantly fed a high-fat diet (HFD), comprising over 60% fat compared to carbohydrates (Figure 3A). Most studies employed young, male C57BL/6J, except for two studies which included females but did not consider biological sex as a variable parameter or specify the number of females per group (Figure 3B).

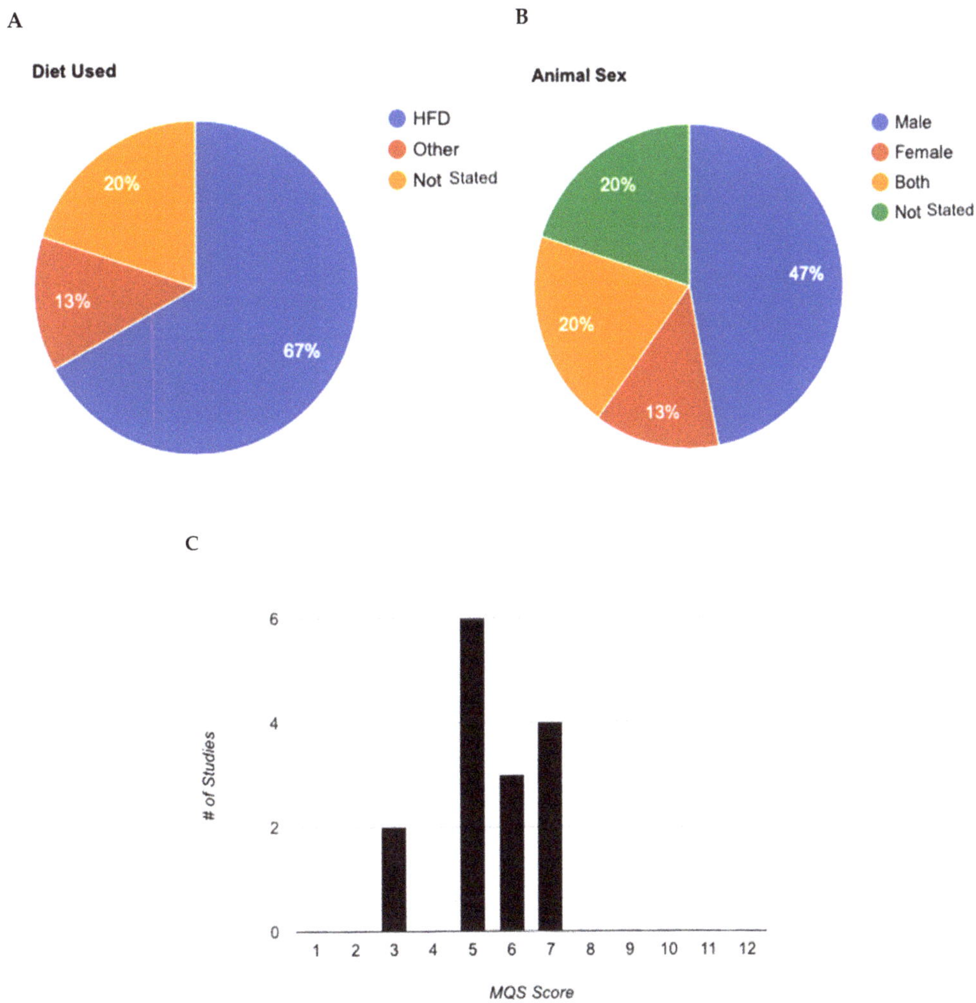

Figure 3. Analysis of experimental characteristics used in animal models for *Akkermansia muciniphila* studies. (**A**): Breakdown of diets used in animal studies. (**B**): Animal sexes used in mouse animal studies. (**C**): Evaluation of methodological quality score for animal studies (max score = 12). MQS, Methodological Quality Score.

All studies measured changes in body weight during Akk intervention. Body composition (lean and fat mass) was assessed in 84% of the studies, highlighting its significance as an outcome measure for Akk intervention. Interestingly, four studies employed antibiotics prior to probiotic administration, likely aimed to create a more favorable intestinal environment for robust Akk colonization. The characteristics of interest for the enrolled studies were ranked from most to least prevalent to provide an overview of the current literature characteristics of selected studies (Table 2).

Table 2. Methodological quality scale reporting elements for *Akkermansia muciniphila* research in type 2 diabetes and obesity, and percentage adherence.

Element	% Adherence
Control of diet	100
Blinding to outcome(s)	87
Complete reporting of infusion parameters	87
Group randomization	80
Includes type 2 diabetes	67
Exclusion statement	60
Conflict of interest statement	47
Use of male and female animals	40
Blinding to type 2 diabetes	40
Includes obesity	33
Blinding to obesity	23
Use of aged animals	0
Sample size calculation	0
A priori study registration	0
Comorbidities	0

3.3. *Quality Assessment*

The methodological quality of these studies was assessed using the STAIR and RIGOR guidelines, specifically designed to evaluate the rigor and robustness of preclinical research, thereby ensuring reliable translation of findings into human studies [28,29]. Of the 15 eligible studies, only 10 employed blinding to minimize detection bias. Reporting on other potential biases varied among the studies. Unfortunately, none of the included studies explicitly mentioned blinding procedures. For outcomes like obesity, which can be visually apparent, it is unclear what specific tools or methods were used to ensure blinding. Future studies should incorporate more rigorous blinding procedures, such as using blinded assessors for subjective outcomes and objective measurement tools for outcomes like obesity, to minimize the risk of bias and enhance the quality of the evidence.

Higher risk of attrition bias and other concerns were noted in studies that: 1. lacked clear methods for handling missing outcome data and outliers (three out of 15 studies); 2. had a short follow-up period (one out of 15 studies); 3. experienced excessive or unbalanced loss of subjects during the study (six out of 15 studies); 4. utilized a small sample size (five out of 15 studies); and 5. had unbalanced baseline characteristics between groups (four out of 15 studies). Nine studies assessed glucose tolerance, a key indicator of the body's ability to regulate blood sugar levels. Additionally, 13 studies measured serum insulin levels, and nine studies assessed fasting blood glucose levels.

3.4. *Analysis of Methodological Quality*

Tables 1 and 2 provide a detailed overview of the methodological quality scale and the analysis of studies incorporating experimental elements. None of the included studies explicitly mentioned the specific randomization and concealment methods used. Future studies should explicitly report randomization and concealment methods to enhance the study quality. Table 3 presents the methodological quality scores (MQS) of the selected studies. The overall median score was 5, indicating low to moderate methodological quality across the studies. Scores ranged from three to seven (out of a maximum of 12 points) as illustrated in Figure 3C. Characteristics of C75BL/6J Mice Model Studies in Akk. All studies, except one, administered Akk immediately after initiating a high-fat diet (HFD) containing 60% of energy from fat. The one exception did not use a HFD but instead administered an antibiotic prior to Akk administration. For studies that included additional supplements, such as metformin or tocotrienol, Akk was administered concurrently with the supplements. In these cases, the mice received either an HFD with 800 mg of tocotrienol or an HFD with 200 mg of metformin, along with Akk.

Table 3. Statistical summary comparison and total percentage of reported MQS elements (✓ = yes, χ = no).

References	Pre-Registration	Exclusion State-ment	Both Sexes	Old Age	Sample Size Calcuation	Group Ran-domization	Comorbidities	Outcome(s) Blinding	Disease Blind-ing	Control of Diet	Infusion Parame-ters	Conflict of Interest	Total Score (Max. 12)
Acharya et al. [30]	χ	χ	χ	χ	χ	✓	χ	✓	✓	✓	✓	✓	6
Anhê et al. [31]	χ	✓	χ	χ	χ	✓	χ	✓	✓	✓	✓	✓	7
Chelakkot et al. [32]	χ	χ	χ	χ	χ	✓	χ	χ	✓	✓	✓	✓	5
Chung et al. [33]	χ	✓	χ	χ	χ	✓	χ	✓	χ	✓	✓	✓	5
Everard et al. [34]	χ	✓	χ	χ	χ	✓	χ	✓	χ	✓	✓	✓	5
Hänninen et al. [35]	χ	χ	✓	χ	χ	χ	χ	✓	✓	✓	✓	χ	5
Okamura et al. [36]	χ	✓	✓	χ	χ	✓	χ	✓	✓	✓	✓	χ	7
Plovier et al. [37]	χ	χ	χ	χ	χ	χ	χ	✓	χ	✓	✓	χ	3
Shin et al. [38]	χ	✓	✓	χ	χ	✓	χ	✓	χ	✓	✓	χ	6
Song et al. [39]	χ	χ	✓	χ	χ	✓	χ	✓	χ	✓	χ	✓	5
Wang et al. [40]	χ	✓	χ	χ	χ	✓	χ	✓	✓	✓	✓	✓	7
Wu et al. [41]	χ	✓	✓	χ	χ	✓	χ	✓	✓	✓	✓	χ	7
Zhai et al. [42]	χ	✓	χ	χ	χ	✓	χ	✓	✓	✓	✓	χ	6
Zhang, J et al. [43]	χ	✓	χ	χ	χ	✓	χ	✓	✓	✓	✓	χ	5
Zhang, L et al. [44]	χ	χ	✓	χ	χ	χ	χ	χ	✓	✓	χ	χ	3
Total (%)	0	60	40	0	0	80	0	87	67	100	87	47	

3.5. Impact of Akk on Body Weight

Ten studies examined changes in body weight during and after Akk administration. One study used rats, while the other nine studies used mice as the animal model. The study on rats showed that Akk supplementation significantly reduced body weight by an average of 25%, likely owing to a greater average body weight in rat models than mice models. In the nine mice studies, an average weight reduction of 3.8 g was observed (Table 4). The total number of mice in the control groups across all studies was 135, compared to 155 in the treatment groups. The average body weight in the Akk groups was 32.2 g, while the average weight of the controls was 36.4 g, suggesting a reduction of average body weight gain by 10.4%.

Normalized effect sizes varied across studies, with most studies showing positive effect sizes, suggesting that the treatment generally had a beneficial effect. However, it is important to note that five out of the nine studies reported non-significant changes in overall body weight compared to baseline. This inconsistency suggests significant variability across the studies, with body weight changes ranging from a 0.08 g increase to an 11.0 g decrease following Akk treatment.

Overall, the weighted mean effect size of 0.33 (95% CI: 0.17–0.48) indicates a statistically significant reduction in body weight gain due to Akk treatment. A forest plot analysis indicated a significant reduction in body weight gain among mice treated with Akk compared to controls ($p < 0.001$, Figure 4A). However, substantial heterogeneity existed among studies ($I^2 = 46\%$), and the funnel plot suggested low publication bias (Figure 4B). The Baujat plot identified the studies by Chung et al. and Wu et al. as primary contributors to this heterogeneity (Figure 4C).

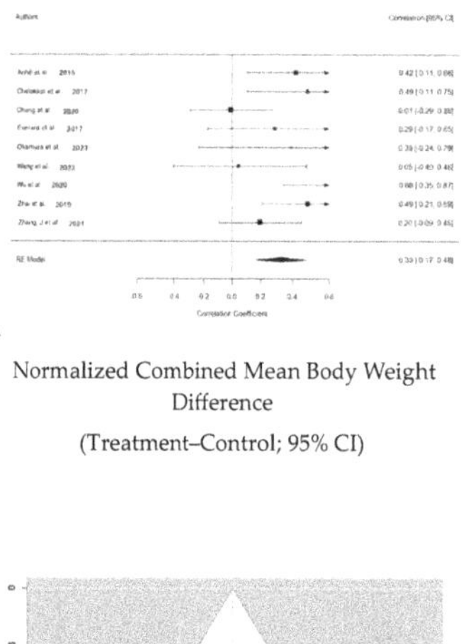

Total = 0.33 [0.17, 0.48]

Heterogeneity: $\chi^2_9 = 14.64$ ($p < 0.0666$), $I^2 = 46\%$

Test for overall effect: $z = 3.8200$ ($p < 0.0001$)

A

Normalized Combined Mean Body Weight Difference

(Treatment–Control; 95% CI)

B **C**

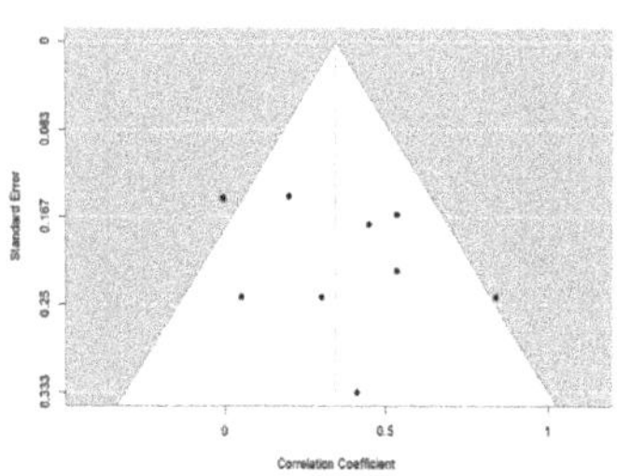

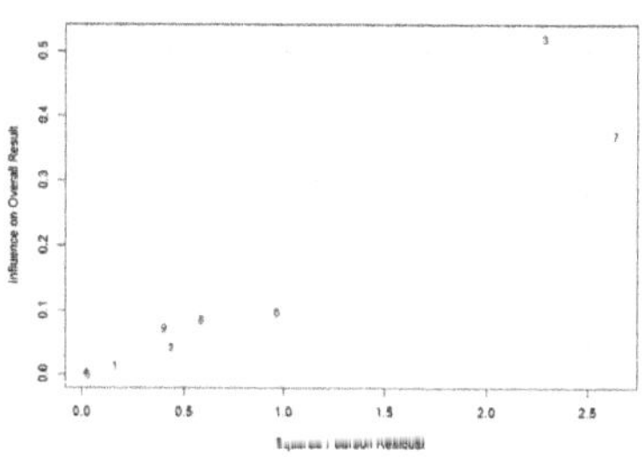

Normalized Combined Mean Body Weight Difference

(Treatment–Control)

Figure 4. Quantitative analysis of studies that assessed body weight using a random-effects meta-analysis. (**A**): Forest plot of studies investigating body weight effects (normalized mean difference ± 95% CI) [31–34,36,40–43]. Effect size estimates were heterogenous, likely owing to study design differences.

(**B**): Funnel plot used to assess publication bias. These results suggest that the studies used in the meta-analysis had relatively low publication bias (i.e., the symmetric distribution of closed circles). (**C**): Baujat plot used to assess the studies that contributed most to heterogeneity. These results suggest that studies Chung et al. 2020 [33] and Wu et al. 2020 [41] likely had moderating variables that contributed the most to the heterogeneity.

Table 4. Descriptive characteristics of studies that assessed body weight.

References	Duration (wk)	Control (n)	Experimental (n)	Control Body Weight (g)	Treatment Body Weight (g)	Normalized Effect Size	95% Confidence Interval
Anhê et al. [31]	8	18	18	27.8	23.5	0.421	0.11, 0.66
Chelakkot et al. [32]	12	12	12	45	40	0.489	0.11, 0.75
Chung et al. [33]	14	24	24	38.44	38.52	−0.008	−0.29, 0.28
Everard et al. [34]	14	10	10	24	21	0.294	−0.17, 0.65
Okamura et al. [36]	16	6	6	48	44	0.391	−0.24, 0.79
Wang et al. [40]	12	10	10	27	26.5	0.049	−0.40, 0.48
Wu et al. [41]	6	10	10	39.5	32.5	0.685	0.35, 0.87
Zhai et al. [42]	14	10	30	55	50	0.489	0.21, 0.69
Zhang, J et al. [43]	20	28	21	31.5	29.5	0.196	−0.09, 0.45
Summary statistic	Median = 13	Σ = 135	Σ = 155	Mean = 36.4	Mean = 32.2	XWeighted = 0.331	XWeighted = 0.17, 0.48

3.6. *Impact of Akk on Glucose Tolerance*

Nine studies evaluated the effect of Akk on glucose tolerance (Table 5). In total, 111 animals were in the control groups, while 123 received treatment. On average, Akk treatment led to a 22.1% improvement in glucose tolerance, as estimated by the 2 h area under the curve (AUC) for blood glucose following a glucose tolerance test. Since the exact AUC values were not provided in all the selected studies, these estimates were derived from the individual study graphs using an image analysis program (https://imagej.nih.gov/ij/, accessed on 10 March 2024). The effect sizes varied. While three studies showed significant reductions in AUC, the majority reported only minor, non-significant decreases.

Overall, a weighted mean effect size of 0.347 (95% CI: 0.18–0.63) indicated a statistically significant reduction in blood glucose levels due to Akk treatment. Forest plot analysis confirmed this, revealing a pooled effect size of 0.43 (95% CI: 0.18–0.63; $p < 0.001$, Figure 5A). A random-effects model was used to account for heterogeneity between studies, which was substantial ($I^2 = 73\%$). Nonetheless, the funnel plot suggested low publication bias (Figure 5B). The study by Shin et al. primarily contributed to the observed heterogeneity (Figure 5C).

A

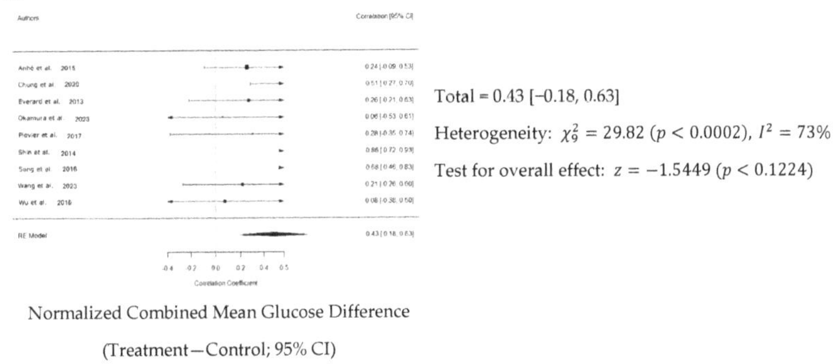

Figure 5. *Cont.*

B C

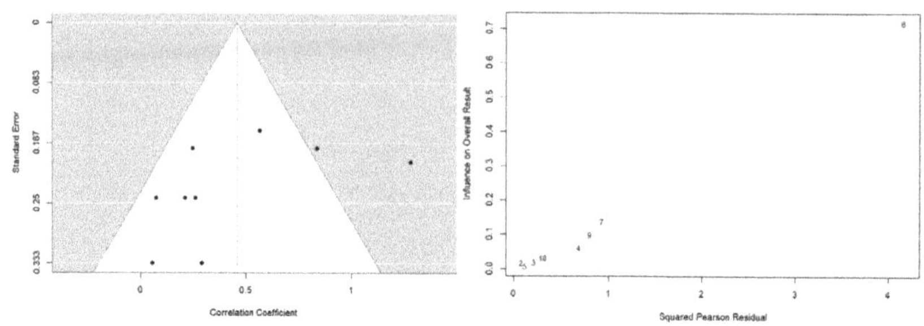

Normalized Combined Mean Glucose Difference

(Treatment—Control)

Figure 5. Quantitative analysis of studies that assessed glucose tolerance using a random-effects meta-analysis. (**A**): Forest plot of studies investigating glucose tolerance (normalized mean difference ±95% CI) [31,33,34,36–41]. Effect size estimates were heterogenous, likely owing to study design differences. (**B**): Funnel plot used to assess publication bias. These results suggest that the studies used in the meta-analysis had relatively low publication bias. (**C**): Baujat plot used to assess the studies that contributed most to heterogeneity. These results suggest that the study Shin et al. 2014 [38] likely had moderating variables that contributed the most to the heterogeneity.

Table 5. Descriptive characteristics of studies that assessed glucose tolerance.

References	Duration (wk)	Control (n)	Experimental (n)	Control Blood Glucose (AUC mg/dL) (120 min)	Treatment Blood Glucose (AUC mg/dL) (120 min)	Normalized Effect Size	95% Confidence Interval
Anhé et al. [31]	8	18	18	10,500	6200	0.245	−0.09, 0.53
Chung et al. [33]	14	24	24	57,000	48,000	0.513	0.27, 0.70
Everard et al. [34]	14	10	10	34,500	30,000	0.257	−0.21, 0.63
Okamura et al. [36]	16	6	6	11,000	10,000	0.057	−0.53, 0.61
Plovier et al. [37]	6	6	6	40,000	35,000	0.285	−0.35, 0.74
Shin et al. [38]	6	15	15	55,000	40,000	0.856	0.72, 0.93
Song et al. [39]	14	12	24	24,000	12,000	0.685	0.46, 0.83
Wang et al. [40]	12	10	10	12,200	8500	0.211	−0.26, 0.60
Wu et al. [41]	6	10	10	11,860	10,530	0.076	−0.38, 0.50
Summary statistic	Median = 12	Σ = 111	Σ = 123	Mean = 28,500	Mean = 22,200	XWeighted = 0.347	XWeighted = 0.18, 0.63

3.7. Impact of Akk on Blood Insulin

Thirteen studies examined circulating insulin hormone levels. As presented in Table 6, the total number of animals in the control groups across all studies was 168, compared to 200 in the treatment groups. The data suggest that Akk treatment stimulated blood insulin production in the animals by 26.9%, as shown by the higher mean level of 2.6 μIU/mL in the treatment groups compared to 1.9 μIU/mL in the control groups.

Normalized effect sizes varied across studies, with most studies showing positive effect sizes, suggesting that the treatment generally had a beneficial effect. Nevertheless, only seven of 13 studies showed that the effect was significant. The weighted mean effect size of 0.827 with a confidence interval of 0.10 to 0.25 indicates a statistically significant reduction in blood glucose levels due to Akk treatment. The forest plot also revealed a significant increase in blood insulin levels in animals administered Akk compared to controls ($p < 0.001$) as shown in Figure 6A. The analysis showed a pooled effect size of 0.18 (95% confidence interval: 0.10–0.25). There was significant variation in the study results ($I^2 = 64\%$). Additionally, the analysis suggests a potential publication bias (Figure 6B). These results indicate that the studies by Shin et al., Song et al. and Wang et al. contributed the most to the observed heterogeneity (Figure 6C).

Table 6. Descriptive characteristics of studies that assessed blood insulin.

References	Duration (wk)	Control (n)	Experimental (n)	Treatment Insulin Levels (µg/mL)	Control Insulin Levels (µg/mL)	Normalized Effect Size	95% Confidence Interval
Acharya et al. [30]	4	7	14	2.5	2.1	0.587	0.02, 0.34
Anhê et al. [31]	8	18	18	0.8	0.6	0.134	−0.01, 0.32
Chelakkot et al. [32]	12	12	12	2.7	2	0.703	0.18, 0.48
Chung et al. [33]	14	24	24	4	2.5	1.406	0.15, 0.47
Everard et al. [34]	14	10	10	2.2	1.9	0.234	0.09, 0.43
Okamura et al. [36]	16	6	6	2.5	2.2	0.469	−0.13, 0.23
Plovier et al. [37]	6	6	6	1.9	1.5	0.469	0.09, 0.42
Shin et al. [38]	6	15	15	2.7	1.9	0.938	−0.18, 0.20
Song et al. [39]	14	12	24	2.8	2	0.938	−0.28, 0.11
Wang et al. [40]	12	10	10	2.9	2.1	0.938	0.21, 0.51
Wu et al. [41]	6	10	10	3	2.2	0.938	−0.14, 0.14
Zhai et al. [42]	14	10	30	3.1	2.1	1.172	−0.01, 0.31
Zhang, J et al. [43]	20	28	21	3.2	1.8	1.641	0.07, 0.40
Summary statistic	Median = 12	Σ = 168	Σ = 200	Mean = 2.6	Mean = 1.9	XWeighted = 0.827	XWeighted = 0.10, 0.25

A

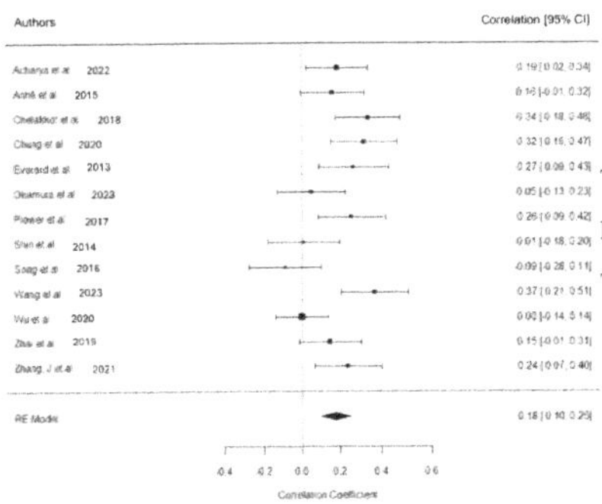

Total = 0.18 [0.10, 0.25]

Heterogeneity: $\chi^2_{13} = 32.95$ ($p < 0.0010$), $I^2 = 64\%$

Test for overall effect: $z = -4.3844$ ($p < 0.0001$)

Normalized Combined Mean Insulin Difference

(Treatment−Control; 95% CI)

B

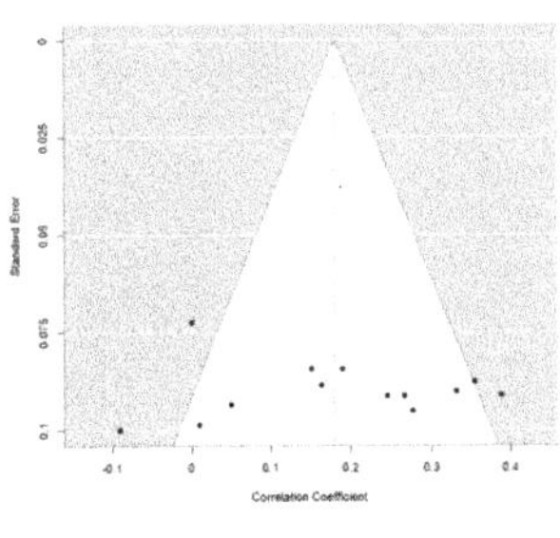

C

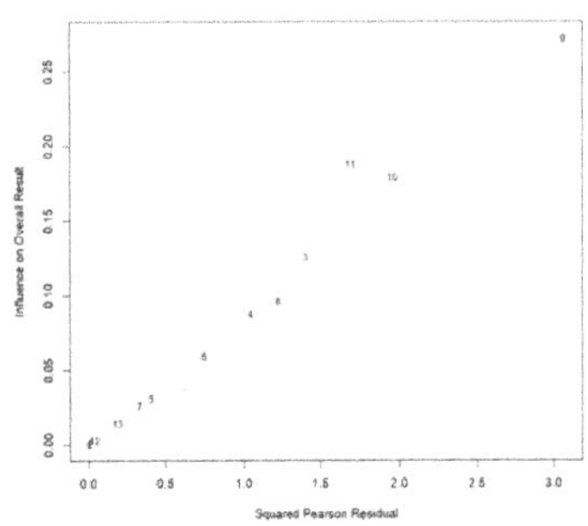

Normalized Combined Mean Insulin Difference

(Treatment−Control)

Figure 6. Quantitative analysis of studies that assessed insulin hormone levels using a random-effects meta-analysis. (**A**): Forest plot of studies investigating insulin levels (normalized mean difference ±95% CI) [30–34,36–43]. Effect size estimates were very heterogenous, likely owing to study design differences and differences in probiotic duration. (**B**): Funnel plot used to assess publication bias. These results suggest that the studies used in the meta-analysis had relatively low publication bias. (**C**): Baujat plot used to assess the studies that contributed most to heterogeneity. These results suggest that studies Shin et al. 2014 [38], Song et al. 2016 [39], and Wang et al. 2023 [40] likely had moderating variables that contributed the most to the heterogeneity.

3.8. Impact of Akk on Fasting Blood Glucose

Nine studies investigated the impact of Akk on fasting blood glucose levels. Detailed information on these assessment methods can be found in Table 7. The analysis revealed that Akk treatment significantly reduced fasting blood glucose levels by 21.2%, as shown by the lower mean level of 114.7 mg/dL in the treatment groups compared to 145.5 mg/dL in the control groups.

Table 7. Descriptive characteristics of studies that assessed fasting blood glucose levels.

References	Duration (wk)	Control (n)	Experimental (n)	Control Fasting Blood Glucose (mg/dL)	Treatment Fasting blood Glucose (mg/dL)	Normalized Effect Size	95% Confidence Interval
Acharya et al. [30]	4	7	14	178	156	0.502	0.04, 0.33
Chung et al. [33]	14	24	24	100	58	0.958	0.14, 0.48
Everard et al. [34]	14	10	10	175	135	0.912	0.08, 0.44
Plovier et al. [37]	6	6	6	260	160	2.281	0.07, 0.43
Shin et al. [38]	6	15	15	122	112	0.228	−0.18, 0.20
Wang et al. [40]	12	10	10	124	114	0.228	0.21, 0.51
Wu et al. [41]	6	10	10	125	115	0.228	−0.18, 0.18
Zhai et al. [42]	14	10	30	126	116	0.228	0.01, 0.30
Zhang, J et al. [43]	20	28	21	99.5	66.5	0.753	0.10, 0.37
Summary statistic	Median = 12	Σ = 120	Σ = 140	Mean = 145.5	Mean = 114.7	XWeighted = 0.623	XWeighted = 0.12, 0.28

Normalized effect sizes varied across studies, with most studies showing positive effect sizes, suggesting that the treatment generally had a beneficial effect. Seven of nine studies showed that the effect was significant. The weighted mean effect size of 0.623 with a confidence interval of 0.12 to 0.28 indicates a statistically significant reduction in blood glucose levels due to Akk treatment. The forest plot also revealed a significant increase in blood insulin levels in animals administered Akk compared to controls ($p < 0.001$) as shown in Figure 7A. The analysis showed a pooled effect size of 0.20 (95% confidence interval: 0.12–0.28). There was significant variation in the study results ($I^2 = 52\%$). However, the analysis suggests a low risk of publication bias, indicating a fair representation of both positive and negative findings (Figure 7B). Three studies by Shin et al., Wang et al. and Wu et al. contributed the most to the observed heterogeneity (Figure 7C).

A

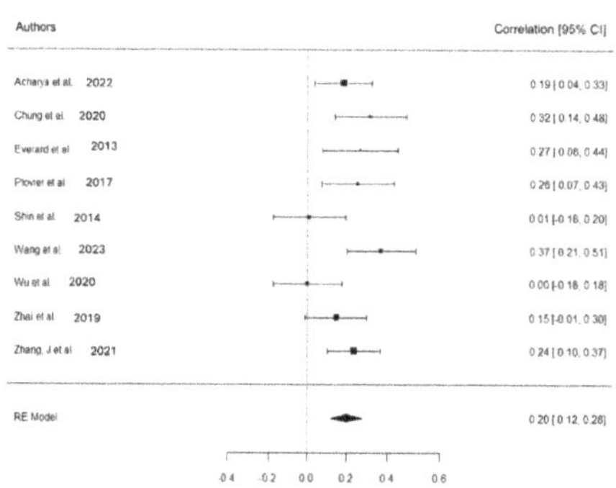

Total = 0.20 [0.12, 0.28]

Heterogeneity: $\chi^2_9 = 16.46$ ($p < 0.0362$), $I^2 = 52\%$

Test for overall effect: $z = 4.8040$ ($p < 0.0001$)

Normalized Combined Mean Fasting Glucose Difference

(Treatment—Control; 95% CI)

Figure 7. *Cont.*

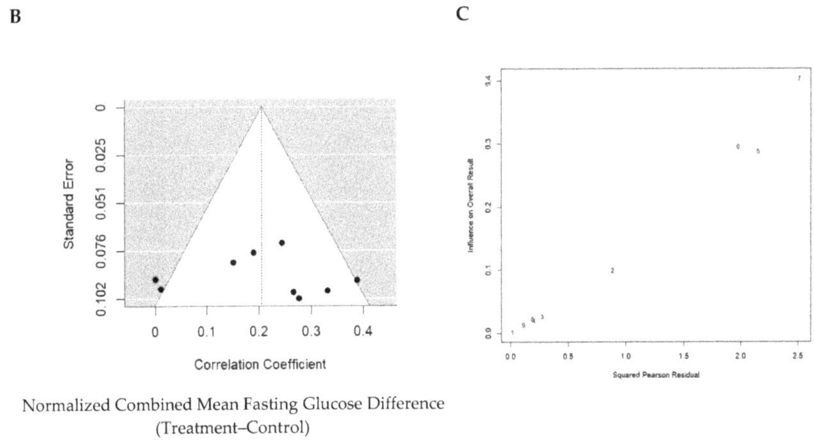

Figure 7. Quantitative analysis of studies that assessed fasting blood glucose using a random-effects meta-analysis. (**A**): Forest plot of studies investigating fasting blood glucose (normalized mean difference ± 95% CI) [30,33,34,37,38,40–43]. Effect size estimates were heterogenous, likely owing to study design differences. (**B**): Funnel plot used to assess publication bias. These results suggest that the studies used in the meta-analysis had relatively low publication bias. (**C**): Baujat plot used to assess the studies that contributed most to heterogeneity. These results suggest that studies Shin et al. 2014 [38], Wang et al. 2023 [40], and Wu et al. 2020 [41] likely had moderating variables that contributed the most to the heterogeneity.

4. Discussion

This meta-analysis underscores the multifaceted benefits of Akk intake in mice subjected to a high-fat diet. Overall, dietary supplementation with Akk, as analyzed from nine selected studies, significantly reduced body weight by an average of 10.4%. The dosage of Akk ranged from 2×10^8 to 5×10^{10} CFU/day, which aligns with the dosages commonly used in most probiotic animal studies. Most of the selected studies on Akk used dosages of 2×10^8 and 1×10^{10} CFU. However, two studies by Wang et al. [40] and Zhang et al. [43] utilized a higher dose of 5×10^{10} CFU in mice. Interestingly, both studies showed that Akk had no effect on body weight, despite other studies with lower doses showing a beneficial effect in reducing body weight gain. These results suggest that there is no dose-dependent relationship of Akk in the prevention of body weight gain. The median duration of Akk treatment across the selected nine animal studies was 14 weeks, ranging from 6 to 20 weeks. The most prominent effects of Akk were observed during treatment durations of 6 to 12 weeks. The results suggest that Akk exerts its effect in reducing body weight gain during the early stages of obesity development (as early as 6 weeks), with the probiotic effect likely diminishing over time. For instance, Zhang's study [43] extended Akk treatment to 20 weeks at higher dose, but showed no inhibiting effect on body weight gain. Obesity is a chronic disease that requires a long-term solution. The current animal studies were all of short duration (less than 20 weeks). Long-term studies are needed to verify Akk's effect on obesity development.

The effect of Akk supplementation on the prevention of type 2 diabetes is reflected in its significant reduction of fasting blood glucose (by 21.2%) and improvement in glucose tolerance (by 22.1%), suggesting that Akk treatment is effective in preventing type 2 diabetes. Nine studies have measured fasting blood glucose. Except for two studies, all others showed a significant reduction in fasting blood glucose with Akk treatment. These two studies had a short treatment duration of 6 weeks, while the others were longer, suggesting that Akk may require more than 6 weeks to demonstrate a significant effect on blood glucose. No dose–response relationship was observed across the tested doses between 2×10^8 and 5×10^{10} CFU/day in the nine studies. It was unclear if and how treatment duration affected the efficiency of the probiotic during administration. Additionally, a discrepancy emerged regarding the inclusion of antibiotics, which was the predominant method. In the study by Acharya et al., the administration of the antibiotic before the probiotic was actually more effective than administering the probiotic by itself [30]. Few authors provided clear justifications for the model choice and dosing parameters utilized in their studies.

Nine studies measured glucose tolerance. The meta-analysis showed that Akk significantly improved glucose tolerance in mice by reducing the 2 h AUC by 22.1%. However, there was substantial variation in the results across studies, as reflected by I^2 = 73%. Indeed, six of nine studies showed modest but non-significant effects. The median duration of Akk treatment across studies was 12 weeks, ranging from 6 to 16 weeks. Shin et al. found that six weeks of Akk treatment significantly reduced DIO mice 2 h AUC by an estimated 27.3%. This mouse study of Akk treatment showed the most prominent effect among the studies with a normalized effect size of 0.856. Plovier et al. also investigated six weeks of Akk treatment on mouse glucose tolerance but with a lower dose (2×10^8 CFU/d versus 1×10^{10} CFU/d in Shin's study) and found no significant effect. The other two studies with significant effects by Akk treatment also used doses at or above 1×10^{10} CFU/d, suggesting that the Akk treatment dose may need to be no less than 1×10^{10} CFU/d to be effective. It should be noted that one study by Wang et al. used a model of FFAR4 knockout mice, which has been shown to cause severely impaired glucose tolerance under high-fat feeding conditions. FFAR4 regulates glucagon-like peptide 1 secretion by modifying Akk abundance. However, our meta-analysis showed that Akk treatment at 5×10^{10} CFU/d for 12 weeks in Wang's study did not significantly improve glucose tolerance. There was substantial heterogeneity among the studies. The studies differed in terms of doses, duration, sample size, and other factors, which could significantly influence the results. Further research is needed to confirm the consistency and magnitude of the effect of Akk on glucose tolerance. Overall, fasting blood glucose decreased by 21.2%, whilst blood insulin increased by 26.9% when comparing control to treatment groups likely because insulin and blood glucose are inversely correlated.

Thirteen studies investigated the effect of Akk treatment on blood insulin levels in animals. The meta-analysis revealed a significant increase in blood insulin levels, from 1.9 to 2.6 μg/mL. Notably, three studies—Zhang et al. [43], Chung et al. [33], and Zhai et al. [42]—demonstrated strong treatment effects, with effect sizes of 1.64, 1.44, and 1.17, respectively. Interestingly, all three studies also reported significant reductions in fasting blood glucose levels. Additionally, some studies explored the anti-inflammatory efficacy of Akk; however, due to the heterogeneity of inflammation biomarkers across blood and tissue, a meta-analysis on the anti-inflammatory effects was not feasible.

One of the primary objectives of this meta-analysis was to identify the variables that contribute to the efficacy of Akk, such as changes in body weight and treatment duration. Surprisingly, the random-effects meta-regression model is not able to determine these expected variables. A random-effects model was selected for meta-regression because of the aforementioned variables in study design, such as probiotic duration, infusion parameters (including temperature, rate volume), and overall methodological quality. Notably, treatment duration which has been a critical determinant of efficacy in previous studies (both preclinical and clinical), did not emerge as a significant factor in our analysis [20,28]. This discrepancy might be due to the limited exploration of treatment durations in the analyzed studies. Only one study specifically investigated the impact of different treatment durations, reporting no significant effect of the probiotic beyond 14 weeks [18].

There are several limitations leading to inclusive results in our meta-regression models. First, the limited number of studies assessing fasting blood glucose levels restricted our ability to conduct a comprehensive meta-regression due to constraints in degrees of freedom [45]. Second, the presence of substantial variability among studies can compromise the power of meta-regression. Our analysis revealed significant variation between studies, as indicated by heterogeneity statistics in our primary endpoints model. This could be due to factors such as system errors among different laboratories, such as experiment duration, sample preparation, and administration parameters of Akk. Third, the animal models used (age, sex, and species) were inconsistent. This significant methodological and model variability among the studies made it challenging to identify clear cause-and-effect relationships. Fourth, most studies employed young, male C57BL/6J mice. Only two studies included female mice, but neither considered biological sex as a variable parameter or specified the number of females per group. Consequently, the potential effects of Akk on female animals remain unclear. Moreover, the inconclusive results regarding microbiota suggest that Akk's influence on gut microbiota might be more critical than its direct metabolic effects on parameters such as blood glucose levels. On the other hand, the current data make it difficult to definitively determine the key factors influencing treatment outcomes.

5. Conclusions

Given the increasing prevalence of metabolic morbidities such as type 2 diabetes and diet-induced obesity, this meta-analysis aimed to evaluate the potential of Akk as a novel therapeutic intervention in animal models. Our findings strongly suggest that Akk is a promising candidate for mitigating these metabolic diseases, demonstrating efficacy in preventing body weight gain and type 2 diabetes. To further elucidate the clinical implications of these findings, future studies should incorporate a broader range of experimental parameters. Factors such as age, sex, and treatment duration may influence treatment outcomes [27,45]. Additionally, comprehensive, long-term outcome assessments are essential for a more complete understanding of Akk's effects on body weight and type 2 diabetes. Therefore, we recommend conducting large-scale animal model validation studies to determine the reliability and generalizability of our meta-analysis findings. These future studies should address the limitations identified in the current literature and contribute to a more comprehensive understanding of the clinical potential of Akk.

Author Contributions: Conceptualization, E.L., X.J. and K.Z.; Data curation, E.L.; Formal analysis, E.L. and K.Z.; Investigation, E.L. and K.Z.; Methodology, E.L., X.J. and K.Z.; Project administration, K.Z.; Resources, K.Z.; Software, E.L.; Supervision, K.Z.; Validation, E.L. and K.Z.; Visualization, K.Z.; Writing—original draft, E.L. and K.Z.; Writing—review and editing, E.L., X.J. and K.Z. All authors have read and agreed to the published version of the manuscript.

Funding: This research received no external funding.

Institutional Review Board Statement: Not applicable.

Informed Consent Statement: Not applicable.

Data Availability Statement: The original contributions presented in this study are included in the article, further inquiries can be directed to the corresponding author.

Conflicts of Interest: The authors declare no conflicts of interest. The funders had no role in the design of this study; in the collection, analyses, or interpretation of data; in the writing of the manuscript; or in the decision to publish the results.

References

1. Bhupathiraju, S.N.; Hu, F.B. Epidemiology of Obesity and Diabetes and Their Cardiovascular Complications. *Circ. Res.* **2016**, *118*, 1723–1735. [CrossRef] [PubMed]
2. Xu, Y.; Wang, N.; Tan, H.Y.; Li, S.; Zhang, C.; Feng, Y. Function of *Akkermansia muciniphila* in Obesity: Interactions With Lipid Metabolism, Immune Response and Gut Systems. *Front. Microbiol.* **2020**, *11*, 219. [CrossRef] [PubMed]
3. Dao, M.C.; Everard, A.; Aron-Wisnewsky, J.; Sokolovska, N.; Prifti, E.; Verger, E.O.; Kayser, B.D.; Levenez, F.; Chilloux, J.; Hoyles, L.; et al. *Akkermansia muciniphila* and Improved Metabolic Health During a Dietary Intervention in Obesity: Relationship with Gut Microbiome Richness and Ecology. *Gut* **2016**, *65*, 426–436. [CrossRef] [PubMed]
4. Arslanian, S.; Bacha, F.; Grey, M.; Marcus, M.D.; White, N.H.; Zeitler, P. Evaluation and Management of Youth-Onset Type 2 Diabetes: A Position Statement by the American Diabetes Association. *Diabetes Care* **2018**, *41*, 2648–2668. [CrossRef] [PubMed]
5. Harsch, I.A.; Konturek, P.C. The Role of Gut Microbiota in Obesity and Type 2 and Type 1 Diabetes Mellitus: New Insights into "Old" Diseases. *Med. Sci.* **2018**, *6*, 32. [CrossRef]

6. Bastos, R.M.C.; Simplício-Filho, A.; Sávio-Silva, C.; Oliveira, L.F.V.; Cruz, G.N.F.; Sousa, E.H.; Noronha, I.L.; Mangueira, C.L.P.; Quaglierini-Ribeiro, H.; Josefi-Rocha, G.R.; et al. Fecal Microbiota Transplant in a Pre-Clinical Model of Type 2 Diabetes Mellitus, Obesity and Diabetic Kidney Disease. *Int. J. Mol. Sci.* **2022**, *23*, 3842. [CrossRef]
7. Dalby, M.J. Questioning the Foundations of the Gut Microbiota and Obesity. *Philos. Trans. R. Soc. Lond. B Biol. Sci.* **2023**, *378*, 20220221. [CrossRef]
8. Liu, B.N.; Liu, X.T.; Liang, Z.H.; Wang, J.H. Gut Microbiota in Obesity. *World J. Gastroenterol.* **2021**, *27*, 3837–3850. [CrossRef]
9. Crovesy, L.; Masterson, D.; Rosado, E.L. Profile of the Gut Microbiota of Adults With Obesity: A Systematic Review. *Eur. J. Clin. Nutr.* **2020**, *74*, 1251–1262. [CrossRef]
10. Malesza, I.J.; Malesza, M.; Walkowiak, J.; Mussin, N.; Walkowiak, D.; Aringazina, R.; Bartkowiak-Wieczorek, J.; Mądry, E. High-Fat, Western-Style Diet, Systemic Inflammation, and Gut Microbiota: A Narrative Review. *Cells* **2021**, *10*, 3164. [CrossRef]
11. Al Bander, Z.; Nitert, M.D.; Mousa, A.; Naderpoor, N. The Gut Microbiota and Inflammation: An Overview. *Int. J. Environ. Res. Public Health* **2020**, *17*, 7618. [CrossRef] [PubMed]
12. Li, J.; Yang, G.; Zhang, Q.; Liu, Z.; Jiang, X.; Xin, Y. Function of *Akkermansia muciniphila* in Type 2 Diabetes and Related Diseases. *Front. Microbiol.* **2023**, *14*, 1172400. [CrossRef] [PubMed]
13. Karamzin, A.M.; Ropot, A.V.; Sergeyev, O.V.; Sechenov, E.O.K. *Akkermansia muciniphila* and Host Interaction Within the Intestinal Tract. *Anaerobe* **2021**, *72*, 102472. [CrossRef] [PubMed]
14. Aron, R.A.C.; Abid, A.; Vesa, C.M.; Nechifor, A.C.; Behl, T.; Ghitea, T.C.; Munteanu, M.A.; Fratila, O.; Andronie-Cioara, F.L.; Toma, M.M.; et al. Recognizing the Benefits of Pre-/Probiotics in Metabolic Syndrome and Type 2 Diabetes Mellitus Considering the Influence of *Akkermansia muciniphila* as a Key Gut Bacterium. *Microorganisms* **2021**, *9*, 618. [CrossRef] [PubMed]
15. Si, J.; Kang, H.; You, H.J.; Ko, G. Revisiting the Role of *Akkermansia muciniphila* as a Therapeutic Bacterium. *Gut Microbes* **2022**, *14*, 2078619. [CrossRef]
16. Sanna, S.; van Zuydam, N.R.; Mahajan, A.; Kurilshikov, A.; Vich Vila, A.; Võsa, U.; Mujagic, Z.; Masclee, A.A.M.; Jonkers, D.; Oosting, M.; et al. Causal Relationships Among the Gut Microbiome, Short-chain Fatty Acids and Metabolic Diseases. *Nat. Genet.* **2019**, *51*, 600–605. [CrossRef]
17. Ley, R.E.; Turnbaugh, P.J.; Klein, S.; Gordon, J.I. Microbial Ecology: Human Gut Microbes Associated With Obesity. *Nature* **2006**, *444*, 1022–1023. [CrossRef]
18. Page, M.J.; McKenzie, J.E.; Bossuyt, P.M.; Boutron, I.; Hoffmann, T.C.; Mulrow, C.D.; Shamseer, L.; Tetzlaff, J.M.; Akl, E.A.; Brennan, S.E.; et al. The PRISMA 2020 Statement: An Updated Guideline for Reporting Systematic Reviews. *BMJ* **2021**, *372*, n71. [CrossRef]
19. Cao, T.T.B.; Wu, K.C.; Hsu, J.L.; Chang, C.S.; Chou, C.; Lin, C.Y.; Liao, Y.M.; Lin, P.C.; Yang, L.Y.; Lin, H.W. Effects of Non-insulin Anti-hyperglycemic Agents on Gut Microbiota: A Systematic Review on Human and Animal Studies. *Front. Endocrinol.* **2020**, *11*, 573891. [CrossRef]
20. Mikolajewicz, N.; Komarova, S.V. Meta-Analytic Methodology for Basic Research: A Practical Guide. *Front. Physiol.* **2019**, *10*, 203. [CrossRef]
21. Higgins, J.P.; Thompson, S.G. Quantifying Heterogeneity in a Meta-analysis. *Stat. Med.* **2002**, *21*, 1539–1558. [CrossRef] [PubMed]
22. Begg, C.B.; Mazumdar, M. Operating Characteristics of a Rank Correlation Test for Publication Bias. *Biometrics* **1994**, *50*, 1088–1101. [CrossRef]
23. Egger, M.; Davey Smith, G.; Schneider, M.; Minder, C. Bias in Meta-analysis Detected by a Simple, Graphical Test. *BMJ* **1997**, *315*, 629–634. [CrossRef] [PubMed]
24. Viechtbauer, W.; López-López, J.A.; Sánchez-Meca, J.; Marín-Martínez, F. A Comparison of Procedures to Test for Moderators in Mixed-effects Meta-regression Models. *Psychol. Methods* **2015**, *20*, 360–374. [CrossRef]
25. McCann, S.K.; Lawrence, C.B. Comorbidity and Age in the Modelling of Stroke: Are We Still Failing to Consider the Characteristics of Stroke Patients? *BMJ Open Sci.* **2020**, *4*, e100013. [CrossRef]
26. Ottman, N.; Reunanen, J.; Meijerink, M.; Pietilä, T.E.; Kainulainen, V.; Klievink, J.; Huuskonen, L.; Aalvink, S.; Skurnik, M.; Boeren, S.; et al. Pili-like Proteins of *Akkermansia muciniphila* Modulate Host Immune Responses and Gut Barrier Function. *PLoS ONE* **2017**, *12*, e0173004. [CrossRef]
27. Meldrum, D.R.; Morris, M.A.; Gambone, J.C. Obesity Pandemic: Causes, Consequences, and Solutions-but Do we Have the Will? *Fertil. Steril.* **2017**, *107*, 833–839. [CrossRef]
28. DerSimonian, R.; Laird, N. Meta-analysis in Clinical Trials. *Control Clin. Trials* **1986**, *7*, 177–188. [CrossRef]
29. Liddle, L.J.; Ralhan, S.; Ward, D.L.; Colbourne, F. Translational Intracerebral Hemorrhage Research: Has Current Neuroprotection Research ARRIVEd at a Standard for Experimental Design and Reporting? *Transl. Stroke Res.* **2020**, *11*, 1203–1213. [CrossRef]
30. Acharya, K.D.; Friedline, R.H.; Ward, D.V.; Graham, M.E.; Tauer, L.; Zheng, D.; Hu, X.; de Vos, W.M.; McCormick, B.A.; Kim, J.K.; et al. Differential Effects of *Akkermansia*-enriched Fecal Microbiota Transplant on Energy Balance in Female Mice on High-fat Diet. *Front. Endocrinol.* **2022**, *13*, 1010806. [CrossRef]
31. Anhê, F.F.; Roy, D.; Pilon, G.; Dudonné, S.; Matamoros, S.; Varin, T.V.; Garofalo, C.; Moine, Q.; Desjardins, Y.; Levy, E.; et al. A Polyphenol-rich Cranberry Extract Protects From Diet-induced Obesity, Insulin Resistance and Intestinal Inflammation in Association With Increased *Akkermansia* spp. Population in the Gut Microbiota of Mice. *Gut* **2015**, *64*, 872–883. [CrossRef] [PubMed]

32. Chelakkot, C.; Choi, Y.; Kim, D.K.; Park, H.T.; Ghim, J.; Kwon, Y.; Jeon, J.; Kim, M.S.; Jee, Y.K.; Gho, Y.S.; et al. *Akkermansia muciniphila*-derived Extracellular Vesicles Influence Gut Permeability Through the Regulation of Tight Junctions. *Exp. Mol. Med.* **2018**, *50*, e450. [CrossRef] [PubMed]
33. Chung, E.; Elmassry, M.M.; Kottapalli, P.; Kottapalli, K.R.; Kaur, G.; Dufour, J.M.; Wright, K.; Ramalingam, L.; Moustaid-Moussa, N.; Wang, R.; et al. Metabolic Benefits of Annatto-extracted Tocotrienol on Glucose Homeostasis, Inflammation, and Gut Microbiome. *Nutr. Res.* **2020**, *77*, 97–107. [CrossRef]
34. Everard, A.; Belzer, C.; Geurts, L.; Ouwerkerk, J.P.; Druart, C.; Bindels, L.B.; Guiot, Y.; Derrien, M.; Muccioli, G.G.; Delzenne, N.M.; et al. Cross-talk Between *Akkermansia muciniphila* and Intestinal Epithelium Controls Diet-induced Obesity. *Proc. Natl. Acad. Sci. USA* **2013**, *110*, 9066–9071. [CrossRef] [PubMed]
35. Hänninen, A.; Toivonen, R.; Pöysti, S.; Belzer, C.; Plovier, H.; Ouwerkerk, J.P.; Emani, R.; Cani, P.D.; De Vos, W.M. *Akkermansia muciniphila* Induces Gut Microbiota Remodelling and Controls Islet Autoimmunity in NOD Mice. *Gut* **2018**, *67*, 1445–1453. [CrossRef] [PubMed]
36. Okamura, T.; Hamaguchi, M.; Nakajima, H.; Kitagawa, N.; Majima, S.; Senmaru, T.; Okada, H.; Ushigome, E.; Nakanishi, N.; Sasano, R.; et al. Milk Protects Against Sarcopenic Obesity Due to Increase in the Genus *Akkermansia* in Faeces of db/db Mice. *J. Cachexia Sarcopenia Muscle* **2023**, *14*, 1395–1409. [CrossRef]
37. Plovier, H.; Everard, A.; Druart, C.; Depommier, C.; Van Hul, M.; Geurts, L.; Chilloux, J.; Ottman, N.; Duparc, T.; Lichtenstein, L.; et al. A Purified Membrane Protein From *Akkermansia muciniphila* or the Pasteurized Bacterium Improves Metabolism in Obese and Diabetic Mice. *Nat. Med.* **2017**, *23*, 107–113. [CrossRef]
38. Shin, N.R.; Lee, J.C.; Lee, H.Y.; Kim, M.S.; Whon, T.W.; Lee, M.S.; Bae, J.W. An Increase in the *Akkermansia* spp. Population Induced by Metformin Treatment Improves Glucose Homeostasis in Diet-induced Obese Mice. *Gut* **2014**, *63*, 727–735. [CrossRef]
39. Song, H.Z.; Chu, Q.; Yan, F.J.; Yang, Y.Y.; Han, W.; Zheng, X.D. Red Pitaya Betacyanins Protects From Diet-induced Obesity, Liver Steatosis and Insulin Resistance in Association With Modulation of Gut Microbiota in Mice. *J. Gastroenterol. Hepatol.* **2016**, *31*, 1462–1469. [CrossRef]
40. Wang, Z.; Cui, S.; Zhang, T.; Wang, W.; Li, J.; Chen, Y.Q.; Zhu, S.L. *Akkermansia muciniphila* Supplementation Improves Glucose Tolerance in Intestinal Ffar4 Knockout Mice During the Daily Light to Dark Transition. *mSystems* **2023**, *8*, e00573-23. [CrossRef]
41. Wu, F.; Guo, X.; Zhang, M.; Ou, Z.; Wu, D.; Deng, L.; Lu, Z.; Zhang, J.; Deng, G.; Chen, S.; et al. An *Akkermansia muciniphila* Subtype Alleviates High-fat Diet-induced Metabolic Disorders and Inhibits the Neurodegenerative Process in Mice. *Anaerobe* **2020**, *61*, 102138. [CrossRef] [PubMed]
42. Zhai, R.; Xue, X.; Zhang, L.; Yang, X.; Zhao, L.; Zhang, C. Strain-specific Anti-inflammatory Properties of Two *Akkermansia muciniphila* Strains on Chronic Colitis in Mice. *Front. Cell. Infect. Microbiol.* **2019**, *9*, 239. [CrossRef] [PubMed]
43. Zhang, J.; Ni, Y.; Qian, L.; Fang, Q.; Zheng, T.; Zhang, M.; Gao, Q.; Zhang, Y.; Ni, J.; Hou, X.; et al. Decreased Abundance of *Akkermansia muciniphila* Leads to the Impairment of Insulin Secretion and Glucose Homeostasis in Lean Type 2 Diabetes. *Adv. Sci.* **2021**, *8*, e2100536. [CrossRef] [PubMed]
44. Zhang, L.; Qin, Q.Q.; Liu, M.N.; Zhang, X.L.; He, F.; Wang, G.Q. *Akkermansia muciniphila* can Reduce the Damage of Gluco/lipotoxicity, Oxidative Stress and Inflammation, and Normalize Intestine Microbiota in Streptozotocin-induced Diabetic Rats. *Pathog. Dis.* **2018**, *76*, fty028. [CrossRef]
45. Langan, D.; Higgins, J.P.; Gregory, W.; Sutton, A.J. Graphical Augmentations to the Funnel Plot Assess the Impact of Additional Evidence on a Meta-analysis. *J. Clin. Epidemiol.* **2012**, *65*, 511–519. [CrossRef]

nutrients

MDPI

Review

Probiotics: A Potential Strategy for Preventing and Managing Cardiovascular Disease

Anallely López-Yerena [1,†], Victoria de Santisteban Villaplana [1,2,†], Lina Badimon [1,3,4], Gemma Vilahur [1,3] and Teresa Padro [1,3,*]

1 Institut Recerca Sant Pau, Sant Quinti 77-79, 08041 Barcelona, Spain; naye.yerena@gmail.com (A.L.-Y.); vsantisteban@santpau.cat (V.d.S.V.); lina.badimon@gmail.com (L.B.); gvilahur@santpau.cat (G.V.)
2 School of Pharmacy and Food Sciences, University of Barcelona (UB), 08036 Barcelona, Spain
3 Centro de Investigación Biomédica en Red Cardiovascular (CIBER-CV), Instituto de Salud Carlos III, 28029 Madrid, Spain
4 Cardiovascular Research Foundation for Health Prevention and Innovation (FICSI), 08017 Barcelona, Spain
* Correspondence: tpadro@santpau.cat
† These authors contributed equally to this work.

Abstract: Probiotics are gaining recognition as a viable strategy for mitigating cardiovascular risk factors. Specifically, recent studies highlight their potential benefits in managing cholesterol levels, blood pressure, and inflammation, which are critical components in the prevention of cardiovascular diseases (CVD). This comprehensive review aims to elucidate the impact of probiotic consumption on major cardiovascular risk factors, including individuals with hypertension, type II diabetes mellitus, metabolic syndrome, hypercholesterolemia, and in secondary prevention in coronary artery disease. Scientific evidence based on human studies suggests that probiotic consumption is associated with positive effects on anthropometric measures, inflammation markers, blood pressure, glucose metabolism markers, lipid profiles, and endothelial function. However, these findings should be interpreted pragmatically and acknowledge the significant variability in results. This variability may be attributed to factors such as probiotic composition (single strain or multiple strains), the characteristics of the delivery matrix (food, capsules, and sachets), the duration of the intervention, the dosage regimen, and baseline health profiles of the participants. Incorporating probiotics as part of a comprehensive and healthy lifestyle approach can be considered a feasible strategy for both the prevention and management of CVD. However, further research is needed on factors influencing the effect of probiotics, such as: (i) optimal probiotic strain(s), (ii) appropriate dosage, (iii) duration of treatment, (iv) optimal delivery vehicle, and (v) sex-specific differences.

Keywords: inflammation; lipid profile; functional foods; blood pressure

1. Introduction

Since its appearance in 1908 by Metchnikoff [1], the term probiotic has been associated with host health benefits. In 2001, The World Health Organization (WHO) and the Food and Agriculture Organization of the United Nations (FAO) considered probiotics as live microorganisms, which when administered in adequate amounts confer a health benefit on the host [2]. In 2014, a consensus panel of the International Scientific Association for Probiotics and Prebiotics (ISAPP) reaffirmed the definition with one minor change: replacing "which" with "that", resulting in "live microorganisms that, when administered in appropriate amounts, confer a health benefit on the host" [3].

To date, numerous studies highlight the fact that, in addition to the antipathogenic, anticancer, antiallergic, and angiogenic activity [4], the probiotic health implications include protection against cardiovascular diseases (CVDs) [5]. Despite milestones in preventive measures and treatment, CVD remains associated with a high burden of morbidity and mortality. There are several established risk factors for CVD that include hypertension, dyslipidemia, diabetes, obesity, smoking, alcohol, diet, and sedentary lifestyle [6]. The gut microbiome has been causally linked with cardiometabolic and cardiovascular disorders and is a potential complementary target to understand and reduce the residual risk of CVD [7]. In fact, the comprehensive characterization of probiotic benefits on cardiovascular risk factors has demonstrated the glycemic control in patients with type two diabetes mellitus (T2DM) [8], improvement in inflammatory markers in coronary artery disease (CAD) patients [9] and in obesity-related markers in obese people [9], among others. In fact, probiotic consumption in healthy populations has recently been shown to be associated with increased protection against atherosclerotic disease [10]. As diet-related risk is the most important behavioral factor influencing global health, it appears to be the best target in the challenge against CVD [11].

The gut microbiota has the capability to generate metabolic products from dietary sources that have the potential to exert an influence on the cardiovascular health of the host [12]. Simultaneously, the consumption of probiotics is accompanied by significant alterations in the composition of the intestinal microbiota [13–17]. Furthermore, in tandem with all of the aforementioned factors, emerging risk factors, such as pro-inflammatory molecules (e.g., C-reactive protein (CRP), interleukins (IL)), adhesion molecules, apolipoproteins, glucose metabolism markers (C-peptide, insulin, hemoglobin A1c (HbA1c)), and cholesterol fractions, have been analyzed and linked to an increased cardiovascular risk, prognosis, and complications of CVD [18] and therefore have also been targeted in clinical interventions trying to ensure the effect of probiotic consumption on these markers.

Although the effect of probiotics on CVD has been summarized in numerous papers, most of these have focused on a target population such as T2DM [19], CVD risk patients [20], or in specific markers [21]. Additionally, existing reviews often evaluate not only the effects of probiotics but also include prebiotics and symbiotics, resulting in a broader and less focused analysis [22,23]. In this comprehensive review, we examine the impact of probiotic consumption on vulnerable populations, including individuals with hypertension, T2DM, metabolic syndrome (MetS), hypercholesterolemia, and in secondary prevention in CAD. For this purpose, only studies conducted in humans since 2015 to date and in the English language were included. Scopus, Pubmed, and Google Scholar were used to search for clinical trials testing the effect of probiotics in individuals with hypertension, T2DM, MetS, hypercholesterolemia, and CAD. The search initially identified a total of 186 studies. However, after applying the inclusion criteria—human studies, English language, and probiotics administered alone (not co-administered)—only 44 articles met the criteria and were included in this review.

2. Probiotics

Probiotics are essential functional foods that play a crucial role in maintaining and improving overall health and well-being. Oral probiotics face several challenges on their journey through the mouth, stomach, intestine, and colon. In specific, many microbial species are adversely affected by harsh gastrointestinal conditions characterized by low pH in the stomach and the presence of bile salts in the small intestine [24,25]. Therefore, one of the most important requirements for probiotics is to survive the environmental conditions in the location where they must be active. Successful colonization of the gastrointestinal tract is key to ensuring that probiotics can interact with the host to achieve the desired health benefits [26]. To date, numerous studies have highlighted all those factors that benefit or limit the effect of probiotics. Food matrix [27,28], probiotic design [29], and doses [30], among others, have a recognized effect (Figure 1).

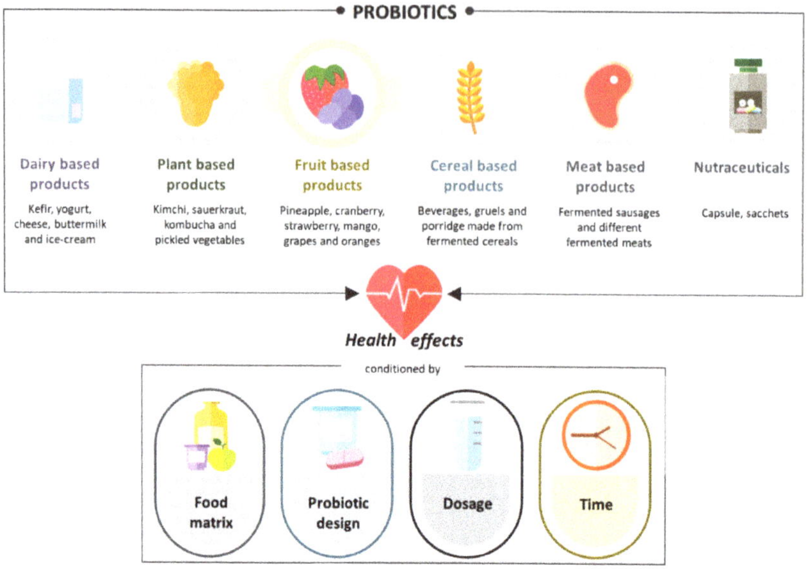

Figure 1. Main probiotic forms.

Probiotic design (monostrain, multistrain, and multispecies probiotics) is raised as an important consideration that can affect the functionality and efficacy of a probiotic [29]. Studies using animal models have shown that multistrain probiotics are more efficient in obesity management [31]. However, to date, very little is known about which preparation has the greatest effect on preventing CVD.

A systematic review and meta-analysis of clinical trials evidenced that the effectiveness of the probiotic is conditioned by the dosage [32]. Regulatory agencies around the world recommend minimum dosages. For example, Health Canada has accepted bacterial species when delivered in food at a level of 1×10^9 colony-forming unit (CFU) per serving, and the Italian Ministry of Health confirmed the use of the word probiotic for food and food supplements under certain conditions, including a minimum number of viable cells (1×10^9 CFU) administered per day [33,34]. However, recent reports have indicated that the dose required for most strains to survive and persist is higher (1×10^{10} CFU) (1×10^{10} CFU) than the doses recommended for probiotics by regulatory agencies [35]. Similarly, in obese postmenopausal women, multispecies probiotic supplementation favorably affects vascular function and reduces arterial stiffness when given at the dose of 1×10^{10} CFU per day [36].

The effect of the probiotics is also conditioned by the time of the intervention [37]. Regarding patients with risk factors for CVD, there is no trend as to whether short- or long-term interventions are more advisable [38].

Foods

Foods are vehicles for delivery of probiotics to the human body and help to buffer the probiotics through the gastrointestinal tract, regulate their colonization, and contain other functional ingredients, such as bioactive components, that can interact with probiotics to alter their functionality and efficacy [28]. In foods, probiotics may be present in fermented dairy products (e.g., yogurt, cheese, and fermented milk), which represent the main vehicle for probiotic delivery (Figure 1). Additionally, many other nondairy probiotic products (both fermented and nonfermented) are gaining popularity among consumers. Currently, a wide range of nondairy probiotic foods on the market, such as soy products, cereal-based products, fruit and vegetable juices, and fermented meat and fish products, are also offered [39,40]. To date, cheese, yogurt, milk (soy, probiotic, or fermented), kefir, and light Yakult are by far the main food vehicles used for the delivery of probiotics.

However, it is important to note that the delivery of probiotics to the host can also be accomplished through other alternatives. In specific, capsules are also a growing trend to use probiotics as nutraceuticals [41]. However, it is important to emphasize that this changing trend in probiotic delivery may result in reduced functional efficacy by eliminating the potential synergistic effect of the food. Probiotics in sachets or capsules are commonly used in studies evaluating their effect in patients at risk of CVD.

3. The Health-Promoting Properties of Probiotics in the Management and Prevention of CVD

There are several established risk factors for CVD that include hypertension, hypercholesterolemia, T2DM, overweight and obesity, smoking, and a sedentary lifestyle [42,43]. Among these risk factors, high blood pressure is associated with the strongest evidence of causality and has a high prevalence of exposure [44]. In recent decades, a growing number of emerging risk factors, such as proinflammatory molecules including CRP, interleukins (IL), adhesion molecules, apolipoproteins, and cholesterol fractions, among others, have been analyzed and associated with increased cardiovascular risk, CVD prognosis, and complications [18].

The relationship between diet and CVD has been the focus of attention for some time. From this perspective, there is growing evidence that functional dietary intervention with probiotics, which maintains or restores the beneficial bacteria of the digestive tract, is a promising therapeutic strategy for intervention in CVD and also reduces the risk of its occurrence [45]. Recently, it was demonstrated that the intervention with *L. plantarum* strains induces beneficial effects on bile acid signature and lipoprotein profile. It reduces ApoB and small LDL levels and LDL susceptibility to oxidation and increases HDL antioxidant capacity in healthy individuals [10].

The following sections summarize the evidence for the effect of probiotic consumption on risk factors for CVD. Figure 2 highlights the key metabolites that act as potential messengers in the molecular and functional processes mediating these beneficial effects. These include short-chain fatty acids (SCFAs) such as acetic, propionic, and butyric acids; bacteriocins with antimicrobial properties; vitamins and essential nutrients (e.g., vitamin K, B vitamins, and aromatic amino acids); organic acids; and cell wall components with immunomodulatory effects [46]. SCFAs play vital roles in regulating the immune system, maintaining gut barrier integrity, improving endothelial function, and modulating cholesterol and glucose metabolism [47]. Although bile acids (BAs) are not directly microbiota-derived, the gut microbiota significantly influences their transformation, playing a key role in cholesterol catabolism [48].

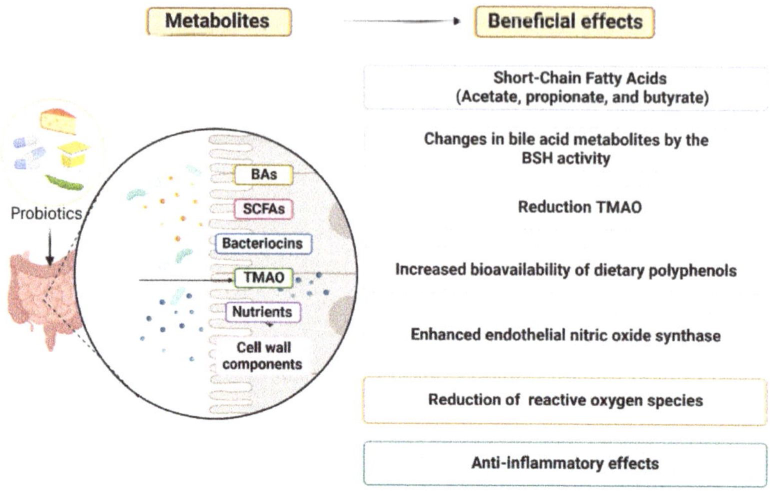

Figure 2. Key metabolites that act as potential messengers in the molecular and functional processes that mediate the health-promoting effects of probiotics.

3.1. *Hypertension*

Hypertension is a leading risk factor for mortality worldwide, accounting for 10.8 million deaths in 2019. Hypertension or high blood pressure, defined as systolic blood pressure (SBP) above 140 mmHg and diastolic blood pressure (DBP) above 90 mmHg in young people, is one of the most important risk factors that predispose an individual to many diseases, including coronary heart disease, cerebral hemorrhage, renal and cardiac failure [49]. Blood pressure is controlled by several complex biochemical pathways. The renin-angiotensin system (RAS) is identified as one of the major controllers of blood pressure and sodium metabolism. In addition, the kinin-nitric oxide, the neutral endopeptidase, and the endothelin-converting enzyme systems have been shown to produce additional vasoregulatory peptides [50].

Probiotics and their fermented products reduce blood pressure by suppressing nitrogen oxide production in the microphages, reducing reactive oxygen species, and improving the absorption of calcium from the diet [51]. More specifically, probiotics enhance endothelial nitric oxide synthase (eNOS) activity, increasing NO bioavailability and promoting vasodilation, which reduces vascular resistance and blood pressure [52,53]. Probiotics also lower oxidative stress and inflammation, protecting NO from degradation and preventing endothelial dysfunction [54]. Additionally, they improve L-arginine availability [55], a key substrate for NO synthesis. Through these mechanisms, probiotics help regulate vascular tone, reduce arterial stiffness, and maintain healthy blood pressure levels, highlighting their therapeutic potential in hypertension management.

A cross-sectional study demonstrated that the exposure to probiotics resulted in a 21% reduction in the odds of hypertension that was evidenced by a significant reduction in SBP and DBP [56]. The rest of the evidence is based on systematic review and meta-analysis focused on human studies [37,57–60]. Despite the enormous concern about the CVD problems associated with hypertension, only five human interventional studies testing the probiotic effects [60–64]. The characteristics of these clinical studies, as well as their main findings, are summarized in Table 1. Of these five studies analyzed, the beneficial effect of probiotic intake on SBP and DBP was evidenced in only two studies of four [61] and eight weeks [60] after regular consumption of cheese with *L. casei* 01 or multistrain capsule.

On the other hand, both SBP and DBP remained unchanged in six- [64], eight- [62], and twelve- [63] week studies.

Table 1. Effect of probiotics supplementation on inflammation markers in patients with hypertension.

Probiotic Strain (Product)	Dose (Intervention Time)	Study Characteristics (*n*)	Parameters Changing	Unchanging Parameters	Ref.
L. casei 01 (Cheese)	Non-specified (4 weeks)	Randomized double-blind pilot trial: Probiotic cheese (15) and conventional cheese (15)	↓ SBP and DBP ↓ TC and TG ↑ HDLc	LDLc	[61]
(1) *L. paracasei* LPC-37 (2) *L. rhamnosus* N001 (3) *L. acidophilus NCFM* (4) *B.lactis* HN019 (Sachet)	(1) 10^9 CFU/day (2) 10^9 CFU/day (3) 10^9 CFU/day (4) 10^9 CFU/day (8 weeks)	Randomized, triple-blind, placebo-controlled trial: Probiotic (19) and placebo (17)	↓ FBG ↓ TC ↑ HDLc	SBP, DBP, TG, VLDLc, LDLc, and hs-CRP,	[62]
L. plantarum DSM 5313 (Sachet)	1×10^9 CFU/day (3 months)	Double-blind, placebo-RCT: Probiotic (44) and placebo (46)		SBP and DBP	[63]
(1) *L.acidophilus* LA-5 (2) B. *Bifidobacterium* B-12 (3) *S.thermophilus* STY-31 (4) *L. bulgaricus* LBY-27 (Capsules)	>4×10^9 CFU/day (8 weeks)	Double-blind, placebo-RCT: Probiotic (32) and placebo (32)	↓ SBP ↓ DBP		[60]
(1) L. *acidophilus* LA-5 (2) B. *lactis* BB-12 (Yogurt and/or capsules)	3×10^9 CFU/day or 6×10^9 CFU/day (6 weeks)	Double-blinded, factorial, parallel study: Yogurt + ProC (40), Yogurt + PlaC (37), CM + ProC (39) and CM + PlaC (40)		SBP, DBP, TC, TG, HDLc and LDLc	[64]

CM: control milk; DBP: diastolic blood pressure; FBG: fasting blood glucose; HDLc: high-density lipoprotein cholesterol; PlaC: placebo capsules; ProC: probiotic capsules; RCT: randomized clinical trial; SBP: systolic blood pressure; TC: total cholesterol; TG: triglycerides; VLDLc: very low-density lipoprotein cholesterol. Downward arrows indicate decreased values. Upward arrows indicate increased values.

3.2. Type 2 Diabetes Mellitus (T2DM)

T2DM is a chronic, non-communicable, multisystem disease that has reached epidemic proportions [65]. T2DM is characterized by dysfunction in pancreatic β-cells, chronic low-grade inflammation, oxidative stress, insulin resistance, and dysregulation of lipid and glucose metabolism [66]. Oxidative stress significantly impacts β-cell health and function in T2DM through mechanisms involving ROS production, antioxidant deficiency, and interactions with metabolic dysregulations, such as insulin resistance and lipotoxicity [67,68]. Addressing these pathways may offer new avenues for diabetes treatment aimed at preserving β-cell function and improving glycemic control.

Multiple molecular mechanisms of gut microbiota contribution to T2DM have recently been summarized, including: (i) modulation of inflammation, (ii) interaction with dietary components, (iii) involvement of intestinal permeability, and (iv) involvement of glucose and lipid metabolism, insulin sensitivity, and overall energy homeostasis in the mammalian host [69,70]. In view of the high incidence of T2DM and its serious consequences, from 2015 to date, a series of human trials have been conducted to evaluate the efficacy of probiotic consumption in patients with this pathology. Specifically, these studies have focused on assessing the effect of probiotic soya milk [71–73], fermented milk [74], or through sachets [75–78] or capsules [38,79–82] on several biomarkers, as is shown in Table 2.

As for anthropometric measures, 50% of the 14 studies included in this review assessed these parameters (Table 2). In a study testing soy milk fortified with *L. plantarum* A7, eight weeks of sustained intake led to a decrease in weight, BMI, and waist–hip ratio [73]. In another study, eight weeks of multiprobiotic "Symbiter" (concentrated biomass of 14 probiotic bacteria genera *Bifidobacterium*, *Lactobacillus*, *Lactococcus*, *Propionibacterium*) administered as a sachet formulation led to a decrease in weight, BMI, and waist circumference [77]. In addition, another study showed that the dose (low vs. high) affects the anthropometric measurements differently, in particular, an increase in weight and BMI was observed in the low group [76]. The remaining studies found no evidence that probiotic consumption induced changes in anthropometric measures in T2DM populations.

Table 2. Effect of probiotics supplementation on metabolic endotoxemia and inflammation markers in patients with T2DM.

Probiotic Strain (Product)	Dose (Intervention Time)	Study Characteristics (*n*)	Parameters Changing	Unchanging Parameters	Ref.
L. plantarum A7 (Soy milk)	4×10^9 CFU/day (8 weeks)	Parallel, RCT: Probiotic (24), Control (24)		MDA	[71]
		Parallel, RCT: Probiotic (20) and control (20)	↓ LDLc ↑ HDLc	FBG, TNF−α, hs−CRP, adiponectin and TG	[72]
		Parallel, RCT: Probiotic (24) and control (24)	↓ Weight ↓ WHR ↓ BMI		[73]
(1) *B. bifidum* W23 (2) *B. lactis* W52 (3) *L. acidophilus* W37 (4) *L. brevis* W63 (5) *L. casei* W56 (6) *L. salivarius* W24 (7) *L. lactis* W19 (8) *L. lactis* W58 (Sachets)	10^{10} CFU/day (12 weeks)	Single-center, double-blind, placebo-RCT: Probiotic (48) and placebo (46)	↓ FBG, insulin, ↓ C−peptide ↓ HOMA−IR ↓ SBP, DBP ↓ TG, TC, LDLc	Weight, BMI, WHR, HDLc and TC/HDLc	[75]
L. casei (Fermented milk)	4×10^{10} CFU/day (16 weeks)	RCT: Probiotic (34) and control (34)	↑ HbA1c ↑ hs−CRP	BMI, FBG, C−peptide, TNF−α, IL−6, adiponectin, TC, TG and HDLc	[74]
L. reuteri DSM 17938 (Tablets)	10^8 CFU/day or 10^{10} CFU/day (12 weeks)	Double-blind, placebo-RCT: Placebo (>12), low (>12) and high (>12)	↑ Weight (low group) ↑ BMI (low group)	WC, FBG, insulin, HbA1c, hs−CRP, adiponectin, leptin, SBP, DPB, TC, TG, HDLc, LDLc	[76]
L. reuteri (Capsules)	ADR-1: 4×10^9 CFU/day ADR-3: 2×10^{10} cells/day (6 months)	Double-blind, placebo-RCT: ADR-1 (22), ADR-3 (24) and placebo (24)	↓ HbA1c ↓ TC ↓ SBP	FBG, insulin, HOMA−IR, C−peptide, hs−CRP, IL−6, IL−10, IL−17, TNF−α, IL−1β, LDLc, HDLc, TG, DBP	[38]
Concentrated of 14 probiotic bacteria genera (1) *Bifidobacterium* (2) *Lactobacillus* (3) *Lactococcus* (4) *Propionibacterium* (5) *Acetobacter* (Sachets)	(1) 10^{11} CFU/day (2) (3) 6×10^{11} CFU/day (4) 3×10^{11} CFU/day (5) 10^7 CFU/day (8 weeks)	Single-center double blind, placebo, parallel, RCT: Probiotic (31) and placebo (22)	↓ Weight, WC, BMI ↓ HOMA−IR ↓ TNF−α ↓ IL−6, IL−8, IL−17, IL−1β	FBG, insulin, HbA1c	[77]
(1) *B. bifidum* W23 (2) *B. lactis* W52 (3) *L. acidophilus* W37 (4) *L. brevis* W63 (5) *L. casei* W56 (6) *L. salivarius* W24 (7) *L.lactis* W19 (8) *L. lactis* W58 (Sachets)	10^{10} CFU (6 months)	Double-blind, placebo-RCT: Probiotic (31) and placebo (30)	↓ FBG ↓ Insulin ↓ HOMA−IR ↓ hs−CRP, ↓ TNF−α, IL−6 ↑ Adiponectin ↓ TG and TC	BMI, WHR, C-peptide, SBP, DBP	[78]
(1) *L.acidophilus* (2) *L.casei* (3) *L. rhamnosus* (4) *L. bulgaricus* (5) *B. breve* (6) *B. longum* (7) *S. thermophilus* (Capsules)	(1) 4×10^9 CFU/day (2) 14×10^9 CFU/day (3) 3×10^9 CFU/day (4) 4×10^8 CFU/day (5) 6×10^{10} CFU/day (6) 14×10^9 CFU/day (7) 3×10^9 CFU/day (6 weeks)	Double-blind, placebo-RCT: Probiotic (30) and placebo (30)	↓ FBG ↑ HDLc	Weight, WC, BMI, insulin, HOMA−IR, TC, TG and LDLc	[79]
L. casei (Capsules)	1×10^8 CFU/day (6 weeks)	Parallel, RCT: Probiotic (20) and placebo (20)	↓ FBG ↓ Insulin ↓ HOMA−IR ↓ TC	HbA1c	[80]
(1) *L. salivarius* BLS22 (2) *L. casei* UBLC42 (3) *L. plantarum* BLP40 (4) *L. acidophilus* UBLA34 (5) *B. breve* UBBr01 (6) *B. coagulans* Unique IS2 (Capsules)	6×10^{10} CFU/day (12 weeks)	Parallel, RCT: Probiotic (40) and placebo (40)	↓ FBG ↓ HbAIc	Weight, insulin, HOMA−IR, TC, TG, LDLc and HDLc	[81]

Table 2. *Cont.*

Probiotic Strain (Product)	Dose (Intervention Time)	Study Characteristics (*n*)	Parameters Changing	Unchanging Parameters	Ref.
(1) *L.acidophilus* (2) *L.plantarum* (3) *L.fermentum* (4) *L.Gasseri* (Capsules)	(1) 5×10^{10} CFU/day (2) 1.5×10^{10} CFU/day (3) 7×10^{9} CFU/day (4) 2×10^{10} CFU/day (8 weeks)	Double-blind, placebo-RCT: Probiotic (34) and placebo (34)	↓ SBP ↓ DBP	TC/HDLc and LDLc/HDLc	[82]

BMI: body mass index; DBP: diastolic blood pressure; FBG: fasting blood glucose; HDLc: high-density lipoprotein cholesterol; HbA1c: glycated hemoglobin; hs-CRP: high-sensitivity C-reactive protein; HOMA-IR: homeostatic model assessment of insulin resistance; IL: interleukin; LDLc: low-density lipoprotein cholesterol; MDA: malondialdehyde; TC: total cholesterol; TG: triglycerides; SBP: systolic blood pressure; TNF−α: tumor necrosis factor−α; WC: waist circumference; WHR: waist-hip ratio. Downward arrows indicate decreased values. Upward arrows indicate increased values.

Regarding changes in the glycemic profile, the following findings were reported. Importantly, a decrease in FBG levels was observed when the probiotic was administered in capsule or sachet forms [75,78–81]. A similar behavior was observed for HOMA-IR, where a decrease was observed when the probiotic was administered mainly in the sachets, regardless of the duration of the study (Table 2). These findings may be directly related to the fact that probiotics administered in capsule or sachet form are usually multistrain compared to foods that are mostly monostrain. Both monostrain and multistrain probiotics have their unique advantages and limitations. However, in the glycemic control of patients with T2DM, evidence would suggest that the multistrain probiotics provide a broader range of benefits through synergistic effects. The level of HbA1c in T2DM patients can accurately reflect the patient's glycemic control [83]. However, there is no pattern of response to probiotic use, with one study showing an increase, three showing a decrease, and three showing no change (Table 2). Another key feature of T2DM is circulating insulin, but in most of the studies evaluating this biomarker, no changes in its concentration were observed. The same trend was observed for C-peptide.

The pathophysiology of T2DM reveals that oxidative stress is one of the factors that play a role in the pathogenesis of insulin resistance, impaired insulin secretion and glucose utilization, and impaired hepatic glucose metabolism, together with the activation of pro-inflammatory cytokines, culminating in T2DM [84]. It is well known that oxidative stress in pancreatic β-cells is induced by high glucose, hyperlipidemia, and inflammatory responses [85]. An established state of oxidative stress leads to increased production of proinflammatory cytokines, such as tumor necrosis factor (TNF) [86]. Given the above, probiotic therapies have been proposed as an alternative therapeutic strategy in the treatment and management of diabetes, specifically for key mediators of insulin resistance, such as TNF−α. Interestingly, a decrease in this proinflammatory marker was observed in two studies [77,78], whereas no changes were observed in three other studies [38,72,74]. It is noteworthy that in those studies where a change was observed, multistrain probiotics were used [77,78], which may suggest that they are more effective compared to mono-strain probiotics.

On the other hand, there is no clear trend between the intake of probiotics and the concentration of hs−CRP and interleukins. hs−CRP remained unchanged after eight weeks [72], twelve weeks [76], and six months [38] of monostrain probiotic intake. However, an increase in this biomarker was observed after four months of monostrain probiotic intake [74] and a reduction with a multistrain probiotic during six months [78]. Similar behavior was observed with interleukins, with multistrain probiotics being more effective.

Regarding the adipocytokines, adiponectin is the most abundant and is known to have a regulatory effect on glucose and lipid metabolism [87]. As shown in Table 2, in most studies there is no association between probiotic consumption and this biomarker. On the other hand, only one study using a multistrain probiotic and lasting six months showed an increase in adiponectin levels [78]. Although leptin, an adipokine whose primary function is to regulate energy balance, has been found to mediate insulin secretion and sensitivity in peripheral tissues [88], only one study evaluated this biomarker and found no change after probiotic supplementation [76].

Patients with T2DM often have comorbidities, including dyslipidemia and hypertension. Diabetes-related changes in plasma lipid levels are among the key factors that are amenable to intervention [89]. Based on the included articles, the lipid profile of patients with T2DM is modestly changed by probiotic supplementation. The most modifiable parameter was total cholesterol, which was reduced in four of the interventional studies. On the other hand, triglycerides and lipoprotein cholesterol (HDLc and LDLc) seemed to be more resistant to change with probiotic supplementation in T2DM patients. TG reduction was only observed in studies using multistrain probiotics [75,78]. On the other hand, no relationship was observed for HDLc and LDLc. Monostrain soy milk lowers LDL and raises HDL [72], and multistrain capsules raise HDL [79].

3.3. Metabolic Syndrome

MetS is a cluster of interrelated risk factors that increase the likelihood of developing CVDs, T2DM, and other health complications [90]. A recent study revealed that MetS and its related cardiometabolic components are highly prevalent worldwide [91]. According to ATP III classification, diagnosis of MetS is established if three out of the following five parameters are pathologically altered: waist circumference (>102 cm for men and >88 cm for women), blood pressure (>135/85 mm/Hg), fasting blood glucose (>6.1 mmol/L), triglyceride (>1.7 mmol/L), and HDLc (<1.03 mmol/L for men and <1.29 mmol/L for women) [92].

Lifestyle modifications, particularly dietary habits, are the main strategy for the prevention and management of MetS [93]. Changes in dietary habits can ameliorate obesity and insulin resistance, which play a key role in these pathological conditions [94]. While probiotics show potential, their effects on MetS markers remain insufficiently understood, limiting their application in the prevention and treatment of MetS in clinical practice [95]. From 2015 to date, the effect of probiotic yogurt [96,97], kefir [96–100], Yakult [101], milk [102,103], and capsules and/or sachets containing strains [16,104] has been studied in MetS patients (Table 3).

Table 3. Effect of probiotics supplementation on metabolic endotoxemia and inflammation markers in patients with metabolic syndrome.

Probiotic Strain (Product)	Dose (Intervention Time)	Study Characteristics (*n*)	Parameters Changing	Unchanging Parameters	Ref.
(1) *L. lactis* ssp. *lactis* (2) *L. lactis* ssp. *cremoris* (3) *L. lactis* ssp. *diacetylactis*, (4) *L. mesenteroides* ssp. *cremoris* (5) *L. kefir* (6) *K.marxianus* (7) *S. unisporus* (Kefir)	180 mL of kefir/day (CFU non-specified) (12 weeks)	Parallel-group, RCT: Kefir (12) and control (10)	↓ Insulin ↓ HOMA–IR ↓ TNF–α ↓ SBP and DBP	BMI, WC, TC, HDLc, LDLc, TG, homocysteine, hs–CRP, IL–6, IL–10, glucose	[99]
Non-specified (Kefir)	Men: 1.6 mL of kefir/kg body weight/day Women: 1.9 mL of kefir/kg body weight/day (CFU non-specified) (12 weeks)	Double-blind placebo-RCT: Kefir (24) and control (24)	↓ SBP and DBP ↓ FBG ↓ LDLc ↓ Non-HDLc, ↓ TG ↓ oxLDL ↑ HDLc (Women)	TC, HDLc (men) and hs-CRP	[98]

Table 3. *Cont.*

Probiotic Strain (Product)	Dose (Intervention Time)	Study Characteristics (*n*)	Parameters Changing	Unchanging Parameters	Ref.
(1) *L. bulgaricus* (2) *S. thermophilus* (3) *B. lactis* Bb12 (4) *L. acidophilus* La5 (Yakult)	First Day of Production: (3) 1.5 × 10^9 CFU/day (4)1.9 × 10^9 CFU/day (2 months)	Double-blind placebo-RCT: Yogurt (22) and control (22)	↓ FBG, CAM-1 ↑ Insulin ↑ HOMA–IR	HOMA-β and ICAM-1	[96]
L. casei Shirota (Milk)	1.95 × 10^{10} CFU/day (12 weeks)	Single-center, prospective, RCT: Probiotic (13) and Control (15)		SBP, DBP, TC, TG, HDLc, LDLc, VLDLc, hs-CRP, sVCAM-1, sICAM-1 and TMAO	[101]
B. lactis HN019 (Milk)	2.72 × 10^{10} CFU/day (45 days)	Randomized Trial: Probiotic (26) and control (25)	↓ BMI ↓ TC and LDLc ↓ TNF–α and IL–6	WC, SBP, DBP, TG, HDLc, glucose, insulin and HOMA–IR	[102]
	2.72 × 10^{10} CFU/day (90 days)	Double-blind placebo-RCT: NoMetS (14) and MetS (19)	↓ IL–6 ↓ Homocysteine ↑ Adiponectin ↑ NO	WC, SBP, DBP, hs-CRP and leptin	[103]
(1) *L. bulgaricus* (2) *S. thermophilus* (3) *B. lactis* Bb12 (4) *L. acidophilus* La5 (Yogurt)	First Day of Production: (3) 1.5×10^9 CFU/day (4) 1.9×10^9 CFU/day (8 weeks)	Double-blind placebo-RCT: Probiotic (22) and control (22)	↓ Uric acid	MDA and oxLDL	[97]
L. reuteri V3401 (Capsule)	5 × 10^9 CFU/day (12 weeks)	Randomized, crossover, placebo-controlled, single-center trial: Group 1 (28) and group 2 (25)		BMI, SBP, DBP, glucose, insulin, HOMA–IR, TC, TG, LDLc, HDLc, hs-CRP, IL–6, IL-8, TNF–α, adiponectin, leptin and sVCAM-1	[16]
(1) *L. helveticus R0052* (2) *B. longum R0175* (Sachets)	1 × 10^{10} CFU/day (8 weeks)	Double-blind, placebo-RCT: Probiotic (27) and placebo (22)		TNF–α, IL–1β, IL–6 and IL–10	[104]
(1) *L. lactis* subsp. *lactis* (2) *L. lactis* subsp. *cremoris* (3) *Ls. lactis* subsp. *diacetylactis* (4) *L. mesenteroides* subsp. *cremoris* (5) *L. kefyr* (6) *K. marxianus* (7) *S.unisporus* (Kefir)	(1), (2), (3), (4), (5) Minimum 10^6 UFC/g/day (6), (7) Minimum 10^5 UFC/g/day (12 weeks)	Randomized controlled clinical trial: Kefir (31) and milk (31)	↓ Homocysteine ↓ TNF–α ↓ IL–6 ↓ IL-10	BMI, WC. SBP, DBP, glucose, insulin, HOMA–IR, TC, TG, HDLc, LDLc, ApoA1, ApoB, Lp(a), hs-CRP	[100]
Bifidobacterium adolescentis CCFM8630 and *Lactobacillus reuteri* CCFM8631	1 × 10^{10} CFU (11 weks)	Randomized, placebo-controlled clinical trial: Probiotic (21) and placebo (19)	↓ FBG ↓ Insuline ↓ TG ↓ LDLc	**TC**	[105]

BMI: body mass index; DBP: diastolic blood pressure; FBG: fasting blood glucose; HDLc: high-density lipoprotein cholesterol; HbA1c: glycated hemoglobin; hs-CRP: high-sensitivity C-reactive protein; HOMA-IR: homeostatic model assessment of insulin resistance; ICAM, intercellular adhesion molecule cell; IL: interleukin; LDLc: low-density lipoprotein cholesterol; MDA: malondialdehyde; TC: total cholesterol; TG: triglycerides; sICAM-1: soluble intercellular adhesion molecule 1; SBP: systolic blood pressure; sVCAM-1: soluble vascular cell adhesion molecule 1; TNF−α: tumor necrosis factor−α; VCAM: vascular cell adhesion molecule cell; WC: waist circumference; WHR: waist-hip ratio. Downward arrows indicate decreased values. Upward arrows indicate increased values.

Based on the findings of the articles included in this review, probiotic consumption leads to only modest changes in the anthropometric characteristics of patients. Only one study found a significant decrease in BMI [102], and no changes in waist circumference were observed. Strain-specific responses could explain these minor changes because different probiotic strains may have variable effects on gut metabolism and microbiota, which could lead to heterogeneous results.

Regarding blood pressure, 50% of the studies found no significant changes following probiotic consumption [16,100–103]. Meanwhile, other studies observed a reduction in both SBP and DBP after three months of daily kefir intake [98,99].

With regard to glucose, three studies showed a clear decrease in its concentration after kefir [98], yogurt [96], and probiotic powder [105] intake (Table 3), while four studies did not show any relationship between glucose levels and probiotic intake [16,99,100,102]. On the other hand, probiotic intake was specifically associated with varying effects on insulin levels and insulin resistance, including reductions [99,105], increases [96], and no significant changes [16,100,102].

Furthermore, even though uric acid is known to correlate with MetS [106], this biomarker has only been measured in one study and was found to decrease after 2 months of daily yogurt intake [97].

Homocysteine has been recognized as a potential marker for atherosclerosis progression [107]. However, very few studies evaluate this marker after sustained probiotic intake. To our knowledge, only three studies followed up on this biomarker, and two of them showed a reduction in its levels [100,103].

Concerning the relationship between probiotic consumption and lipid profile (see Table 3), the circulating levels of both total cholesterol and triglycerides remain unchanged in most of the studies. A decrease in total cholesterol [102] and triglycerides [105] was observed. As for lipoprotein-cholesterol, a positive relationship between probiotic consumption and a reduction in LDLc was observed in three studies using kefir [98], probiotic yogurt [102], and probiotic powder [105], though in other studies the levels remained significantly unchanged [16,99–101]. However, HDLc levels appear to be less responsive to probiotic consumption in patients with MetS [16,98–102].

It is important to note that in the 12-week intervention study with kefir carried out by da Silva Ghizi et al. [98], differences in HDLc levels were observed only in women. Likewise, daily intake of Yakult for 12 weeks did not induce changes in VLDLc levels [101].

Many of the adipokines exert multiple actions in a variety of cellular processes, leading to a complex array of abnormal characteristics in MetS [108]. For this reason, adipokines are target markers for assessing the effects of probiotic consumption in MetS patients.

Regarding TNF–α, the daily intake of kefir [99,100] and probiotic milk [102] leads to its decrease. However, consumption of a probiotic freeze-dried *L. helveticus* R0052 and *B. longum* R0175 (CNCM strain I-3470) bacteria does not affect the content of this marker after two months [104], and *L. reuteri* V3401 does not do so after three months [16].

With respect to IL–6, as presented in Table 3, three studies reported a significant reduction in this biomarker following the daily intake of probiotic milk [102,103] and kefir [100]. However, no changes in plasma levels of IL–1β and IL–8 were observed in the evaluated interventional studies. In addition, a reduction in plasma levels of IL-10 was found only in one 12-week study [100]. Circulating leptin levels showed no change, whereas adiponectin levels tended to increase after a daily intake of 80 mL of probiotic milk over 45 days [103], though no changes were detected in another study [16].

Levels of hs-CRP remain unchanged, regardless of probiotic type, dose, time of intervention, and sex in patients with MetS. A similar trend was observed for ICAM-1, sVCAM-1, and sICAM-1 (Table 3).

Although there is evidence of a positive association between circulating levels of TMAO and MetS [109], only one study evaluated this biomarker, showing that probiotic intake did not produce changes in its levels after 12 weeks [101].

3.4. Hypercholesterolemia

Hypercholesterolemia is one of the most important risk factors of atherosclerosis. Hypercholesterolemia is mostly defined by levels of total cholesterol > 200 mg/dL and LDLc ≥ 130 mg/dL (≥3.4 mmol/L) and/or non-HDLc ≥ 160 mg/dL (≥4.1 mmol/L) [110,111]. Hypercholesterolemia is also characterized by elevated levels of triglycerides and/or low HDLc levels. Due to the benefits of LDLc lowering in cardiovascular risk reduction, the principal's goals of CVD prevention for LDLc are <1.8 mmol/L (<70 mg/dL), <2.6 mmol/L (<100 mg/dL), and <3.0 mmol/L (<116 mg/dL) in high, moderate and low cardiovascular risk [110,112–114], respectively.

The first steps for achieving a cholesterol-lowering effect involve lifestyle and nutritional modifications. Thus, the use of supplements and functional foods for the treatment of dyslipidemias is rising as a good option in individuals considered to be at low cardiovascular risk who are in a stage prior to requiring drug treatment or even in patients treated with pharmacological drugs who have not reached guideline-recommended LDLc levels [115]. In this sense, probiotics have been raised as a non-pharmacological tool for the management of dyslipidemia [116,117].

To the best of our knowledge, only six clinical trials conducted from 2015 to date [118–123] have evaluated the efficacy of probiotics on subjects defined as hypercholesterolemic but without other CVD risk factors or clinical conditions (Table 4). In these clinical trials, the administered probiotic bacteria belonged to lactic acid species known for their cholesterol-lowering capacity [116], except for one study that used the probiotic bacteria *S. boulardii* [121].

Table 4. Studies evaluating the effect of probiotic supplementation in hypercholesterolemic patients.

Probiotic Strain (Product)	Dose (Intervention Time)	Study Characteristics (*n*)	Parameters Changing	Unchanging Parameters	Ref.
(1) *L. acidophilus* La5 (2) *L. casei* TMC (3) *B. lactis* Bb12 (Skimmed milk drink)	(1) 1.2 × 10^8 CFU/day (2) 1.2 × 10^8 CFU/day (3) 1.2 × 10^8 CFU/day (10 weeks)	Double-blind, placebo-RCT: Probiotic (20) and placebo (20)	↑ LDL-OXI lag time ↓ TC and LDLc	BMI, body weight, HDLc	[118]
L. plantarum ECGC 13110402 (Capsules)	4 × 10^9 CFU/day (12 weeks)	Single-center, prospective, randomized, placebo-controlled, parallel-group: Probiotic (23) and placebo (23)	↓ LDLc ↓ TC ↓ TG ↑ HDLc ↓ SBP	Body weight, BMI, waist, DBP, IL-6, TNF-α, CRP and IL-10.	[119]
L. Paracasei TISTR 2593 (Capsules)	3.675 × 10^9 CFU/day (90 days)	Single-center, prospective, randomized, double-blind, placebo-controlled, parallel-group trial: Probiotic (21) and placebo (21)	↓ LDLc ↓ MDA ↓ TNF-α ↑ Adiponectin ↑ ApoE	BMI, SBP, DBP, FBG, TC, TG, HDLc, IL-10, IL-6	[120]
S. boulardii (Capsules)	1.12 × 10^{11} CFU/day (8 weeks)	Single-arm, open-label pilot study: (11)	↓ VLDLp ↓ ILDp	BMI, TC, LDLc, HDLc, TG, VLDLp, LDLp, HDLp, non-HDLp, ApoB-100, Lp(a), hs-CRP, insulin, homocysteine	[121]
L. reuteri (Capsules)	Week 1 and 2: 3 × 10^9 CFU/day Week 3: 6 × 10^9 CFU/day Week 4: 9 × 10^9 CFU/day	Pilot, randomized, dose-escalation design: Standard capsules-SC (5) and delayed release capsules-DC (5)	↓ LDLc with DC	TC, HDLc, TG	[122]

Table 4. *Cont.*

Probiotic Strain (Product)	Dose (Intervention Time)	Study Characteristics (*n*)	Parameters Changing	Unchanging Parameters	Ref.
S. thermophilus YIT 2001 (Fermented milk)	1×10^{11} CFU/day (12 weeks)	Randomized, double-blind, placebo-controlled: Probiotic (29) and placebo (30)	↓ MDA-LDL, ↓ MDA-LDL/LDLc ↓ SBP and DBP	TC, LDLc, HDLc and TG	[123]

Apo: apolipoprotein; BMI: body mass index; DBP: diastolic blood pressure; FBG: fasting blood glucose; HDLc: high-density lipoprotein cholesterol; HbA1c: glycated hemoglobin; hs-CRP: high-sensitivity C-reactive protein; HOMA-IR: homeostatic model assessment of insulin resistance; ICAM, intercellular adhesion molecule cell; IL: interleukin; LDLc: low-density lipoprotein cholesterol; MDA: malondialdehyde; OXI: oxidation; P: particles. TC: total cholesterol; TG: triglycerides; sICAM-1: soluble intercellular adhesion molecule 1; SBP: systolic blood pressure; sVCAM-1: soluble vascular cell adhesion molecule 1; TNF−α: tumor necrosis factor−α; VCAM: vascular cell adhesion molecule cell; WC: waist circumference; WHR: waist-hip ratio. Downward arrows indicate decreased values. Upward arrows indicate increased values.

The lipid profile was thoroughly analyzed in the six clinical trials. Daily intake of multistrain milk (*Lactobacillus* and *Bifidobacterium* strains) for ten weeks reduced total cholesterol by 8.1% [118] as did the consumption of *L. plantarum* ECGC 13110402 [119]. However, the other four probiotic bacteria showed no impact on plasmatic cholesterol levels [120–123]. Regarding LDLc levels, a critical target for reducing cardiovascular risk, probiotic intake appears to be an effective strategy. Significant reductions were reported in four clinical trials [118–120,122], with reductions reaching up to 10.4% when a mix of three acid lactic bacteria was administered [118]. However, *Streptococcus thermophilus* YIT 2001 and *S. boulardii* failed to reduce LDLc levels [121,123]. In contrast, HDLc and triglyceride levels proved more challenging to modify through probiotic intervention. Only the study that used *L. plantarum* ECGC 13110402 strain achieved an increase in HDLc levels [119]. Triglyceride levels, on the other hand, were elevated after probiotic intervention in the single clinical trial that used a probiotic multistrain [118] but reduced after administration of *L. plantarum* ECGC 13110402 [119]. Additionally, probiotic intake was associated with a reduction in the concentration of VLDL and intermediate density lipoprotein (IDLc) particles [121]. As shown in Table 4, probiotics generally show a greater effect on LDLc reduction than HDLc elevation due to more defined mechanisms like bile acid metabolism, cholesterol assimilation, and SCFA production. Bile salt hydrolase (BSH) activity reduces cholesterol absorption by deconjugating BAs and promoting their excretion [124]. A decrease in BAs triggers an increase in de novo BA synthesis from cholesterol to restore balance. The conversion of cholesterol into BAs represents a major pathway for reducing serum cholesterol levels. Certain probiotics can also directly assimilate cholesterol into their cell membranes, limiting intestinal absorption. Additionally, some strains can convert cholesterol into coprostanol, a compound that is poorly absorbed and readily excreted in feces [125,126]. In contrast to the LDLc, HDLc modulation relies more on anti-inflammatory pathways and metabolic signaling, which are less direct and strain dependent [127]. The variability in outcomes underscores the importance of strain specificity, individual health status, and baseline cholesterol levels in determining the lipid-modulating effects of probiotics.

It is well known that hypercholesterolemic patients exhibit elevated levels of inflammatory markers [128]. Probiotics reduce inflammatory markers by modulating gut microbiota, strengthening gut barrier integrity, and decreasing systemic endotoxins. They lower levels of pro-inflammatory cytokines (e.g., TNF-α, IL-6, IL-1β) while increasing anti-inflammatory cytokines (e.g., IL-10) [129]. However, the effects remain inconsistent and are closely related to the probiotic strain and the health or disease status of the individual. Thus, in the included clinical trials, probiotic intake did not affect IL-10, IL-6 [119,120], CRP [119–121], and Lp(a) [121] levels. Nonetheless, TNFα levels were reduced with prolonged intake of *L. paracasei* TISTR 2593 [120], though no reduction was observed with *L. plantarum* ECGC

13110402 [119]. Regarding oxidation markers, probiotic intake was associated with reductions in malondialdehyde (MDA) [120] and MDA-LDL levels [123], as well as an increase in resistance to LDL oxidation [118].

3.5. Secondary Prevention in Coronary Artery Disease

CAD, also termed as coronary heart disease or ischemic heart disease, is one of the major CVDs affecting the world's population and has atherosclerosis as the primary underlying cause [130]. CAD is the leading single cause of mortality and disability-adjusted life years worldwide. Much of this burden falls on low- and middle-income countries, accounting for nearly 7 million deaths and 129 million DALYs annually [131,132]. Since 2015, numerous human studies have been conducted to evaluate the effects of probiotic consumption on inflammation, glucometabolic parameters, and lipid markers in patients with established CAD [133–138]. The characteristics of the studies as well as the main findings are summarized in Table 5.

Table 5. Studies evaluating the effect of probiotic supplementation in CAD patients.

Probiotic Strain (Product)	Dose (Intervention Time)	Study Characteristics (*n*)	Parameters Changing	Unchanging Parameters	Ref.
L. rhamnosus (Capsules)	1.6×10^9 CFU/day (12 weeks)	Double-blind, placebo-RCT: LGG (22), Placebo (22)	↓ IL–1β ↓ LPS	IL–10	[133]
L. rhamnosus (Capsules)	1.6×10^9 CFU/day (2 months)	Double-blind, placebo-RCT in end-stage renal disease patients: Probiotic (24), Placebo (24)	↓ SBP ↓ TC ↓ LPS ↓ TNF–α	DBP, LDLc, HDLc, TG, IL–10 and hs–CRP	[138]
L. rhamnosus (Sachet)	3×10^{10} CFU/day (6 months)	Double-blind, placebo-RCT: Probiotic (36), Placebo (24)	↓ IL–6 ↓ LDLc	Creatinine	[134]
(1) *B. bifidum* (2) *L. casei* (3) *L. acidophilus* (Capsules)	(1), (2), (3) 2×10^9 CFU/day (12 weeks)	Double-blind, placebo-RCT in patients with 2- and 3-vessel CHD: Probiotic (30), Placebo (30)	↓ FBG, insulin ↓ HOMA-IR ↓ TC/HDLc ratio ↓ hs–CRP ↓ NO ↑ HDLc	VLDLc, LDLc, TC, TG, SBP and DBP	[135]
L. plantarum 299v (Juice drink)	2×10^{10} CFU/day (6 weeks)	Non-randomized intervention in coronary angiography patients: Lp299v (20)	↓ SBP ↓ IL–8 and IL–12 ↓ Leptin	DBP, TC, TG, LDLc and HDLc	[136]
L. plantarum 299v (Juice drink)	2×10^{10} CFU/day (6 weeks)	Non-randomized intervention in coronary angiography patients: Lp299v (15)	↓ Leptin ↓ IL–8 and IL–12	DBP, SBP, FBG, TC, TG, HDLc and LDLc	[137]

BMI: body mass index; DBP: diastolic blood pressure; FBG: fasting blood glucose; HDLc: high-density lipoprotein cholesterol; HbA1c: glycated hemoglobin; hs-CRP: high-sensitivity C-reactive protein; HOMA-IR: homeostatic model assessment of insulin resistance; IL: interleukin; LDLc: low-density lipoprotein cholesterol; LPS: lipopolysaccharide; MDA: malondialdehyde, NO: nitric oxide; TC: total cholesterol; TG: triglycerides; SBP: systolic blood pressure; TNF−α: tumor necrosis factor−α; WC: waist circumference; WHR: waist-hip ratio. Downward arrows indicate decreased values. Upward arrows indicate increased values.

Two studies have evidenced that SBP responds more readily than DBP, with reductions observed after six [136] and eight weeks [138] of probiotic consumption in patients with coronary angiography and end-stage renal disease, respectively. In contrast, other studies lasting six and sixteen weeks found no changes in blood pressure following daily probiotic intake [135,137].

Dyslipidemia, a predominant cause and modifiable risk factor for CAD, is particularly significant, with 56% of CAD related to abnormal cholesterol levels [139]. As shown in

Table 5, only in one study in patients with end-stage renal disease reported a decrease in total cholesterol after two months of probiotic intervention with one capsule containing 1.9×10^9 CFU of *L. rhamnosus* per day [138]. In contrast, six [136,137], eight [133,138], and sixteen [135] weeks of probiotic supplementation do not seem to be sufficient to improve LDLc levels. However, a longer intervention time (6 months) led to a significant reduction in LDLc [134]. A similar trend was observed for HDLc. No changes were observed after six [136,137] and eight [138] weeks, but an increase was observed when the probiotic intervention was prolonged in time to six months [134]. In the four studies assessing triglyceride levels, no changes were observed at six [136,137], eight [138], or sixteen weeks [135].

Although leptin is essential for the maintenance of homeostasis in the cardiovascular system, only two of the five analyzed studies included this marker. The results showed that after daily intake of 80 mL of a probiotic with *L. plantarum* 299v for six weeks, leptin levels significantly decreased in participants with CAD [136,137]. Regarding the interleukins (IL-1β, IL–6, IL–8 and IL–12), these markers appear to be more easily modified, as a decrease in their content was observed (Table 5). In contrast, the anti-inflammatory IL-10 showed no change in its concentration in clinical trials lasting two months [133,138]. The immunomodulatory effects of probiotics on pro-inflammatory and anti-inflammatory pathways have been widely studied, as extensively reviewed by Cristofori et al. [129]. However, whether probiotics primarily target pro-inflammatory cytokines while leaving anti-inflammatory pathways largely unaffected remains a topic of debate. Probiotics predominantly reduce pro-inflammatory cytokines (e.g., TNF-α, IL-6, IL-1β) by modulating immune pathways such as NF-κB and MAPK, thereby decreasing systemic inflammation. They also produce SCFAs and other metabolites that further suppress inflammatory responses. While some strains (*Lactobacillus reuteri, Bifidobacterium bifidum*) can upregulate anti-inflammatory cytokines like IL-10, evidence for this effect remains less consistent and highly strain-dependent.

4. Final Remarks/Conclusions

This review, for the first time, compiles existing evidence from human studies on the effects of probiotic intake in vulnerable populations, including individuals with hypertension, T2DM, MetS, and hypercholesterolemia, and in secondary prevention in CAD. With the existing evidence, it could be suggested that, in populations at risk of CVD, probiotics may serve as a potential intervention tool in the prevention of CVD. Improvements have been observed in anthropometric measures, inflammation, blood pressure, markers of glucose metabolism, lipid profiles, and endothelial function. Nevertheless, it is crucial to adopt a pragmatic approach, given the heterogeneity of findings. These divergences may be attributed to factors such as probiotic composition (mono- or multistrain), characteristics of the delivery matrix (food, capsules, and sachets), intervention duration, dosage regimen, and the baseline health profiles of participants.

Further research is warranted to comprehensively elucidate the precise mechanisms by which probiotics exert their beneficial effects in the context of CVD. In addition, the evaluation of other factors that have an impact on the effect of probiotics needs further investigation, such as: (i) determining the optimal probiotic strain or strains, (ii) appropriate dosage, (iii) treatment duration, and (iv) optimal delivery vehicle. Moreover, exploring sex-specific differences is crucial, as current evidence in populations with cardiovascular risk factors remains limited in this area.

Funding: This work was supported by the "Fundacio la Marato"—project number 202329-10 to TP, Spanish Ministry of Economy and Competitiveness of Science and Agencia Estatal de Investigación PID2021-128891OB-I00 to G.V. and AEI/10.13039/501100011033-[PID2019-107160RB-I00] to L.B.;

CIBERCV to G.V. A.L.-Y. gratefully acknowledges financial support through the "Juan de la Cierva-Formación" programme funded by MCIN (MCIN/AEI/10.13039/501100011033) and by the European Union (NextGenerationEU/PRTR).

Conflicts of Interest: L.B. declares to have served as a SAB member of Sanofi, Ionnis, Pfizer, and NovoNordisk; to have received a research grant from AstraZeneca; to have received speaker fees from Sanofi, Bayer and AB-BIOTICS S.A.; and to have founded the Spin-Off Ivastatin Therapeutics S.L. (which is not associated with this research). T.P. discloses to have received speaker fees from AB-BIOTICS S.A. and to be a co-founder of Spin-off Ivastatin Therapeutics S.L. (both unrelated to this study). G.V. discloses to be a co-founder of Spin-off Ivastatin Therapeutics S.L. (both unrelated to this study). The remaining authors have no competing interests to declare.

References

1. Metchnikoff, E.; Metchnikoff, I.I. *The Prolongation of Life: Optimistic Studies*; G.P. Putnam's Sons: New York, NY, USA, 1908; ISBN 0826118763.
2. World Health Organization; Food and Agricultural Organization of the United Nations. *Health and Nutritional Properties of Probiotics in Food Including Powder Milk with Live Lactic Acid Bacteria*; World Health Organization: Geneva, Switzerland, 2001.
3. Hill, C.; Guarner, F.; Reid, G.; Gibson, G.R.; Merenstein, D.J.; Pot, B.; Morelli, L.; Canani, R.B.; Flint, H.J.; Salminen, S.; et al. The International Scientific Association for Probiotics and Prebiotics Consensus Statement on the Scope and Appropriate Use of the Term Probiotic. *Nat. Rev. Gastroenterol. Hepatol.* **2014**, *11*, 506–514. [CrossRef] [PubMed]
4. George Kerry, R.; Patra, J.K.; Gouda, S.; Park, Y.; Shin, H.S.; Das, G. Benefaction of Probiotics for Human Health: A Review. *J. Food Drug Anal.* **2018**, *26*, 927–939. [CrossRef] [PubMed]
5. Thushara, R.M.; Gangadaran, S.; Solati, Z.; Moghadasian, M.H. Cardiovascular Benefits of Probiotics: A Review of Experimental and Clinical Studies. *Food Funct.* **2016**, *7*, 632–642. [CrossRef] [PubMed]
6. Timmis, A.; Townsend, N.; Gale, C.P.; Torbica, A.; Lettino, M.; Petersen, S.E.; Mossialos, E.A.; Maggioni, A.P.; Kazakiewicz, D.; May, H.T.; et al. European Society of Cardiology: Cardiovascular Disease Statistics 2019. *Eur. Heart J.* **2020**, *41*, 12–85. [CrossRef]
7. Chakaroun, R.M.; Olsson, L.M.; Bäckhed, F. The Potential of Tailoring the Gut Microbiome to Prevent and Treat Cardiometabolic Disease. *Nat. Rev. Cardiol.* **2022**, *20*, 217–235. [CrossRef]
8. Rittiphairoj, T.; Pongpirul, K.; Janchot, K.; Mueller, N.T.; Li, T. Probiotics Contribute to Glycemic Control in Patients with Type 2 Diabetes Mellitus: A Systematic Review and Meta-Analysis. *Adv. Nutr.* **2021**, *12*, 722–734. [CrossRef]
9. Song, E.J.; Han, K.; Lim, T.J.; Lim, S.; Chung, M.J.; Nam, M.H.; Kim, H.; Nam, Y. Do Effect of Probiotics on Obesity-Related Markers per Enterotype: A Double-Blind, Placebo-Controlled, Randomized Clinical Trial. *EPMA J.* **2020**, *11*, 31–51. [CrossRef]
10. Padro, T.; Santisteban, V.; Huedo, P.; Puntes, M.; Aguiló, M.; Espadaler-Mazo, J.; Badimon, L. *Lactiplantibacillus plantarum* Strains KABP011, KABP012, and KABP013 Modulate Bile Acids and Cholesterol Metabolism in Humans. *Cardiovasc. Res.* **2024**, *120*, 708–722. [CrossRef]
11. Ravera, A.; Carubelli, V.; Sciatti, E.; Bonadei, I.; Gorga, E.; Cani, D.; Vizzardi, E.; Metra, M.; Lombardi, C. Nutrition and Cardiovascular Disease: Finding the Perfect Recipe for Cardiovascular Health. *Nutrients* **2016**, *8*, 363. [CrossRef]
12. Oniszczuk, A.; Oniszczuk, T.; Gancarz, M. Role of Gut Microbiota, Probiotics and Prebiotics in the Cardiovascular Diseases. *Molecules* **2021**, *26*, 1172. [CrossRef]
13. Bagarolli, R.A.; Tobar, N.; Oliveira, A.G.; Araújo, T.G.; Carvalho, B.M.; Rocha, G.Z.; Vecina, J.F.; Calisto, K.; Guadagnini, D.; Prada, P.O.; et al. Probiotics Modulate Gut Microbiota and Improve Insulin Sensitivity in DIO Mice. *J. Nutr. Biochem.* **2017**, *50*, 16–25. [CrossRef] [PubMed]
14. Plaza-Díaz, J.; Fernández-Caballero, J.Á.; Chueca, N.; García, F.; Gómez-Llorente, C.; Sáez-Lara, M.J.; Fontana, L.; Gil, Á. Pyrosequencing Analysis Reveals Changes in Intestinal Microbiota of Healthy Adults Who Received a Daily Dose of Immunomodulatory Probiotic Strains. *Nutrients* **2015**, *7*, 3999–4015. [CrossRef] [PubMed]
15. Toscano, M.; De Grandi, R.; Miniello, V.L.; Mattina, R.; Drago, L. Ability of Lactobacillus Kefiri LKF01 (DSM32079) to Colonize the Intestinal Environment and Modify the Gut Microbiota Composition of Healthy Individuals. *Dig. Liver Dis.* **2017**, *49*, 261–267. [CrossRef] [PubMed]
16. Tenorio-Jiménez, C.; Martínez-Ramírez, M.J.; Del Castillo-Codes, I.; Arraiza-Irigoyen, C.; Tercero-Lozano, M.; Camacho, J.; Chueca, N.; García, F.; Olza, J.; Plaza-Díaz, J.; et al. *Lactobacillus reuteri* V3401 Reduces Inflammatory Biomarkers and Modifies the Gastrointestinal Microbiome in Adults with Metabolic Syndrome: The PROSIR Study. *Nutrients* **2019**, *11*, 1761. [CrossRef]
17. Wang, C.; Nagata, S.; Asahara, T.; Yuki, N.; Matsuda, K.; Tsuji, H.; Takahashi, T.; Nomoto, K.; Yamashiro, Y. Intestinal Microbiota Profiles of Healthy Pre-School and School-Age Children and Effects of Probiotic Supplementation. *Ann. Nutr. Metab.* **2015**, *67*, 257–266. [CrossRef]

18. Badimon, L.; Chagas, P.; Chiva-Blanch, G. Diet and Cardiovascular Disease: Effects of Foods and Nutrients in Classical and Emerging Cardiovascular Risk Factors. *Curr. Med. Chem.* **2017**, *26*, 3639–3651. [CrossRef]
19. Hendijani, F.; Akbari, V. Probiotic Supplementation for Management of Cardiovascular Risk Factors in Adults with Type II Diabetes: A Systematic Review and Meta-Analysis. *Clin. Nutr.* **2018**, *37*, 532–541. [CrossRef]
20. Dixon, A.; Robertson, K.; Yung, A.; Que, M.; Randall, H.; Wellalagodage, D.; Cox, T.; Robertson, D.; Chi, C.; Sun, J. Efficacy of Probiotics in Patients of Cardiovascular Disease Risk: A Systematic Review and Meta-Analysis. *Curr. Hypertens. Rep.* **2020**, *22*, 74. [CrossRef]
21. Sun, J.; Buys, N. Effects of Probiotics Consumption on Lowering Lipids and CVD Risk Factors: A Systematic Review and Meta-Analysis of Randomized Controlled Trials. *Ann. Med.* **2015**, *47*, 430–440. [CrossRef]
22. Olas, B. Probiotics, Prebiotics and Synbiotics—A Promising Strategy in Prevention and Treatment of Cardiovascular Diseases? *Int. J. Mol. Sci.* **2020**, *21*, 9737. [CrossRef]
23. Ghanbari, F.; Hasani, S.; Aghili, Z.S.; Asgary, S. The Potential Preventive Effect of Probiotics, Prebiotics, and Synbiotics on Cardiovascular Risk Factors through Modulation of Gut Microbiota: A Review. *Food Sci. Nutr.* **2024**, *12*, 4569–4580. [CrossRef] [PubMed]
24. Derrien, M.; van Hylckama Vlieg, J.E.T. Fate, Activity, and Impact of Ingested Bacteria within the Human Gut Microbiota. *Trends Microbiol.* **2015**, *23*, 354–366. [CrossRef] [PubMed]
25. Plaza-Diaz, J.; Ruiz-Ojeda, F.J.; Gil-Campos, M.; Gil, A. Mechanisms of Action of Probiotics. *Adv. Nutr.* **2019**, *10*, S49–S66. [CrossRef]
26. Alp, D.; Kuleaşan, H. Adhesion Mechanisms of Lactic Acid Bacteria: Conventional and Novel Approaches for Testing. *World J. Microbiol. Biotechnol.* **2019**, *35*, 156. [CrossRef] [PubMed]
27. Flach, J.; van der Waal, M.B.; van den Nieuwboer, M.; Claassen, E.; Larsen, O.F.A. The Underexposed Role of Food Matrices in Probiotic Products: Reviewing the Relationship between Carrier Matrices and Product Parameters. *Crit. Rev. Food Sci. Nutr.* **2018**, *58*, 2570–2584. [CrossRef]
28. Ranadheera, R.D.C.S.; Baines, S.K.; Adams, M.C. Importance of Food in Probiotic Efficacy. *Food Res. Int.* **2010**, *43*, 1–7. [CrossRef]
29. Timmerman, H.M.; Koning, C.J.M.; Mulder, L.; Rombouts, F.M.; Beynen, A.C. Monostrain, Multistrain and Multispecies Probiotics—A Comparison of Functionality and Efficacy. *Int. J. Food Microbiol.* **2004**, *96*, 219–233. [CrossRef]
30. Wu, L.; Sun, D. Consumption of Yogurt and the Incident Risk of Cardiovascular Disease: A Meta-Analysis of Nine Cohort Studies. *Nutrients* **2017**, *9*, 315. [CrossRef]
31. Alard, J.; Lehrter, V.; Rhimi, M.; Mangin, I.; Peucelle, V.; Abraham, A.L.; Mariadassou, M.; Maguin, E.; Waligora-Dupriet, A.J.; Pot, B.; et al. Beneficial Metabolic Effects of Selected Probiotics on Diet-Induced Obesity and Insulin Resistance in Mice Are Associated with Improvement of Dysbiotic Gut Microbiota. *Environ. Microbiol.* **2016**, *18*, 1484–1497. [CrossRef]
32. Kazemi, A.; Soltani, S.; Ghorabi, S.; Keshtkar, A.; Daneshzad, E.; Nasri, F.; Mazloomi, S.M. Effect of Probiotic and Synbiotic Supplementation on Inflammatory Markers in Health and Disease Status: A Systematic Review and Meta-Analysis of Clinical Trials. *Clin. Nutr.* **2020**, *39*, 789–819. [CrossRef]
33. Government of Canada. Natural Health Products Ingredients Database. Available online: https://webprod.hc-sc.gc.ca/nhpid-bdipsn/ (accessed on 22 December 2024).
34. Ministero della Salute. *Guidelines on Probiotics and Prebiotics*; Ministero della Salute: Rome, Italy, 2018; pp. 1–4.
35. Morelli, L.; Pellegrino, P. A Critical Evaluation of the Factors Affecting the Survival and Persistence of Beneficial Bacteria in Healthy Adults. *Benef. Microbes* **2021**, *12*, 321–331. [CrossRef] [PubMed]
36. Szulińska, M.; Łoniewski, I.; Skrypnik, K.; Sobieska, M.; Korybalska, K.; Suliburska, J.; Bogdański, P. Multispecies Probiotic Supplementation Favorably Affects Vascular Function and Reduces Arterial Stiffness in Obese Postmenopausal Women—A 12-Week Placebo-Controlled and Randomized Clinical Study. *Nutrients* **2018**, *10*, 1672. [CrossRef] [PubMed]
37. Qi, D.; Nie, X.L.; Zhang, J.J. The Effect of Probiotics Supplementation on Blood Pressure: A Systemic Review and Meta-Analysis. *Lipids Health Dis.* **2020**, *19*, 79. [CrossRef] [PubMed]
38. Hsieh, M.C.; Tsai, W.H.; Jheng, Y.P.; Su, S.L.; Wang, S.Y.; Lin, C.C.; Chen, Y.H.; Chang, W.W. The Beneficial Effects of *Lactobacillus reuteri* ADR-1 or ADR-3 Consumption on Type 2 Diabetes Mellitus: A Randomized, Double-Blinded, Placebo Controlled Trial. *Sci. Rep.* **2018**, *8*, 16791. [CrossRef]
39. Ranadheera, C.S.; Vidanarachchi, J.K.; Rocha, R.S.; Cruz, A.G.; Ajlouni, S. Probiotic Delivery through Fermentation: Dairy vs. Non-Dairy Beverages. *Fermentation* **2017**, *3*, 67. [CrossRef]
40. Damián, M.R.; Cortes-Perez, N.G.; Quintana, E.T.; Ortiz-Moreno, A.; Noguez, C.G.; Cruceño-Casarrubias, C.E.; Pardo, M.E.S.; Bermúdez-Humarán, L.G. Functional Foods, Nutraceuticals and Probiotics: A Focus on Human Health. *Microorganisms* **2022**, *10*, 1065. [CrossRef]
41. Companys, J.; Pla-Pagà, L.; Calderen-Pérez, L.; Llaurade, E.; Solà, R.; Pedret, A.; Valls, R.M. Fermented Dairy Products, Probiotic Supplementation, and Cardiometabolic Diseases: A Systematic Review and Meta-Analysis. *Adv. Nutr.* **2020**, *11*, 834–863. [CrossRef]

42. Kazemian, N.; Mahmoudi, M.; Halperin, F.; Wu, J.C.; Pakpour, S. Gut Microbiota and Cardiovascular Disease: Opportunities and Challenges. *Microbiome* **2020**, *8*, 36. [CrossRef]
43. Appelman, Y.; van Rijn, B.B.; ten Haaf, M.E.; Boersma, E.; Peters, S.A.E. Sex Differences in Cardiovascular Risk Factors and Disease Prevention. *Atherosclerosis* **2014**, *241*, 211–218. [CrossRef]
44. Fuchs, F.D.; Whelton, P.K. High Blood Pressure and Cardiovascular Disease. *Hypertension* **2020**, *75*, 285–292. [CrossRef]
45. Vasquez, E.C.; Pereira, T.M.C.; Peotta, V.A.; Baldo, M.P.; Campos-Toimil, M. Probiotics as Beneficial Dietary Supplements to Prevent and Treat Cardiovascular Diseases: Uncovering Their Impact on Oxidative Stress. *Oxid. Med. Cell. Longev.* **2019**, *2019*, 3086270. [CrossRef] [PubMed]
46. Pelton, R. Postbiotic Metabolites: How Probiotics Regulate Health. *Integr. Med. A Clin. J.* **2020**, *19*, 25.
47. Du, Y.; He, C.; An, Y.; Huang, Y.; Zhang, H.; Fu, W.; Wang, M.; Shan, Z.; Xie, J.; Yang, Y. The Role of Short Chain Fatty Acids in Inflammation and Body Health. *Int. J. Mol. Sci.* **2024**, *25*, 7379. [CrossRef]
48. Vourakis, M.; Mayer, G.; Rousseau, G. The Role of Gut Microbiota on Cholesterol Metabolism in Atherosclerosis. *Int. J. Mol. Sci.* **2021**, *22*, 8074. [CrossRef]
49. Upadrasta, A.; Madempudi, R.S. Probiotics and Blood Pressure: Current Insights. *Integr. Blood Press. Control* **2016**, *9*, 33–42.
50. FitzGerald, R.J.; Murray, B.A.; Walsh, D.J. Hypotensive Peptides from Milk Proteins. *J. Nutr.* **2004**, *134*, 980S–988S. [CrossRef]
51. Daliri, E.B.M.; Lee, B.H.; Oh, D.H. Current Perspectives on Antihypertensive Probiotics. *Probiotics Antimicrob. Proteins* **2017**, *9*, 91–101. [CrossRef]
52. Adams, C.; Sawh, F.; Green-Johnson, J.M.; Taggart, H.J.; Strap, J.L. Characterization of Casein-Derived Peptide Bioactivity: Differential Effects on Angiotensin-Converting Enzyme Inhibition and Cytokine and Nitric Oxide Production. *J. Dairy Sci.* **2020**, *103*, 5805–5815. [CrossRef]
53. Gómez-Guzmán, M.; Toral, M.; Romero, M.; Jiménez, R.; Galindo, P.; Sanchez, M.; Zarzuelo, M.J.; Olivares, M.; Gálvez, J.; Duarte, J. Antihypertensive Effects of Probiotics *Lactobacillus* Strains in Spontaneously Hypertensive Rats. *Mol. Nutr. Food Res.* **2015**, *59*, 2326–2336. [CrossRef]
54. Friques, A.G.F.; Arpini, C.M.; Kalil, I.C.; Gava, A.L.; Leal, M.A.; Porto, M.L.; Nogueira, B.V.; Dias, A.T.; Andrade, T.U.; Pereira, T.M.C. Chronic Administration of the Probiotic Kefir Improves the Endothelial Function in Spontaneously Hypertensive Rats. *J. Transl. Med.* **2015**, *13*, 390. [CrossRef]
55. Kim, D.Y.; Park, J.Y.; Gee, H.Y. *Lactobacillus plantarum* Ameliorates NASH-Related Inflammation by Upregulating L-Arginine Production. *Exp. Mol. Med.* **2023**, *55*, 2332–2345. [CrossRef] [PubMed]
56. Lau, E.; Neves, J.S.; Ferreira-Magalhães, M.; Carvalho, D.; Freitas, P. Probiotic Ingestion, Obesity, and Metabolic-Related Disorders: Results from NHANES, 1999–2014. *Nutrients* **2019**, *11*, 1482. [CrossRef] [PubMed]
57. Lewis-Mikhael, A.M.; Davoodvandi, A.; Jafarnejad, S. Effect of Lactobacillusplantarum Containing Probiotics on Blood Pressure: A Systematic Review and Meta-Analysis. *Pharmacol. Res.* **2020**, *153*, 104663. [CrossRef] [PubMed]
58. Chi, C.; Li, C.; Wu, D.; Buys, N.; Wang, W.; Fan, H.; Sun, J. Effects of Probiotics on Patients with Hypertension: A Systematic Review and Meta-Analysis. *Curr. Hypertens. Rep.* **2020**, *22*, 34. [CrossRef]
59. Ejtahed, H.S.; Ardeshirlarijani, E.; Tabatabaei-Malazy, O.; Hoseini-Tavassol, Z.; Hasani-Ranjbar, S.; Soroush, A.R.; Larijani, B. Effect of Probiotic Foods and Supplements on Blood Pressure: A Systematic Review of Meta-Analyses Studies of Controlled Trials. *J. Diabetes Metab. Disord.* **2020**, *19*, 617–623. [CrossRef]
60. Hajifaraji, M.; Jahanjou, F.; Abbasalizadeh, F.; Aghamohammadzadeh, N.; Abbasi, M.M.; Dolatkhah, N. Effect of Probiotic Supplementation on Blood Pressure of Females with Gestational Diabetes Mellitus: A Randomized Double Blind Controlled Clinical Trial. *Iran. Red. Crescent Med. J.* **2017**, *19*, 1–10. [CrossRef]
61. Sperry, M.F.; Silva, H.L.A.; Balthazar, C.F.; Esmerino, E.A.; Verruck, S.; Prudencio, E.S.; Neto, R.P.C.; Tavares, M.I.B.; Peixoto, J.C.; Nazzaro, F.; et al. Probiotic Minas Frescal Cheese Added with L. Casei 01: Physicochemical and Bioactivity Characterization and Effects on Hematological/Biochemical Parameters of Hypertensive Overweighted Women–A Randomized Double-Blind Pilot Trial. *J. Funct. Foods* **2018**, *45*, 435–443. [CrossRef]
62. Romão Da Silva, L.D.F.; De Oliveira, Y.; De Souza, E.L.; De Luna Freire, M.O.; Braga, V.D.A.; Magnani, M.; De Brito Alves, J.L. Effects of Probiotic Therapy on Cardio-Metabolic Parameters and Autonomic Modulation in Hypertensive Women: A Randomized, Triple-Blind, Placebo-Controlled Trial. *Food Funct.* **2020**, *11*, 7152–7163. [CrossRef]
63. Xu, J.; Lazou Ahrén, I.; Olsson, C.; Jeppsson, B.; Ahrné, S.; Molin, G. Oral and Faecal Microbiota in Volunteers with Hypertension in a Double Blind, Randomised Placebo Controlled Trial with Probiotics and Fermented Bilberries. *J. Funct. Foods* **2015**, *18*, 275–288. [CrossRef]
64. Ivey, K.L.; Hodgson, J.M.; Kerr, D.A.; Thompson, P.L.; Stojceski, B.; Prince, R.L. The Effect of Yoghurt and Its Probiotics on Blood Pressure and Serum Lipid Profile; a Randomised Controlled Trial. *Nutr. Metab. Cardiovasc. Dis.* **2015**, *25*, 46–51. [CrossRef]
65. Faselis, C.; Katsimardou, A.; Imprialos, K.; Deligkaris, P.; Kallistratos, M.; Dimitriadis, K. Microvascular Complications of Type 2 Diabetes Mellitus. *Curr. Vasc. Pharmacol.* **2019**, *18*, 117–124. [CrossRef] [PubMed]

66. Tanase, D.M.; Gosav, E.M.; Neculae, E.; Costea, C.F.; Ciocoiu, M.; Hurjui, L.L.; Tarniceriu, C.C.; Maranduca, M.A.; Lacatusu, C.M.; Floria, M.; et al. Role of Gut Microbiota on Onset and Progression of Microvascular Complications of Type 2 Diabetes (T2DM). *Nutrients* **2020**, *12*, 3719. [CrossRef] [PubMed]
67. Leenders, F.; Groen, N.; de Graaf, N.; Engelse, M.A.; Rabelink, T.J.; de Koning, E.J.P.; Carlotti, F. Oxidative Stress Leads to β-Cell Dysfunction through Loss of β-Cell Identity. *Front. Immunol.* **2021**, *12*, 690379. [CrossRef] [PubMed]
68. Robertson, R.P.; Harmon, J.; Tran, P.O.T.; Poitout, V. β-Cell Glucose Toxicity, Lipotoxicity, and Chronic Oxidative Stress in Type 2 Diabetes. *Diabetes* **2004**, *53*, S119–S124. [CrossRef] [PubMed]
69. Aw, W.; Fukuda, S. Understanding the Role of the Gut Ecosystem in Diabetes Mellitus. *J. Diabetes Investig.* **2018**, *9*, 5–12. [CrossRef]
70. Gurung, M.; Li, Z.; You, H.; Rodrigues, R.; Jump, D.B.; Morgun, A.; Shulzhenko, N. Role of Gut Microbiota in Type 2 Diabetes Pathophysiology. *EBioMedicine* **2020**, *51*, 102590. [CrossRef]
71. Miraghajani, M.; Zaghian, N.; Mirlohi, M.; Feizi, A.; Ghiasvand, R. The Impact of Probiotic Soy Milk Consumption on Oxidative Stress Among Type 2 Diabetic Kidney Disease Patients: A Randomized Controlled Clinical Trial. *J. Ren. Nutr.* **2017**, *27*, 317–324. [CrossRef]
72. Feizollahzadeh, S.; Ghiasvand, R.; Rezaei, A.; Khanahmad, H.; Sadeghi, A.; Hariri, M. Effect of Probiotic Soy Milk on Serum Levels of Adiponectin, Inflammatory Mediators, Lipid Profile, and Fasting Blood Glucose Among Patients with Type II Diabetes Mellitus. *Probiotics Antimicrob. Proteins* **2017**, *9*, 41–47. [CrossRef]
73. Miraghajani, M.; Zaghian, N.; Dehkohneh, A.; Mirlohi, M.; Ghiasvand, R. Probiotic Soy Milk Consumption and Renal Function Among Type 2 Diabetic Patients with Nephropathy: A Randomized Controlled Clinical Trial. *Probiotics Antimicrob. Proteins* **2019**, *11*, 124–132. [CrossRef]
74. Sato, J.; Kanazawa, A.; Azuma, K.; Ikeda, F.; Goto, H.; Komiya, K.; Kanno, R.; Tamura, Y.; Asahara, T.; Takahashi, T.; et al. Probiotic Reduces Bacterial Translocation in Type 2 Diabetes Mellitus: A Randomised Controlled Study. *Sci. Rep.* **2017**, *7*, 12115. [CrossRef]
75. Sabico, S.; Al-Mashharawi, A.; Al-Daghri, N.M.; Yakout, S.; Alnaami, A.M.; Alokail, M.S.; McTernan, P.G. Effects of a Multi-Strain Probiotic Supplement for 12 Weeks in Circulating Endotoxin Levels and Cardiometabolic Profiles of Medication Naïve T2DM Patients: A Randomized Clinical Trial. *J. Transl. Med.* **2017**, *15*, 249. [CrossRef] [PubMed]
76. Mobini, R.; Tremaroli, V.; Ståhlman, M.; Karlsson, F.; Levin, M.; Ljungberg, M.; Sohlin, M.; Bertéus Forslund, H.; Perkins, R.; Bäckhed, F.; et al. Metabolic Effects of *Lactobacillus reuteri* DSM 17938 in People with Type 2 Diabetes: A Randomized Controlled Trial. *Diabetes Obes. Metab.* **2017**, *19*, 579–589. [CrossRef] [PubMed]
77. Kobyliak, N.; Falalyeyeva, T.; Mykhalchyshyn, G.; Kyriienko, D.; Komissarenko, I. Effect of Alive Probiotic on Insulin Resistance in Type 2 Diabetes Patients: Randomized Clinical Trial. *Diabetes Metab. Syndr. Clin. Res. Rev.* **2018**, *12*, 617–624. [CrossRef]
78. Sabico, S.; Al-Mashharawi, A.; Al-Daghri, N.M.; Wani, K.; Amer, O.E.; Hussain, D.S.; Ahmed Ansari, M.G.; Masoud, M.S.; Alokail, M.S.; McTernan, P.G. Effects of a 6-Month Multi-Strain Probiotics Supplementation in Endotoxemic, Inflammatory and Cardiometabolic Status of T2DM Patients: A Randomized, Double-Blind, Placebo-Controlled Trial. *Clin. Nutr.* **2019**, *38*, 1561–1569. [CrossRef]
79. Razmpoosh, E.; Javadi, A.; Ejtahed, H.S.; Mirmiran, P.; Javadi, M.; Yousefinejad, A. The Effect of Probiotic Supplementation on Glycemic Control and Lipid Profile in Patients with Type 2 Diabetes: A Randomized Placebo Controlled Trial. *Diabetes Metab. Syndr. Clin. Res. Rev.* **2019**, *13*, 175–182. [CrossRef]
80. Khalili, L.; Alipour, B.; Jafar-Abadi, M.A.; Faraji, I.; Hassanalilou, T.; Abbasi, M.M.; Vaghef-Mehrabany, E.; Sani, M.A. The Effects of *Lactobacillus casei* on Glycemic Response, Serum Sirtuin1 and Fetuin-A Levels in Patients with Type 2 Diabetes Mellitus: A Randomized Controlled Trial. *Iran. Biomed. J.* **2019**, *23*, 68–77. [CrossRef]
81. Madempudi, R.S.; Ahire, J.J.; Neelamraju, J.; Tripathi, A.; Nanal, S. Efficacy of UB0316, a Multi-Strain Probiotic Formulation in Patients with Type 2 Diabetes Mellitus: A Double Blind, Randomized, Placebo Controlled Study. *PLoS ONE* **2019**, *14*, e0225168. [CrossRef]
82. Ahmadian, F.; Razmpoosh, E.; Ejtahed, H.S.; Javadi, M.; Mirmiran, P.; Azizi, F. Effects of Probiotic Supplementation on Major Cardiovascular-Related Parameters in Patients with Type-2 Diabetes Mellitus: A Secondary-Data Analysis of a Randomized Double-Blind Controlled Trial. *Diabetol. Metab. Syndr.* **2022**, *14*, 52. [CrossRef]
83. Tao, Y.W.; Gu, Y.L.; Mao, X.Q.; Zhang, L.; Pei, Y.F. Effects of Probiotics on Type II Diabetes Mellitus: A Meta-Analysis. *J. Transl. Med.* **2020**, *18*, 30. [CrossRef]
84. Rehman, K.; Akash, M.S.H. Mechanism of Generation of Oxidative Stress and Pathophysiology of Type 2 Diabetes Mellitus: How Are They Interlinked? *J. Cell. Biochem.* **2017**, *118*, 3577–3585. [CrossRef]
85. Dinarello, C.A.; Donath, M.Y.; Mandrup-Poulsen, T. Role of IL-1β in Type 2 Diabetes. *Curr. Opin. Endocrinol. Diabetes Obes.* **2010**, *17*, 314–321. [CrossRef] [PubMed]
86. Oguntibeju, O.O. Type 2 Diabetes Mellitus, Oxidative Stress and Inflammation: Examining the Links. *Int. J. Physiol. Pathophysiol. Pharmacol.* **2019**, *11*, 45–63. [PubMed]

87. Aleidi, S.; Issa, A.; Bustanji, H.; Khalil, M.; Bustanji, Y. Adiponectin Serum Levels Correlate with Insulin Resistance in Type 2 Diabetic Patients. *Saudi Pharm. J.* **2015**, *23*, 250–256. [CrossRef] [PubMed]
88. Moonishaa, T.; Nanda, S.; Shamraj, M.; Sivaa, R.; Sivakumar, P.; Ravichandran, K. Evaluation of Leptin as a Marker of Insulin Resistance in Type 2 Diabetes Mellitus. *Int. J. Appl. Basic. Med. Res.* **2017**, *7*, 176–180. [CrossRef]
89. Mooradian, A.D. Dyslipidemia in Type 2 Diabetes Mellitus. *Nat. Clin. Pract. Endocrinol. Metab.* **2009**, *5*, 150–159. [CrossRef]
90. Tune, J.D.; Goodwill, A.G.; Sassoon, D.J.; Mather, K.J. Cardiovascular Consequences of Metabolic Syndrome. *Transl. Res.* **2017**, *183*, 57–70. [CrossRef]
91. Noubiap, J.J.; Nansseu, J.R.; Lontchi-Yimagou, E.; Nkeck, J.R.; Nyaga, U.F.; Ngouo, A.T.; Tounouga, D.N.; Tianyi, F.L.; Foka, A.J.; Ndoadoumgue, A.L.; et al. Geographic Distribution of Metabolic Syndrome and Its Components in the General Adult Population: A Meta-Analysis of Global Data from 28 Million Individuals. *Diabetes Res. Clin. Pract.* **2022**, *188*, 109924. [CrossRef]
92. Cleeman, J.I. Executive Summary of the Third Report of the National Cholesterol Education Program (NCEP) Expert Panel on Detection, Evaluation, and Treatment of High Blood Cholesterol in Adults (Adult Treatment Panel III). *J. Am. Med. Assoc.* **2001**, *285*, 2486–2497. [CrossRef]
93. Castro-Barquero, S.; Ruiz-León, A.M.; Sierra-Pérez, M.; Estruch, R.; Casas, R. Dietary Strategies for Metabolic Syndrome: A Comprehensive Review. *Nutrients* **2020**, *12*, 2983. [CrossRef]
94. Hoyas, I.; Leon-Sanz, M. Nutritional Challenges in Metabolic Syndrome. *J. Clin. Med.* **2019**, *8*, 1301. [CrossRef]
95. Xavier-Santos, D.; Bedani, R.; Lima, E.D.; Saad, S.M.I. Impact of Probiotics and Prebiotics Targeting Metabolic Syndrome. *J. Funct. Foods* **2020**, *64*, 103666. [CrossRef]
96. Rezazadeh, L.; Gargari, B.P.; Jafarabadi, M.A.; Alipour, B. Effects of Probiotic Yogurt on Glycemic Indexes and Endothelial Dysfunction Markers in Patients with Metabolic Syndrome. *Nutrition* **2019**, *62*, 162–168. [CrossRef] [PubMed]
97. Rezazadeh, L.; Alipour, B.; Jafarabadi, M.A.; Behrooz, M.; Gargari, B.P. Daily Consumption Effects of Probiotic Yogurt Containing *Lactobacillus acidophilus* La5 and *Bifidobacterium lactis* Bb12 on Oxidative Stress in Metabolic Syndrome Patients. *Clin. Nutr. ESPEN* **2021**, *41*, 136–142. [CrossRef] [PubMed]
98. Ghizi, A.C.d.S.; de Almeida Silva, M.; Moraes, F.S.d.A.; da Silva, C.L.; Endringer, D.C.; Scherer, R.; Lenz, D.; de Lima, E.M.; Brasil, G.A.; Maia, J.F.; et al. Kefir Improves Blood Parameters and Reduces Cardiovascular Risks in Patients with Metabolic Syndrome. *PharmaNutrition* **2021**, *16*, 100266. [CrossRef]
99. Bellikci-Koyu, E.; Sarer-Yurekli, B.P.; Akyon, Y.; Aydin-Kose, F.; Karagozlu, C.; Ozgen, A.G.; Brinkmann, A.; Nitsche, A.; Ergunay, K.; Yilmaz, E.; et al. Effects of Regular Kefir Consumption on Gut Microbiota in Patients with Metabolic Syndrome: A Parallel-Group, Randomized, Controlled Study. *Nutrients* **2019**, *11*, 2089. [CrossRef]
100. Bellikci-Koyu, E.; Sarer-Yurekli, B.P.; Karagozlu, C.; Aydin-Kose, F.; Ozgen, A.G.; Buyuktuncer, Z. Probiotic Kefir Consumption Improves Serum Apolipoprotein A1 Levels in Metabolic Syndrome Patients: A Randomized Controlled Clinical Trial. *Nutr. Res.* **2022**, *102*, 59–70. [CrossRef]
101. Tripolt, N.J.; Leber, B.; Triebl, A.; Köfeler, H.; Stadlbauer, V.; Sourij, H. Effect of *Lactobacillus casei* Shirota Supplementation on Trimethylamine-N-Oxide Levels in Patients with Metabolic Syndrome: An Open-Label, Randomized Study. *Atherosclerosis* **2015**, *242*, 141–144. [CrossRef]
102. Bernini, L.J.; Simão, A.N.C.; Alfieri, D.F.; Lozovoy, M.A.B.; Mari, N.L.; de Souza, C.H.B.; Dichi, I.; Costa, G.N. Beneficial Effects of *Bifidobacterium lactis* on Lipid Profile and Cytokines in Patients with Metabolic Syndrome: A Randomized Trial. Effects of Probiotics on Metabolic Syndrome. *Nutrition* **2016**, *32*, 716–719. [CrossRef]
103. Bernini, L.J.; Simão, A.N.C.; De Souza, C.H.B.; Alfieri, D.F.; Segura, L.G.; Costa, G.N.; Dichi, I. Effect of *Bifidobacterium lactis* HN019 on Inflammatory Markers and Oxidative Stress in Subjects with and without the Metabolic Syndrome. *Br. J. Nutr.* **2018**, *120*, 645–652. [CrossRef]
104. Kazemi, A.; Noorbala, A.A.; Azam, K.; Djafarian, K. Effect of Prebiotic and Probiotic Supplementation on Circulating Pro-Inflammatory Cytokines and Urinary Cortisol Levels in Patients with Major Depressive Disorder: A Double-Blind, Placebo-Controlled Randomized Clinical Trial. *J. Funct. Foods* **2019**, *52*, 596–602. [CrossRef]
105. Xiao, R.; Chen, Y.; Zhu, X.; Wang, L.; Tian, P.; Jin, X.; Liang, M.; Chen, Z.; Zhang, T.; Qian, L. A Randomised Double-Blind Placebo-Controlled Trial of a Probiotic Combination for Manipulating the Gut Microbiota and Managing Metabolic Syndrome. *Food Biosci.* **2024**, *59*, 104076. [CrossRef]
106. Babio, N.; Martínez-González, M.A.; Estruch, R.; Wärnberg, J.; Recondo, J.; Ortega-Calvo, M.; Serra-Majem, L.; Corella, D.; Fitó, M.; Ros, E.; et al. Associations between Serum Uric Acid Concentrations and Metabolic Syndrome and Its Components in the PREDIMED Study. *Nutr. Metab. Cardiovasc. Dis.* **2015**, *25*, 173–180. [CrossRef] [PubMed]
107. Sreckovic, B.; Sreckovic, V.D.; Soldatovic, I.; Colak, E.; Sumarac-Dumanovic, M.; Janeski, H.; Janeski, N.; Gacic, J.; Mrdovic, I. Homocysteine Is a Marker for Metabolic Syndrome and Atherosclerosis. *Diabetes Metab. Syndr. Clin. Res. Rev.* **2017**, *11*, 179–182. [CrossRef] [PubMed]
108. Kumari, R.; Kumar, S.; Kant, R. An Update on Metabolic Syndrome: Metabolic Risk Markers and Adipokines in the Development of Metabolic Syndrome. *Diabetes Metab. Syndr. Clin. Res. Rev.* **2019**, *13*, 2409–2417. [CrossRef]

109. Barrea, L.; Annunziata, G.; Muscogiuri, G.; Di Somma, C.; Laudisio, D.; Maisto, M.; de Alteriis, G.; Tenore, G.C.; Colao, A.; Savastano, S. Trimethylamine-N-Oxide (TMAO) as Novel Potential Biomarker of Early Predictors of Metabolic Syndrome. *Nutrients* **2018**, *10*, 1971. [CrossRef]
110. Mach, F.; Baigent, C.; Catapano, A.L.; Koskina, K.C.; Casula, M.; Badimon, L.; Chapman, M.J.; De Backer, G.G.; Delgado, V.; Ference, B.A.; et al. 2019 ESC/EAS Guidelines for the Management of Dyslipidaemias: Lipid Modification to Reduce Cardiovascular Risk. *Atherosclerosis* **2019**, *290*, 140–205. [CrossRef]
111. Civeira, F.; Arca, M.; Cenarro, A.; Hegele, R.A. A Mechanism-Based Operational Definition and Classification of Hypercholesterolemia. *J. Clin. Lipidol.* **2022**, *16*, 813–821. [CrossRef]
112. Bhatnagar, D.; Soran, H.; Durrington, P.N. Hypercholesterolaemia and Its Management. *BMJ* **2008**, *337*, 503–508. [CrossRef]
113. El-Tantawy, W.H.; Temraz, A. Natural Products for Controlling Hyperlipidemia: Review. *Arch. Physiol. Biochem.* **2019**, *125*, 128–135. [CrossRef]
114. De Ferranti, S.D.; Rodday, A.M.; Mendelson, M.M.; Wong, J.B.; Leslie, L.K.; Sheldrick, R.C. Prevalence of Familial Hypercholesterolemia in the 1999 to 2012 United States National Health and Nutrition Examination Surveys (NHANES). *Circulation* **2016**, *133*, 1067–1072. [CrossRef]
115. Hunter, P.M.; Hegele, R.A. Functional Foods and Dietary Supplements for the Management of Dyslipidaemia. *Nat. Rev. Endocrinol.* **2017**, *13*, 278–288. [CrossRef] [PubMed]
116. Tsai, C.C.; Lin, P.P.; Hsieh, Y.M.; Zhang, Z.Y.; Wu, H.C.; Huang, C.C. Cholesterol-Lowering Potentials of Lactic Acid Bacteria Based on Bile-Salt Hydrolase Activity and Effect of Potent Strains on Cholesterol Metabolism In Vitro and In Vivo. *Sci. World J.* **2014**, *2014*, 690752. [CrossRef] [PubMed]
117. Ma, C.; Zhang, S.; Lu, J.; Zhang, C.; Pang, X.; Lv, J. Screening for Cholesterol-Lowering Probiotics from Lactic Acid Bacteria Isolated from Corn Silage Based on Three Hypothesized Pathways. *Int. J. Mol. Sci.* **2019**, *20*, 2073. [CrossRef] [PubMed]
118. Chiu, H.F.; Fang, C.Y.; Shen, Y.C.; Venkatakrishnan, K.; Wang, C.K. Efficacy of Probiotic Milk Formula on Blood Lipid and Intestinal Function in Mild Hypercholesterolemic Volunteers: A Placebo-Control, Randomized Clinical Trial. *Probiotics Antimicrob. Proteins* **2021**, *13*, 624–632. [CrossRef]
119. Costabile, A.; Buttarazzi, I.; Kolida, S.; Quercia, S.; Baldini, J.; Swann, J.R.; Brigidi, P.; Gibson, G.R. An in Vivo Assessment of the Cholesterol-Lowering Efficacy of *Lactobacillus plantarum* ECGC 13110402 in Normal to Mildly Hypercholesterolaemic Adults. *PLoS ONE* **2017**, *12*, e0187964. [CrossRef]
120. Khongrum, J.; Yingthongchai, P.; Boonyapranai, K.; Wongtanasarasin, W.; Aobchecy, P.; Tateing, S.; Prachansuwan, A.; Sitdhipol, J.; Niwasabutra, K.; Thaveethaptaikul, P.; et al. Safety and Effects of *Lactobacillus paracasei* TISTR 2593 Supplementation on Improving Cholesterol Metabolism and Atherosclerosis-Related Parameters in Subjects with Hypercholesterolemia: A Randomized, Double-Blind, Placebo-Controlled Clinical Trial. *Nutrients* **2023**, *15*, 661. [CrossRef]
121. Ryan, J.J.; Hanes, D.A.; Schafer, M.B.; Mikolai, J.; Zwickey, H. Effect of the Probiotic *Saccharomyces boulardii* on Cholesterol and Lipoprotein Particles in Hypercholesterolemic Adults: A Single-Arm, Open-Label Pilot Study. *J. Altern. Complement. Med.* **2015**, *21*, 288–293. [CrossRef]
122. Martoni, C.J.; Labbe, A.; Ganopolsky, J.G.; Prakash, S.; Jones, M.L. Changes in Bile Acids, FGF-19 and Sterol Absorption in Response to Bile Salt Hydrolase Active *L. reuteri* NCIMB 30242. *Gut Microbes* **2015**, *6*, 57–65. [CrossRef]
123. Ito, M.; Kusuhara, S.; Yokoi, W.; Sato, T.; Ishiki, H.; Miida, S.; Matsui, A.; Nakamori, K.; Nonaka, C.; Miyazaki, K. *Streptococcus thermophilus* Fermented Milk Reduces Serum MDA-LDL and Blood Pressure in Healthy and Mildly Hypercholesterolaemic Adults. *Benef. Microbes* **2017**, *8*, 171–178. [CrossRef]
124. Kumar, M.; Nagpal, R.; Kumar, R.; Hemalatha, R.; Verma, V.; Kumar, A.; Chakraborty, C.; Singh, B.; Marotta, F.; Jain, S. Cholesterol-lowering Probiotics as Potential Biotherapeutics for Metabolic Diseases. *J. Diabetes Res.* **2012**, *2012*, 902917. [CrossRef]
125. Juste, C.; Gérard, P. Cholesterol-to-Coprostanol Conversion by the Gut Microbiota: What We Know, Suspect, and Ignore. *Microorganisms* **2021**, *9*, 1881. [CrossRef] [PubMed]
126. Liong, M.T.; Shah, N.P. Bile Salt Deconjugation and BSH Activity of Five *Bifidobacterial* Strains and Their Cholesterol Co-Precipitating Properties. *Food Res. Int.* **2005**, *38*, 135–142. [CrossRef]
127. Yao, Y.; Hong, Q.; Ding, S.; Cui, J.; Li, W.; Zhang, J.; Sun, Y.; Yu, Y.; Yu, M.; Mi, L. Meta-Analysis of the Effects of Probiotics on Hyperlipidemia. *Curr. Res. Food Sci.* **2024**, *9*, 100885. [CrossRef] [PubMed]
128. Collado, A.; Marques, P.; Domingo, E.; Perello, E.; González-Navarro, H.; Martinez-Hervás, S.; Real, J.T.; Piqueras, L.; Ascaso, J.F.; Sanz, M.J. Novel Immune Features of the Systemic Inflammation Associated with Primary Hypercholesterolemia: Changes in Cytokine/Chemokine Profile, Increased Platelet and Leukocyte Activation. *J. Clin. Med.* **2019**, *8*, 18. [CrossRef]
129. Cristofori, F.; Dargenio, V.N.; Dargenio, C.; Miniello, V.L.; Barone, M.; Francavilla, R. Anti-Inflammatory and Immunomodulatory Effects of Probiotics in Gut Inflammation: A Door to the Body. *Front. Immunol.* **2021**, *12*, 578386. [CrossRef]
130. Malakar, A.K.; Choudhury, D.; Halder, B.; Paul, P.; Uddin, A.; Chakraborty, S. A Review on Coronary Artery Disease, Its Risk Factors, and Therapeutics. *J. Cell Physiol.* **2019**, *234*, 16812–16823. [CrossRef]

131. Moran, A.E.; Oliver, J.T.; Mirzaie, M.; Forouzanfar, M.H.; Chilov, M.; Anderson, L.; Morrison, J.L.; Khan, A.; Zhang, N.; Haynes, N.; et al. Assessing the Global Burden of Ischemic Heart Disease: Part 1: Methods for a Systematic Review of the Global Epidemiology of Ischemic Heart Disease in 1990 and 2010. *Glob. Heart* **2012**, *7*, 315–329. [CrossRef]
132. Nowbar, A.N.; Howard, J.P.; Finegold, J.A.; Asaria, P.; Francis, D.P. 2014 Global Geographic Analysis of Mortality from Ischaemic Heart Disease by Country, Age and Income: Statistics from World Health Organisation and United Nations. *Int. J. Cardiol.* **2014**, *174*, 293–298. [CrossRef]
133. Moludi, J.; Kafil, H.S.; Qaisar, S.A.; Gholizadeh, P.; Alizadeh, M.; Vayghyan, H.J. Effect of Probiotic Supplementation along with Calorie Restriction on Metabolic Endotoxemia, and Inflammation Markers in Coronary Artery Disease Patients: A Double Blind Placebo Controlled Randomized Clinical Trial. *Nutr. J.* **2021**, *20*, 47. [CrossRef]
134. Sun, B.; Ma, T.; Li, Y.; Yang, N.; Li, B.; Zhou, X.; Guo, S.; Zhang, S.; Kwok, L.-Y.; Sun, Z.; et al. *Bifidobacterium lactis* Probio-M8 Adjuvant Treatment Confers Added Benefits to Patients with Coronary Artery Disease via Target Modulation of the Gut-Heart/-Brain Axes. *mSystems* **2022**, *7*, e0010022. [CrossRef]
135. Raygan, F.; Rezavandi, Z.; Bahmani, F.; Ostadmohammadi, V.; Mansournia, M.A.; Tajabadi-Ebrahimi, M.; Borzabadi, S.; Asemi, Z. The Effects of Probiotic Supplementation on Metabolic Status in Type 2 Diabetic Patients with Coronary Heart Disease IRCT2017082733941N5 IRCT. *Diabetol. Metab. Syndr.* **2018**, *10*, 51. [CrossRef] [PubMed]
136. Malik, M.; Suboc, T.M.; Tyagi, S.; Salzman, N.; Wang, J.; Ying, R.; Tanner, M.J.; Kakarla, M.; Baker, J.E.; Widlansky, M.E. *Lactobacillus plantarum* 299v Supplementation Improves Vascular Endothelial Function and Reduces Inflammatory Biomarkers in Men with Stable Coronary Artery Disease. *Circ. Res.* **2018**, *123*, 1091–1102. [CrossRef] [PubMed]
137. Hofeld, B.C.; Puppala, V.K.; Tyagi, S.; Ahn, K.W.; Anger, A.; Jia, S.; Salzman, N.H.; Hessner, M.J.; Widlansky, M.E. *Lactobacillus plantarum* 299v Probiotic Supplementation in Men with Stable Coronary Artery Disease Suppresses Systemic Inflammation. *Sci. Rep.* **2021**, *11*, 3972. [CrossRef] [PubMed]
138. Moludi, J.; Khedmatgozar, H.; Nachvak, S.M.; Abdollahzad, H.; Moradinazar, M.; Tabaei, A.S. The Effects of Co-Administration of Probiotics and Prebiotics on Chronic Inflammation, and Depression Symptoms in Patients with Coronary Artery Diseases: A Randomized Clinical Trial. *Nutr. Neurosci.* **2022**, *25*, 1659–1668. [CrossRef] [PubMed]
139. Vinay, B.C.; Shastry, C.S.; Kodangala, S.; Mateti, U.V.; Bhat, K. Association of Diet and Lipid Profile among Coronary Heart Disease Patients. *Clin. Epidemiol. Glob. Health* **2020**, *8*, 1321–1324. [CrossRef]

nutrients

MDPI

Review

Health-Promoting and Functional Properties of Fermented Milk Beverages with Probiotic Bacteria in the Prevention of Civilization Diseases

Milena Alicja Stachelska [1,*], Piotr Karpiński [1] and Bartosz Kruszewski [2,*]

[1] Faculty of Health Sciences, University of Lomza, Akademicka 14, 18-400 Łomża, Poland; pkarpinski@al.edu.pl
[2] Department of Food Technology and Assessment, Institute of Food Sciences, Warsaw University of Life Sciences—SGGW, Nowoursynowska 159 C, 02-776 Warsaw, Poland
* Correspondence: mstachelska@al.edu.pl (M.A.S.); bartosz_kruszewski@sggw.edu.pl (B.K.)

Abstract: Background/Objectives: There is scattered information in the scientific literature regarding the characterization of probiotic bacteria found in fermented milk beverages and the beneficial effects of probiotic bacteria on human health. Our objective was to gather the available information on the use of probiotic bacteria in the prevention of civilization diseases, with a special focus on the prevention of obesity, diabetes, and cancer. Methods: We carried out a literature review including the following keywords, either individually or collectively: lactic acid bacteria; probiotic bacteria; obesity; lactose intolerance; diabetes; cancer protection; civilization diseases; intestinal microbiota; intestinal pathogens. Results: This review summarizes the current state of knowledge on the use of probiotic bacteria in the prevention of civilization diseases. Probiotic bacteria are a set of living microorganisms that, when administered in adequate amounts, exert a beneficial effect on the health of the host and allow for the renewal of the correct quantitative and qualitative composition of the microbiota. Probiotic bacteria favorably modify the composition of the intestinal microbiota, inhibit the development of intestinal pathogens, prevent constipation, strengthen the immune system, and reduce symptoms of lactose intolerance. As fermented milk beverages are an excellent source of probiotic bacteria, their regular consumption can be a strong point in the prevention of various types of civilization diseases. Conclusions: The presence of lactic acid bacteria, including probiotic bacteria in fermented milk beverages, reduces the incidence of obesity and diabetes and serves as a tool in the prevention of cancer diseases.

Keywords: lactic acid bacteria; probiotic bacteria; obesity; lactose intolerance; diabetes; cancer protection; civilization diseases; intestinal microbiota; intestinal pathogens

1. Introduction

Fermented milk beverages are produced based on lactic acid fermentation, which, at the same time, is a method of milk preservation. The classification of this group of products is based on the type of basic microflora used in the production of fermented milk beverages, which is divided into thermophilic and mesophilic due to the optimal temperature of their growth. The typical thermophilic bacteria are *Lactobacillus delbrueckii* ssp. *bulgaricus* and *Streptococcus salivarius* ssp. *thermophilus*. These are the typical starter microflora used in the production of yogurt. For the production of kefir, in addition to mesophilic bacterial species, yeast is used, and then the production of fermented milk beverages is carried out through mixed lacto-alcohol fermentation [1]. Products formed as a result of lactic fermentation are characterized by a pure sour taste, given by lactic acid, and enriched by the main flavor components in the form of diacetyl and acetaldehyde [2]. When using mixed starters, which contain yeast in addition to lactic fermentation bacteria, used for the production of kefir, the additionally formed ethyl alcohol and carbon dioxide give a specific, slightly sharp, yeasty flavor. Fermented dairy beverages have a special nutritional importance. They are valued not only for their great palatability but also for their unique nutritional, preventive, and medicinal properties [3].

The main dairy products made with pure bacterial cultures include traditional fermented beverages such as yogurt, kefir, acidophilic milk, and new-generation dairy products. The first of them is produced with selected lactic acid bacteria, while the second group uses bacterial strains isolated from the digestive tract of healthy humans, mainly *Bifidobacterium*. Among the new generation of dairy products, bio-yogurts, which are popular in the Polish market, deserve special attention. Both of these groups of dairy products have specific effects on our body [4]. The lactic acid bacteria present in traditional dairy beverages are very sensitive, and most of them die in the digestive tract due to the bactericidal effect of gastric juice. Bacteria introduced with new-generation beverages easily overcome the acidic stomach environment by settling in the mucous membranes of the digestive tract. There, their rapid multiplication takes place, which has an extremely beneficial effect on the state of our internal bacterial flora [5].

Fermented milk beverages are an extremely valuable source of nutrients with high nutritional and biological value. They contain high-quality proteins with a balanced amino acid composition and are also a source of easily digestible calcium, phosphorus, and potassium [6]. These products are characterized by very high digestibility. Bacterial enzymes contained in these products cause the initial digestion of proteins and the release of free amino acids that are essential for our body. The presence of lactic acid contributes to the degradation of the main protein of milk-casein in the form of small particles, which significantly facilitates the digestion process. The digestion of fat also increases as a result of bacterial enzymes. For these reasons, these products are especially recommended for the elderly and people with gastrointestinal ailments. Fermented beverages contain substances with antibacterial properties that inhibit the growth and activity of putrefactive bacteria. In addition, the microorganisms contained in milk contribute to the additional biosynthesis of important vitamins of the B group for our body [7].

The biological value of food is closely related to the nutrient content in the food and its bioavailability. Fermented milk beverages contain similar amounts of nutrients that are in the milk from which they are made. However, due to the processes of lactic fermentation, they are better absorbed by the human body in the digestive process. Milk proteins are broken down into simpler and more easily digested compounds in the form of low-molecular-weight peptides and free amino acids. Lactic acid bacteria produce lipolytic enzymes that break down fats to glycerol and free fatty acids. Lipolysis processes help improve the digestibility of milk fat, which is present in fermented milk beverages [3].

The best source of probiotic bacteria is fermented milk beverages (yogurt, kefir, and acidophilus milk). Probiotic bacteria are primarily used in the dairy industry as starter cultures to carry out acid coagulation, i.e., the formation of curd in the manufacturing of yogurt or kefir. The metabolic products of probiotic microorganisms give fermented milk beverages their health-promoting properties and shape the appropriate organoleptic characteristics. The term "probiotic" comes from the Greek "pro bios", meaning "for life". The current definition of a probiotic is provided by the World Health Organization (WHO). According to it, probiotics constitute specific species that, when provided to humans (or animals) in an appropriate dose, exert a beneficial effect on the organisms. They are well-defined microorganisms that help improve the balance of the microflora inhabiting different areas of the human body and thus have a beneficial health effect. Probiotic microorganisms are lactic acid bacteria, meaning they produce lactic acid and mainly belong to the genera *Lactobacillus* and *Bifidobacterium*. The most important representatives of probiotic bacteria with documented health-promoting properties are *Lactobacillus acidophilus*, *Lacticaseibacillus rhamnosus*, and *Lactobacillus delbrueckii* ssp. *bulgaricus*, *Lactiplantibacillus plantarum*, *Lacticaseibacillus casei* and *Bifidobacterium bifidum* [5].

The probiotic microflora that primarily inhabits our digestive system is constantly being destroyed due to the overuse of antibiotics, consumption of processed foods, acid-forming products, food preservatives, alcohol, and some medications, which can lead to intestinal imbalance. Probiotics, by colonizing and multiplying in our large intestine, ensure the maintenance of the proper balance of intestinal microbiota and the body's natural balance by having a beneficial effect on our digestive tract. The human digestive system is also inhabited by undesirable microorganisms, including pathogenic ones, whereby probiotic bacteria inhabiting our digestive tract in large numbers defend our body from the action of unfavorable bacteria. They inhibit the growth of unfavorable bacteria in the intestine. They produce bacteriostatic substances, as well as bactericidal substances, including lactic acid, which leads to a lowering of the pH in the intestines, and thus, many pathogenic microorganisms are killed. Consumption of more and more highly processed foods (fast food), often containing too much fat and not enough vegetables, is also a factor that adversely modifies the composition of human gut microorganisms. Probiotic bacteria play a huge role in the prevention of civilization diseases and aging and contribute to the overall improvement of human health. Probiotic bacteria favorably modify the composition of the intestinal microbiota, inhibit the development of intestinal pathogens, protect against cancer, lower bad cholesterol, prevent constipation, strengthen the immunological system, decrease the occurrence of obesity, and reduce symptoms of lactose intolerance [8–10].

There is scattered information in the scientific literature regarding the characterization of probiotic bacteria found in fermented milk beverages and their beneficial effects on human health. The objective of this review was to gather available information on the use of probiotic bacteria in the prevention of civilization diseases, with a special focus on the properties of probiotic bacteria in the prevention of obesity, diabetes, and cancer.

2. Modification of the Composition of the Intestinal Microbiota

The term "microbiota" should be understood as all microorganisms, i.e., bacteria, fungi, eukaryotes, and viruses that populate the human body. It is known that up to 1014 different bacteria make up the entire human microbiota. Also, it is known that 70% of the microflora inhabits the large intestine. The role of the microflora relies on protection against infections, digestion of long-chain carbohydrates and dietary fibers, production of short-chain fatty acids and synthesis of vitamins, as well as regulation of the immune response and metabolic balance. Microbiota imbalances are at the root of many diseases, including allergies, diabetes, obesity, inflammatory bowel disease, functional gastrointestinal diseases, neurodegenerative diseases, depression, and autism. Thus, consuming fermented milk beverages containing strains of probiotic bacteria can help prevent many diseases. The intestinal microbiota can be effectively modified through the use of probiotics, prebiotics, and synbiotics.

The results of recent studies have shown that the development of the gut microbiota begins already during prenatal life. Still, intensive colonization of the gastrointestinal tract occurs at the time of delivery, during exposure to bacteria of the birth tract (in the case of natural childbirth), or to bacteria residing in the skin area if delivery is by cesarean section [11]. The mode of feeding during the neonatal period is also important for regulating the composition of the microbiota, with a very significant advantage in the case of natural feeding with breast milk, which, in addition to its nutritional value, contains proteins with antibacterial properties against pathogens, secretory immunoglobulin A, bacteria (in naturally fed children, *Bifidobacterium* and *Lactobacillus* predominate in the gastrointestinal tract) and oligosaccharides with prebiotic effects. The latter promotes the growth of commensal bacteria and prevents the colonization of the gastrointestinal tract by pathogens [12,13]. However, an infant's microbiota is highly unstable and characterized by low microbial diversity.

The physiological role of the microbiota is very broad. It includes protection against gastrointestinal infections, maturation of the immune system, regulation of host metabolic pathways, digestion of long-chain carbohydrates or dietary fiber, as well as the formation of short-chain fatty acids and vitamins [14,15]. However, in light of recent studies, the impact of intestinal microbiota on such functions of the central nervous system as the formation of cognitive functions and basic behavioral patterns, social interactions, or coping with stress should also be emphasized with full emphasis. In view of the important role played by the microbiota, the term "bacterial organ" given to it seems appropriate. This organ is a component of the brain-gut-microbiota axis, which structurally includes the central nervous system, the neuroendocrine and neuroimmune systems, the parasympathetic and sympathetic parts of the autonomic nervous system, the visceral nervous system, and, most importantly, the microbiota. The components of the axis maintain a two-way communication of signal networks; those from the brain affect motility, sensation, and secretion, while visceral signals from the gut exert influence on central functions [16–18].

The term "dysbiosis" refers to disorders in the composition, proportion, and function of the microbes that make up the microbiota. The etiopathogenesis of many diseases is linked to disorders of the microbiota, although in most cases, they are not the sole etiological factor. The specific "pattern" of microbiota disorders attributed to a given disease entity has not been clearly established. However, dysbiosis is known to play a role in the pathogenesis of inflammatory bowel disease (IBD), functional gastrointestinal diseases headed by irritable bowel syndrome, allergic diseases, diabetes and obesity, steatohepatic disease, atherosclerosis, as well as in neurodegenerative diseases, depression, autism, and schizophrenia [19–22]. The most consistent feature accompanying diseases is lower diversity of the microbiota, as it is known that genetic diversity of the microbiome is an important factor affecting the health of the host organism. For many decades, the belief prevailed that the composition and structure of the microbiota in a given host is constant from childhood to old age. In light of the results of modern research, it is known that it can undergo changes, including those going in the direction of dysbiosis, which can be led by a great many factors. They include diet, infectious diseases, the use of antibiotic therapy and drugs such as proton pump inhibitors or non-steroidal anti-inflammatory drugs, and the level of hygiene in a given environment or exposure to stressful situations [23,24].

Recognition of the role of the microbiota in the maintenance of homeostasis and its disorder in the pathogenesis of many diseases has led to tremendous interest in methods of modification. Among the very important methods for modifying the composition of the intestinal microbiota is the use of probiotics and prebiotics. Probiotics are live microorganisms that, when administered in adequate amounts, exert a beneficial health effect on the host body. Prebiotics, per contra, are food elements that are not digested but selectively stimulate the growth or metabolic activity of specific beneficial bacteria in the large intestine and thus have a beneficial effect on human health. Synbiotics consist of probiotics with prebiotics used together. The pursuit of beneficial modification of the intestinal microbiota as a prophylaxis or treatment of many diseases has generated tremendous interest in the potential use of probiotics. The definition of probiotics given above was developed in 2001 and confirmed by the International Scientific Association for Probiotics and Prebiotics (ISAPP) [25].

When selecting the use of a probiotic preparation, it is very important to know the taxonomic identification of microorganisms and to know that each of them should be identified not only by genus and species but also by strain. This is because the properties of probiotics are strictly strain-dependent, and each strain requires separate studies to determine its properties and efficacy in a specific clinical situation. The results of studies conducted on one specific strain and at a specific dose cannot then be extrapolated to other related but untested strains and doses [26,27]. Thus, in characterizing the "ideal" optimal probiotic strain, it should be emphasized that it is of human origin, non-pathogenic, resistant to gastric juice, pancreatic enzymes, and bile acids, survivable and active despite technological and manufacturing processes, able to adhere to intestinal mucosal epithelial cells, antagonistic to pathogens, beneficial to host metabolism and, as emphasized above, clinically tested.

In addition to single-strain probiotic preparations, there are also multi-strain preparations, the clinical effects of which should also be evaluated in a reliable clinical trial since the effects of the joint action of individual strains can be both synergistic and antagonistic [26]. At this point, it should also be mentioned that it is currently impossible to give general rules for the dosage of probiotics, and it is appropriate to apply such a dose that in a reliable study in humans, using the necessary strain for implementation showed a beneficial effect [27]. The mechanisms of action of probiotics are still the subject of research and discussion. It should be noted that it is not possible to consider a single mechanism of action common to all probiotic strains. ISAAP experts have distinguished three main directions of probiotic activity: (1) mechanisms that are common and shared by many types of probiotics, such as the production of short-chain fatty acids; (2) common mechanisms shared by individual species, such as the metabolism of bile acid salts; and (3) rare mechanisms specific only to individual strains (e.g., production of bioactive factors, endocrine and neurogenic effects, effects on the immune response) [26].

Clinically effective, i.e., beneficial modification of the microbiota with probiotics in the light of evidence-based medicine, as shown by analysis of randomized trials or their meta-analysis in recent years, has been shown to treat acute infectious diarrhea in children and (according to the World Gastroenterology Organization [WGO]) also in adults, reducing diarrhea by one day [26–28] and preventing diarrhea associated with antibiotic use in both adults and children [29,30]. In the latter indication, the role of *Saccharomyces boulardii* and *Lactobacillus* GG is best documented [31–33]. For diarrhea caused by *Clostridium difficile* infection, which accounts for up to 25% of antibiotic-associated diarrhea episodes, the results of several meta-analyses have shown that the prophylactic use of probiotics (evaluated together) reduces the risk of diarrhea caused by this infection, with an emphasis on probiotic use within the first 2 days of antibiotic therapy [34,35].

Among the potentially effective strains are *Bifidobacterium infantis* 35,624 and *L. plantarum* 299v, and in children, *Lactobacillus* GG [36–38]. Probiotic therapy has been evaluated in clinical trials among patients with IBD. While their efficacy in Crohn's disease has not been confirmed, in moderate and mild forms of ulcerative colitis, the addition of probiotics can achieve a faster response and maintain remission than conventional therapy alone. Beneficial effects have also been obtained in moderate intestinal reservoir inflammation after colectomy and prevention of recurrence of this inflammation [39]. According to the Food and Drug Administration (FDA), which has granted probiotics "generally recognized as safe" (GRAS, generally recognized as safe) status, they are safe and well tolerated. In European Union countries, probiotics have been granted "qualified presumption of safety" (QPS) status. However, caution in administration and consideration of the appropriateness of use should be exercised in patients with immunodeficiencies, in severe clinical conditions, and treated in intensive care units.

3. Reducing the Risk of Obesity

Obesity is a disease that results from excessive body fat (the body's natural store of excess energy stored in it). Thus, it is a chronic disease with no tendency to subside on its own. Its occurrence in the modern world is steadily increasing, and it affects children, adolescents, and adults alike. It has been shown that fermented milk products can be utilized as adjuvant care in order to decrease total cholesterol, LDL cholesterol, and triglycerides in the blood. Yogurt may significantly contribute to the reduction of weight because it contains probiotics, has a high protein and calcium content, and has a low glycemic index [9]. There are many reasons for the occurrence of obesity, but the most common causes are environmental factors, including excess food intake and too little physical activity. Endocrine, metabolic, and psychological disorders (such as depression) and genetic factors are also among the causes. However, all of these factors provide no explanation for the magnitude of disorders affecting human metabolism. Increasingly, the scientific world is paying attention to the involvement of the microbiota in metabolic and energy disorders. Ongoing research has already established the role of the intestinal microbiota in the process of digestion and obtaining energy from food. It is known that gut bacteria are proven to be responsible for the growth as well as differentiation of intestinal epithelium, fermentation of undigested nutrients, synthesis of B vitamins and vitamin K as well as amino acids (such as lysine and threonine), metabolism of dietary cholesterol and bile acids, and absorption of micronutrients [40].

However, the question still remains as to what composition of bacteria in the gastrointestinal tract protects it and what promotes metabolic disorders. Indeed, each person has its own unique diversity of the intestinal microbiota ecosystem. This ecosystem includes about 1000 phylotypes (weighing 1–1.5 kg), which constitute different taxonomic units: strains, species, and genera. Previous experimental studies to assess the trophic function of the microbiota have been conducted on gnotobiotic germ-free (free of detectable microorganisms and parasites) mice. Transplantation of gut bacteria from obese mice or from obese individuals resulted in rapid obesity and insulin resistance in germ-free mice [41]. This is explained by more efficient absorption of energy from food under the influence of the transplanted microbiota and a higher content of energy-rich short-chain fatty acids in their digestive tract [42]. One study has shown that some bacterial strains have the ability to synthesize glycoside hydrolases, enzymes necessary to break down plant polysaccharides previously considered impossible to digest in the human body (such as insoluble fiber). This process can increase the energy amount provided to the host by 80–200 kcal (i.e., 4–10% of 24-h energy) [40]. It has also been found that through hydrolysis and fermentation of short-chain fatty acids (propionic acid, acetic acid, and butyric acid) and following their absorption, microbiota can increase the host's energy intake by 150 kcal/day. Based on other studies, it has been shown that short-chain fatty acids can affect host appetite through the Gpr41 receptor, GLP-1 secretion, and the FFAR2 receptor. It also alters intestinal passage time or energy recovery and utilization, and this translates into increased human energy balance [43]. Fatty acid SCFAs also affect G proteins produced by gut endocrine cells, which stimulate the release of the molecular appetite controllers GLP-1 (glucagon-like peptide-1) and peptide YY. Peptide YY is a hormone that has been of particular interest to researchers in recent years. This is because it decreases intestinal motility and slows intestinal passage, and thus may increase nutrient absorption time and the delivery of energy value to the host [44].

Information that the intestinal microbiota is differentiated in slim and obese people has prompted research into the use of targeted bacterial genera and strains for the prevention and treatment of obesity and comorbidities. The genera *Lactobacillus* and *Bifidobacterium*, in particular, have been shown to have beneficial effects in this regard. This is because they reduce the intensity of inflammation in the intestine, improve the efficiency of the intestinal barrier, and reduce, as well as, what is most important, maintain reduced body weight. *Bifidobacterium* has been found to increase the expression of genes encoding the proteins of tight junctions between enterocytes [45,46]. In contrast, *Lactobacillus* has been found to reduce visceral fat and adipocyte size [47–49], improve insulin sensitivity, affect leptin secretion and the synthesis of fatty acids, as well as inhibit lipoprotein lipase activity [50,51]. In an intervention study, a probiotic containing *Lactobacillus gasseri SBT2055* was administered to patients for 12 weeks. In overweight patients, it caused a significant reduction in their body weight, as well as a reduction in subcutaneous and visceral fat, BMI (body mass index), waist and hip circumference, and on top of that, adiponectin levels increased in their blood [52]. Obese patients, on the other hand, achieved reductions in weight, BMI, waist and hip circumference, and body fat [53]. Meanwhile, in a randomized, double-blind study, a strain of *L. rhamnosus CGMCC1.3724* was administered to obese women and resulted in a reduction in body weight, body fat, and serum leptin levels [54].

People who drank the most whole-fat yogurt were significantly less prone to develop metabolic syndrome components such as abdominal obesity, hypertriglyceridemia, low HDL cholesterol, high blood pressure, and high fasting plasma glucose, according to Babio et al. [55]. Yogurt consumption was strongly associated with a lower chance of gaining weight, according to a study that examined three large cohorts of people for up to 20 years and included 120,877 obese men and women free of chronic conditions at the start of the trial. The authors concluded that the bacteria that live in the digestive tract could be responsible for observed variations in weight [9]. The promising therapeutic effects of probiotic yogurt consumption in humans in the treatment of obesity are presented in Table 1.

Prebiotics should also be considered in the therapy of conditions such as overweight and obesity. Their primary function is to selectively stimulate the growth and activity of selected types of intestinal microbiota. In experiments on animal models, prebiotics, i.e., inulin and fructooligosaccharides, stimulated the growth of *Bifidobacteria*, *Bacteroidetes*, *Prevotella*, and *Roseburia* and decreased the population of *Firmicutes* [56,57]. In contrast, after inulin was used for 3 months in obese women, beneficial changes in the intestinal ecosystem were observed in the form of an increase in *Bifidobacterium* and *Faecalibacterium prausnitzii* and a decrease in *Bacteroidetes* and *Propionibacterium*. Probiotics administration usually has positive effects on reducing weight in people. However, some studies have shown contrasting results. Different *Lactobacillus* species are connected with various effects on weight modification that are host-specific. *L. acidophilus* administration resulted in significant weight gain in humans and animals (SMD 0.15; 95% confidence intervals 0.05–0.25). Results were consistent in humans and animals. *Lactobacillus fermentum* and *Lactobacillus ingluviei* were associated with weight gain in animals. *L. plantarum* was associated with weight loss in animals, and *L. gasseri* was associated with weight loss both in obese humans and in animals [58]. What is more, ready-for-consumption remedial food containing probiotic organisms gave similar results for weight gain and the treatment of malnutrition compared to conventional remedial food without probiotics. As an effect, early shaping of gut microbiota composition through the management of probiotics presumably results in raised weight gain [59].

Table 1. Promising therapeutic effects of probiotics consumption in the treatment of human obesity.

Activity	Effect	References
Reduction of body weight	In an intervention study, a probiotic containing *L. gasseri SBT2055* was administered to patients for 12 weeks. In overweight patients, it caused a significant reduction in their body weight, as well as a reduction in subcutaneous and visceral fat, BMI, waist and hip circumference, and on top of that, adiponectin levels increased in their blood.	[52]
Reduction of body weight	Obese patients achieved reductions in weight, BMI, waist and hip circumference, and body fat.	[53]
Reduction of body weight	The strain of *L. rhamnosus* CGMCC1.3724 was administered to obese women and caused a reduction of body weight, body fat, and serum leptin levels.	[54]
Prevention of abdominal obesity and accompanying symptoms	Drinking whole-fat yogurt significantly decreased the risk of development of metabolic syndrome factors like abdominal obesity, high blood pressure, hypertriglyceridemia, high fasting plasma glucose, or low HDL cholesterol.	[55]
Prevention of gaining weight	Yogurt drinking was strongly associated with a lower possibility of increasing weight in people not exceeding 20 years with obesity but without chronic conditions at the start of the tests.	[9]
Weight loss in overweight and obese populations	Consumption of probiotics or synbiotics can cause significant weight decreases, either by maintaining usual lifestyle habits or together with energy restriction and/or enhanced physical activity for a period of 12 weeks. Strains within the genera *Lactobacillus* and *Bifidobacterium* were the most utilized and exhibited the best results in reducing body weight.	[60]
Reduction of body weight	Results showed that the probiotic supplementation was significantly effective in reducing weight. Better effects on BW occurred when the duration of supplementation was higher than 8 weeks and on obese persons. BMI was significantly impacted as well in participants with metabolic syndrome and when the supplementation period lasted for more than 12 weeks.	[61]
No significant effect of probiotics on weight and BMI after bariatric surgery (BS)	The possibility of probiotics usage as an accompaniment to bariatric surgery (BS) is disputable. Results showed a statistically significant difference during probiotics consumption in the decrease in waist circumference at 12 months after BS. However, probiotics were not effective in weight and BMI both within 3 months and at 12 months postoperation. Probiotics help people with morbid obesity in order to achieve waist circumference improvement after BS, with no impact on weight and BMI.	[62]
No significant effects on birth weight or weight gain during pregnancy and infancy	Probiotics and synbiotics did not demonstrate any profitable result on weight and BMI in pregnant women by 6.6×10^5–6.6×10^{10} CFU/day of probiotics during 1–25 weeks and 1×10^9–112.5×10^9 CFU/capsule of synbiotics during 4–8 weeks. The result of biotics on weight and BMI in the case of infants was non-significant. Prebiotics and probiotics used in infancy were from 0.15 to 0.8 g/dL and 2×10^6–6×10^9 CFU/day for 2–24 weeks, respectively. They had no significant effects on birth weight or weight gain during pregnancy and infancy.	[63]
Significant weight gain as well as weight loss in humans and animals	*L. acidophilus* management emerged in meaningful weight gain in both humans and animals. Effects were coherent in humans and animals. *L. fermentum* and *L. ingluviei* were connected with weight gain in animals. *L. plantarum* was connected with weight loss in animals. *L. gasseri* was linked with weight loss in all subjects.	[58]
Weight gain in children with malnutrition, weight loss in people with obesity	Revised knowledge about the capacity of specific probiotics to gain energy from the host diet might introduce the development of new therapies for obesity and malnutrition. Probiotics and antibiotics contribute to weight gain or weight loss in human beings. Ready-to-use remedial food led to weight gain in children and limited the commonness of malnutrition.	[59]

In other studies, prebiotics improved appetite control by affecting the stimulation of GLP-1 and peptide YY secretion and reducing the production of ghrelin, thus contributing to the reduction of body weight, adipocyte size, and the amount of adipose tissue. Moreover, they counteracted the accumulation of fatty acids in the liver, which may prevent liver steatosis [64,65]. In contrast, in obese women with dyslipidemia, the use of oligofructose for 120 days reduced body weight, BMI, and waist circumference and lowered serum total cholesterol and LDL fractions [66]. Prebiotics (oligofructose, arabi-noxylose) have also been credited with reducing intestinal inflammation, improving intestinal barrier integrity, stimulating GLP-2 secretion, and improving glucose tolerance [67]. Both probiotics and synbiotics have the prospective implications of aiding in weight reduction for overweight and obese populations [60]. The findings demonstrated that probiotic supplementation was significantly effective in decreasing weight [61]. It seems that probiotic products could have beneficial effects as an adjunct therapy for the care and management of obesity when used in high doses [68]. Another study demonstrates that oral probiotics supplementation can be a complementary treatment for improving the fitness of postmenopausal women with overweight and obesity [69]. Probiotics are effective in generating body weight loss in patients who are overweight or obese with connected metabolic diseases [70–72]. However, more quality clinical studies are needed to confirm the efficacy and safety of probiotics and address a number of practical issues before the routine clinical use of probiotics in adults with obesity undergoing BS [62]. Some studies showed that probiotics and synbiotics did not demonstrate any beneficial effect on weight and body mass index (BMI) in pregnant women by 6.6×10^5–6.6×10^{10} CFU/day of probiotics during 1–25 weeks and 1×10^9–112.5×10^9 CFU/capsule of synbiotics during 4–8 weeks. The effect of biotics on weight and BMI in infants was predominantly non-significant. Prebiotics and probiotics used in infancy were from 0.15 to 0.8 g/dL and 2×10^6–6×10^9 CFU/day for 2–24 weeks, respectively. They had no significant effects on birth weight or weight gain during pregnancy and infancy [63]. In the treatment of obesity and metabolic disorders, it is worthwhile to use probiotics or live bacteria, which have beneficial effects on human health. They should provide a diverse, well-functioning gut microbiota, which is supposed to support optimal recovery of energy from food and its proper storage in the body. It is also supposed to increase the efficiency of the gut barrier, thereby decreasing internal endotoxemia.

4. Reducing Symptoms of Lactose Intolerance

Lactose is a disaccharide containing the monosaccharides glucose and galactose. Lactose occurs naturally and almost exclusively in milk from mammals, where it is the main carbohydrate and is often referred to as "milk sugar". The average lactose content of cow's milk is about 4.5%. Lactose can be hydrolyzed to glucose and galactose (its constituent monosaccharides) under the action of the enzyme ß-galactosidase (lactase). Lactose intolerance is an abnormal reaction of the human body after consuming products that contain lactose. It can be caused by a deficiency or complete absence of the digestive enzyme lactase, which breaks down lactose into simple sugars: glucose and galactose. If there is not enough of this enzyme in the human body, then non digested lactose ferments in the large intestine under the influence of bacteria. This, in turn, causes the formation of acids and gases that cause unpleasant digestive discomfort. People who suffer from lactose intolerance experience stomach problems when they drink milk or consume milk products because they do not produce enough lactase amount in their small intestines to digest the milk sugar, which is lactose [73]. Fortunately, many studies have demonstrated that people who do not tolerate lactose can consume fermented milk products like yogurt, kefir, or acidophilic milk. Lactic acid bacteria contained in fermented milk beverages are able to produce lactase, which breaks down lactose in the digestive system. Studies have shown that probiotics such as *Lactobacillus* spp., *B. longum*, and *B. animalis* possess a beneficial influence on people suffering from lactose intolerance when they consume a probiotic yogurt comprising *L. acidophilus* and *Bifidobacterium* spp. [74]. Another study proved that probiotic yogurt supplemented with *L. acidophilus* and *Bifidobacterium* spp. may significantly decrease lactose intolerance symptoms. This means that the consumption of probiotic yogurt may serve as the therapy of choice for lactose intolerance in patients [75]. Low levels of the enzyme lactase cause lactose intolerance, which makes it difficult to digest lactose contained in dairy products. Yogurt has less lactose than non-fermented milk because lactic acid bacteria used as a bacterial starter for yogurt production digests some amount of lactose, so its level in yogurt is lower compared to milk that is not fermented [76].

Symptoms of lactose intolerance occur when the ability to break down lactose to galactose and glucose is reduced, most often due to reduced lactase activity in the small intestine. Depending on the cause, four main types of lactose intolerance can be distinguished: primary, secondary, congenital, and developmental [77]. Secondary lactose intolerance is attributable to a partial, rarely complete decrease in lactase activity in the course of diseases, leading to damage to the small intestinal mucosa or a reduction in its surface area. Congenital lactose intolerance is extremely rare. The underlying cause of the disease is a complete or almost complete lack of the ability to synthesize lactase. Developmental lactose intolerance results from immaturity of the small intestinal mucosa and occurs in premature infants born before 34 weeks of gestation. The most frequently met form of lactose intolerance is primary lactose intolerance (adult-type hypolactasia), which is inherited in an autosomal recessive manner and, in the Caucasian population, is associated with a C/T polymorphism of the lactase gene [78,79]. Both the age at which lactase activity is reduced and the prevalence of lactose intolerance in adulthood depends on ethnicity. It is worth noting that in a certain percentage of people, lactase activity remains relatively high throughout life.

The lactose content of dairy products varies and depends mainly on how they are produced. Dairy products produced by fermentation contain less lactose, which is a substrate for bacteria. As a result of their action, lactose is transformed into lactic acid as well as other substances (e.g., diacetyl, acetic acid, ethanol, carbon dioxide), giving dairy products their characteristic sensory properties. It is important to try to include low-lactose dairy products with a high calcium content in the diet of a person with lactose intolerance. Such products include hard cheese and molded cheese, as well as fermented milk beverages. It is worth noting that the lactose content of hard cheeses is inversely proportional to their ripening time. Lactose tolerance depends on many factors, including how and when dairy products are consumed. A specific portion of lactose consumed at one time may produce significant clinical symptoms while spreading it over several meals, and especially consumed in the company of other products, may lead to leveling or even disappearance of clinical symptoms. The degree of lactose tolerance also depends on the rate of gastric emptying and passage time through the small intestine [80].

It is well known that people with lactose intolerance can consume fermented dairy products better than dairy products that are not fermented with lactic acid bacteria. The concentration of lactose before the fermentation process in the mixture used to prepare yogurt, depending on the additives used, is about 6%. One of the changes that occurs as a result of fermentation is a 20–30% reduction in lactose content. It is broken down by lactase, produced by bacterial microflora. However, the final change in lactose content may not be as significant when powdered milk is used as an additive in yogurt. Other factors are also important. The same amount of lactose contained in yogurt is better tolerated than in milk. Bacteria included in the microflora of yogurt, such as *L. bulgaricus* or *S.*

thermophilus, produce lactase, increase the pool of its activity in the intestine, and thus support the digestion of lactose. Products containing live bacterial cultures are therefore recommended. Lactase is relatively resistant to environmental factors. However, heating yogurt significantly reduces its activity. Thus, heat-treated yogurts are less beneficial for people with lactose intolerance. The increased tolerance of lactose consumed with yogurt may also be explained by a direct increase in lactase activity in the small intestine. Animal studies indicate that lactic acid bacteria can induce lactase activity in intestinal epithelial cells. The supply of a lactic-fermented beverage to mice has been shown to stimulate the regeneration of intestinal villi, as well as an increase in lactase activity [81]. The management of probiotics was efficient at improving adult lactose intolerance, and it is expected that the results of this study could help improve the nutritional status of adults by increasing their consumption of milk and dairy products in the future [82]. Lactose-free dairy products could be recommended as alternatives for the alleviation of lactose intolerance and for the promotion of human health and wellness [83]. Another study also demonstrated that the consumption of ice cream containing high or low concentrations of *B. bifidum* 900,791 improves lactose tolerance in hypolactasic subjects [84]. Accumulating evidence has indicated that probiotic bacteria present in milk products can be used to reduce the clinical signs of lactose intolerance [74,85]. Another study highlighted the importance of selected probiotics and vitamin B6 to alleviate symptoms and gut dysbiosis in lactose-intolerant patients with persistent functional gastrointestinal symptoms [86]. However, there are some limitations regarding the wide heterogeneity between the studies examining the effect of probiotics consumption on reducing the symptoms of lactose intolerance [87]. The promising therapeutic influence of probiotic yogurt intake to reduce symptoms of lactose intolerance is presented in Table 2.

Table 2. Promising therapeutic effects of probiotic yogurt consumption in decreasing signs of lactose intolerance.

Subject	Effect	References
Human	The studies have shown that probiotics such as *Lactobacillus* spp., *Bifidobacterium longum*, and *Bifidobacterium animalis* possessed profitable influence on people suffering from lactose intolerance when they consumed a yoghurt including *L. acidophilus* and *B. bifidum*.	[74]
Human	The study proved that yogurt containing *L. acidophilus* and *Bifidobacterium* spp. is capable of significantly decreasing lactose intolerance symptoms. This means that the consumption of probiotic yogurt may serve as the treatment for lactose intolerance in patients.	[75]
Human	Bacteria included in the microflora of yogurt, such as *L. bulgaricus* or *S. thermophilus*, produce lactase, increase the pool of its activity in the intestine, and thus support the digestion of lactose.	[80]
Mice	The supply of a lactic-fermented beverage to mice has been shown to stimulate the regeneration of intestinal villi, as well as an increase in lactase activity.	[81]
Human	The study showed that probiotic management mitigated the symptoms of lactose intolerance.	[82]
Human	Probiotics and fermented milk products influence the metabolic work of colonic microbiota and may diminish the symptoms of lactose intolerance.	[83]
Human	This study demonstrated that the consumption of ice creams with the application of *B. bifidum* 900,791 at high and low levels has improved lactose tolerance in hypolactasic persons.	[84]
Human	The wide heterogeneity between the research studies is shown in this review. One research study inspects the profits of probiotic and prebiotic supplementation, which is why additional clinical trials should be carried out in order to gather more evidence.	[87]

5. Reducing the Risk of Diabetes

Dairy products, especially fermented milk beverages, constitute a great origin of vitamins, calcium, phosphorus, magnesium, vitamin D, and some fatty acids. It is proved that the consumption of milk products is connected with a decreased occurrence of type 2 diabetes [88]. A special role in the prevention of type 2 diabetes is played by probiotic yogurt intake. Everyday yogurt consumption can also reduce the risk of the incidence of type 2 diabetes and cardiovascular disease [89,90]. It is well known that probiotic bacteria in fermented milk can reduce inflammation or promote insulin effectiveness. Moreover, the consumption of probiotic yogurt may reduce the intestinal flora imbalance and help patients with chronic liver disease experience. Subjects in the tested group consumed three times per day for 2 weeks probiotic yogurt with *B. bifidum*, *L. acidophilus*, *L. delbrueckii* subsp. *bulgaricus*, and *S. thermophilus*. Such treatment of patients successfully reduced liver conditions, particularly in diabetes [91]. The research proved that because of the probiotic yogurt with high nutritional characteristics and low glycemic index, yogurt may help treat diabetes [92].

Insulin resistance and type II diabetes are the most common disorders of carbohydrate metabolism in the world. They are associated with abnormal production of the hormone insulin by the pancreas or lack of tissue sensitivity to it. In Poland, an average of 2 million people have diabetes, but about 25% of sufferers are undiagnosed. According to the Central Statistical Office, 5073 people died of diabetes in 2018 and 10,834 in 2022 [93]. The data show an upward trend in deaths despite the widely used pharmacotherapy for diabetes. Many clinical studies suggest a positive effect of probiotic therapy in slowing the progress of resistance insulin and, thus, type II diabetes [94].

Moreover, scientific reports suggest that probiotic therapy may offset the negative effects of pharmacotherapy, commonly used during type II diabetes. Insulin is a secretory hormone of the β cells of the pancreatic islets (Langerhans). It is composed of proinsulin (insulin precursor), which is composed of amino acid chains A, B, and C. Insulin secretion in the body occurs continuously. Its highest concentration is recorded in the morning hours. Glucose increases insulin production. Rapid insulin secretion from β-cells occurs when blood glucose levels rise suddenly [95].

Reduced sensitivity of tissues to insulin (insulin resistance) results in the inability of glucose isolated by meal consumption to be absorbed into tissues in combination with insulin. Specific glucose transporters (GLUTs), which are located on the surface of peripheral tissues, do not catch the presence of insulin, which impedes the absorption of glucose into cells. This condition leads to hyperglycemia [96]. It results in the relentless production of insulin, causing pancreatic β-cell hypertrophy.

In the long term, this situation can lead to their death, leading to type II diabetes. Proper insulin function is also dependent on hormones. Excessive insulin secretion activates the secretion of factor IGF-1, which is produced under the influence of growth hormone. The activity shown prevents hypoglycemia caused by excessive insulin secretion. This hormone inhibits insulin secretion and synthesis of glycogen in the liver, as well as increases the uptake of circulating glucose in the peripheral blood [97]. Glucagon, glucocorticosteroids, and catecholamines also act synergistically with insulin, inhibiting insulin secretion and glucose synthesis [98]. Insulin resistance is a metabolic disorder in which pathological sensitivity of adipocytes (adipose tissue cells) and cardiomyocytes (cardiac muscle cells) to insulin is observed [97]. It results from impaired working and alarming of insulin receptors, elevated levels of insulin-binding antibodies, or incorrect structure of the insulin molecule. The main factor in the onset of insulin resistance is obesity. It is also found that the risk of this metabolic disorder increases with age [99,100].

Insulin resistance is a condition that premises the onset of type II diabetes. The disorder is characterized by excessive insulin secretion by pancreatic β cells, leading to hyperinsulinemia. This condition is compounded by a diet that is rich in fats and carbohydrates. If pancreatic β-cells are damaged, insulin is no longer produced by them, resulting in the development of a prediabetic state and subsequent type II diabetes. In the course of insulin resistance, as a rule, pharmacotherapy is not used. A patient with this disorder should change his eating habits and lifestyle. Weight reduction, increased physical activity, and the introduction of a low glycemic index diet are recommended. Reducing the energy supply of the diet may be more effective with the help of synbiotic supplementation. They affect the hormones adiponectin and leptin. These hormones are produced by so-called white adipose tissue. Adiponectin acts to increase insulin sensitivity. It also has anti-inflammatory properties that affect weight reduction or minimize the risk of type II diabetes. Leptin reduces hunger and affects insulin secretion in the pancreas. In obesity, which often occurs along with insulin resistance, the action of the aforementioned hormones can be affected [101].

Excessively high levels of leptin in the blood can cause tissue resistance to its action, resulting in excessive appetite and weight gain [102]. Noormohammadi et al. carried out a comprehensive analysis that looked at whether synbiotics affect the levels of the aforementioned hormones. They found that synbiotics can reduce blood leptin levels by decreasing its release by adipocytes, as well as indirect activation of peroxisome proliferator-activated receptor (PPAR), which reduces food intake and leads to weight reduction. This effect reduces tissue sensitivity to insulin. In addition, probiotic bacteria of the genera *Lactobacillus* and *Bifidobacterium* reduce the hydrolysis of leptin in the colon, which increases its concentration. Too high a concentration of leptin affects the activation of oxytocin in the hypothalamus. Activation of oxytocin and its long-term elevated concentration increases leptin resistance, which is very often observed among obese patients. Probiotic bacteria, such as *Lactobacillus reuteri*, have been shown to increase oxytocin production, leading to improved regulation of its homeostasis and affecting weight normalization [101].

Adiponectin has anti-inflammatory, antiatherosclerotic, and anti-diabetic effects. Its elevated levels in the body improve tissue sensitivity to insulin. Kim et al. [103] demonstrated that a strain of *L. rhamnosus* GG administered to mice for 13 weeks increased adiponectin production and activated the adenosine monophosphate-activated protein kinase (AMP-activated protein kinase or AMPK) signaling pathway and thus improved tissue sensitivity to insulin. On the other hand, Raji et al. [104] proved that adiponectin levels in overweight or obese women increased after synbiotic therapy and a low-calorie diet.

An interesting study was conducted at the University of Cambridge. The scientists tested whether a typical Western diet, characterized by high-fat products, while supported by probiotics, can affect the occurrence of syndromes, including resistance to insulin. To this end, the study group consumed a high-fat diet along with a probiotic containing the bacterial species *L. casei*. The control group did not consume the probiotic. The results obtained support the thesis that changing the composition of the intestinal microbiota effectively inhibits the appearance of immunity to insulin in human beings [105].

It was found that despite the consumption of a high fat diet, fasting blood glucose remained in the typical range in the group of people consuming the probiotics. In addition, probiotic therapy with *L. casei* did not cause cellular resistance to insulin despite the subjects' consumption of about 270 g of fat per day. Conclusions were drawn that supporting a typically Western diet with probiotics may reduce the possibility of insulin resistance. However, such an intervention should not replace changes in dietary habits in overweight or obese individuals, and probiotic therapy may be a supportive element in changing dietary habits [105].

Type II diabetes is a consequence of insulin resistance. It is characterized by hyperglycemia that results from a defect in insulin secretion. The pathogenesis of type II diabetes centers on insufficient insulin production by pancreatic β cells. The disease most often affects people over the age of 40 and is more common in overweight individuals than in normal-weight individuals [94,106]. Risk factors that influence the development of type II diabetes, in addition to obesity and overweight, include genetic predisposition, low physical activity, hypertension, elevated HDL cholesterol and triglycerides, and in women, a history of gestational diabetes and polycystic ovary syndrome. Individuals diagnosed with fasting glucose levels indicative of pre-diabetes should be introduced to appropriate physical exercises together with dietary treatment to affect weight reduction. Scientific reports suggest the effect of probiotics on reducing the risk of type II diabetes. Zhang et al. tested the effect of *L. casei* bacteria on the influx of chloride ions to reduce susceptibility to diabetes. The mouse study confirmed that high chloride ion concentrations in the pancreas are necessary for β-cell cell membrane activity and insulin release from the cells [107].

However, some studies have revealed that probiotic consumption has not contributed to a significant health effect in the treatment of diabetes. The study assessed the effectiveness of probiotics on glycemic control in type 2 diabetes patients. 16-week probiotic supplementation (25 mL of beverage containing over 10^8 CFU/mL of *Lactobacillus*, four times per day) resulted in no profitable effects on glycemic control, profile of lipids, as well as weight [108].

The examples of therapeutic effects of probiotics intake in reducing the risk of diabetes are presented in Table 3.

Table 3. Promising therapeutic effects of probiotics consumption in decreasing the occurrence of diabetes.

Subject	Effect	References
Human	The intervention group of 40 subjects consumed probiotic yogurt with *B. bifidum*, *L. acidophilus*, *L. delbrueckii* subsp. *bulgaricus*, and *S. thermophilus* three times per day for 14 days. Such treatment of patients successfully lowered liver symptoms, particularly in diabetes.	[91]
Human	The research proved that because of the probiotic yogurt's high nutritional content and low glycemic index, yogurt may help treat diabetes.	[92]
Human	Many clinical studies suggest a positive effect of probiotic therapy in slowing the progress of insulin resistance and, thus, type II diabetes.	[94]
Human	Probiotic bacteria, such as *L. reuteri*, have been shown to increase oxytocin production, leading to improved regulation of its homeostasis and affecting weight normalization.	[101]
Mice	*L. rhamnosus* GG administered to mice for 13 weeks increased adiponectin production and activated the AMP-activated protein kinase (AMPK) signaling pathway, thus improving tissue sensitivity to insulin.	[103]
Human	Adiponectin amount in overweight or obese women studied rose after synbiotic therapy and a low-calorie diet.	[104]
Human	To this end, the study group consumed a high-fat diet along with a probiotic containing the bacterial species *L. casei*. The control group did not consume the probiotic. The results obtained support the thesis that changing the composition of the intestinal microbiota effectively inhibits the progress of insulin resistance in humans.	[105]
Human	Ingestion of *L. casei* bacteria in the form of a probiotic causes an influx of chloride ions, which possess an inhibitory influence on the occurrence of type II diabetes.	[107]
Human	*Lb. rhamnosus*, *Lactobacillus paracasei*, *Lb. plantarum* and *Bifidobacterium* species were mentioned in many clinical studies providing facts about their anti-diabetic influence. However, anti-diabetic supplements are at the stage of clinical trials, so there is no such product on the market at the moment.	[109]

Table 3. *Cont.*

Subject	Effect	References
Human	The usage of hypoglycemic drugs has some limitations and side effects, while probiotics are recognized as safe, economical, and effective. Probiotics, through their good application prospects in the remodeling of intestinal microecological health, are becoming a hot topic of diabetes prevention and treatment.	[110]
Human	The study showed that *L. paracasei* HII01 has a role as an adjuvant treatment in type 2 diabetes by improving hyperglycemia and inflammatory markers. *L. paracasei* positively influences gut microbiota and subsequently improves leaky gut and endotoxemia.	[111]
Mice	The study showed that *L. paracasei* IMC 502 transforms short-chain fatty acids and next increases the secretion of downstream hormones with beneficial outcomes in the gut microbiome.	[112]
Mice	Fourteen probiotic bacteria were identified from fermented camel milk. Blood glucose and lipid parameters were significantly improved, as well as the morphological changes of the pancreas, liver, and kidney.	[113]
Mice	*L. plantarum* HAC01 reduced hyperglycemia and type 2 diabetes mellitus by regulating glucose metabolism in the liver, protecting the islet β-cell mass, and restoring the gut microbiota. *L. plantarum* HAC01 may thus be an effective therapeutic agent for type 2 diabetes mellitus.	[114]
Human	The results of the study suggest that *L. plantarum* Y15 may serve as a potential agent for ameliorating type 2 diabetes through the regulation of the expression rate of genes responsible for pathways of increasing inflammation and insulin.	[115]
Human	The study assessed the effectiveness of probiotics on glycemic control in type 2 diabetes patients. 16-week probiotic supplementation (25 mL of beverage containing over 10^8 CFU/mL of Lactobacillus, four times per day) resulted in no profitable effects on glycemic control, profile of lipids, as well as weight.	[108]

The effect of *L. casei* bacteria causes the release of lipopolysaccharides into the blood through a mechanism that regulates chloride production [107]. Kupffer cells, located in the liver, are composed of a chloride channel coupled to glycine. Glycine is an amino acid classified as a glycine receptor agonist. Their activation affects, among other things, Kupffer cells by reducing their sensitivity to pro-inflammatory factors (TNF-alpha). Ingestion of *L. casei* bacteria in the form of a probiotic causes an influx of chloride ions, which have an inhibitory effect on the development of type II diabetes. The authors focus attention on the fact that the loss of chloride ions in tissues, which affects the pathogenesis of type II diabetes, may also be related to comorbidities in the course of diabetes, such as insulin sensitivity, myotonia, and kidney stones [107]. Overweight and obesity directly affect the risk of insulin resistance. In turn, insulin resistance is the first step toward the development of type II diabetes. Proper prevention and use of probiotics may lead to health benefits.

The risk of insulin resistance among obese patients who consume a typical high-fat diet can be minimized by probiotic therapy with *L. casei*. These bacteria have a protective effect on the onset of cellular resistance to insulin. Increased appetite can be influenced by concentrations of leptin, the satiety hormone, that are too high. In turn, concentrations that are too high influence the increase in food consumption, leading to obesity and, consequently, immunity to insulin. In patients already diagnosed, it is worthwhile to use probiotic therapy with *Lactobacillus* and *Bifidobacterium*, which reduce the hydrolysis of leptin in the colon, which lowers the leptin concentration. In addition, the *L. rhamnosus* GG strain increases adiponectin levels, which can improve tissue sensitivity to insulin.

In patients at risk of developing type II diabetes, it is recommended to include probiotic therapy with *L. casei*. The consumption of metformin affects the gastrointestinal tract by decreasing the amount of these bacteria. In turn, pharmacotherapy with drugs from the α-glucosidase inhibitor group can cause a decrease in the number of bacteria from the *Firmicutes* cluster. The disturbed ratio causes dysbiosis manifested by diarrhea. In patients treated with α-glucosidase inhibitors, it is worth introducing probiotic therapy recommended for diarrhea. These strains include *L. rhamnosus* GG and *S. boulardii* [107]. Diabetes cannot be completely cured. However, there are various methods to control diabetes. A promising strategy is the use of probiotics for diabetes intervention [109]. As a potential new intervention target for the treatment of diabetes, probiotics may participate in the regulation of energy metabolism through various mechanisms, namely, reducing chronic low-grade inflammation, regulating intestinal flora, reducing oxidative stress, increasing bacterial bioactive peptides and improving insulin resistance, to achieve the purpose of regulating blood glucose. Probiotics are considered economical and safe alternatives to treat chronic diseases and improve human health [110]. The administration of *L. paracasei* HII01 was shown to be effective in the improvement of metabolic variables in diabetes [111]. Another study showed that *L. paracasei* IMC 502 significantly decreased blood glucose and lipid levels, improved insulin resistance and glucose intolerance, and repaired pancreatic and hepatic tissue damage. This probiotic conferred beneficial outcomes in the gut microbiome of diabetic mice, which induced the transformation of short-chain fatty acids (SCFAs), further enhanced the secretion of downstream hormones, and ultimately ameliorated the inflammatory response [112]. Probiotics significantly improved blood glucose and blood lipid parameters, as well as the morphological changes of the pancreas, liver, and kidney in diabetic mice [113]. One of the important incretins in the improvement of diabetes is glucagon-like peptide (GLP-1), which is secreted by the gut and reduces the apoptosis of pancreatic β-cells and improves insulin sensitivity. The study showed that probiotics and resveratrol significantly decreased ($p < 0.001$) glucose and insulin resistance and increased ($p < 0.001$) GLP1 and total antioxidant capacity compared to the diabetic group. Treatment with probiotics and resveratrol also returned intestinal histological changes in diabetic rats to normal [116]. The consumption of probiotics could be a useful intervention to improve cardiometabolic outcomes through reduced inflammation and oxidative stress in patients with prediabetes and type 2 diabetes [117–119]. The study showed that *L. plantarum* HAC01 was efficient in treating hyperglycemia and type 2 diabetes mellitus in mice with high-fat diets and streptozotocin-induced diabetes [114]. *L. plantarum* Y15 administration to type 2 diabetes mice could improve the biochemical indexes related to diabetes and reduce the production of pro-inflammatory cytokines. *L. plantarum* Y15 administration could reshape the structure of gut microbiota. *L. plantarum* Y15 administration could also regulate the expression levels of the inflammation and insulin signaling pathway-related genes [115]. The results of many studies suggested that probiotics may serve as potential agents for ameliorating type 2 diabetes [120–126].

6. Inhibition of the Growth of Intestinal Pathogens

Probiotics are living microorganisms that constitute the natural human intestinal microbiota and ensure its homeostasis. They have the ability to adhere to the intestinal epithelium, colonize the intestine, and antagonize the action of typical pathogens of the gastrointestinal tract. At the same time, they do not exhibit toxic and pathogenic effects on the host organism. Probiotic properties are possessed by strains of lactic acid bacteria, such as *Bifidobacterium*, *Lactobacillus*, *Enterococcus*, *Propionibacterium*, *Lactococcus*, *Saccharomyces*, *Bifidus* or *Streptococcus salivarius*, and the yeast *S. boulardii*. In the gastrointestinal tract, they have the ability to inhibit the growth of pathogenic bacteria through the production of organic acids and hydrogen peroxide and by a competitive mechanism of microbial adhesion to the intestinal epithelium. Organic acids formed in the gastrointestinal tract during the metabolism of probiotics, such as pyroglutamic acid, inhibit the growth of

Gram-negative bacteria, such as *Pseudomonas* and *Enterobacter*. In turn, hydroxyl radicals produced by *Lactobacillus lactis* inhibit the growth of *Staphylococcus aureus*. In addition, the acidification of intestinal contents by probiotics inhibits the growth of certain pathogenic bacteria.

In the lumen of the digestive tract, probiotics compete with other microorganisms for nutrients; probiotics consuming simple sugars inhibit the growth of *C. difficile*. In the digestive tract, they also increase the secretion of mucins, which are glycoproteins that have a protective effect in intestinal infections. Such an effect has been proven for the *L. acidophilus*. In the gastrointestinal tract, probiotics are characterized by a very wide range of actions. At the cellular level, their involvement in increasing the phagocytic activity of macrophages and lymphocytes and activating natural cytotoxic cells is highlighted [127].

Numerous clinical trials are currently being conducted to determine the beneficial effects of probiotics in conditions such as bacterial infectious diarrhea, viral infectious diarrhea, post-antibiotic diarrhea, and "traveler's" diarrhea. Acute infectious diarrhea causes about 5% of hospitalizations of children in Poland. Their cause is most often rotavirus or adenovirus, less often bacteria such as *Salmonella*, *Shigella*, *Yersinia*, *E. coli*, or parasites such as *Giardia* [128,129]. There have been a number of studies that show that the supply of certain probiotics can shorten the duration of diarrhea. Isolauri et al. [130] showed that *Lactobacillus* GG significantly reduces the duration of rotavirus diarrhea, while Majama et al. [131] compared the effectiveness of their treatment with different types of lactic acid bacteria. The duration of diarrhea in patients receiving *Lactobacillus* GG was 1.8 days, significantly shorter than those receiving *L. rhamnosus* (2.8 days) and *S. thermophilus* (2.6 days). Another probiotic showing a beneficial effect on the duration of diarrhea in children was *L. reuteri* [132].

Saavedra et al. [133], on the other hand, showed the beneficial effects of *B. bifidum* and *S. thermophilus* in preventing rotavirus diarrhea in infants. Their incidence was significantly lower in infants receiving probiotics (7%) than in the placebo group (35%). Diarrhea associated with antibiotic use occurs in about 11–40% of pediatric patients [134] and depends on the type of antibiotic used (the highest risk is with beta-lactam antibiotics). The cause of post-antibiotic diarrhea is the regrouping of the intestinal microbiota and the compounds it synthesizes. As a result, there is an excessive accumulation of undesirable microorganisms, such as *C. difficile*, *Clostridium perfringens*, and *Staphylococcus aureus* [129]. Avrola et al. [135] demonstrated that the incidence of post-antibiotic diarrhea diminished twofold in children receiving a preparation containing *Lactobacillus* GG ($n = 61$) compared to the group receiving placebo ($n = 58$). Vanderhoof et al. [136] described an even greater protective potential of probiotics. Incidents of diarrhea in the children studied, thanks to the supply of *Lactobacillus* GG, occurred more than three times less often in comparison to the control group ($n = 188$). In contrast, Piątkowska et al. [137] showed that supplementation with *Saccharomyces boulardi* reduced the risk of diarrhea in children by more than 10%. Similar results regarding the use of *Saccharomyces boulardi* in children were obtained by Kotowska et al. [138]. Szamański et al. [139] proved that the supply of *B. longum*, *L. rhamnosus*, and *L. plantarum* to patients aged 5 months to 16 years has an effect on reducing the number of stools per day.

The modulation of the gut microbiota through reshaping host–microbiota interactions can be achieved with strategies such as probiotics and personalized nutrition as adjunctive therapy. Pathogenic microorganisms alter the homeostasis of the gut microbiota, leading to an increased risk of related diseases. Probiotics inhibit these pathogens by stimulating epithelial barrier function, secreting anti-microbial components, competitively excluding pathogens by binding sites, and limiting their access to nutrients [140]. Many studies implied that a small number of genetic mutations or even a single-nucleotide variant in the microbial genome could significantly alter the pathogenic behavior of gut bacteria and affect host health. The study demonstrated that probiotic consumption can lead to widespread single-nucleotide variants in the native microbiota. The study substantially extended the understanding of the co-evolution of the probiotics and the indigenous gut microbiota, highlighting the importance of assessment of probiotics efficacy and safety in an integrated manner [141]. The study showed that probiotics can interact with pathogens in foods and in the hosts. Probiotics use different mechanisms to control enteric pathogen colonization. They are able to produce organic acids, bacteriocins, and hydrogen peroxide, which have an inhibitory effect on the growth of many pathogens in the gut [142]. The promising therapeutic effects of probiotic yogurt consumption in the inhibition of the growth of intestinal pathogens are presented in Table 4.

Table 4. Promising therapeutic effects of probiotic yogurt consumption in the inhibition of the growth of intestinal pathogens in humans.

No.	Effect	References
1	*Lactobacillus GG* significantly shortens the length of rotavirus diarrhea.	[130]
2	The duration of diarrhea in patients receiving *Lactobacillus GG* was 1.8 days, significantly shorter than those receiving *L. casei rhamnosus* (2.8 days) and *S. thermophilus* (2.6 days).	[131]
3	The study showed the beneficial effects of *B. bifidum* and *S. thermophilus* in preventing rotavirus diarrhea in infants. Their incidence was significantly lower in infants receiving probiotics (7%) than in the *placebo* group (35%).	[133]
4	Incidents of diarrhea in the children studied, thanks to the supply of *Lactobacillus GG*, occurred more than three times less often compared to the control group.	[135]
5	Supplementation with *Saccharomyces boulardi* reduced the risk of diarrhea in children by more than 10%.	[137]
6	The supply of *B. longum*, *L. rhamnosus*, and *L. plantarum* to patients aged 5 months to 16 years has an effect on reducing the number of stools per day.	[139]
7	The review showed that pathogenic microorganisms alter the homeostasis of the gut microbiota, leading to an increased risk of related diseases. The study demonstrated that probiotics inhibit these pathogens by stimulating epithelial barrier function, secreting anti-microbial components, competitively excluding pathogens by binding sites, and limiting their access to nutrients.	[140]
8	The article demonstrated that even a small number of genetic mutations or even a single-nucleotide variant in the microbial genome can significantly alter the pathogenic behavior of gut bacteria and affect host health. The study highlighted that probiotic consumption can significantly impede the proliferation of intestinal pathogenic bacteria.	[141]
9	The study showed that probiotics can interact with pathogens in foods and in the hosts. They are able to produce organic acids, bacteriocins, and hydrogen peroxide, which have an inhibitory effect on the growth of many pathogens in the gut.	[142]

7. Protection Against Cancer

The composition of the gut microflora remains dependent on various factors, such as age, dietary habits, physical activity levels, drug treatment, and surgical procedures. The intestinal microbiota contributes to the process of cancer formation. Intestinal dysbiosis, or microflora imbalance, is otherwise known as qualitative and quantitative changes in the intestinal microbiota, which are observed in cancer. Increased amounts of *Fusobacterium nucleatum*, *Bacteroides fragilis*, *Enterococcus faecalis*, *Streptococcus bovis*, and *Peptostreptococcus anaerobius* have been reported in colon cancer patients. Studies show that the abundance of several specific bacteria, such as *Lactobacillus*, *Escherichia*, *Shigella*, *Nitrospirae*, *Burkholderia fungorum*, and *Lachnospiraceae*, is increased in patients with gastric cancer.

The main bacterial clusters residing in the human gastrointestinal tract are *Firmicutes* (64%), *Bacteroidetes* (23%), *Proteobacteria* (8%), and *Actinobacteria* (3%) [143]. The environment of the gastrointestinal tract and its conditions are variable, so the type and density of individual microorganisms depend on the location [144]. The composition of the microbiota varies depending on the gastrointestinal tract section. The oral cavity is dominated by bacteria, including *Streptococcus*, *Peptococcus*, *Staphylococcus*, *Bifidobacterium*, *Lactobacillus*, and *Fusobacterium* [145]. The stomach has an acidic pH, which means that there can be few microorganisms capable of surviving in such an environment, such as *Helicobacter pylori* and *L. plantarum* 299v. The small intestine is dominated by Gram-positive and Gram-negative anaerobic bacteria. In contrast, the large intestine is a place where numerous bacteria can thrive, and Gram-negative aerobic bacteria predominate [144].

Intestinal dysbiosis is defined as a disorder in the quantitative and qualitative composition of the gastrointestinal microbiota [144]. These disorders can contribute to a number of diseases, including inflammatory bowel disease (Crohn's disease, ulcerative colitis), chronic kidney disease, and gastrointestinal cancers. The carcinogenic activity of the intestinal microbiota is associated with negative metabolic transformations induced by intestinal microorganisms. As a result of these transformations, toxic, mutagenic, and carcinogenic substances can be formed [145]. The gastric microbiota is mainly composed of bacteria: *Firmicutes*, *Bacteroidetes*, *Fusobacteria*, *Actinobacteria*, and *Proteobacteria* [146]. Increased amounts of *Lactobacillus*, *Escherichia*, *Shigella*, *Nitrospirae*, *Burkholderia fungorum*, and *Lachnospiraceae* are observed in patients with gastric cancer [145,146].

The pathogenesis of colorectal cancer also includes disturbances in the composition and activity of the intestinal microbiota. Bacteria involved in the carcinogenesis of colorectal cancer are *Fusobacterium nucleatum*, *B. fragilis*, *Escherichia coli*, *Enterococcus faecalis*, *S. bovis*, and *Pept. anaerobius*. The effect of individual bacteria as carcinogens varies. For example, a major part of the enterotoxigenic pathogenicity of *B. fragilis* (ETBF) is the synthesis of *B. fragilis* toxin (BFT) [147]. This toxin activates signal transducer and activator of transcription 3 (STAT3) proteins. STAT proteins are a family of transcription factors involved in the transduction of extracellular signals and the direct regulation of transcription [147,148]. The function of these proteins is to control the expression of genes involved in cell survival, proliferation, chemoresistance, and angiogenesis. STAT3 protein is a latent cytoplasmic transcription factor activated by cytokines and growth factors, among others. STAT3 protein is involved in the generation of cells responsible for inflammation: Th17. Th17 cells produce IL-17 and activate the transcription factor NF-kB and the Wnt signaling pathway. Abnormalities in the Wnt pathway are observed in many diseases, including but not limited to cancer [149].

Probiotic strains have anti-cancer properties by, among other things, binding carcinogens, inhibiting the activity of bacterial nitroreductases, lowering the concentration of secondary bile acids, and inhibiting the synthesis of fecal enzymes (e.g., p-glucuronidase) [150]. The gastrointestinal microbiota can be modified not only with probiotics but also with prebiotics and synbiotics [151]. Prebiotics stimulate the growth or activity of one or a specific number of bacterial genera in the colon and benefit the health of the host [152,153]. Prebiotics include inulin, lactulose, and fructooligosaccharides, among others. It should be noted that prebiotics provide a medium for probiotics and stimulate their growth, but unlike them, they do not have microorganisms in their composition [152]. Synbiotics exert a beneficial effect on the gastrointestinal microbiota by stimulating probiotics with prebiotics and impeding the proliferation of pathogenic bacteria. Synbiotics inactivate nitrosamines and carcinogens [152].

Today, colorectal cancer is the third most common cancer worldwide. Etiopathogenesis includes genetic and environmental factors, such as a poor diet (with high saturated fatty acids, consumption of red meat, and low dietary fiber intake) and a sedentary lifestyle [154]. Most colorectal cancers are sporadic and not genetically determined. Familial polyposis syndrome and Lynch syndrome (hereditary colorectal cancer unrelated to polyposis) account for 5% of all cases. Genetic disorders, usually inherited in an autosomal dominant manner, contribute to the growth of such kinds of cancer [154,155].

Counteracting colorectal cancer includes chemoprevention and screening, so-called screening tests [154]. Vitamins may have a potential chemopreventive effect. So far, regular consumption of acetylsalicylic acid has been shown to reduce the risk of developing adenomas and colorectal cancer. However, acetylsalicylic acid increases the incidence of gastrointestinal bleeding and hemorrhagic stroke [155]. Chemopreventive factors also include a diet with little red meat and plenty of vegetables, fruits, and dietary fiber. Probiotic strains can also be used in the control of colorectal cancer [154]. In the in vitro studies, probiotics have been observed to exhibit a number of anti-cancer properties, including inactivation of mutagens and carcinogens, lowering of intestinal pH, inhibition of tyrosine kinase pathway activity, immunomodulation and modification of the gastrointestinal microbiota [156].

In an animal model study, *Ligilactobacillus salivarius* strain UCC118 was shown to reduce levels of enterococci and *C. perfringens* [157]. It should be noted that *C. perfringens* does not infect healthy cells but produces toxins and extracellular enzymes responsible for pathogenicity. To date, 20 *C. perfringens* toxins have been described, which can be divided into four main categories: cell membrane-damaging, pore-forming, intracellular toxins, and hydrolytic enzymes. Strains of *C. perfringens* are divided into five subtypes: A-E. However, subtype A is the most common cause of food poisoning [158]. On the other hand, a study by Horie et al. [159] reported that a mixture of pro-biotic strains (*Streptococcus faecalis, Clostridium butyricum, Bacillus mesentericus*) reduced the formation of DNA adducts in the colonic epithelium.

The *L. plantarum* strain reduces the enzymatic activity of different bacteria and the concentration of bile acids in feces. *L. rhamnosus* 231 reduces the activity of fecal nitroreductase, nitroreductase, and glutathione S-transferase. It also causes an increase in glutathione reductase activity. *L. acidophilus* KFRI342 reduces fecal *Escherichia coli*, glucuronidase, and glucosidase, as well as triglyceride levels [160]. In vitro studies have also confirmed the antinociceptive effects of synbiotics and prebiotics. A synbiotic containing *Bifidobacterium lactis* and resistant starch exerts a pro-apoptotic effect in response to a carcinogen. In vivo studies also confirm the antitumor activity of probiotics [156]. The probiotic strain *S. boulardii* prevents epidermal growth factor (EGF)-induced proliferation and enhances apoptosis in vitro and in vivo. In contrast, the *Bifidobacterium polyfermenticus* strain inhibits ErbB2 and ErbB3 activity [161]. ErbB2 is a trans-membrane receptor tyrosine kinase encoded by a gene located in chromosomal region 17q12. Overexpression of ErbB2 and ErbB3 plays an important role in oncogenesis [162].

Clinical studies with patients have shown that probiotics administered in the preoperative period, as well as during chemotherapy, reduced treatment side effects and modified the gastrointestinal microbiota. In a study by Hattak et al. [163], it was observed that the administration of a probiotic mixture (*L. rhamnosus* LC705, *Propionibacterium freudenreichii* ssp. *shermanii* JS) reduced glucosidase activity and modified the gastrointestinal microbiota. In an animal model study, Jacouton et al. [164] showed that *L. casei* strain BL23 prevents the development of colorectal cancer, as it has immunomodulatory properties (reduces anti-inflammatory interleukin-IL-22) and has antiproliferative effect by regulating caspases (7 and 9) and the pro-apoptotic protein Bik.

The other study highlights the pivotal role of probiotics in preventing and alleviating colon cancer. Probiotics are able to use the diverse mechanisms through which they contribute to mitigating colon cancer, including inhibiting cell proliferation and promoting apoptosis, enhancing the immune response, regulating the intestinal microbiota and their metabolic processes, strengthening the intestinal barrier, and boosting antioxidant effects. Probiotics themselves exhibit anticancer activity, and the metabolites they produce, such as bacteriocins and short-chain fatty acids, possess the capacity to inhibit colon cancer [165]. Probiotics have shown promising anticancer effects, which, combined with their ability to fight the side effects of synthetic drugs, may provide potentially useful treatments in the future. The studies at the cellular level revealed the occurrence of apoptosis under the effect of the probiotic mix. Collectively, the experimental data show that probiotics have the ability to efficiently fight cancer proliferation. Further studies should reveal their efficiency in vivo and eventually in clinical settings [166]. Daily consumption of the probiotic *L. casei* strain was shown to impair tumor growth. This effect could be attributed to the production of Th1 immunostimulatory cytokines and secretion of chemoattractant molecules in tumor tissue, accompanied by a migration of cytotoxic T cells in the tumor [167]. Treatment with *L. coryniformis* MXJ32 could significantly inhibit the total number of tumors and the average tumor diameter [168]. The effects of the probiotic mixture on proliferation and metastasis of mouse colon cancer CT26 cells were assessed by probiotics and cells co-culture assay, Cell Counting Kit-8 assay, colony formation assay, wound-healing assay, as well as migration and invasion assays. The probiotic mixture significantly inhibited the proliferation, invasion, and migration ability of CT26 cells compared to the control cells [169]. The promising therapeutic effects of probiotics administration in the protection against cancer are presented in Table 5.

However, some studies have revealed that probiotics consumption has not contributed to a significant health effect in the treatment of cancer. Although probiotics have shown success in preventing the development of experimental colitis-associated colorectal cancer (CRC), the beneficial effects of interventional treatment are relatively unknown. The study showed that interventional treatment with VSL#3 probiotics alters the luminal and mucosally adherent microbiota but does not protect against inflammation or tumorigenesis in mouse models [170]. Evidence from in vitro and animal studies supports the potential chemopreventive properties of prebiotics and probiotics. However, human studies using pro and prebiotics have not provided consistent results in support of their efficacy in preventing cancer. More randomized controlled human trials need to be conducted with a wide range of populations with stringent controls. These control measures are difficult because genetics and immune response potential are varied throughout the population [171].

Table 5. Promising therapeutic effects of probiotics administration in the protection against cancer.

Subject	Effect	References
Human	Probiotic strains have anti-cancer properties by, among other things, binding carcinogens, inhibiting the activity of bacterial nitroreductases, lowering the concentration of secondary bile acids, and inhibiting the synthesis of fecal enzymes (e.g., β glucuronidase).	[150]
Human	*B. lactis* and resistant starch exert a pro-apoptotic effect in response to a carcinogen. In vivo studies also confirm the antitumor activity of probiotics.	[156]
Human	Administration of a probiotic mixture (*L. rhamnosus* LC705, *Propionibacterium freudenreichii* sp. *shermanii* JS) reduced glucosidase activity and modified the gastrointestinal microbiota.	[163]

Table 5. *Cont.*

Subject	Effect	References
Mice	In an animal model study, Jacouton et al. showed that *L. casei* strain BL23 prevents the development of colorectal cancer, as it has immunomodulatory properties (reduces anti-inflammatory interleukin-IL-22) and has an antiproliferative effect by regulating caspases (7 and 9) and the pro-apoptotic protein Bik.	[164]
Human	The other study highlights the pivotal role of probiotics in preventing and alleviating colon cancer. Probiotics themselves exhibit anticancer activity, and the metabolites they produce, such as bacteriocins and short-chain fatty acids, possess the capacity to inhibit colon cancer.	[165]
In vitro study	Probiotics have shown promising anticancer effects, which, combined with their ability to fight the side effects of synthetic drugs, may provide potentially useful treatments in the future. The studies at the cellular level revealed the occurrence of apoptosis under the effect of the probiotic mix.	[166]
Mice	Daily consumption of the probiotic *L. casei* strain was shown to impair tumor growth. This effect could be attributed to the production of Th1 immunostimulatory cytokines and secretion of chemoattractant molecules in tumor tissue, accompanied by a migration of cytotoxic T cells in the tumor. However, due to the limitations of pre-clinical mouse models, caution should be taken when interpreting these findings for clinical application; further work in that direction is needed.	[167]
Mice	Treatment with *L. coryniformis* MXJ32 could significantly inhibit the total number of tumors and the average tumor diameter. This probiotic administration prevented the damage to intestinal barrier function by enhancing the expression of tight junction proteins (Occludin, Claudin-1, and ZO-1) and recovering the loss of goblet cells.	[168]
Mice	Colorectal cancer (CRC) is one of the most common cancers, and supplementation of probiotics may be a promising intervention method. *Lactiplantibacillus plantarum* KX041 could significantly inhibit inflammation and tumor formation and induce tumor cell apoptosis.	[172]
Mice	The study showed that interventional treatment with VSL#3 probiotics alters the luminal and mucosally adherent microbiota but does not protect against inflammation or tumorigenesis in mouse models.	[170]
In vitro study	Evidence from in vitro and animal studies supports the potential chemopreventive properties of prebiotics and probiotics. However, human studies using pro and prebiotics have not provided consistent results in support of their efficacy in preventing cancer.	[171]

Probiotics have applications not only at the stage of cancer prevention but also can significantly improve the results of standard anticancer treatment. In addition, they reduce the side effects of enteral feeding, and with long-term probiotic therapy, they can potentially improve the nutritional status of the patient. Probiotic strains also have an immunomodulatory effect, influencing the immune system, and in patients in the postoperative period, they reduce the risk of infection.

8. The Efficacy of Probiotic Therapy in the Eradication of *Helicobacter pylori* Infection

Probiotic strains have also been tried for the treatment of peptic ulcer disease, in whose pathogenesis the role of *H. pylori* is well known and documented. Indeed, more and more effective treatment regimens are still being sought. Currently, the most commonly used is a three-drug therapy consisting of a proton pump inhibitor and two antibiotics [129,137,173]. Numerous studies have been conducted to test the efficacy of probiotics in both inhibiting the growth of *H. pylori* and reducing side effects associated with eradication treatment (Table 6). However, the results of clinical trials evaluating the efficacy of probiotics in *H. pylori* eradication are inconclusive. However, the role of probiotics in reducing the incidence of side effects associated with the treatment of the infection is well documented [174]. In a study conducted by Czerwionka-Szaflarska et al. [173], it was proven that the supply of probiotics during *H. pylori* eradication therapy statistically reduces the number of symptoms, such as abdominal pain, nausea, and vomiting, compared to the group not receiving the probiotic ($n = 60$). A study by Sykora et al. [175] using a placebo confirmed the efficacy of *L. casei* in reducing the incidence of side effects of eradication therapy (excluding loose stools) in study patients ($n = 86$). Nista et al. [176] showed that a probiotic preparation containing *Bacillus clausii* significantly reduced the frequency and severity of nausea, abdominal pain, and loose stools as adverse impacts of *H. pylori* removal treatment in patients ($n = 120$).

The efficacy of probiotic therapy in the eradication treatment of *H. pylori* infection has also been confirmed, particularly emphasizing the improved tolerability of treatment due to the lower risk of side effects of the combined antibiotic combination. However, specific probiotic strains should only be selected on the basis of demonstrated clinical efficacy. The best-documented effect has been shown for *S. boulardii* [177]. Modification of the microbiota through the use of probiotics is also a therapeutic pathway in functional diseases, especially irritable bowel syndrome (IBS). In patients with this syndrome, there was a reduction in the severity of symptoms, bloating sensation, and frequency of intestinal gas evacuation as a result of probiotic therapy [178]. The authors suggest the need to administer probiotics in patients with IBS not only "more than 7 days" but at least 4 weeks [179].

However, the most important species responsible for the formation of gastric cancer is *H. pylori*. Gastric cancer is the fifth most common cancer worldwide. The incidence of this cancer is declining, but it remains a relatively common cause of death in Poland, the United States, and Japan [174]. The first-order carcinogen is the bacterium described above, *H. pylori*. There are many different classifications of gastric cancer. Clinically, gastric cancer can be divided into early gastric cancer (EGC) and advanced gastric cancer (AGC). However, the most useful histological division includes two types: Lauren 1 and Lauren 2. It is worth noting that the histological type of cancer is important for the patient's prognosis [180].

H. pylori causes inflammation of the mucosa, mucosal atrophy, and, consequently, the development of gastric cancer. There are several therapeutic methods that can be successfully used to change the composition and activity of the intestinal microbiota. One of them is the administration of probiotic strains, prebiotics, and synbiotics. Probiotics can be administered to prevent the development of gastric and colorectal cancer, which has been shown in many in vivo and in vitro studies. Probiotics reduce the incidence of diarrhea associated with enteral feeding. Probiotic bacterial strains can be included as adjunctive therapy in the treatment of *H. pylori* infection. Probiotics reduce the incidence of postoperative infections, abdominal pain, and radiation diarrhea. This means that probiotics can be used to prevent the development of cancer and can significantly improve the effectiveness of standard cancer therapy [181].

However, *H. pylori* (a Gram-negative, microaerophilic, spiral- or sigmoid-shaped bacillus) is the main pathogenic bacterium responsible for the formation of gastric cancer [176]. Its length is about 2.5–5 pm, and its width is about 0.5–1 pm. It shows the ability to move due to the presence of cilia arranged in a polar pattern. Approximately 70% of people from developing countries and about 30% of people in developed countries are infected with this bacterium [182]. *H. pylori* is one of the main contributors to gastritis and duodenal ulcers [183].

In counteracting gastric cancer, *Helicobacter pylori* eradication is particularly important. A study by Namkin et al. [184] evaluated the efficacy of *S. boulardii* CNCM I-745 in the eradication of *H. pylori* in children. The subjects ($n = 28$) were divided into two groups; the first received the probiotic at a dose of 250 mg/day for one month, and the control group received a placebo. There was no statistically significant difference in achieving eradication between the study groups. Another study observed that oral supplementation of *S. boulardii* CNCM I-745 at a dose of 250 mg, two times/day for 2 weeks, reduced the incidence of diarrhea, an adverse influence of standard removal treatment [185]. Similar results were obtained in a systematic review and meta-analysis by Szajewska et al. [186]. Probiotic strains *L. reuteri* and *L. gasseri*, in combination with proton pump inhibitors, increase the eradication speed of *H. pylori* [186]. The results of a meta-analysis by Tong et al. [187] involving 14 studies also confirmed that probiotics are effective in increasing this rate. Previous studies show that probiotic strains cannot be used as the sole eradication agent, but they are an adjunctive therapy during standard treatment and reduce the side effects of antibiotic therapy [188].

Table 6. Promising therapeutic effects of probiotics in the eradication of *H. pylori* infection.

No.	Effect	References
1	The supply of probiotics during *H. pylori* eradication therapy statistically reduces the number of symptoms, such as abdominal pain, nausea, and vomiting, compared to the group not receiving the probiotic.	[173]
2	The probiotic preparation containing *Bacillus clausii* significantly reduced the frequency and severity of nausea, abdominal pain, and loose stools, which are side effects of *H. pylori* eradication therapy in patients.	[176]
3	Probiotic bacterial strains can be included as adjunctive therapy in the treatment of *H. pylori* infection. Probiotics reduce the incidence of postoperative infections, abdominal pain, and radiation diarrhea. This means that probiotics can be used to prevent the development of cancer and can significantly improve the effectiveness of standard cancer therapy.	[186]
4	Probiotic strains *L. reuteri* and *L. gasseri*, in combination with proton pump inhibitors, increase the eradication rate of *H. pylori*.	[187]

9. Conclusions

Fermented milk beverages are a very important food category in the structure of the Polish diet. They have health-promoting effects on the human body. The scientific studies cited in this article confirm the health-promoting benefits associated with the consumption of fermented milk beverages. The presence of lactic acid bacteria, including probiotic bacteria in yogurts and kefirs, supports the maintenance of immunity, reduces the incidence of obesity and diabetes, and serves as a weapon in the prevention of cancer. The consumption of fermented milk beverages containing probiotic bacteria, therefore, contributes to the overall improvement of human health and is an essential point in preventing the occurrence of civilization diseases. Probiotic bacteria regulate the immune system, maintain the integrity of the intestinal epithelium, protect the host body from pathogens, and produce a number of metabolites that possess a beneficial influence on human health. Fermented milk drinks are one of the richest sources of probiotic bacteria, which is why it is so important to consume them daily, especially in the context of preventing the development of cancer diseases.

Author Contributions: Conceptualization, M.A.S. and B.K.; methodology, M.A.S. and P.K.; software, B.K.; investigation, M.A.S., B.K. and P.K.; data curation, M.A.S. and P.K.; writing—original draft preparation, M.A.S. and B.K.; writing—review and editing, M.A.S. and B.K.; visualization, P.K. and B.K.; supervision, M.A.S.; project administration, M.A.S.; funding acquisition, M.A.S. All authors have read and agreed to the published version of the manuscript.

Funding: This research received no funding.

Data Availability Statement: This review is based on the reported literature search, with no original data presented.

Conflicts of Interest: The authors declare no conflicts of interest.

References

1. Salama, H.H.; Bhattacharya, S. Advancement of yogurt production technology. In *Advances in Dairy Microbial Products*; Singh, J., Vyas, A., Eds.; Woodhead Publishing: Delhi, India, 2022; pp. 117–131. [CrossRef]
2. Hadjimbei, E.; Botsaris, G.; Chrysostomou, S. Beneficial effects of yoghurts and probiotic fermented milks and their functional food potential. *Foods* **2022**, *11*, 2691. [CrossRef] [PubMed]
3. Dimidi, E.; Cox, S.R.; Rossi, M.; Whelan, K. Fermented foods: Definitions and characteristics, impact on the gut microbiota and effects on gastrointestinal health and disease. *Nutrients* **2019**, *11*, 1806. [CrossRef] [PubMed]
4. Marsh, A.J.; Hill, C.; Ross, R.P.; Cotter, P.D. Fermented beverages with health-promoting potential: Past and future perspectives. *Trends Food Sci. Technol.* **2014**, *38*, 113–124. [CrossRef]
5. Gaba, K.; Anand, S. Incorporation of probiotics and other functional ingredients in dairy fat-rich products: Benefits, challenges, and opportunities. *Dairy* **2023**, *4*, 630–649. [CrossRef]
6. Ravyts, F.; De, V.L.; Leroy, F. Bacterial diversity and functionalities in food fermentations. *Eng. Life Sci.* **2012**, *12*, 356–367. [CrossRef]
7. Markowiak, P.; Śliżewska, K. The role of probiotics, prebiotics and synbiotics in animal nutrition. *Gut Pathog.* **2018**, *10*, 21–30. [CrossRef] [PubMed]
8. Ziaei, R.; Ghavami, A.; Khalesi, S.; Ghiasvand, R.; Mokari, Y. The effect of probiotic fermented milk products on blood lipid concentrations: A systematic review and meta-analysis of randomized controlled trials. *Nutr. Metab. Cardiovasc. Dis.* **2021**, *31*, 997–1015. [CrossRef] [PubMed]
9. Mozaffarian, D.; Hao, T.; Rimm, E.B.; Willett, W.C.; Hu, F.B. Changes in diet and lifestyle and long-term weight gain in women and men. *N. Engl. J. Med.* **2011**, *364*, 2392–2404. [CrossRef]
10. Sen, M. Role of probiotics in health and disease—A review. *Int. J. Adv. Life Sci. Res.* **2019**, *2*, 1–11. [CrossRef]
11. Vargas, M.H.; Del-Razo-Rodríguez, R.; López-García, A.; Lezana-Fernández, J.L.; Chávez, J.; Furuya, M.E.Y.; Marín-Santana, J.C. Effect of oral glycine on the clinical, spirometric and inflammatory status in subjects with cystic fibrosis: A pilot randomized trial. *BMC Pulm. Med.* **2017**, *17*, 206. [CrossRef]
12. Albenberg, L.G.; Wu, G.D. Diet and the intestinal microbiome: Associations, functions, and implications for health and disease. *Gastroenterology* **2014**, *146*, 1564–1572. [CrossRef] [PubMed]
13. Wopereis, H.; Oozeer, R.; Knipping, K.; Belzer, C.; Knol, J. The first thousand days—Intestinal microbiology of early life: Establishinga symbiosis. *Pediatr. Allergy Immunol.* **2014**, *25*, 428–438. [CrossRef] [PubMed]
14. Nishida, A.; Inoue, R.; Inatomi, O.; Bamba, S.; Naito, Y.; Andoh, A. Gut microbiota in the pathogenesis of inflammatory bowel disease. *Clin. J. Gastroenterol.* **2018**, *11*, 1–10. [CrossRef] [PubMed]
15. Donohoe, D.R.; Garge, N.; Zhang, X.; Sun, W.; O'Connell, T.M.; Bunger, M.K.; Bultman, S.J. The microbiome and butyrate regulate energy metabolism and autophagy in the mammalian colon. *Cell Metab.* **2011**, *13*, 517–526. [CrossRef]
16. Mayer, E.A. Gut feelings: The emerging biology of gut-brain communication. *Nat. Rev. Neurosci.* **2011**, *12*, 453–466. [CrossRef]
17. Grenham, S.; Clarke, G.; Cryan, J.F.; Dinan, T.G. Brain-gut-microbe communication in health and disease. *Front. Physiol.* **2011**, *2*, 94. [CrossRef] [PubMed]
18. Montiel-Castro, A.J.; Gonzalez-Cervantes, R.M.; Bravo-Ruiseco, G.; Pacheco-López, G. The microbiota-gut-brain axis: Neurobehavioral correlates, health and sociality. *Front. Integr. Neurosci.* **2013**, *7*, 70. [CrossRef] [PubMed]
19. Dinan, T.G.; Stilling, R.M.; Stanton, C.; Cryan, J.F. Collective unconscious: How gut microbes shape human behavior. *J. Psychiatr. Res.* **2015**, *63*, 1–9. [CrossRef]
20. de Vos, W.M.; de Vos, E.A.J. Role of the intestinal microbiome in health and disease: From correlation to causation. *Nutr. Rev.* **2012**, *70* (Suppl. S1), 845–856. [CrossRef] [PubMed]
21. Lynch, S.V.; Pedersen, O. The human intestinal microbiome in health and disease. *N. Engl. J. Med.* **2016**, *375*, 2369–2379. [CrossRef]
22. Rudzki, L.; Frank, M.; Szulc, A.; Gałęcka, M.; Szachta, P.; Barwinek, D. Od jelit do depresji-rola zaburzeń ciągłości barieryjelitowej i następcza aktywacja układu immunologicznego w zapalnej hipotezie depresji. *Neuropsychiatr. Neuropsychol.* **2012**, *2*, 76–84.
23. Duca, F.A.; Lam, T.K.T. Gut microbiota, nutrient sensing and energy balance. *Diabetes Obes. Metab.* **2014**, *16* (Suppl. S1), 68–76. [CrossRef] [PubMed]
24. Mayer, E.A.; Savidge, T.; Shulman, R.J. Brain-gut microbiome interactions and functional bowel disorders. *Gastroenterology* **2014**, *146*, 1500–1512. [CrossRef]
25. Hill, C.; Guarner, F.; Reid, G.; Gibson, G.R.; Merenstein, D.J.; Pot, B.; Morelli, L.; Canani, R.B.; Flint, H.J.; Salminen, S.; et al. Expert consensus document. The International Scientific Association for Probiotics and Prebiotics consensus statement on thescope and appropriate useof the term probiotic. *Nat. Rev. Gastroenterol. Hepatol.* **2014**, *11*, 506–514. [CrossRef]
26. Szajewska, H. Probiotyki aktualny stan wiedzy i zalecenia dla praktyki klinicznej. *Med. Prakt.* **2017**, *7–8*, 1–10.
27. Floch, M.H.; Walker, W.A.; Guandalini, S.; Hibberd, P.; Gorbach, S.; Surawicz, C.; Sanders, M.E.; Garcia-Tsao, G.; Quigley, E.M.M.; Isolauri, E.; et al. Recommendations for probiotic use—2008. *J. Clin. Gastroenterol.* **2008**, *42* (Suppl. S2), 104–108. [CrossRef]

28. Szajewska, H.; Guarino, A.; Hojsak, I.; Indrio, F.; Kolacek, S.; Shamir, R.; Vandenplas, Y.; Weizman, Z. European Society for Pediatrie Gastroenterology, Hepatology, and Nutrition. Use of probiotics for management of acute gastroenteritis: A position paper by the ESPGHAN Working Group for Probiotics and Prebiotics. *J. Pediatr. Gastroenterol. Nutr.* **2014**, *58*, 531–539. [CrossRef]
29. Riddle, M.S.; DuPont, H.L.; Connor, B.A. ACG Clinical Guideline: Diagnosis, Treatment, and Prevention of Acute Diarrheal Infections in Adults. *Am. J. Gastroenterol.* **2016**, *111*, 602–622. [CrossRef] [PubMed]
30. Szajewska, H.; Canani, R.B.; Guarino, A.; Hojsak, I.; Indrio, F.; Kolacek, S.; Orel, R.; Shamir, R.; Vandenplas, Y.; van Goudoever, J.B.; et al. ESPGHAN Working Group for Probiotics Prebiotics. Probiotics for the prevention of antibiotic- -associated diarrhea in children. *J. Pediatr. Gastroenterol. Nutr.* **2016**, *62*, 495–506. [CrossRef] [PubMed]
31. Szajewska, H.; Kołodziej, M. Systematic review with meta-analysis: *Saccharomyces boulardii* in the prevention of antibiotic-associated diarrhea. *Aliment. Pharmacol. Ther.* **2005**, *42*, 793–801. [CrossRef]
32. Draper, K.; Ley, C.; Parsonnet, J. Probiotic guidelines and physician practice: A cross-sectional survey and overview of the literature. *Benef. Microbes* **2017**, *8*, 507–519. [CrossRef]
33. Szajewska, H.; Kołodziej, M. Systematic review with meta-analysis: *Lactobacillus rhamnosus* GG in the prevention of antibiotic-associated diarrhoea in children and adults. *Aliment. Pharmacol. Ther.* **2015**, *42*, 1149–1157. [CrossRef]
34. Shen, N.T.; Maw, A.; Tmanova, L.L.; Pino, A.; Ancy, K.; Crawfors, C.V.; Simon, M.S.; Evans, A.T. Timely Use of Probiotics in Hospitalized Adults Prevents *Clostridium difficile* Infection: A Systematic Review With Meta-Regression Analysis. *Gastroenterology* **2017**, *152*, 1889–1900.e9. [CrossRef]
35. Lau, C.S.; Chamberlain, R.S. Probiotics are effective at preventing *Clostridium difficile*-associated diarrhea: A systematic review and meta-analysis. *Int. J. Gen. Med.* **2016**, *9*, 27–37. [CrossRef]
36. Whorwell, P.I.; Altringer, L.; Morel, J.; Bond, Y.; Chabonneau, D.; O'Mahony, L.; Kiely, B.; Shanahan, F.; Quigley, E. Efficacy of an encapsulated probiotic *Bifidobacterium infantis* 35624 in women with irritable bowel syndrome. *Am. J. Gastroenterol.* **2006**, *101*, 1581–1590. [CrossRef]
37. Ducrotte, P.; Sawant, P.; Jayanthi, V. Clinical trial: *Lactobacillus plantarum* 299v (DSM 9843) improves symptoms of irritable bowel syndrome. *World J. Gastroenterol.* **2012**, *18*, 4012–4018. [CrossRef] [PubMed]
38. Horvath, A.; Dziechciarz, P.; Szajewska, H. Meta-analysis: *Lactobacillus rhamnosus* GG for abdominal pain-related functional gastrointestinal disorders in childhood. *Aliment. Pharmacol. Ther.* **2011**, *33*, 1302–1310. [CrossRef] [PubMed]
39. Guarner, F.; Sanders, M.E.; Szajewska, H.; Cohen, H.; Eliakim, R.; Herrera-deGuise, C.; Karakan, T.; Merenstein, D.; Piscoya, A.; Ramakrishna, B.; et al. Probiotics and prebiotics. In *World Gastroenterology Organisation Global Guidelines*; World Gastroenterology Organisation: Milwaukee, WI, USA, 2017; pp. 1–34. [CrossRef]
40. Harris, K.; Kassis, A.; Major, G. Is the gut microbiota a new factor contributing to Obesity and its Metabolic disorders. *J. Obes.* **2012**, *2012*, 879151. [CrossRef]
41. Blaut, M.; Klaus, S. Intestinal microbiota and Obesity. *Handb. Exp. Pharmacol.* **2012**, *209*, 251–273. [CrossRef]
42. Tumbaugh, P.; Ley, R.; Mahowald, M. An Obesity-associated gut microbiome with increased capacity for Energy harvest. *Nature* **2006**, *444*, 1027–1031. [CrossRef]
43. Ostrowska, L. Mikrobiota jelitowa a zaburzenia metaboliczne i otyłość—Punkt widzenia internisty i dietetyka. *Gastroenterol. Klin.* **2016**, *8*, 1–12.
44. Grudell, A.B.; Camilleri, M. The role of peptide YY in integrative gut physiology and potential role in obesity. *Curr. Opin. Endocrinol. Diabetes Obes.* **2007**, *14*, 52–57. [CrossRef] [PubMed]
45. Amar, J.; Chabo, C.; Waget, A.; Klopp, P.; Vachoux, C.; Bermudez-Humaran, L.G.; Smirnova, N.; Berge, M.; Sulpice, T.; Lahtinen, S.; et al. Intestinal mucosal adherence and translocation of commensal bacteria at the early onset oftype 2 diabetes: Molecular mechanism and probiotic treatment. *EMBO Mol. Med.* **2011**, *3*, 559–572. [CrossRef]
46. Cani, P.D.; Neyrinck, A.M.; Fava, F.; Knauf, C.; Burcelin, R.G.; Tuohy, K.M.; Gibson, G.R.; Delzenne, N.M. Selective increases of bifidobacteria in gut microflora improve high-fat-diet-induced diabetes in mice through a mechanism associated with endotoxaemia. *Diabetologia* **2007**, *50*, 2374–2383. [CrossRef] [PubMed]
47. Lee, H.Y.; Park, J.H.; Seok, S.H.; Baek, M.W.; Kim, D.J.; Lee, K.E.; Paek, K.S.; Lee, Y.; Park, J.H. Human originated bacteria, *Lactobacillus rhamnosus* PL60, produce conjugated linoleic acid and show anti-obesity effects in diet-induced obese mice. *Biochim. Biophys. Acta* **2006**, *1761*, 736–744. [CrossRef]
48. Lee, K.; Paek, K.; Lee, H.Y.; Park, J.H.; Lee, Y. Antiobesity effect of trans-10,cis-12-conjugated linoleic acid-producing *Lactobacillus plantarum* PL62 on diet-induced obese mice. *J. Appl. Microbiol.* **2007**, *103*, 1140–1146. [CrossRef]
49. Sato, M.; Uzu, K.; Yoshida, T.; Hamad, E.M.; Kawakami, H.; Matsuyama, H.; Abd El-Gawad, I.A.; Imaizumi, K. Effects ofmilk fermented by *Lactobacillus gasseri* SBT2055 on adipocyte size in rates. *Br. J. Nutr.* **2008**, *99*, 1013–1017. [CrossRef] [PubMed]
50. Tomaro-Duchesneau, C.; Saha, S.; Malhotra, M.; Jones, M.L.; Labbe, A.; Rodes, L.; Kahouli, I.; Prakash, S. Effect of orally administered L fermentum NCIMB 5221 on markers of metabolic syndrome: An in vivo analysis using ZDF rats. *Appl. Microbiol. Biotechnol.* **2014**, *98*, 115–126. [CrossRef]

51. Nerstedt, A.; Nilsson, E.C.; Ohlson, K.; Hakansson, J.; Svensson, T.; Lowenadler, B.; Svensson, Y.K.; Mahlapuu, M. Administration of *Lactobacillus* evokes coordinated changes in the intestinal expression profile ofgenes regulating energy homeostasis and immune phenotype in mice. *Br. J. Nutr.* **2007**, *97*, 1117–1127. [CrossRef] [PubMed]
52. Kadooka, Y.; Sato, M.; Imaizumi, K.; Ogawa, A.; Ikuyama, K.; Akai, Y.; Okano, M.; Kagoshima, M.; Tsuchida, T. Regulation of abdominal adiposity by probiotics (*Lactobacillus gasseri* SBT2055) in adults with obese tendencies in a randomized controlled trial. *Eur. J. Clin. Nutr.* **2010**, *64*, 636–643. [CrossRef]
53. Kadooka, Y.; Sato, M.; Ogawa, A.; Miyoshi, M.; Uenish, H.; Ogawa, H.; Ikuyama, K.; Kagoshima, M.; Ysuchida, T. Effect of *Lactobacillus gasseri* SBT2055 in fermented milk on abdominal adiposity in adults in a randomised controll trial. *Br. J. Nutr.* **2013**, *110*, 1696–1703. [CrossRef] [PubMed]
54. Sanchez, M.; Darimont, C.; Drapeau, V.; Emady-Azar, S.; Lepage, M.; Rezzonico, E.; Ngom-Bru, C.; Berger, B.; Philippe, L.; Ammon-Zuffrey, C.; et al. Effect of *Lactobacillus rhamnosus* CGMCC1.3724 supplementation on weight loss and maintenance in obese men and women. *Br. J. Nutr.* **2014**, *111*, 1507–1519. [CrossRef]
55. Babio, N.; Becerra-Tomas, N.; Martinez-Gonzalez, M.A.; Corella, D.; Estruch, R.; Ros, E.; Sayon-Orea, C.; Fito, M.; Serra-Majem, L.; Aros, F.; et al. Consumption of yogurt, low-fat milk, and other low-fat dairy products is associated with lower risk of metabolic syndrome incidence in an elderly Mediterranean population. *J. Nutr.* **2015**, *145*, 2308–2316. [CrossRef] [PubMed]
56. Neyrinck, A.M.; Possemiers, S.; Druart, C.; Van de Wiele, T.; De Backer, F.; Cani, P.D.; Larondelle, Y.; Delzenne, N.M. Prebiotic effects of wheat arabinoxylan related to the increase in *Bifidobacteria, Roseburia* and *Bacteroides/Prevotella* in diet-induced obese mice. *PLoS ONE* **2011**, *6*, 20944. [CrossRef]
57. Parnell, J.A.; Reimer, R.A. Prebiotic fibres dose-dependently increase satiety hormones and alter Bacteroidetes and Firmicutes in lean and obese JCR: LA-cprats. *Br. J. Nutr.* **2012**, *107*, 601–613. [CrossRef] [PubMed]
58. Million, M.; Angelakis, E.; Paul, M.; Armougom, F.; Leibovici, L.; Raoult, D. Comparative meta-analysis of the effect of *Lactobacillus* species on weight gain in humans and animals. *Microb. Pathog.* **2012**, *53*, 100–108. [CrossRef]
59. Angelakis, E.; Merhej, V.; Raoult, D. Related actions of probiotics and antibiotics on gut microbiota and weight modification. *Lancet Infect. Dis.* **2013**, *13*, 889–899. [CrossRef]
60. Alvarez-Arrano, V.; Martin-Pelaez, S. Effects of probiotics and synbiotics on weight loss in subjects with overweight or obesity: A systematic review. *Nutrients* **2021**, *13*, 3627. [CrossRef] [PubMed]
61. Musazadeh, V.; Zarezadeh, M.; Ghalichi, F.; Ahrabi, S.S.; Jamilian, P.; Jamilian, P.; Ghoreishi, Z. Anti-obesity properties of probiotics; a considerable medical nutrition intervention: Findings from an umbrella meta-analysis. *Eur. J. Pharmacol.* **2022**, *928*, 175069. [CrossRef] [PubMed]
62. Zhang, Y.; Yan, T.; Xu, C.; Yang, H.; Zhang, T.; Liu, Y. Probiotics can further reduce waist circumference in adults with morbid obesity after bariatric surgery: A systematic review and meta-analysis of randomized controlled trials. *Evid.-Based Complement. Altern. Med.* **2021**, *2021*, 5542626. [CrossRef]
63. Niloufar Rasaei, N.; Heidari, M.; Esmaeili, F.; Khosravi, S.; Baeeri, M.; Tabatabaei-Malazy, O.; Emamgholipour, S. The effects of prebiotic, probiotic or synbiotic supplementation on overweight/obesity indicators: An umbrella review of the trials' meta-analyses. *Front. Endocrinol.* **2024**, *15*, 1277921. [CrossRef]
64. Cani, P.D.; Neyrinck, A.M.; Maton, N.; Delzenne, N.M. Oligo-fructose promotes satiety in rats fed a high-fat diet: Involvement of glucagon-like Peptide-1. *Obes. Res.* **2005**, *13*, 1000–1007. [CrossRef]
65. Cani, P.D.; Daubioul, C.A.; Reusens, B.; Remacle, C.; Catillon, G.; Delzenne, N.M. Involvement of endogenous glucagon-like peptide-1 (7-36) amide on glycaemia-lowering effect of oligofructose in streptozotocin-treated rats. *J. Endocrinol.* **2005**, *185*, 457–465. [CrossRef]
66. Genta, S.; Cabrera, W.; Habib, N.; Pons, J.; Carillo, I.M.; Grau, A.; Sanchez, A. Yacon syrup: Beneficial effects on obesity and insulin resistance in humans. *Clin. Nutr.* **2009**, *28*, 182–187. [CrossRef] [PubMed]
67. Cani, P.D.; Possemiers, S.; Van de Wiele, T.; Guiot, Y.; Everard, A.; Rottier, O.; Geurts, L.; Naslain, D.; Neyrinck, A.; Lambert, D.M.; et al. Changes in gut microbiota control inflammation in obese mice through a mechanism involving GLP-2 driven improvement ofgut permeability. *Gut* **2009**, *58*, 1091–1103. [CrossRef] [PubMed]
68. Shirvani-Rad, S.; Tabatabaei-Malazy, O.; Mohseni, S.; Hasani-Ranjbar, S.; Soroush, A.-R.; Hoseini-Tavassol, Z.; Ejtahed, H.-S.; Larijani, B. Probiotics as a complementary therapy for management of obesity: A systematic review. *Evid. Based Complement. Alternat. Med.* **2021**, *2021*, 6688450. [CrossRef] [PubMed]
69. Li, Z.; Li, Y.; Pan, B.; Wang, X.; Wu, Y.; Guo, K.; Yang, M.; Ma, M.; Qiao, C.; Yang, K. The effects of oral probiotic supplementation in postmenopausal women with overweight and obesity: A systematic review and meta-analysis of randomized controlled trials. *Probiotics Antimicrob. Proteins* **2022**, *15*, 1567–1582. [CrossRef]
70. Perna, S.; Ilyas, Z.; Giacosa, A.; Gasparri, C.; Peroni, G.; Faliva, M.A.; Rigon, C.; Naso, M.; Riva, A.; Petrangolini, G.; et al. Is probiotic supplementation useful for the management of body weight and other anthropometric measures in adults affected by overweight and obesity with metabolic related diseases? A systematic review and meta-analysis. *Nutrients* **2021**, *13*, 666. [CrossRef]

71. Mayta-Tovalino, F.; Diaz-Arocutipa, C.; Piscoya, A.; Hernandez, A.V. Effects of probiotics on intermediate cardiovascular outcomes in patients with overweight or obesity: A systematic review and meta-analysis. *J. Clin. Med.* **2023**, *12*, 2554. [CrossRef]
72. Hadi, A.; Alizadeh, K.; Hajianfar, H.; Mohammadi, H.; Miraghajani, M. Efficacy of synbiotic supplementation in obesity treatment: A systematic review and meta-analysis of clinical trials. *Crit. Rev. Food Sci. Nutr.* **2020**, *60*, 584–596. [CrossRef]
73. Deng, Y.; Misselwitz, B.; Dai, N.; Fox, M. Lactose intolerance in adults: Biological mechanism and dietary management. *Nutrients* **2015**, *7*, 8020–8035. [CrossRef]
74. Oak, S.J.; Jha, R. The effects of probiotics in lactose intolerance: A systematic review. *Crit. Rev. Food Sci. Nutr.* **2019**, *59*, 1675–1683. [CrossRef] [PubMed]
75. Masoumi, S.J.; Mehrabani, D.; Saberifiroozi, M.; Fattahi, M.R.; Moradi, F.; Najafi, M. The effect of yogurt fortified with *Lactobacillus acidophilus* and *Bifidobacterium* sp. probiotic in patients with lactose intolerance. *Food Sci. Nutr.* **2021**, *9*, 1704–1711. [CrossRef] [PubMed]
76. Savaiano, D.A. Lactose digestion from yogurt: Mechanism and relevance. *Am. J. Clin. Nutr.* **2014**, *99*, 1251S–1255S. [CrossRef]
77. Heyman, M.B. Committee on Nutrition. Lactose intolerance in infants, children, and adolescents. *Pediatrics* **2006**, *118*, 1279–1286. [CrossRef] [PubMed]
78. Sahi, T.; Isokoski, M.; Jussila, J.; Launiala, K.; Pyorala, K. Recessive inheritance of adult-type lactose malabsorption. *Lancet* **1973**, *13*, 823–826. [CrossRef]
79. Enattah, N.S.; Sahi, T.; Savilahti, E.; Terwilliger, J.D.; Peltonen, L.; Jarvela, I. Identification of a variant associated with adult-type hypolactasia. *Nat. Genet.* **2002**, *30*, 233–237. [CrossRef] [PubMed]
80. Adolfsson, O.; Meydani, S.N.; Russell, R.M. Yogurt and gut function. *Am. J. Clin. Nutr.* **2004**, *80*, 245–256. [CrossRef] [PubMed]
81. Thoreux, K.; Balas, D.; Bouley, C.; Senegas-Balas, F. Diet supplemented with yoghurt or milk fermented by *Lactobacillus casei* DN-114 001 stimulates growth and brush-border enzyme activities in mouse small intestine. *Digestion* **1998**, *59*, 349–359. [CrossRef]
82. Ahn, S.; Kim, M.S.; Park, D.G.; Han, B.K.; Kim, Y.J. Effects of probiotics administration on lactose intolerance in adulthood: A meta-analysis. *J. Dairy Sci.* **2023**, *106*, 4489–4501. [CrossRef] [PubMed]
83. Ibrahim, S.A.; Gyawali, R.; Awaisheh, S.S.; Krastanov, A.I. Fermented foods and probiotics: An approach to lactose intolerance. *J. Dairy Res.* **2021**, *88*, 357–365. [CrossRef]
84. Aguilera, G.; Cárcamo, C.; Soto-Alarcón, S.; Gotteland, M. Improvement in lactose tolerance in hypolactasic subjects consuming ice creams with high or low concentrations of *Bifidobacterium bifidum* 900791. *Foods* **2021**, *10*, 2468. [CrossRef]
85. Gingold-Belfer, R.; Levy, S.; Layfer, O.; Pakanaev, L.; Niv, Y.; Dickman, R.; Perets, T. Use of a novel probiotic formulation to alleviate lactose intolerance symptoms—A pilot study. *Probiotics Antimicrob. Proteins* **2020**, *12*, 112–118. [CrossRef] [PubMed]
86. Vitellio, P.; Celano, G.; Bonfrate, L.; Gobbetti, M.; Portincasa, P.; De Angelis, M. Effects of *Bifidobacterium longum* and *Lactoibacillus rhamnosus* on Gut Microbiota in Patients with Lactose Intolerance and Persisting Functional Gastrointestinal Symptoms: A Randomised, Double-Blind, Cross-Over Study. *Nutrients* **2019**, *11*, 886. [CrossRef]
87. Leis, R.; de Castro, M.; de Lamas, C.; Couce, M.L. Effects of Prebiotic and Probiotic Supplementation on Lactase Deficiency and Lactose Intolerance: A Systematic Review of Controlled Trials. *Nutrients* **2020**, *2*, 1487. [CrossRef]
88. Gijsbers, L.; Ding, E.L.; Malik, V.S.; De Goede, J.; Geleijnse, J.M.; Soedamah-Muthu, S.S. Consumption of dairy foods and diabetes incidence: A dose-response meta-analysis of observational studies. *Am. J. Clin. Nutr.* **2016**, *103*, 1111–1124. [CrossRef] [PubMed]
89. Ivey, K.L.; Lewis, J.R.; Hodgson, J.M.; Zhu, K.; Dhaliwal, S.S.; Thompson, P.L.; Richard, P. Association between yogurt, milk, and cheese consumption and common carotid artery intima-media thickness and cardiovascular disease risk factors in elderly women. *Am. J. Clin. Nutr.* **2011**, *94*, 234–239. [CrossRef] [PubMed]
90. Margolis, K.L.; Wei, F.; de Boer, I.H.; Howard, B.V.; Liu, S.; Manson, J.E.; Mossavar-Rahmani, Y.; Phillips, L.S.; Shikany, J.M.; Tinker, L.F.; et al. A diet high in low-fat dairy products lowers diabetes risk in postmenopausal women. *J. Nutr.* **2011**, *141*, 1969–1974. [CrossRef] [PubMed]
91. Liu, J.E.; Zhang, Y.; Zhang, J.; Dong, P.L.; Chen, M.; Duan, Z.P. Probiotic yogurt effects on intestinal flora of patients with chronic liver disease. *Nurs. Res.* **2010**, *59*, 426–432. [CrossRef]
92. Salas-Salvado, J.; Guasch-Ferre, M.; Diaz-López, A.; Babio, N. Yogurt and diabetes: Overview of recent observational studies. *J. Nutr.* **2017**, *147*, 1452S–1461S. [CrossRef]
93. Available online: www.stat.gov.pl (accessed on 11 November 2024).
94. Pokrzywnicka, P.; Gumprecht, J. "Mikrobiota i jej związek z cukrzycą typu 2 i otyłością" Szpital Miejski w Zabrzu, Katedra i Klinika Chorób Wewnętrznych, Diabetologii i Nefrologii, Śląski Uniwersytet Medyczny w Zabrzu. *Diabetol. Prakt.* **2016**, *2*, 190–199.
95. Konturek, S. *Fizjologia Człowieka Podręcznik dla Studentów Medycyny*; Edra Urban & Partner: Wrocław, Poland, 2013; pp. 533–535.
96. Stawerska, R.; Łupińska, A.; Bieniek, E.; Lewiński, A. Insulinooporność i stan przedcukrzycowy. *Lekarz POZ* **2021**, *5*, 358–365.
97. Sadagurski, M.; White, M.F. Integrating metabolism and longevity through insulin and IGF1 signaling. *Endocrinol. Metab. Clin. N. Am.* **2013**, *42*, 127–148. [CrossRef] [PubMed]

98. Nowosad, K. *Rola diety i Stylu Życia w Leczeniu Insulinooporności*; Polskie Towarzystwo Przyrodników im. Kopernika wydawnictwo KOSMOS: Kraków, Poland, 2021; Volume 70, pp. 731–739. [CrossRef]
99. Gołąbek, K.D.; Regulska-Ilow, B. Dietary support in insulin resistance: An overview of current scientific reports. *Adv. Clin. Exp. Med.* **2019**, *28*, 1577–1585. [CrossRef] [PubMed]
100. Ostrowska, L.; Witczak, K.; Adamska, E. Czy istnieją środowiskowe uwarunkowania insulinooporności? *Forum Zaburzeń Metab.* **2012**, *3*, 85–93.
101. Noormohammadi, M.; Ghorbani, Z.; Löber, U.; Mahdavi-Roshan, M.; Bartolomaeus, T.U.P.; Kazemi, A.; Shoaibinobarian, N.; Forslund, S.K. The effect of probiotic and synbiotic supplementation on appetite-regulating hormones and desire to eat: A systematic review and meta-analysis of clinical trials. *Pharmacol. Res.* **2023**, *187*, 106614. [CrossRef]
102. Stachowicz, M.; Janas-Kozik, M.; Olszanecka-Glinianowicz, M.; Chudek, J. Rola leptyny w zaburzeniach odżywiania się—Współczesne poglądy. *Psychiatr. Pol.* **2013**, *47*, 897–907.
103. Kim, S.W.; Park, K.Y.; Kim, B.; Kim, E.; Hyun, C.K. *Lactobacillus rhamnosus* GG improves insulin sensitivity and reduces adiposity in high-fat diet-fed mice through enhancement of adiponectin production. *Biochem. Biophys. Res. Commun.* **2013**, *431*, 258–263. [CrossRef] [PubMed]
104. Raji Lahiji, M.; Zarrati, M.; Najafi, S.; Yazdani, B.; Cheshmazar, E.; Razmpoosh, E.; Janani, L.; Lahiji, M.R.; Shidfar, F. Effects of synbiotic supplementation on serum adiponectin and inflammation status of overweight and obese breast cancer survivors: A randomized, triple-blind, placebo-controlled trial. *Support. Care Cancer* **2021**, *29*, 4147–4157. [CrossRef] [PubMed]
105. Hulston, C.J.; Churnside, A.A.; Venables, M.C. Probiotic supplementation prevents high-fat, overfeeding-induced insulin resistance in human subjects. *Br. J. Nutr.* **2015**, *113*, 596–602. [CrossRef]
106. Elbere, I.; Silamikelis, I.; Dindune, I.I.; Kalnina, I.; Ustinova, M.; Zaharenko, L.; Silamikele, L.; Rovite, V.; Gudra, D.; Konrade, I.; et al. Baseline gut microbiome composition predicts metformin therapy short-term efficacy in newly diagnosed type 2 diabetes patients. *PLoS ONE* **2020**, *15*, e0241338. [CrossRef]
107. Zhang, Y.; Guo, X.; Guo, J.; He, Q.; Li, H.; Song, Y.; Zhang, H. *Lactobacillus casei* reduces susceptibility to type 2 diabetes via microbiota-mediated body chloride ion influx. *Sci. Rep.* **2014**, *4*, 5654. [CrossRef] [PubMed]
108. Peng, X.; Xian, H.; Ge, N.; Hou, L.; Tang, T.; Xie, D.; Gao, L.; Yue, J. Effect of probiotics on glycemic control and lipid profiles in patients with type 2 diabetes mellitus: Arandomized, double blind, controlled trial. *Front. Endocrinol.* **2024**, *15*, 1440286. [CrossRef] [PubMed]
109. Li, S.; Liu, Z.; Zhang, Q.; Su, D.; Wang, P.; Li, Y.; Shi, W.; Zhang, Q. The Antidiabetic Potential of Probiotics: A Review. *Nutrients* **2024**, *16*, 2494. [CrossRef] [PubMed]
110. Shen, X.; Ma, C.; Yang, Y.; Liu, X.; Wang, B.; Wang, Y.; Zhang, G.; Bian, X.; Zhang, N. The Role and Mechanism of Probiotics Supplementation in Blood Glucose Regulation: A Review. *Foods* **2024**, *13*, 2719. [CrossRef] [PubMed]
111. Toejing, P.; Khampithum, N.; Sirilun, S.; Chaiyasut, C.; Lailerd, N. Influence of *Lactobacillus paracasei* HII01 Supplementation on Glycemia and Inflammatory Biomarkers in Type 2 Diabetes: A Randomized Clinical Trial. *Foods* **2021**, *10*, 1455. [CrossRef]
112. Gu, Y.X.; Chen, H.R.; Li, X.; Li, D.; Sun, Y.; Yang, L.; Ma, Y.; Chan, E.C.Y. *Lactobacillus paracasei* IMC 502 ameliorates type 2 diabetes by mediating gut microbiota-SCFA-hormone/inflammation pathway in mice. *J. Sci. Food Agric.* **2023**, *103*, 2949–2959. [CrossRef]
113. Wang, Y.M.; Dilidaxi, D.; Wu, Y.C.; Sailike, J.; Sun, X.; Nabi, X.H. Composite probiotics alleviate type 2 diabetes by regulating intestinal microbiota and inducing GLP-1 secretion in db/db mice. *Biomed. Pharmacother.* **2020**, *125*, 109914. [CrossRef]
114. Lee, Y.S.; Lee, D.; Park, G.S.; Ko, S.H.; Park, J.; Lee, Y.K.; Kang, J. *Lactobacillus plantarum* HAC01 ameliorates type 2 diabetes in high-fat diet and streptozotocin-induced diabetic mice in association with modulating the gut microbiota. *Food Funct.* **2021**, *12*, 6363–6373. [CrossRef] [PubMed]
115. Liu, Y.; Zheng, S.J.; Cui, J.L.; Guo, T.T.; Zhang, J.T. Lactiplantibacillus plantarum Y15 alleviate type 2 diabetes in mice via modulating gut microbiota and regulating NF-κB and insulin signaling pathway. *Braz. J. Microbiol.* **2022**, *53*, 935–945. [CrossRef]
116. Pegah, A.; Abbasi-Oshaghi, E.; Khodadadi, I.; Mirzaei, F.; Tayebinai, H. Probiotic and resveratrol normalize GLP-1 levels and oxidative stress in the intestine of diabetic rats. *Metab. Open* **2021**, *10*, 100093. [CrossRef]
117. Naseri, K.; Saadati, S.; Ghaemi, F.; Ashtary-Larky, D.; Asbaghi, O.; Sadeghi, A.; Afrisham, R.; de Courten, B. The effects of probiotic and synbiotic supplementation on inflammation, oxidative stress, and circulating adiponectin and leptin concentration in subjects with prediabetes and type 2 diabetes mellitus: A GRADE-assessed systematic review, meta-analysis, and meta-regression of randomized clinical trials. *Eur. J. Nutr.* **2023**, *62*, 543–561. [CrossRef]
118. Zhao, J.Y.; Wang, L.H.; Cheng, S.S.; Zhang, Y.; Yang, M.; Fang, R.X.; Li, H.X.; Man, C.X.; Jiang, Y.J. A Potential Synbiotic Strategy for the Prevention of Type 2 Diabetes: *Lactobacillus paracasei* JY062 and Exopolysaccharide Isolated from *Lactobacillus plantarum* JY039. *Nutrients* **2022**, *14*, 377. [CrossRef]
119. Xiao, R.; Wang, L.L.; Tian, P.J.; Jin, X.; Zhao, J.X.; Zhang, H.; Wang, G.; Zhu, M.M. The Effect of Probiotic Supplementation on Glucolipid Metabolism in Patients with Type 2 Diabetes: A Systematic Review and Meta-Analysis. *Nutrients* **2023**, *15*, 3240. [CrossRef] [PubMed]

120. Rodrigues, R.R.; Gurung, M.; Li, Z.P.; García-Jaramillo, M.; Greer, R.; Gaulke, C.; Bauchinger, F.; You, H.; Pederson, J.W.; Vasquez-Perez, S.; et al. Transkingdom interactions between Lactobacilli and hepatic mitochondria attenuate western diet-induced diabetes. *Nat. Commun.* **2021**, *12*, 101. [CrossRef]
121. Jiang, H.R.; Cai, M.M.; Shen, B.Y.; Wang, Q.; Zhang, T.C.; Zhou, X. Synbiotics and Gut Microbiota: New Perspectives in the Treatment of Type 2 Diabetes Mellitus. *Foods* **2022**, *11*, 2438. [CrossRef] [PubMed]
122. Gulnaz, A.; Nadeem, J.; Han, J.H.; Lew, L.C.; Son, J.D.; Park, Y.H.; Rather, I.A.; Hor, Y.Y. *Lactobacillus* sps in Reducing the Risk of Diabetes in High-Fat Diet-Induced Diabetic Mice by Modulating the Gut Microbiome and Inhibiting Key Digestive Enzymes Associated with Diabetes. *Biology* **2021**, *10*, 348. [CrossRef] [PubMed]
123. Zhou, X.R.; Shang, G.S.; Tan, Q.; He, Q.; Tan, X.Y.; Park, K.Y.; Zhao, X. Effect of *Lactobacillus fermentum* TKSN041 on improving streptozotocin-induced type 2 diabetes in rats. *Food Funct.* **2021**, *12*, 7938–7953. [CrossRef]
124. Archer, A.C.; Muthukumar, S.P.; Halami, P.M. *Lactobacillus fermentum* MCC2759 and MCC2760 Alleviate Inflammation and Intestinal Function in High-Fat Diet-Fed and Streptozotocin-Induced Diabetic Rats. *Probiotics Antimicrob. Proteins* **2021**, *13*, 1068–1080; Erratum in *Probiotics Antimicrob. Proteins* **2023**, *15*, 1078. [CrossRef]
125. Koczarski, M. The Effect of Probiotic Supplementation on Glycemic Control in Women with Gestational Diabetes Mellitus A Systematic Review. *Top. Clin. Nutr.* **2020**, *35*, 270–276. [CrossRef]
126. Wu, L.; Gao, Y.; Su, Y.; Li, J.; Ren, W.C.; Wang, Q.H.; Kuang, H.X. Probiotics with anti-type 2 diabetes mellitus properties: Targets of polysaccharides from traditional Chinese medicine. *Chin. J. Nat. Med.* **2022**, *20*, 641–655. [CrossRef] [PubMed]
127. Maciorkowska, E.; Ryszczuk, E.; Kaczmarski, M. Rola probiotyków i prebiotyków w apoptozie przewodu pokarmowego. *Przegląd Gastroenterol.* **2010**, *5*, 88–93. [CrossRef]
128. Ignyś, I.; Piątkowska, P.; Cichy, W. Probiotyki i prebiotyki w żywieniu i leczeniu dzieci. *Ped. Pol.* **2008**, *83*, 68–75. [CrossRef]
129. Cichy, W.; Ignyś, I.; Piątkowska, P. Współczesne poglądy na profilaktyczne i terapeutyczne zastosowanie probiotyków u dzieci. *Świat Med. Farm.* **2006**, *9*, 34–37.
130. Isolauri, E.; Juntunen, M.; Rautanen, T.; Sillanaukee, P.; Koivula, T. A human *Lactobacillus* strain (*Lactobacillus casei* sp. Strain GG) promotes recovery from acute diarrhoea in children. *Pediatrics* **1991**, *88*, 90–97. [PubMed]
131. Majamaa, H.; Isolauri, E.; Saxelin, M.; Vesikari, T. Lactic acid bacteria in the treatment of acute rotavirus gastroenteritis. *J. Pediatr. Gastroenterol. Nutr.* **1995**, *20*, 333–338. [CrossRef] [PubMed]
132. Shornikova, A.V.; Isolauri, E.; Casas, I.A.; Vesikari, T. *Lactobacillus reuteri* effectively colonises GI tract and shortens acute diarrhoea in children. *J. Pediatr. Gastroenterol. Nutr.* **1996**, *22*, 410. [CrossRef]
133. Saavedra, J.M.; Bauman, N.A.; Perman, J.A.; Yolken, R.H.; Saavedra, J.M.; Bauman, N.A.; Oung, I. Feeding of *Bifidobacterium bifidum* and *Streptococcus thermophilus* to infants in hospital for prevention of diarrhoea and sheeding of rotavirus. *Lancet* **1994**, *344*, 1046–1049. [CrossRef]
134. Ruszczyński, M.; Szajewska, H. Probiotyki w zapobieganiu biegunce związanej ze stosowaniem antybiotyków—Aktualizacja metaanalizy badań z randomizacją. *Pediatr. Współcz.* **2008**, *10*, 96–104.
135. Arvola, T.; Laiho, K.; Torkkeli, S.; Mykkanen, H.; Salminen, S.; Maunula, L.; Isolauri, E. Prophylactic *Lactobacillus* GG reduces antibiotic-assosiated diarrhea in children with respiratory infections: A randomized study. *Pediatrics* **1999**, *104*, e64. [CrossRef]
136. Vanderhoof, J.A.; Whitnej, D.B.; Antonson, D.L.; Hanner, T.L.; Lupo, J.V.; Young, R.J. *Lactobacillus* GG in the prevention of antibiotic-associated diarrhea in children. *J. Pediatr.* **1999**, *135*, 564–568. [CrossRef]
137. Piątkowska, P.; Ignyś, I.; Roszak, D.; Cichy, W. Probiotyki a antybiotykoterapia u dzieci. *Świat Med. Farm.* **2007**, *5*, 36–37.
138. Kotowska, M.; Albrecht, P.; Szajewska, H. *Saccharomyces boulardii* in the prevention of antibiotic-associated diarrhoea in children: A randomized double-blind placebo-controlled trial. *Aliment. Pharmacol. Ther.* **2005**, *21*, 583–590. [CrossRef]
139. Szamański, H.; Armańska, M.; Kowalska-Duplaga, K.; Szajewska, H. *Bifidobacterium longum* PL03, *Lactobacillus rhamnosus* KL53A and *Lactobacillus plantarum* PL02 in the prevention of antibiotic-associated diarrhoea in children: A randomized controlled pilot trial. *Digestion* **2008**, *78*, 13–17. [CrossRef]
140. Chandrasekaran, P.; Weiskirchen, S.; Weiskirchen, R. Effects of Probiotics on Gut Microbiota: An Overview. *Int. J. Mol. Sci.* **2024**, *25*, 6022. [CrossRef]
141. Ma, C.; Zhang, C.; Chen, D.; Jiang, S.; Shen, S.; Huo, D.; Huang, S.; Zhai, Q.; Zhang, J. Probiotic consumption influences universal adaptive mutations in indigenous human and mouse gut microbiota. *Commun. Biol.* **2021**, *4*, 1198. [CrossRef] [PubMed]
142. Khaneghah, A.M.; Abhari, K.; Eş, I.; Soares, M.B.; Oliveira, R.B.A.; Hosseini, H.; Rezaei, M.; Balthazar, C.F.; Silva, R.; Cruz, A.G.; et al. Interactions between probiotics and pathogenic microorganisms in hosts and foods: A review. *Trends Food Sci. Technol.* **2020**, *95*, 205–218. [CrossRef]
143. D'Argenio, V.; Salvatore, F. The role of the gut microbiome in the healthy adult status. *Clin. Chim. Acta* **2015**, *451*, 97–102. [CrossRef]
144. Sun, J.; Chang, E.B. Exploring gut microbes in human health and disease: Pushing the envelope. *Genes Dis.* **2014**, *1*, 132–139. [CrossRef]

145. Javanmard, A.; Ashtari, S.; Sabet, B.; Davoodi, S.H.; Rostami-Nejad, M.; Akbari, M.E.; Niaz, A.; Mortazavian, A.M. Probiotics and their role in gastrointestinal cancer prevention and treatment: An overview. *Gastroenterol. Hepatol. Bed Bench* **2018**, *11*, 284–295. [PubMed] [PubMed Central]
146. Wang, L.; Zhou, J.; Xin, Y.; Geng, C.; Tian, Z.; Yu, X.; Zibin, Y.; Xinjuan, Y.; Quanjiang, D. Bacterial overgrowth and diversification of microbiota in gastric cancer. *Eur. J. Gastroenterol. Hepatol.* **2016**, *3*, 262–266. [CrossRef] [PubMed]
147. Dai, Z.; Zhang, J.; Wu, Q.; Chen, J.; Liu, J.; Wang, L.; Chen, C.; Xu, J.; Zhang, H.; Shi, C. The role of microbiota in the development of colorectal cancer. *Int. J. Cancer* **2018**, *8*, 2032–2041. [CrossRef]
148. Kaźmierczak-Siedlecka, K.; Ruszkowski, J.; Folwarski, M.; Obara, K.; Makarewicz, W.; Lebiedzińska, A. Zastosowanie fitoterapii w leczeniu wrzodziejącego zapalenia jelita grubego. *Bromatol. Chem. Toksykol.* **2019**, *LII*, 41–48.
149. Koziński, K.; Dobrzyń, A. Szlak sygnałowy Wnt i jego rola w regulacji metabolizmu komórki. *Postępy Hig. Med. Doświadczalnej* **2013**, *67*, 1098–1108. [CrossRef] [PubMed]
150. Kuśmierska, A.; Fol, M. Właściwości immunomodulacyjne i terapeutyczne drobnoustrojów probiotycznych. *Probl. Hig. Epidemiol.* **2014**, *3*, 529–540.
151. Yu, A.; Li, L. The Potential Role of Probiotics in Cancer Prevention and Treatment. *Nutr. Cancer* **2016**, *4*, 535–544. [CrossRef] [PubMed]
152. Mojka, K. Probiotyki, prebiotyki i synbiotyki—Charakterystyka i funkcje. *Probl. Hig. Epidemiol.* **2014**, *3*, 541–549.
153. Holscher, H.D. Dietary fiber and prebiotics and the gastrointestinal microbiota. *Gut Microbes* **2017**, *2*, 172–184. [CrossRef] [PubMed]
154. Siepsiak, M.; Połom, A.; Adrych, K. Profilaktyka raka jelita grubego. *Farm Współ.* **2015**, *8*, 1–5.
155. Rothwell, P.M.; Wilson, M.; Elwin, C.E. Long-term effect of aspirin on colorectal cancer incidence and mortality: 20-year follow-up of five randomised trials. *Lancet* **2010**, *9754*, 1741–1750. [CrossRef] [PubMed]
156. Ambalam, P.; Raman, M.; Purama, R.K.; Doble, M. Probiotics, Prebiotics and Colorectal Cancer Prevention. *Best Pract. Res. Clin. Gastroenterol.* **2016**, *1*, 119–131. [CrossRef] [PubMed]
157. O'Mahony, L.; Feeney, M.; O'Halloran, S.; Murphy, L.; Kiely, B.; Fitzgibbon, J.; Lee, G.; O'Sullivan, L.G.; Shanahan, F.; Collins, J.K. Probiotic impact on microbial flora, inflammation and tumour development in IL-10 knockout mice. *Aliment. Pharmacol. Ther.* **2001**, *8*, 1219–1225. [CrossRef]
158. Kozieł, N.; Kukier, E.; Kwiatek, K. *Clostridium perfringens*—Znaczenie epidemiologiczne i diagnostyka zachorowań. *Med. Weter.* **2019**, *75*, 5. [CrossRef]
159. Horie, H.; Zeisig, M.; Hirayama, K.; Midtvedt, T.; Moller, L.; Rafter, J. Probiotic mixture decreases DNA adduct formation in colonic epithelium induced by the food mutagen 2-amino-9H-pyrido[2,3-b]indole in a human-flora associated mouse model. *Eur. J. Cancer Prev.* **2003**, *2*, 101–107. [CrossRef] [PubMed]
160. Bertkova, I.; Hijova, E.; Chmelarova, A.; Mojzisova, G.; Petrasova, D.; Strojny, L.; Bomba, A.; Zitnan, R. The effect of probiotic microorganisms and bioactive compounds on chemically induced carcinogenesis in rats. *Neoplasma* **2010**, *5*, 422–428. [CrossRef]
161. Ma, E.L.; Choi, Y.J.; Choi, J.; Pothoulakis, C.; Rhee, S.H.; Im, E. The anticancer effect of probiotic Bacillus polyfermenticus on human colon cancer cells is mediated through ErbB2 and ErbB3 inhibition. *Int. J. Cancer* **2010**, *4*, 780–790. [CrossRef] [PubMed]
162. Bertucci, F.; Borie, N.; Ginestier, C.; Groulet, A.; Charafe-Jauffret, E.; Adélaïde, J.; Geneix, J.; Bachelart, L.; Finetti, P.; Koki, A.; et al. Identification and validation of an ERBB2 gene expression signature in breast cancers. *Oncogene* **2004**, *23*, 2564–2575. [CrossRef]
163. Hatakka, K.; Holma, R.; El-Nezami, H.; Suomalainen, T.; Kuisma, M.; Saxelin, M.; Poussa, T.; Mykkanen, H.; Korpela, R. The influence of *Lactobacillus rhamnosus* LC705 together with Propionibacterium freudenreichii ssp. shermanii JS on potentially carcinogenic bacterial activity in human colon. *Int. J. Food Microbiol.* **2008**, *2*, 406–410. [CrossRef] [PubMed]
164. Jacouton, E.; Chain, F.; Sokol, H.; Langella, P.; Bermudez-Humaran, G.L. Probiotic Strain *Lactobacillus casei* BL23 Prevents Colitis-Associated Colorectal Cancer. *Front. Immunol.* **2017**, *8*, 1553. [CrossRef]
165. Deng, X.; Yang, J.; Zhang, Y.; Chen, X.; Wang, C.; Suo, H.; Song, J. An Update on the Pivotal Roles of Probiotics, Their Components, and Metabolites in Preventing Colon Cancer. *Foods* **2023**, *12*, 3706. [CrossRef]
166. Budu, O.; Banciu, C.; Pinzaru, I.; Sarău, C.; Lighezan, D.; Șoica, C.; Dehelean, C.; Drăghici, G.; Dolghi, A.; Prodea, A. A combination of two probiotics, *Lactobacillus sporogenes* and *Clostridium butyricum*, inhibits Colon Cancer Development: An In Vitro Study. *Microorganisms* **2022**, *10*, 1692. [CrossRef] [PubMed]
167. Aindelis, G.; Tiptiri-Kourpeti, A.; Lampri, E.; Spyridopoulou, K.; Lamprianidou, E.; Kotsianidis, I.; Ypsilantis, P.; Pappa, A.; Chlichlia, K. Immune responses raised in an experimental colon carcinoma model following oral administration of *Lactobacillus casei*. *Cancers* **2020**, *12*, 368. [CrossRef] [PubMed]
168. Wang, T.; Zhang, L.; Wang, P.; Liu, Y.; Wang, G.; Shan, Y.; Yi, Y.; Zhou, Y.; Liu, B.; Wang, X. *Lactobacillus coryniformis* MXJ32 administration ameliorates azoxymethane/dextran sulfate sodium-induced colitis-associated colorectal cancer via reshaping intestinal microenvironment and alleviating inflammatory response. *Eur. J. Nutr.* **2022**, *61*, 85–99. [CrossRef] [PubMed]
169. Shang, F.; Jiang, X.; Wang, H.; Chen, S.; Wang, X.; Liu, Y.; Guo, S.; Li, D.; Yu, W.; Zhao, Z. The inhibitory effects of probiotics on colon cancer cells: In vitro and in vivo studies. *J. Gastrointest. Oncol.* **2020**, *11*, 1224. [CrossRef]

170. Janelle, A.C.; Raad, Z.G.; Joshua, M.U.; Perez-Chanona, E.; Sha, W.; Tomkovich, S.; Mühlbauer, M.; Fodor, A.A.; Jobin, C. VSL#3 probiotic modifies mucosal microbial composition but does not reduce colitis-associated colorectal cancer. *Sci. Rep.* **2013**, *3*, 2868. [CrossRef]
171. Sunkata, R.; Herring, J.; Walker, L.T.; Verghese, M. Chemopreventive Potential of Probiotics and Prebiotics. *Food Nutr. Sci.* **2014**, *5*, 18. [CrossRef]
172. Wang, T.; Wang, P.; Yin, L.; Wang, X.; Shan, Y.; Yi, Y.; Zhou, Y.; Liu, B.; Wang, X.; Lü, X. Dietary *Lactiplantibacillus plantarum* KX041 attenuates colitis-associated tumorigenesis and modulates gut microbiota. *Food Sci. Hum. Wellness* **2023**, *12*, 1626–1636. [CrossRef]
173. Czerwionka-Szaflarska, M.; Kuczyńska, R.; Mierzwa, G.; Bała, G.; Murawska, S. Ocena wpływu bakterii probiotycznych na tolerancję terapii eradykacyjnej zakażeń *Helicobacterpylori* u dzieci i młodzieży. *Ped. Pol.* **2006**, *81*, 334–341.
174. Szajewska, H. Rola probiotyków w zapobieganiu i leczeniu chorób przewodu pokarmowego. *Pediatr. Współcz.* **2005**, *7*, 53–60.
175. Sykora, J.; Valeckova, K.; Amlerova, J.; Siala, K.; Dedek, P.; Watkins, S.; Varvarovska, J.; Stozicky, F.; Pazdiora, P.; Schwarz, J. Effects of a specially de- signed fermented milk product containing probiotic *Lactobacillus casei* DN-114 001 and the eradication of *H. pylori* in children: A pro- spective randomized double-blind study. *J. Clin. Gastroenterol.* **2005**, *39*, 692–698. [CrossRef]
176. Nista, E.C.; Candelli, M.; Cremonini, F.; Cazzato, I.A.; Zocco, M.A.; Franceschi, F.; Cammarota, G.; Gasbarrini, G.; Gasbarrini, A. *Bacillus clausi* therapy to reduce side-effects of anti-*Helicobacter pylori* treatment: Randomiz- ded, double-blind, placebo controlled trial. *Aliment. Pharmacol. Ther.* **2004**, *20*, 1181–1188. [CrossRef] [PubMed]
177. Malfertheiner, P.; Megraud, F.; O'Morain, C.A.; Gisbert, J.P.; Kuipers, E.J.; Axon, A.T.; Bazzoli, F.; Gasbarrini, A.; Artherton, J.; Graham, D.Y.; et al. European Helicobacter and microbiota study group and concensus panel. *Management of Helicobacter pylori infection—The Mastricht V/Florence Consensus Report. Gut* **2017**, *66*, 6–30. [CrossRef]
178. Ford, A.C.; Quigley, E.M.M.; Lacy, B.E.; Lembo, A.; Saito, Y.; Schiller, L.R.; Soffer, E.; Spiegel, B.; Moayyedi, P. Efficacy of prebiotics, probiotics, and synbiotics in irritable bowel syndrome and chronic idiopathic constipation: Systematic review and meta-analysis. *Am. J. Gastroenterol.* **2014**, *109*, 1547–1561. [CrossRef] [PubMed]
179. Hungin, A.P.S.; Mitchell, C.R.; Whorwell, P.; Mulligan, C.; Cole, O.; Agreus, L.; Fracasso, P.; Lionis, C.; Mendive, J.; Philippart de Foy, J.-M.; et al. Systematic review: Probiotics in the management of lower gastrointestinal symptoms—An updated evidence-based International consensus. *Aliment. Pharmacol. Ther.* **2018**, *47*, 1054–1070. [CrossRef]
180. Strzelec, B.; Stuła, M.; Chmielewski, P.; Taboła, R. Profilaktyka i leczenie raka żołądka—Aktualny problem interdyscyplinarny. *Pol. Nurs.* **2018**, *2*, 188–195. [CrossRef]
181. Yu, G.; Hu, N.; Wang, L.; Wang, C.; Han, X.Y.; Humpry, M.; Ravel, J.; Abnet, C.C.; Taylor, P.R.; Goldstein, A.M. Gastric microbiota features associated with cancer risk factors and clinical outcomes: A pilot study in gastric cardia cancer patients from Shanxi, China. *Int. J. Cancer* **2017**, *1*, 45–51. [CrossRef]
182. Dyrla, P.; Gil, J.; Wojtuń, S.; Korszun, K.; Kasińska, E.; Mackiewicz, A. Zakażenie *Helicobacter pylori*. Diagnostyka i leczenie. *Pediatr. Med. Rodz.* **2015**, *1*, 68–74. [CrossRef]
183. Castano-Rodriquez, N.; Goh, K.L.; Fock, K.M.; Hazel, M.M.; Nadeem, O.K. Dysbiosis of the microbiome in gastric cancer. *Sci. Rep.* **2017**, *7*, 15957. [CrossRef]
184. Namkin, K.; Zardast, M.; Basirinejad, F. *Saccharomyces boulardii* in *Helicobacter pylori* eradication in children: A randomized trial from Iran. *Iran. J. Pediatr.* **2016**, *1*, e3768. [CrossRef] [PubMed]
185. Bin, Z.; Ya-Zheng, X.; Zhao-Hui, D.; Bo, C.; Li-Rong, J.; Vandenplas, Y. The efficiency of *Saccharomyces boulardii* CNCM I-745 in addition to standard *Helicobacter pylori* eradication treatment in children. *Pediatr. Gastroenterol. Hepatol. Nutr.* **2015**, *1*, 17–22. [CrossRef] [PubMed]
186. Szajewska, H.; Horvath, A.; Kołodziej, M. Systematic review and meta-analysis: *Saccharomyces boulardii* supplementation and eradication of *Helicobacter pylori* infection. *Aliment. Pharmacol. Ther.* **2015**, *12*, 1237–1245. [CrossRef] [PubMed]
187. Tong, J.L.; Ran, Z.H.; Shen, J.; Zhang, C.X.; Xiao, S.D. Meta-analysis: The effect of supplementation with probiotics on eradication rates and adverse events during *Helicobacter pylori* eradication therapy. *Aliment. Pharmacol. Ther.* **2007**, *25*, 155–168. [CrossRef]
188. Eslami, M.; Yousefi, B.; Kokhaei, P.; Moghadas, A.J.; Moghadam, B.S.; Arabkari, V.; Niazi, Z. Are Probiotics Useful for Therapy of *Helicobacter pylori* Diseases? *Comp. Immunol. Microbiol. Infect. Dis.* **2019**, *64*, 99–108. [CrossRef]

nutrients

Review

Intestinal Barrier Impairment, Preservation, and Repair: An Update

Ayah Matar †, John A. Damianos †, Kara J. Jencks and Michael Camilleri *

Clinical Enteric Neuroscience Translational and Epidemiological Research (CENTER), Division of Gastroenterology and Hepatology, Mayo Clinic, Rochester, MN 55905, USA; matar.ayah@mayo.edu (A.M.); damianos.john@mayo.edu (J.A.D.)
* Correspondence: camilleri.michael@mayo.edu; Tel.: +1-507-266-2305
† These authors contributed equally to this work.

Abstract: Background/Objectives: Our objective was to review published studies of the intestinal barrier and permeability, the deleterious effects of dietary components (particularly fat), the impact of altered intestinal permeability in disease models and human diseases, the role of the microbiome and epigenomics in control of barrier function, and the opportunities to restore normal barrier function with dietary interventions and products of the microbiota. Methods: We conducted a literature review including the following keywords alone or in combination: intestinal barrier, permeability, microbiome, epigenomics, diet, irritable bowel syndrome, inflammatory bowel disease, probiotics. Results: Intestinal permeability is modified by a diet including fat, which increases permeability, and nutrients such as fiber, glutamine, zinc, vitamin D, polyphenols, emulsifiers, and anthocyanins, which decrease permeability. There is significant interaction of the microbiome and barrier function, including the inflammatory of luminal/bacterial antigens, and anti-inflammatory effects of commensals or probiotics and their products, including short-chain fatty acids. Epigenomic modification of barrier functions are best illustrated by effects on junction proteins or inflammation. Detailed documentation of the protective effects of diet, probiotics, prebiotics, and microbiota is provided. Conclusion: intestinal permeability is a critical factor in protection against gastrointestinal diseases and is impacted by nutrients that preserve or heal and repair the barrier and nurture anti-inflammatory effects.

Keywords: permeability; fat; emulsifier; tight junctions; epigenomics; inflammation

1. Introduction

The objective of this review is to provide information regarding the intestinal barrier and permeability, the deleterious effects of dietary components (particularly fat), the impact of altered intestinal permeability in disease models or human diseases, the role of the microbiome and epigenomics in the control of barrier function, the opportunities to restore normal barrier function with dietary interventions, and products of microbiota.

Intestinal Barrier and Permeability

The gastrointestinal tract features one of the longest barriers between the environment and the systemic circulation, spanning up to 40 square meters. This barrier is composed of a mucus layer, commensal microbiota, the intestinal epithelium, and immune cells situated in the lamina propria [1–3]. The mucus layer over the intestinal epithelium safeguards it from contents within the intestinal lumen [4]. Commensal microbiota support barrier function, shape intestinal and systemic immune responses, and inhibit pathogenic bacteria by directly stimulating epithelial cells, producing nutrients and metabolites that are essential for enterocyte health, and influencing the priming of the immune system [5]. The epithelial semi-permeable barrier contributes to maintaining intestinal homeostasis by selectively allowing nutrients to cross from the intestinal lumen into the internal milieu, to reach the systemic circulation, while controlling the passage of bacterial pathogens, allergens, and toxins [2].

The epithelial cells are organized into a single layer of cells from four primary lineages: enterocytes (the most abundant), goblet cells, enteroendocrine cells, and Paneth cells [4,6,7]. Enterocytes are chiefly involved in absorption of nutrients, water and electrolytes from the lumen, goblet cells secret mucus that adds protection to the barrier layer, enteroendocrine cells secrete hormones that have diverse regulatory functions, and Paneth cells release antimicrobial peptides [2,6,8]. These cells function synergistically to maintain the gut barrier's integrity [6].

Tight junctions (TJs) are a series of transmembrane proteins that connect intestinal epithelial cells and are essential for maintaining barrier integrity, particularly when the intestines are distended [4]. The recent literature has reported three main proteins that make up TJs and contribute to their function. Proteins found in the cytoplasm beneath the TJ membrane include cingulin (CGN), guanine nucleotide exchange factors (GEFs), GTPase-activating proteins (GAPs), and zonula occludens proteins (ZOs) including ZO-1, ZO-2, and ZO-3 (which are also known as TJP1, TJP2, and TJP3, respectively) [9,10]. Other proteins that contribute to the permeability/barrier function of TJs comprise claudin polymers that are either barrier-forming or channel-forming. It is important to note that further interactions between claudin isoforms also exist but have yet to be established [9,11]. Additionally among the proteins that contribute to the permeability, barrier, and adhesion function of TJs, there is junctional adhesion molecule A (JAM-A, also known as F11R) [9].

These junctions are also crucial for regulating the transport of substances between the intestinal lumen and systemic circulation [12]; such transport is mediated in part by the permeability of TJs, leading to three types of functional gaps with different properties: pore pathway, leak pathway, and restricted pathway [13]. The pore pathway is of high capacity and charge-selective, permitting the passage of small ions and uncharged molecules (typically <8 Å); the leak pathway is low-capacity and nonselective (<100 Å); on the other hand, the unrestricted pathway is independent of the TJ and results from epithelial damage [9,12,14]. Damage to these pathways alters the barrier integrity and may contribute to the development of disease [15,16].

Intestinal permeability refers to the functional properties of the intestinal barrier and is characterized primarily by paracellular and transcellular transport mechanisms [7]. The paracellular route, regulated by tight junctions, allows the passage of ions, water, and large hydrophilic compounds [17], while the transcellular route facilitates the passage of proteins, sugars, amino acids, and bacteria [18], typically by carrier-mediated transport. Disruption in either route can affect barrier homeostasis, alter permeability and potentially lead to disease [3,18,19].

Various factors, including dietary components, genetic predisposition, medications (e.g., NSAIDs and antibiotics), alcohol consumption, strenuous physical activity, psychological or environmental stress, pregnancy, pathogens, systemic diseases, inflammatory conditions and cytokines, metabolic disorders including obesity, and surfactants (e.g., bile acids and emulsifiers) can alter barrier homeostasis [3,17–20] and increase permeability, leading to "leaky gut" [18,21]. This "leakiness" allows passage of microorganisms, allergens, and toxins inciting inflammation locally in the gut, and passage into the systemic circulation [3,21]. "Leaky gut" has been implicated in a wide range of systemic diseases (including type 2 diabetes mellitus, obesity), neuropsychiatric diseases (e.g., Alzheimer disease, Parkinson disease, autism spectrum disorders, major depressive disorder), and autoimmune disease (e.g., psoriasis, rheumatologic diseases, and uveitis), in addition to intestinal diseases (e.g., inflammatory bowel disease (IBD), irritable bowel syndrome (IBS), celiac disease) [1,4,18,20,22].

2. Epigenetic Mechanisms Related to Intestinal Permeability

Recent data suggest epigenetic mechanisms are involved in regulating intestinal permeability. Epigenetic mechanisms include how the environment alters the expression of DNA without changing DNA nucleotides. Examples of epigenetic mechanisms include DNA methylation, histone modification, non-coding RNA activity, and chromatin remodeling, which all affect how genes are expressed. Environmental exposures, stress, toxins, medications, development, aging, and diet can induce epigenetic changes. Environmental states with increased levels of stress are thought to effect change via epigenetic mechanisms, related to the corticotropin releasing factor/hypothalamic-pituitary-adrenal axis [23]. The published data on epigenetic changes on intestinal permeability are primarily from stressed animal models which have increased intestinal paracellular permeability and visceral hypersensitivity [23]. In a chronic preclinical stress model, which is relevant to pathophysiological states like irritable bowel syndrome, the mice had increased levels of cytokine IL-6, which is pro-inflammatory, and correlated to a decrease in tight junction proteins in the colon, documented by an inverse correlation of IL-6 level and the expression of occludins [24]. IL-6 acted via epigenetic mechanisms (as evidenced by increased methylation of the repressive histone H3K9) with an observed increase in paracellular permeability [24]. In biopsies taken from patients with diarrhea-predominant irritable bowel syndrome, there were increased levels of micro-RNA 29A and B and reduced levels of claudin-1 (CLDN1) and nuclear factor-kB-repressing factor (NKRF), which was replicated in a knockout animal model that documented the fact that increased micro-RNA 29A and B decreased the levels of CLDN1 and NKRF mRNA [25].

Network enrichment analysis of RNA-sequencing data in a chronic stress model of rats identified that super enhancers play an important role in intestinal barrier dysfunction [26]. Super enhancers are sites in the genome with increased areas for transcription factors to bind (enhancers) and enhance genetic expression of an associated gene up to one million base pairs away. Super enhancers have recently been considered an epigenetic mechanism as they regulate gene expression without modifying DNA. In particular, in the rat chronic stress model, it was shown that super enhancers played a role in the downregulation of adherens and intestinal epithelial tight junction genes (e-cadherin (CDH1), tight junction protein 3 or ZO-3 (TJP3), p-cadherin (CDH3), m-cadherin (CDH15), claudin-2 (CLDN2), claudin-3 (CLDN3), claudin-7 (CLDN7), and tight junction associated protein 1 or 4 (TJAP1)), which are linked to increased paracellular permeability [26]. The microRNAs involved in intestinal permeability include microRNA-16 (downregulated in IBS), microRNA 125b (downregulated in jejunal IBS-D tissue), microRNA 144 (upregulated in a colon IBS_D rat model), and microRNA-29a (upregulated in colon and duodenum of IBS and rat models) [23,27–31].

Irritable bowel syndrome is not the only phenotype where intestinal permeability and epigenetic mechanisms have been studied. Paracellular membrane permeability was influenced by DNA methyltransferase 3A activity (which is involved in DNA methylation) in the colon epithelial cells from patients with IBD in studies conducted in vitro [32]. Colon tissue samples and organoids from patients with ulcerative colitis had increased levels of IL1B mRNA and microRNA 200C-3p that decreased the expression of occludin and increased intestinal permeability [33]. In patients with systemic lupus erythematosus, there is also evidence of association of possibly increased intestinal permeability, with DNA methylation levels being highest in 926 CpG sites [34]

Additionally, the microbiome is also thought to contribute to local changes in intestinal permeability and maintenance of membrane barrier function [35–37]. Increased intestinal permeability can result from altered expression of tight junction related proteins with changes in intestinal microbiota profiles [38]. The host phenotype is influenced by the epigenome–microbiome axis. This includes how the environment and host genotype affect both the host epigenotype and the microbiome composition and activity. It is also known that the microbiome and epigenotype contribute to the host phenotype [39]. Microbiota can induce modification of gene expression through epigenetic mechanisms [39]. For example, disruption to the barrier function was repaired though the activation of epithelial histone deacetylase 3 (HDAC3) via microbiota-derived IP3 (inositol triphosphate) in a murine model and intestinal organoid model [37]. Histone deacetylases remove acetyl groups from histones (and non-histones), decreasing transcription. Short chain fatty acids (SCFAs) like butyrate, acetate, and propionate inhibit host histone deacetylases, leading to silencing of transcription, chromatin condensation, histone acylation, and DNA methylation [39].

Chronic stress and the microbiome are not the only ways via which epigenetic modulation affects intestinal permeability. Ingested substances (discussed more extensively in subsequent sections and Table 1 also influence epigenetic mechanisms. For example, anthocyanins, which are part of the flavonoid group of polyphenols, naturally occur in many colorful fruits and vegetables. Anthocyanins appear to play a role in epigenetic modulation of the expression of key membrane integrity proteins, such as ZO-1 and occludins, in animal models [40]. Zinc also influences the gene expression of tight junction proteins, claudin 1 and 2, through histone deacetylase activity and chromatin remodeling [41,42].

Table 1. Effects of high-fat diet on intestinal barrier function in humans in vivo or in vitro (adapted and updated from Camilleri and Vella [2]).

Participants	Treatment/Duration/Method	Main Results	Ref.
1015 healthy people randomly recruited; in vivo	Three-day food record; plasma LPS tested in 201 male participants.	Association between food intake (positively correlated with fat intake) and plasma LPS.	Amar et al., 2008 [43]
20 healthy adults (mean age 25 ± 3.2 y); in vivo	Control diet (olive oil, 20%) HFD with omega-3 (fish oil, 35%) HFD with omega-6 (grape seed oil, 35%); diet rich in saturated fat (coconut oil, 35%); serum endotoxin concentration	Serum endotoxin concentration increased during postprandial period after consumption of a high-saturated-fat meal, but decreased after the meal with omega-3.	Lyte et al., 2016 [44]
13 normal weight, sedentary adult males (mean age 22.2 ± 1.6 y); all weight-stable; in vivo	Two-week control diet [55% CHO, 30% fat (9% saturated), and 15% protein]; HFD for 5 days [55% fat (25% saturated fat), 30% CHO, and 15% protein]; HFM challenge [820 kcal: 25% CHO, 12% protein, 63% fat (~26% saturated fat)] pre- and post-5-day HFD; urine excretion of probe molecules.	No significant changes in gastroduodenal, small intestinal (p = 0.084 LM ratio), or colonic permeability following HFD.	Bowser et al., 2020 [45]
M-cell monolayers, human Peyer's patches	Soluble NSP and food emulsifiers. Polysorbate-80 at 0.01% and 0.1%vol/vol *E. coli* translocation.	Polysorbate-80 increased *E. coli* translocation across M cells and human Peyer's patches.	Roberts et al., 2010 [46]

CHO: carbohydrate; LPS: lipopolysaccaride, HFD: high-fat diet, HFM: high-fat meal, LM ratio: lactulose–mannitol ratio; NSP: non-starch polysaccaride.

3. Effect of Food Substances and Disease States on Intestinal Permeability

3.1. Food Substances That Decrease Intestinal Barrier Integrity or Increase Permeability

In view of the most recent extensive literature regarding the deleterious effect of fats on intestinal barrier function, and the associations of Western diet on diverse diseases, Table 1 summarizes the effects of high-fat diet on intestinal barrier function [21,43–46]. The table shows that, in vivo, fat intake is associated with serological markers of increased permeability such as plasma lipopolysaccharide and serum endotoxin; in addition, there was a trend to increased permeability measured using the ratio of the urinary excretion of oral sugar probe molecules (lactulose and mannitol). There is also evidence, based on in vitro studies of modulators from human Peyer's patches, that the emulsifier polysorbate-80 increased translocation of *E. coli*.

3.2. Altered Permeability and Disease States

Altered permeability has been investigated in vivo in preclinical models of disease, as well as in human disease states, and these are summarized in Tables 2 and 3 and elaborated further in Section 4 [21,47–55].

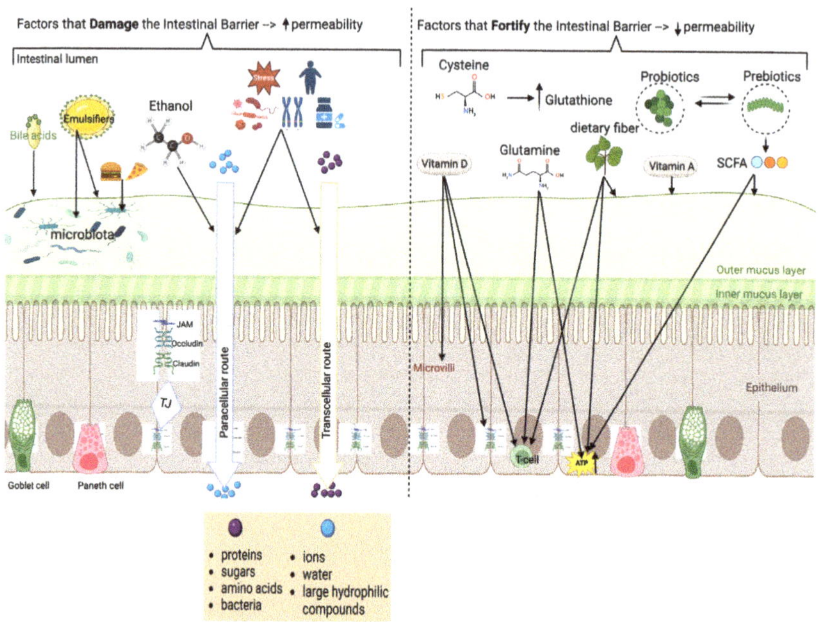

Figure 1. Composition of barrier, physiology of permeability, and factors which help or harm permeability (created in BioRender. matar, a. (2024) BioRender.com/m56y070 (accessed on 10 October 2024)). The left side of the figure summarizes the factors that damage the intestinal barrier resulting in increased permeability; the right side summarizes factors that enhance the intestinal barrier resulting in reduced intestinal permeability. Several amino acids, exemplified by glutamine in the figure, are associated with fortification of the intestinal barrier (as detailed in the text).

Table 2. Summary of preclinical models of altered permeability investigated in vivo (adapted and updated from Khoshbin and Camilleri [42]).

Component	Preclinical Models	Effects in Preclinical Models	Reference
	Dietary Component		
Dietary Fiber	- Resistant oligosaccharides: Mistry et al. (male mice on Western-type diet, in vivo); - Non-starch polysaccharides: in vivo study with inulin (healthy male volunteers); - Resistant starches: Gondalia et al., in vivo study (healthy adults with high- vs. low-amylose wheat).	Supplementation reduced bodyweight gain, fat accumulation, insulin resistance, altered gut microbiota, lowered lactulose/mannitol ratio and serum zonulin, increased mucosal GLP-2; Similar effects on fecal output and SCFA excretion; HAW-R increased fecal butyrate.	Mistry et al., 2020 [47] Camilleri et al., 2022 [21]

Table 2. *Cont.*

Component	Preclinical Models	Effects in Preclinical Models	Reference
Vitamin D	- VDR-deficient mice, in vivo:	Increased susceptibility to bacteria and LPS, weakened tight junctions.	Yamamoto et al., 2020 [49]
Minerals: Zinc	- Zinc deficiency: Omry et al., in vivo study (chicks); - Zinc deficiency [51]; - Zinc overdose: chronic exposure in mice, in vivo study.	Mixed evidence on potential to upregulate "leaky" junctions in some contexts; Reduced microbial diversity, impaired nutrient uptake.	Yamamoto et al., 2020 [49] Koren et al.,2020 [51]
Others: polyphenols, flavanones, anthocyanins	- Urolithins: Administration of Uro-A and Uro-B in rats (in vivo study) on a high-fat diet.	Altered gut microbiota, decreased microbes associated with weight and inflammation.	Abdulrahman et al., 2021 [53]
Arabinoxylans	Overweight and obesity	Effects on gut health detailed in the body of the text.	
Probiotics	Obesity; primary sclerosing cholangitis and IBD.		
Synbiotics	Indomethacin-induced increased permeability; obesity.		
Prebiotics	Non-obese diabetic mice; Western diet induced increased intestinal permeability in mice; aspirin-induced intestinal permeability in humans; children with type 1 diabetes mellitus; pre-term infants; burns.		
	Macronutrients		
Protein	Protein-restricted diet or dexamethasone-induced permeability in chickens; Dietary meat and fish (and fat) in epidemiological studies of IBD.	Increased permeability and bacterial translocation; Increased risk of IBD.	Khoshbin et al., 2020 [42]
Sulfur-containing AAs: cysteine & methionine	Rats infected with *Salmonella enteritidis*; ischemia-reperfusion injury in rats; high-fat diet with methionine restriction in mice.	Effects on gut health detailed in Figure 1.	
Other AAs: Glutamine, L-tryptophan, Arginine	- Glycyl-glutamine (GlyGln): in vivo study with weaned piglets; - Ala-Gln and glutamine (Gln): in vivo study in mice with DSS-induced colitis; - Tryptophan: colitis in mice. - Arginine: intestinal injury induced by heat stress; ischemia reperfusion; methotrexate; NASH or intestinal obstruction in rodents; mouse colitis.	Improved ileum morphology, reduced inflammation, enhanced oxidative status, Both improved colitis symptoms, with Ala-Gln showing superior efficacy; Evidence suggests benefits in gut health and barrier function.	Xu et al., 2021 [54] Xu et al., 2021 [55]
Fat:	Fat-restricted diets.	Alterations in microbiota and further explanations in Table 1.	
Alcohol	Alcohol abuse and alcoholic liver disease.	Increased permeability and bacterial translocation.	Khoshbin et al., 2020 [42]

Table 2. *Cont.*

Component	Preclinical Models	Effects in Preclinical Models	Reference
		Intraluminal Emulsifiers	
Endogenous bile acid	Mammalian colon	Detergent effects with increased permeability measured by PEG 400 and scanning EM.	Khoshbin et al., 2020 [42]
Dietary emulsifiers	Mouse colon permeability and inflammatory changes.	Effects on gut health detailed in the text.	
		Receptors Associated with Intraluminal Factors	
Aryl hydrocarbon receptor	Diverse animal models of immune diseases.	Anti-inflammatory	Khoshbin et al., 2020 [42]

AA: amino acids; DSS: dioctyl sodium sulfosuccinate; EM electron microscopy; IBD: inflammatory bowel disease; IBS-D: diarrhea-predominant irritable bowel syndrome; Ala-Gln: alanyl glutamine; DSS: dextran sodium sulfate; GLP-2: glucagon-like peptide 2; Gln: glutamine; GlyGln: glycyl-glutamine; HAW R: high-amylose wheat resistant starch; NAFLD: non-alcoholic fatty liver disease; NASH: non-alcoholic steatohepatitis; Uro-A: urolithin A; Uro-B: urolithin B; VDR: vitamin D receptor.

Table 3. Summary of preclinical models investigating human disease states of altered permeability (adapted and updated from Khoshbin and Camilleri [42]).

Component	Human Diseases	Effects in Human Diseases	Reference
	Dietary Component		
Dietary Fiber	Effect on metabolic markers and gut health detailed in text.		Gondalia et al., 2022 [48]
Vitamin D	In vivo study with high levels of active vitamin D.	Associated with gut bacteria producing butyrate, enhancing intestinal barrier; Mixed evidence on potential to upregulate "leaky" junctions in some contexts.	Thomas et al., 2020 [50] Yamamoto et al., 2020 [49]
Minerals: Zinc	Zinc deficiency linked to gastrointestinal disorders; appropriate dosing improves gut bacteria biodiversity and barrier integrity.	Increased oxidative stress, compromised barrier integrity.	Skalny et al., 2021 [52]
Others: polyphenols, flavanones, anthocyanins	Limited direct studies on permeability.	Polyphenols show general gut health benefits (see text).	
		Macronutrients	
Protein	Dietary meat and fish (and fat) in epidemiological studies of IBD.	Increased risk of IBD	Khoshbin et al., 2020 [42]
Other AAs: Glutamine, L-tryptophan, Arginine	Limited direct studies.	Evidence suggests benefits in gut health and barrier function	Xu et al., 2021 [55]
Fat.	Fat-restricted diets.	Alterations in microbiota and further explanations in Table 1	Xu et al., 2021 [54]
Alcohol	Alcohol abuse and alcoholic liver disease.	Increased permeability and bacterial translocation	Khoshbin et al., 2020 [42]

AA: amino acids; IBD: inflammatory bowel disease.

4. Effects of Dietary Components That Enhance or Damage the Intestinal Barrier

4.1. Nutrients

Table 4 provide a summary of the nutrients that either increase or decrease intestinal permeability as well as the mechanisms proposed for the changes in intestinal permeability

Table 4. Summary of nutrients increasing or decreasing intestinal permeability and proposed mechanisms.

Nutrient	Proposed Mechanisms	Factors That Decrease Permeability	Factors That Increase Permeability	References
Dietary fiber	- Fermentation by gut microbiota produces SCFAs (e.g., acetate, butyrate, propionate); - SCFAs enhance tight junction integrity and modulate inflammation.	- SCFAs increase production of mucins and enhance epithelial cell function; - Butyrate supports mucosal health and decreases inflammation.	- Inadequate fiber intake can lead to reduced SCFA production and compromised barrier function.	[21,47,48,56–62]
Polyphenols	- Antioxidant properties; - Modulation of gut microbiota; - Reduction in oxidative stress and inflammation.	- Urolithin A and B reduce inflammation and oxidative stress, improving barrier function; - Anthocyanins provide antioxidant protection.	- Variable metabolism of polyphenols leading to inconsistent effects across individuals.	[53,63–67]
Glutamine	- Supports synthesis of tight junction proteins; - Enhances gut microbiota diversity and function; - Reduces inflammation.	- GlyGln and Gln supplementation improves intestinal morphology and barrier integrity; - Support for mucosal health and reduction in inflammation.	- High doses of supplementation could disrupt balance and exacerbate inflammation.	[54,55]
Vitamin D	- Enhances expression of tight junction proteins (e.g., ZO-1, occludin, claudin-1); - Upregulates antimicrobial peptides.	- Adequate levels of active vitamin D strengthen the epithelial barrier; - Supports microbiota associated with butyrate production.	- Potential to upregulate "leaky" junctions in some cases; - Over-supplementation may disrupt barrier function.	[49,50,68]

Table 4. *Cont.*

Nutrient	Proposed Mechanisms	Factors That Decrease Permeability	Factors That Increase Permeability	References
Zinc	- Influences tight junction protein expression; - Modulates gut microbiota diversity; - Affects immune responses.	- Optimal zinc levels improve barrier integrity and gut microbiota diversity; - Enhances nutrient uptake and reduces permeability.	- Zinc deficiency leads to dysbiosis and compromised barrier function; - Overdosing induces oxidative stress and disrupts barrier integrity.	[51,52,69,70]
SCFAs	- Produced from fermentation of dietary fiber by gut microbiota; - SCFAs (acetate, butyrate, propionate) enhance tight junction integrity and reduce inflammation.	- Butyrate is particularly beneficial in reducing inflammation, supporting mucosal health, and increasing tight junction protein expression; - SCFAs lower colonic pH, inhibiting pathogenic bacteria.	- Reduced SCFA production due to low fiber intake can compromise barrier integrity and gut health.	[58–62]

SCFAs: short-chain fatty acids, GLN: glutamine; GLY: glycine; ZO-1: zonula occludens.

4.1.1. Substances That Help Increase Intestinal Barrier Integrity

Numerous strategies have been suggested to address gut barrier dysfunction, such as direct immune therapies, blocking signaling factors, introducing specific microbes, fecal microbiota transplantation, using microbial metabolites, probiotics, targeting disease-induced regulatory factors, hormone treatments, treating underlying conditions, dietary supplementation, and maintaining a healthy diet and overall wellness [71]. This section focuses on dietary factors and microbial metabolites and nutrients, based on a review of the recent literature and updated versions of reports written by Khoshbin and Camilleri [42] and Camilleri and Vella [21].

4.1.2. Dietary Fiber

Dietary fiber is a carbohydrate polymer made up of 10 or more monomers that are neither absorbed nor digested in the small intestine [56,57]. The four subgroups of dietary fiber that research primarily focuses on are resistant oligosaccharides, non-starch polysaccharides, resistant starches, and associated substances [57]. Dietary sources of resistant oligosaccharides include various legumes, vegetables, fruits, and specific plant products like chicory root and soybeans. Non-starch polysaccharides, such as cellulose, hemicellulose, and pectins are found in cereals, grains, fruits, and vegetables, while resistant starches come from foods like grains, green bananas, and processed products. Additionally, associated non-carbohydrate substances like lignin, waxes, and chitins are present in cereal grain outer layers, insect secretions, and the exoskeletons of crustaceans. These types of fiber are considered as prebiotics since stimulate bacteria beneficial for the gut health and aid in the increase of short chains of fatty acids (SCFAs) which also enhances the integrity of the intestinal barrier [47].

SCFAs, produced from dietary fiber fermentation by gut microbiota, play a crucial role in colon health and microbiota–gut–brain communication, providing 5–10% of human basal energy needs [58,59]. Research has focused around three SCFAs: acetate, butyrate, and propionate [60]. Acetate, the most abundant SCFA, supports ATP production, while SCFAs overall lower colon pH to inhibit pathogenic bacteria and modulate inflammation through various cellular mechanisms [60,61]. Butyrate, in particular, has significant health benefits, including cancer prevention, while propionate may reduce blood cholesterol, and both contribute to communication along the microbiota–gut–brain axis due to their neuro-active properties [62].

Resistant oligosaccharides include fructo-oligosaccharides (short chain inulin), which are β-(2 → 1) linear fructans derived from enzymatic hydrolysis of long-chain inulin or synthesized from sucrose [58]. Galacto-oligosaccharides consist of two to eight saccharide units with glucose and galactose and can be found in human milk or synthesized from lactose [58]. Other resistant oligosaccharides include non-digestible types like konjac oligosaccharide. Incorporating a wide range of fruits, vegetables, various legumes, and soybeans (resistant oligosaccharide products) can go along way toward enhancing gut health, especially considering recent Westernized diets that have become widely popular. Mistry et al. showed in an in vivo study on male mice fed a Western-type diet that resistant oligosaccharide supplementation significantly reduced bodyweight gain, fat accumulation, insulin resistance, and plasma cholesterol levels, while also altering gut microbiota composition in a way that may benefit metabolic health. These findings suggest that resistant oligosaccharides could have therapeutic potential for improving metabolic markers and reducing the risk of metabolic syndrome [47].

Non-starch polysaccharides include cellulose, the main structural component of plant cell walls, and hemicelluloses, which are diverse cell-wall polysaccharides found in fruits, vegetables, and cereals [58]. Pectins, found in plant cell walls, and various gums and mucilages from plants, microbes, and seaweed, are also key non-starch polysaccharides. Additionally, β-glucans and β-fructans, such as inulin from chicory roots, are non-digestible fibers that are resistant to enzymatic digestion but fermentable in the colon [58]. In an in vivo study with healthy male volunteers, inulin was shown to lower the lactulose–mannitol (L/M) ratio and serum zonulin while increasing mucosal GLP-2 after 8 weeks [21]. However, the study's methods were suboptimal, including the use of inappropriate sugar probes, limited urine collection time, and serum levels that may not have accurately indicated intestinal permeability.

Resistant starches (RS) come in various forms, including physically inaccessible starch (RS1), granular native starch (RS2), retrograded starch (RS3), chemically modified starch (RS4), and resistant maltodextrins like Nutriose (RS5) [58]. Gondalia et al. [48] showed that in an in vivo study of 80 healthy adults who were either given high-amylose wheat (HAW) product or low-amylose wheat (LAW) product, HAW and LAW had similar effects on fecal output and total SCFA excretion, but the HAW-R group showed 38% higher fecal butyrate excretion and more SCFA-producing bacteria at 4 weeks. While LAW-R increased fecal p-cresol levels, which disrupts the epithelial barrier function, and also increased the abundance of a p-cresol-producing bacterium (*Clostridium difficile, Clostridium scatologenes, Clostridium bolteae*), these were reduced by HAW-R, with no impact on fecal consistency or digestive comfort from the amylose level [48].

4.1.3. Polyphenols, Anthocyanins, and Ellagitannins

Recent studies have focused on polyphenols, particularly flavonoids (such as anthocyanins, flavonols, and flavanols), condensed and hydrolysable tannins (like ellagitannins), phenolic acids, stilbenes, and lignans, due to their potential benefits for the intestinal barrier [63–65]. These polyphenols are predominantly found in various types of berries, including blueberries, strawberries, and blackberries [65]. Berries are a rich source of flavonoids, particularly anthocyanins, which give them their vibrant colors and have strong antioxidant properties [65]. These pigments, along with flavonols and flavan-3-ols, are not only capable of crossing the blood–brain barrier but also offer potential health benefits, including cardioprotective, neuroprotective, anti-inflammatory, and anticancer effects [65].

Ellagitannins (ETs) are hydrolysable tannins abundantly found in raspberries, walnuts, strawberries, and pomegranate [64]. They are hydrolyzed in the intestinal lumen and release ellagic acid (EA), which is then further metabolized with ellagitannins into urolithins [64,66]. Due to the interindividual variability of metabolization of ETs, three Uro metabotypes (UM) that are microbiome-specific have been identified and are most relevant to this paper, metabotype A, metabotype B, and metabotype 0, yielding UM-A, UM-B, and UM-0, respectively [65,66].

Urolithin A (Uro-A) and to a lesser extent Urothilin B (Uro-B) exhibit anti-inflammatory, neuroprotective, cardioprotective, and anti-obesity activites, as well as improving gut microbiota and tight junction protein expression, cognitive function, and muscle function, while also demonstrating potential in reducing oxidative stress, protecting against organ damage, and modulating the immune response in various animal models [67]. A recent in vivo study found that administering Uro-A and Uro-B intraperitoneally for 4 weeks in rats on a high-fat diet altered gut microbiota composition, leading to a decrease in microbes associated with body weight, lipid metabolism issues, and inflammation [53].

4.1.4. Glutamine

In an in vivo study investigating the effects of dietary glycyl-glutamine (GlyGln) supplementation, weaned piglets were given either a basal diet or the same diet supplemented with 0.25% GlyGln for 3 weeks [54]. Following intraperitoneal injections of lipopolysaccharide (LPS) to induce inflammation, the GlyGln-supplemented piglets showed improved ileum morphology, reduced inflammation, and enhanced oxidative status, with increased levels of interleukin 10 and tight junction proteins, as well as higher superoxide dismutase activity [54]. Additionally, GlyGln supplementation restored gut microbiota diversity and function, enriching beneficial bacteria and short-chain fatty acid producers, and improving intestinal integrity and microbial balance disrupted by the LPS challenge [54].

In another study that investigated the effects of oral supplementation with Ala-Gln and glutamine (Gln) on dextran sulfate sodium (DSS)-induced colitis in mice [55], both supplements significantly improved colitis symptoms, such as bodyweight loss and colon damage, reduced inflammation markers and tissue apoptosis, and enhanced gut microbiota diversity and function, with Ala-Gln demonstrating superior efficacy over Gln in preserving intestinal integrity and microbiota composition [55].

4.1.5. Vitamin D

Research shows that vitamin D is essential for maintaining gut barrier integrity, with VDR-deficient mice study displaying increased susceptibility to bacteria and LPS in vivo due to weakened tight junctions [49]. Vitamin D supplementation strengthens the epithelial barrier by enhancing the expression of tight junction proteins like ZO-1, occludin, and claudin-1, as demonstrated in studies where 1,25(OH)2D3 treatment partially rescued these proteins' reduced expression in DSS-treated Caco-2 cells [49,68]. Additionally, vitamin D upregulates antimicrobial peptides, which are crucial for maintaining a balanced microbiome and preventing harmful bacterial colonization [68]. Thomas et al. conducted an in vivo study where 567 men provided stool samples, to study their microbiome and correlate it with vitamin D metabolite levels. This study showed that men with the highest levels of active vitamin D (1,25(OH)2D) or activation ratios were more likely to have gut bacteria associated with butyrate production, which helps increase the integrity of the intestinal barrier, whereas serum 25(OH)D levels showed no strong association with microbiota diversity or specific bacteria [50]. This suggests that the regulation of vitamin D metabolism, rather than overall body stores of vitamin D, may have more significant health implications.

It is worth noting that Yamamoto et al. showed that improper regulation of vitamin D, whether through deficiency or excessive supplementation, can result in "leaky" junctions, which may partially contribute to the development of colitis [49]. They highlighted the importance of balancing vitamin D levels to ensure a therapeutic effect and not a damaging one [49]. However, more evidence is needed to fully understand the extent of vitamin D's role in this process.

4.1.6. Zinc

Recent studies have shown that zinc is a double-edged sword. In other words, both the deficiency and the overdosing of zinc can cause dysbiosis in the gut microbiome [69]. The deficiency of zinc has been correlated with multiple gastrointestinal disorders such as gastric cancer, Crohn's disease, impaired intestinal permeability, and irritable bowel syndrome [51,70]. Omry et al. show in an in vivo study with chicks divided into two treatment groups based on sex and body weight, "high Zn" and "low Zn," that Zn deficiency led to significant changes in microbial taxonomy, reduced species richness and diversity, and substantial reductions in KEGG pathways for nutrient uptake and beneficial short-chain fatty acids, which can impair optimal host Zn availability [51].

Consequently, supplementation with the appropriate dose of Zn has been shown to increase gut bacteria biodiversity, improve intestinal barrier integrity, and thereby limit the number of bacteria that can pass through the barrier into the systemic circulation [52]. The overdosing of Zn has been hypothesized to be related to the presence of "free flowing" Zn, thus altering immunity and causing dysbiosis [52]. An in vivo study in mice of chronic toxic exposure to ZnSO4 for 7 weeks showed reduced body and organ weight and increased AST activity [52]. Thus, excessive Zn doses can induce oxidative stress, compromise barrier integrity, and increase intestinal permeability, leading to a higher risk of the progression of other diseases [52,70]. Therefore, the right dosage of Zn should be provided and monitored to ensure its beneficial outcomes.

4.1.7. Emulsifiers

Emulsifiers, commonly known as surfactants, are widely used as food additives in the food industry and are highly prevalent in ultra-processed foods [42]. Previous research conducted primarily on mice in vitro indicated that emulsifiers increased intestinal permeability and were proinflammatory [72–75]. The study details were as follows:

Levine et al. [72] and Bancil et al. [74] conducted reviews of the existing literature, including both in vivo and in vitro studies, which showed that emulsifiers such as carboxymethylcellulose (CMS) and polysorbate 80 (P80) disrupt the intestinal mucosal layer leading to increased intestinal permeability or "leaky gut".

Naimi et al. studied the effects of CMC and P80 on the gut microbiota using in vitro fermentation of healthy human fecal samples. This study showed that exposure to either CMC or P80 caused a reduction in microbial diversity, an increase in pro-inflammatory bacteria (*Proteobacteria*), a decrease in butyrate production, decreased barrier integrity, and increased permeability in an in vitro epithelial model.

Ogulur et al. [75] conducted both in vitro and in vivo studies with polysorbate 20 (P20) and P80. In vitro studies were carried out on human intestinal epithelial cell lines (Caco-2 and HT29 cells), indicating that P80 and P20 compromised barrier function and disrupted TJ proteins. In vivo studies were conducted on mice and also showed an increase in intestinal permeability.

However, a recent in vivo and in vitro study by Fitzpatrick et al. involving 22 healthy adults who were fed either a high- or low-emulsifier diet (CMC, P80) produced unexpected results [76]. The study found that, based on diverse measurements (specifically, 2 h urinary lactulose–rhamnose ratio, serum concentrations of lipopolysaccharide-binding protein, soluble CD14, markers of epithelial injury and inflammation), diets high in emulsifiers actually improved intestinal barrier function in unstressed conditions, but increased sensitivity of intestinal permeability in response to stress [76]. Neither effect was associated with signs of inflammation [76]. More studies should be conducted to further solidify this finding and to appraise the interaction of experimental stress and exposure to emulsifiers.

4.2. Microbial Nutrients and Metabolites

4.2.1. Prebiotics

Descriptions and Mechanisms of Action: Prebiotics are defined as "substrate[s] that [are] selectively utilized by host microorganisms conferring a health benefit" [77]. While many different classes of compounds function as prebiotics, the most common types are poorly or non-digestible carbohydrates that are resistant to endogenous intestinal digestive enzymes. Non-digestible oligosaccharides represent a broader category that includes any oligosaccharides that are not digested nor absorbed in the small intestine; this group encompasses resistant or non-resistant oligosaccharides from the perspective of microbial fermentation. These oligosaccharides, such as fructans and galactans, reach the colon and are selectively metabolized by beneficial bacteria such as bifidobacteria. For instance, fructo-oligosaccharides (FOSs) and galacto-oligosaccharides (GOSs) are not digestible by human enzymes and can serve as substrates for fermentation by beneficial gut bacteria. Thus, they are degraded by β-fructanosidase and β-galactosidase enzymes, respectively. This selective utilization results in the production of short-chain fatty acids (SCFAs) such as acetate, propionate, and butyrate, which are crucial for maintaining intestinal health and can influence metabolic activities, immune functions, and overall homeostasis. Other examples of prebiotics include human milk oligosaccharides (HMOs), which are vital for the development of the newborn intestinal microbiota and immune system. HMOs are selectively utilized by specific *Bifidobacterium* species, promoting the growth of beneficial bacteria and protecting against pathogens. Plant polyphenols are another class of compounds that meet prebiotic criteria, undergoing extensive biotransformation in the colon to produce health-promoting metabolites [77].

Prebiotics exert significant protective effects on the intestinal barrier through multiple mechanisms. One primary effect is the modulation of microbial communities within the gut. Fermentation of prebiotic fibers leads to the production of SCFAs, which play a crucial role in maintaining the integrity of the intestinal barrier. Butyrate, in particular, is a key energy source for colonocytes and helps strengthen the epithelial barrier by promoting mucus production and secretion. This mucus layer acts as a protective shield, preventing microbial invasion and reducing susceptibility to infections and inflammatory conditions. Additionally, acetate and propionate support goblet cell function and mucin production, further enhancing the barrier function [78]. Prebiotics can also enhance the intestinal microenvironment in mechanisms independent of SCFAs. For instance, fiber can bind and transport essential minerals like calcium, zinc, and copper to the distal gut, where they are released for absorption. This process not only supports the microbiota but also improves mineral bioavailability for the host. Moreover, fiber may facilitate interactions between bacteria and biomolecules such as bile acids, enhancing microbial metabolism [78]. In addition to a large body of pre-clinical evidence detailing the mechanisms of prebiotics, there is also considerable pre-clinical evidence that these effects are anti-inflammatory in the intestines. For example, numerous studies have found that prebiotics can reduce inflammation in animal models of colitis [79]. A comprehensive summary of clinical trials that have assessed the effects of prebiotics on intestinal permeability is presented in Table 5 [3,80–92].

Table 5. Study characteristics and findings of clinical trials of prebiotics where effects on intestinal permeability were among the outcomes assessed.

Sample	Treatment/Duration	Main Results	Ref.
Formula-fed infants and exclusively breast-fed infants	Formula supplementation with a prebiotic mixture of galacto-oligosaccharides and inulin for 10 weeks	Reduced IP (assessed using the lactulose-to-mannitol ratio) and improved microbiota profiles	Francavilla et al., 2006 [80]

Table 5. *Cont.*

Sample	Treatment/Duration	Main Results	Ref.
Preterm infants	Enteral supplementation with a prebiotic mixture (1.5 g per kg per day of small-chain galacto-oligosaccharides, long-chain fructo-oligosaccharides, and nonhuman milk acidic oligosaccharides) for 30 days	No effect on IP (L:M ratio)	Westerbeek et al., 2010 [81]
Children with type 1 diabetes	8 g of oligofructose-enriched inulin (chicory root) for three months	Reduced IP (L:M ratio), increased C-peptide levels, induced favorable changes in gut microbiota composition	Ho et al., 2019 [82]
Adult burn patients	6 g of oligofructose for 15 days	No effect on IP (L:M ratio and sucrose excretion)	Olguin et al., 2005 [83]
Healthy young men	Inulin-enriched pasta for 5 weeks	Reduced IP (L:M ratio) and decreased serum levels of zonulin and GLP-2	Russo et al., 2012 [84]
Adults with overweight or obesity	Arabinoxylan (7.5 or 15 g per day) for 6 weeks	No effect on IP (multi-sugar test), but upregulation of gene transcription of tight junction proteins, decreased microbiome diversity (though without compositional change), decreased fecal pH, increased fecal concentrations of total SCFAs, acetate, propionate and butyrate, decreased TNFα production	Salden et al., 2018 [85]
Adults with slow gastrointestinal transit without constipation	15 g of wheat bran extract arabinoxylan–oligosaccharide (AXOS) for 12 weeks	No effect on IP (multi-sugar test), improved stool consistency, increased *Bifidobacterium* levels, no effect on whole-gut transit time or energy metabolism	Müller et al., 2020 [86]
Elderly adults	12 g per day oat β-glucan or wheat arabinoxylan for 6 weeks	No effect on indomethacin-induced increase in IP (multi-sugar test) or microbiota composition	Ganda Mall et al., 2020 [87]
Adults with overweight or obesity	25 g of yacon flour (rich in phenolic compounds and fructooligosaccharides) plus an energy-restricted diet for 6 weeks	No effect on IP (multi-sugar test), increased plasma antioxidant capacity, deceased oxidative stress markers, no effect on fecal short-chain fatty acids or inflammation markers	Machado et al., 2020 [88]
Adult men with type II diabetes	5.5 g per day of galacto-oligosaccharides for 12 weeks	No effect on IP (by urinary recovery of oral 51Cr-EDTA), glucose tolerance, or microbial community structure	Pedersen et al., 2016 [89]

Table 5. *Cont.*

Sample	Treatment/Duration	Main Results	Ref.
Adults at risk for type II diabetes	10 g per day of inulin for 6 weeks	No effect on IP (multi-sugar test), reduced fasting insulin levels, improved HOMA-IR, increased fecal Bifidobacteria, no effect on plasma endotoxin concentrations or lipopolysaccharide-binding protein concentrations	Mitchell et al., 2021 [90]
Adults with metabolic syndrome	Dietary Guidelines for Americans (DGA)-based diet incorporating potatoes (17.5 g per day of resistant starch) for 2 weeks	Reduced small IP (L:M ratio) and postprandial endotoxemia, no changes in cardiometabolic markers	Cao et al., 2022 [91]
Women with obesity and major depressive disorder	10 g per day of inulin	No effect on IP, depressive symptoms, inflammatory biomarkers, or weight	Vaghef-Mehrabani et al., 2023 [92]
Systematic review	Chicory inulin	Reduced IP	Nascimento et al., 2024 [3]

IP = intestinal permeability.

In summary, the evidence for prebiotics to reduce intestinal permeability is mixed. Some studies, such as those involving formula-fed infants and healthy young men, demonstrated significant reductions in intestinal permeability with prebiotic supplementation. However, other studies, particularly those involving vulnerable populations like preterm infants, burn patients, and individuals with type 2 diabetes or obesity, showed no significant improvements in intestinal permeability. The methodologies for assessing intestinal permeability varied across studies, with most involving the lactulose–mannitol ratio or other sugar-based tests. Other heterogeneity among the studies resulted from study design, population variability, and differences in prebiotic formulations (as well as dosing and duration). While prebiotics show promise in reducing intestinal permeability, further research is needed to identify which populations benefit most and the optimal prebiotic formulation for the given indication.

4.2.2. Probiotics

Descriptions and Mechanisms of Action: Probiotics are defined as "live microorganisms which when administered in adequate amounts confer a health benefit on the host" [93]. They encompass a wide range of single and multi-strain formulations of microorganisms (usually bacteria and/or fungi). While many of the specific health benefits derived from probiotics are strain-specific, there are general mechanisms thought to be shared among the most common probiotic organisms. These include the production of active metabolites (such as short-chain fatty acids, SCFAs), secretion of compounds (such as secretory IgA), interaction with the immune system, contribution to digestion and bile acid metabolism, manufacturing of systemically active molecules (such as serotonin), communication with the endogenous gut microbiota, and maintenance of the gut epithelial barrier [94]. Probiotics influence intestinal barrier function by modulating tight junction (TJ) proteins in intestinal epithelial cells (IECs), which are crucial for maintaining barrier integrity and preventing pathogen entry. Certain probiotics such as *Lactobacillus reuteri* and *Lactobacillus rhamnosus* enhance the expression and localization of TJ proteins such as ZO1, occludin, and claudin, thereby improving intestinal permeability and barrier function. They also regulate immune responses by promoting the maturation of dendritic cells, enhancing IgA secretion, and modulating inflammatory pathways. Additionally, probiotics can alter the gut microbiome composition, increase beneficial bacteria, and produce metabolites like SCFAs that further support barrier function and immune regulation [95]. The evidence for effects on intestinal permeability comes mainly from pre-clinical models. *Lacticaseibacillus rhamnosus* GG (LGG) normalizes intestinal permeability in rats with cow's milk-induced increase in permeability [96], and it also normalizes the increased permeability caused by acute alcohol exposure [97]. This effect may be mediated in part by LGG's propensity to adhere to the intestinal mucus layer with the adhesive protein LGG-0186 and its pili [98]. A systematic review and meta-analysis of nine studies found that probiotics and synbiotics significantly reduces serum zonulin levels, indicating improved intestinal permeability [99]. A summary of clinical trials of probiotics that have evaluated their effects on intestinal permeability is presented in Table 6 [100–132].

Table 6. Study characteristics and findings of clinical trials of probiotics where effect on intestinal permeability was among the outcomes assessed. Specific information about the microbiota in diverse, commercial formulations is included in the Supplementary Material.

Sample	Treatment/Duration	Main Results	Ref.
Preterm Infants	Fortification of formula with *Bifidobacter lactis* (2×10^7 cfu/g of dry milk) for 30 days	Reduced IP (L:M ratio) and increased head growth	Stratiki et al., 2007 [100]
Children with rotavirus or cryptosporidial diarrhea	Culturelle *Lacticaseibacillus rhamnosus* GG (ATCC 53103) (1×10^{10} CFU) for 4 weeks	Reduced IP (L:M ratio) and improved clinical outcomes	Sindhu et al., 2014 [101]
Children with Crohn disease	Valio LGG (1×10^{10} CFU twice daily) for 6 months	Reduced IP (double sugar test) and improved Crohn disease severity scores	Gupta et al., 2000 [102]
Children with atopic dermatitis	*Lactobacillus rhamnosus* 19070-2 (1×10^{10} CFU) and *L reuteri* DSM 12246 (1×10^{10} CFU) for 6 weeks	Reduced IP (L:M ratio), improved gastrointestinal symptoms; association between improved permeability and reduced eczema.	Rosenfeldt et al., 2004 [103]
Children with short bowel syndrome	Culturelle LGG (1×10^9 CFU) for 4 weeks	No effect on IP (L:M ratio), fecal *Lactobacillus* colonization, or small intestinal bacterial overgrowth	Sentongo et al., 2008 [104]
Healthy adults	Dairy product containing live or heat-inactivated *Lactobacillus GG* (>10^7/mL), *Lactobacillus helveticus* (>10^7/mL), and *Lactobacillus acidophilus* (>10^7/mL) (2.4×10^9 CFU) for 10 days	Live but not heat-killed probiotics reduced indomethacin-induced alterations in GP (urinary excretion of sucrose and L:M ratio) but did not affect IP	Gotteland, Cruchet, and Verbeke 2008 [105]
Healthy adults	De Simone formulation probiotic (900 billion bacteria per day) for 21 days	Reduced fecal calprotectin concentrations during indomethacin therapy	Montalto et al., 2010 [106]
Healthy adults	Yogurt enriched with *Lactobacillus gasseri* OLL2716 (1×10^9 CFU) for 16 weeks	Reduced IP (urinary sucrose excretion) and the likelihood of a positive fecal occult blood test after both high and low doses of aspirin	Akama et al., 2011 [107]

Table 6. *Cont.*

Sample	Treatment/Duration	Main Results	Ref.
Healthy adults	Lallemand *Lacticaseibacillus rhamnosus* R0011 and *Lactobacillus helveticus* R0052 (at least 4 billion CFU)	Did not prevent the increase in gastroduodenal permeability (urinary sucrose excretion) induced by an acute aspirin challenge	Judkins et al., 2024 [108]
Adults with Crohn disease in remission	Floratil *Saccharomyces boulardii* (4×10^8 CFU 3 times per day) for three months	Reduced IP (L:M ratio), although did not normalize it	Garcia Vilela et al., 2008 [109]
Adults with ulcerative colitis in remission	Ecologic 825 formulation (1.5×10^{10} CFU) for 12 weeks	No effect on IP (multi-sugar test), serum zonulin, fecal zonulin, inflammation markers, or stool characteristics	Wegh et al., 2019 [110]
Adults with diarrhea-predominant IBS	Probiotic fermented milk for 4 weeks	Reduced small IP (L:M ratio) and reduced IBS symptoms, though did not affect colonic permeability (sucralose excretion)	Zeng et al., 2008 [111]
Adults with IBS	Zircombi *Bifidobacterium longum* BB536 (4 billion CFU), *Lactobacillus rhamnosus* HN001 (1 billion CFU), and vitamin B6 for 30 days	Reduced IP (sucralose excretion), improved IBS symptoms, and favorably modified the gut microbiota and metabolome	Bonfrate et al., 2020 [112]
Adults with IBS	De Simone formulation (900 billion CFU) for 4 or 8 weeks	Reduced IP (multi-sugar test) and improved IBS symptoms	Boonma et al., 2021 [113]
Adults with IBS-D and confirmed increased permeability	Lactibiane Tolérance formulation (1×10^{10} CFU twice per day) for 30 days	Reduced (81.5%) or normalized (37%) IP (radionucleotide tracers) and improved IBS symptoms, including abdominal pain and stool consistency, while also enhancing QOL	Ait Abdellah et al., 2023 [114]
Adults with IBS-D	Lactibiane Tolérance formulation (10×10^9 CFU twice daily) for 4 weeks	While IP (urinary lactulose excretion) remained unchanged, the probiotic improved IBS symptoms, QOL, and gut microbiota. In responders with reduced diarrhea, transcellular permeability significantly decreased, and paracellular permeability trended toward a decrease, though overall permeability showed no significant change.	Marchix et al., 2023 [115]
Meta-analysis of patients with small intestinal bacterial overgrowth	Various	No effect on intestinal permeability	Zhong et al., 2017 [116]

Table 6. *Cont.*

Sample	Treatment/Duration	Main Results	Ref.
Adults with metabolic syndrome	Yakult (milk beverage fortified with 10^8 CFU/mL *Lactobacillus casei* Shirota) three bottles per day for 3 months	No effect on intestinal permeability (sugar absorption test and diaminooxidase serum levels), endotoxin levels, or neutrophil function	Leber et al., 2012 [117]
Systematic review of 12 animal and 14 clinical studies in obesity	Various, especially with *Bifidobacterium*, *Lactobacillus*, and *Akkermansia*	Often reduces IP in obesity, although clinical results are inconsistent	DiMattia et al., 2014 [118]
Adult patients with cirrhosis and a hepatic venous pressure gradient > 10	De Simone formulation (3600 billion bacteria daily) for 2 months	No effect on IP (L:M ratio, sucrose and sucralose tests) or portal pressure	Tandon et al., 2009 [119]
		No effect on IP (endotoxin levels), cytokine levels, microbiota or HVPG, but decrease in aldosterone	Jayakumar et al., 2013 [120]
Adults with chronic liver disease	Duolac Gold formulation (5×10^9 CFU twice daily) for 4 weeks	No effect on IP (L:M ratio), alleviated SIBO, improved GI symptoms	Kwak et al., 2014 [121]
Adults with cirrhosis primary and secondary analysis	Ecologic Barrier formulation (1.5×10^{10} CFU per day) for 6 months	No effect on IP (L:M ratio) or bacterial translocation, but did improve some immune and liver function, seen by increased serum neopterin levels and enhanced neutrophil reactive oxygen species production	Horvath et al., 2016 [122]
		Reduced IP (increased neopterin and decreased fecal zonulin), enriched the gut microbiota, and increased levels of beneficial bacteria	Horvath et al., 2020 [123]
Adults with metabolic dysfunction-associated steatotic liver disease	HEXBIO Microbial Cell Preparation (30 billion CFU twice daily) for 6 months	No effect on IP (zonulin and zonula occluden-1 (ZO-1) levels) or gut microbial diversity, although did induce changes in microbiota composition and decreases in IFN-γ and TNF-α	Ayob et al., 2023 [124]
Adults with acute pancreatitis	Enteral feeding supplemented with *Lactobacillus plantarum* (1×10^8 CFU) for 7 days	Reduced IP (L:M ratio) and improved clinical outcomes including reduced colonization by pathogenic organisms and fewer septic complications	Qin et al., 2008 [125]

Table 6. *Cont.*

Sample	Treatment/Duration	Main Results	Ref.
Adults with severe acute pancreatitis	Ecologic 641 formulation (1×10^{10} CFU twice daily) for 28 days	No effect on IP (PEG permeability test), increased enterocyte damage and bacterial translocation among those with organ failure (a subsequent study showed increased mortality with this probiotic in acute pancreatitis) [122]	Besselink et al., 2009 [126]
Critically ill adults	Proviva oatmeal and fruit drink containing 5×10^7 CFU/mL of *Lactobacillus plantarum* 299v 500 mL per day until hospital discharge or patient preference to discontinue	No effect on IP L:M ratio), gastric microbiota composition, endotoxin levels, sepsis morbidity or mortality, but reduced serum IL-6 levels	McNaught et al., 2005 [127]
Critically ill adults	De Simone formulation 900 billion CFU twice daily or inactivated probiotic sonicates	No effect on IP (L:M ratio), but increased systemic IgA and IgG in live but not dead bacteria group	Alberda et al., 2007 [128]
Adults with HIV on antiretroviral therapy	De Simone formulation 900 billion CFU once daily for 4 weeks followed by twice daily to 26 weeks	No effect on IP (assessed by colonic biopsies measuring CD4+ cells, IL-17+ cells, and myeloperoxidase), systemic inflammation, or cellular markers of inflammation, although it did alter the microbiome by increasing beneficial species and reducing *Gammaproteobacteria*	Presti et al., 2021 [129]
Pregnant women with overweight	*Bifidobacterium animalis* ssp. *lactis* 420 (1×10^{10} CFU) and *Lactobacillus rhamnosus* HN00 (1×10^{10} CFU) and/or LC-PUFA for 21 weeks (on average)	No protective effect on the increase in IP during pregnancy (serum zonulin and LPS)	Mokkala et al., 2018 [130]
Elderly adults	*Lactobacillus paracasei* HII01 (2×10^{10} CFU), *Bifidobacterium breve* (2×10^{10} CFU), and *Bifidobacterium longum* (1×10^{10} CFU)	Reduced IP (assessed using a colorimetric urine analysis), enhanced HDL-cholesterol levels, and positively affected obesity-related biomarkers and short-chain fatty acids	Chaiyasut et al., 2022 [131]
Adults with migraine	Ecologic barrier formulation 5×10^9 CFU daily for 12 weeks	No effect on IP (L:M ratio and fecal and serum zonulin levels) or migraine severity or frequency	de Roos et al., 2017 [132]

IP = intestinal permeability; GP = gastric permeability GI = gastrointestinal QOL = quality of life.

In summary, the evidence for probiotics in reducing intestinal permeability is mixed. Heterogeneity deriving from differences in study protocols, target population or disease state, probiotic formulation (as well as dosing and duration), and assessment of intestinal permeability makes it challenging to draw definitive conclusions regarding probiotics and permeability. Further large-scale, well-designed trials are needed to clarify the role of different probiotic formulations, optimal doses, and intervention durations in improving intestinal permeability across specific populations.

4.2.3. Synbiotics

Descriptions and Mechanisms of Action: Synbiotics are defined as "mixture[s] comprising live microorganisms and substrate(s) selectively utilized by host microorganisms that confers a health benefit on the host" [133]. Synbiotics can be categorized into two types: complementary and synergistic. Complementary synbiotics involve a mixture where the probiotic and prebiotic components work independently to provide health benefits, whereas synergistic synbiotics involve a specific substrate that enhances the effects of the co-administered live microorganism. To be considered a synbiotic, the formulation must show evidence of health benefits when compared against a placebo and demonstrate either selective utilization by the endogenous microbiota or the administered microorganism [133].

Synbiotics support the gut epithelial barrier and intestinal permeability through multiple mechanisms, derived from their combined pre- and probiotic constituents. They enhance microbial balance by providing beneficial microorganisms (probiotics) and substrates (prebiotics), which promote the growth of beneficial bacteria and protection against pathogens. This balance leads to the production SCFAs like butyrate, which serve as an energy source for epithelial cells, enhance mucin production, and maintain tight junctions, thereby reducing intestinal permeability. Synbiotics may also regulate tight junction proteins, support mucosal immunity, reduce inflammation, and competitively exclude pathogens. These combined effects help protect and strengthen the gut barrier, ensuring its integrity and proper function [134]. A summary of clinical trials of synbiotics where effects on intestinal permeability were assessed is displayed in Table 7 [90,135–148].

Table 7. Study characteristics and findings of clinical trials of synbiotics where effects on intestinal permeability were among the outcomes assessed. Specific information about the microbiota in diverse, commercial formulations is included in the Supplementary Material.

Sample	Treatment/Duration	Main Results	Ref.
Critically ill adults	Trevis probiotic (4×10^9 of *Lactobacillus acidophilus* La5, *Bifidobacterium lactis* Bb 12, *Streptococcus thermophilus*, *Lactobacillus bulgaricus*) plus 7.5 g of oligofructose twice daily for 8 days	No effect on IP (L:M ratio), septic complications, or mortality, but reduced the incidence of potentially pathogenic bacteria in nasogastric aspirates.	Jain et al., 2004 [90]
Adults undergoing elective colorectal surgery	Mechanical bowel preparation, neomycin, and Trevis probiotic three times per day plus 15 g oligofructose twice daily	No effect on small IP (L:M ratio), whole gut permeability (sucralose excretion), inflammatory response, or sepsis morbidity, but there was significantly reduced fecal *Enterobacteriaceae* and bacterial translocation.	Reddy et al., 2007 [135]
Adult critically ill trauma patients	Synbiotic 2000 (4×10^{10} CFU) plus 2.5 g of each of β glucan, inulin, pectin, and resistant starch for 7 days	Reduced IP (L:M ratio) and incidence of infections, including pneumonia.	Spindler-Vesel et al., 2007 [136]
Adults with acute pancreatitis	2.5 billion CFU of *Lactobacillus acidophilus*, *Bifidobacterium longus*, *Bifidobacterium bifidum*, and *Bifidobacterium infantalis* with 25 mg of fructo-oligosaccharide for 7 days	No effect on IP (L:M ratio), endotoxemia, duration of hospital or intensive care unit stay, or mortality, but decreased levels of C-reactive protein and immunoglobulins.	Sharma et al., 2011 [137]

Table 7. *Cont.*

Sample	Treatment/Duration	Main Results	Ref.
Healthy adults	Biosource Gut Balance (2×10^9 CFU) plus 200 mg immunoglobulin, 50 mg lactoferrin, 90 mg raftiline, and 10 mg raftilose) for 21 days	No effect on IP (uncertain how this was assessed apart from some measure via fecal and urine samples), fecal SCFAs, or markers of mucosal immunity.	West et al., 2012 [138]
Adults with esophageal cancer undergoing esophagectomy	Yakult 400 (at least 4×10^{10} *Lactobacillus casei* Shirota) Yakult Honsha (at least 1×10^{10} *Bifidobacterium breve* Yakult), and 15 g galacto-oligosaccharides for 7 days following surgery	Reduced IP (indirectly assessed via reduced bacterial translocation to mesenteric lymph nodes and reduced incidence of postoperative bacteremia).	Yokoyama et al., 2014 [139]
Healthy adults	Ecologic 825 (6 g per day) combined with 10 g per day fructooligosaccharides for 2 weeks	No effect on IP (multi-sugar test) at baseline or after indomethacin, though stool frequency increased.	Wilms et al., 2016 [140]
Adults with overweight	*Bifidobacterium animalis* ssp. *lactis* 420 B420 1×10^{10} CFU per day combined with 12 g of ultra polydextrose for 6 months	Reduced effect on IP (plasma zonulin levels; reduction in zonulin correlated with reductions in trunk fat mass), reduced body fat mass, waist circumference, and energy intake, increased fecal SCFAs.	Stenman et al., 2016 [141]
Adults with MASLD	Nestle Fiber Mais Flora *Lactobacillus reuteri* 1×10^8 CFU plus 4 g of guar gum and inulin twice daily combined with nutritional counseling for three months	No effect on IP (L:M ratio) or LPS levels, but reduced hepatic steatosis, weight, BMI, and waist circumference.	Ferolla et al., 2016 [142]
Adults with IBS-D	OMNi-BiOTiC Stress Repair (6×10^{10} CFU) plus corn starch, maltodextrin, inulin, fructooligosaccharides, and amylases) for 4 weeks	Reduced IP (fecal zonulin levels), improved IBS symptoms, increased microbial diversity in the upper GI tract, reduced CD4+ T cells in the ascending colon, and elevated fecal SCFAs.	Moser et al., 2018 [143]
Adults on long-term proton pump inhibitor therapy	OMNi-BiOTiC PPI (24×10^9 CFU) in a prebiotic matrix (composed of corn starch, maltodextrin, fructo-oligosaccharide P6, inulin P2, and vegetable protein) for 3 months	Reduced IP (reflected by a reduction in fecal zonulin) in those with increased permeability at baseline, which was maintained three months post-intervention; no significant changes were observed in other markers of IP, including lipopolysaccharide, lipopolysaccharide-binding protein, and sCD14 levels.	Horvath et al., 2020 [144]

Table 7. *Cont.*

Sample	Treatment/Duration	Main Results	Ref.
Adults with obesity and type II diabetes	Ecologic barrier formulation with fructo-oligosaccharides P6, and konjac glucomannan P13 for 6 months	Reduced IP (serum zonulin), lipoprotein (a), and hip circumference, with no changes in glucose metabolism.	Horvath et al., 2020 [145]
Adults with stage III–IV chronic kidney disease	NATUREN G (4.8 × 10^9 CFU), 2.5 g fructoligosaccharides, 2.5 g inulin, and antioxidants quercetin, resveratrol, and proanthocyanidins for 2 months	Reduced small IP (assessed using urinary recovery of oligosaccharide probes after oral administration), alleviated GI symptoms, and reduced free serum indoxyl sulfate..	Cosola et al., 2021 [146]
Adult women with migraine	Familact (1 × 10^9 CFU) plus 21 mg fructooligosaccharides for 12 weeks	Reduced IP (serum zonulin), frequency of migraine attacks, painkiller use, GI symptoms, and CRP.	Ghavami et al., 2021 [147]
Adults with coronary artery disease	Inulin 15 mg or LGG 1.9 × 10^9 CFU or their combination for 60 days	Reduced IP (LPS), IL-6, and TLR-4 levels while increasing serum total antioxidant capacity.	Liu et al., 2024 [148]

IP = intestinal permeability; GI = gastrointestinal.

The available evidence on synbiotics to reduce intestinal permeability shows varied results depending on the population and condition studied. Several studies have reported improvements in intestinal permeability with synbiotic interventions, while others have found no significant effects. Once again, interpretation is limited by considerable heterogeneity among study methodologies, target population or disease state, intervention (including dosing and duration), and assessment of intestinal permeability. Further well-designed, large-scale trials with standardized methods are needed to better understand the efficacy of synbiotics in enhancing intestinal permeability and to establish clearer guidelines for the use of specific formulations in specific conditions.

5. Recommendations and Conclusions

Intestinal permeability is an important component of the barrier between intraluminal antigens and the establishment of diseases of the gastrointestinal tract as well as other organs. It is significantly modified by diet, including fat and emulsifiers that increase permeability, and nutrients such as fiber, glutamine, zinc, vitamin D, polyphenols, and anthocyanins that decrease permeability. There is significant interaction of the microbiome and barrier function, including the inflammatory effects of luminal/bacterial antigens and the anti-inflammatory effects of commensals or probiotics and their products including short chain fatty acids. Epigenomic modifications of barrier functions are best illustrated by effects on junction proteins or inflammation. Further understanding of the barrier function and its potential amelioration by dietary, microbial, or, in the future, pharmacological agents will have the potential to reverse the pathobiology underpinning gastrointestinal diseases, as well as the multitude of other systemic diseases that are attributed to the leaky gut phenomenon. It is essential to use accurate measurements of intestinal permeability, particularly in vivo, and to ascertain the longitudinal changes in the barrier that occur with perturbations, disease, and amelioration through treatment.

Supplementary Materials: The following supporting information can be downloaded at: https://www.mdpi.com/article/10.3390/nu16203494/s1, File S1.

Author Contributions: A.M.: literature review, writing and revising manuscript; J.A.D.: literature review, writing and revising manuscript; K.J.J.: literature review, writing and revising manuscript; M.C.: conceptualization, senior author, revising manuscript. All authors have read and agreed to the published version of the manuscript.

Funding: R01-DK135440 grant from National Institutes of Health to Michael Camilleri.

Data Availability Statement: This narrative review is based on the reported literature search, with no original data presented.

Acknowledgments: The authors thank Cindy Stanislav for excellent secretarial assistance.

Conflicts of Interest: The authors have no relevant conflicts of interest.

References

1. Barbara, G.; Barbaro, M.R.; Fuschi, D.; Palombo, M.; Falangone, F.; Cremon, C.; Marasco, G.; Stanghellini, V. Inflammatory and microbiota-related regulation of the intestinal epithelial barrier. *Front. Nutr.* **2021**, *8*, 718356. [CrossRef] [PubMed]
2. Farré, R.; Fiorani, M.; Rahiman, S.A.; Matteoli, G. Intestinal permeability, inflammation and the role of nutrients. *Nutrients* **2020**, *12*, 1185. [CrossRef]
3. de Souza Marinho do Nascimento, D.; Costa Campos Mota, A.C.; da Cruz Carvalho, M.C.; de Oliveira Andrade, E.D.; de Oliveira, E.P.S.F.; Galvão, L.L.P.; Maciel, B.L.L. Can diet alter the intestinal barrier permeability in healthy people? A systematic review. *Nutrients* **2024**, *16*, 1871. [CrossRef] [PubMed]
4. Allam-Ndoul, B.; Castonguay-Paradis, S.; Veilleux, A. Gut microbiota and intestinal trans-epithelial permeability. *Int. J. Mol. Sci.* **2020**, *21*, 6402. [CrossRef]
5. Ahern, P.P.; Maloy, K.J. Understanding immune–microbiota interactions in the intestine. *Immunology* **2020**, *159*, 4–14. [CrossRef]
6. Allaire, J.M.; Crowley, S.M.; Law, H.T.; Chang, S.-Y.; Ko, H.-J.; Vallance, B.A. The intestinal epithelium: Central coordinator of mucosal immunity. *Trends Immunol.* **2018**, *39*, 677–696. [CrossRef]
7. Dunleavy, K.A.; Raffals, L.E.; Camilleri, M. Intestinal barrier dysfunction in inflammatory bowel disease: Underpinning pathogenesis and therapeutics. *Dig. Dis. Sci.* **2023**, *68*, 4306–4320. [CrossRef] [PubMed]
8. Yao, Y.; Shang, W.; Bao, L.; Peng, Z.; Wu, C. Epithelial-immune cell crosstalk for intestinal barrier homeostasis. *Eur. J. Immunol.* **2024**, *54*, e2350631. [CrossRef]
9. Citi, S.; Fromm, M.; Furuse, M.; González-Mariscal, L.; Nusrat, A.; Tsukita, S.; Turner, J.R. A short guide to the tight junction. *J. Cell Sci.* **2024**, *137*, jcs261776. [CrossRef]
10. Imafuku, K.; Iwata, H.; Natsuga, K.; Okumura, M.; Kobayashi, Y.; Kitahata, H.; Kubo, A.; Nagayama, M.; Ujiie, H. Zonula occludens-1 distribution and barrier functions are affected by epithelial proliferation and turnover rates. *Cell Prolif.* **2023**, *56*, e13441. [CrossRef]
11. AlMarzooqi, S.K.; Almarzooqi, F.; Sadida, H.Q.; Jerobin, J.; Ahmed, I.; Abou-Samra, A.-B.; Fakhro, K.A.; Dhawan, P.; Bhat, A.A.; Al-Shabeeb Akil, A.S. Deciphering the complex interplay of obesity, epithelial barrier dysfunction, and tight junction remodeling: Unraveling potential therapeutic avenues. *Obes. Rev.* **2024**, *25*, e13766. [CrossRef] [PubMed]
12. Horowitz, A.; Chanez-Paredes, S.D.; Haest, X.; Turner, J.R. Paracellular permeability and tight junction regulation in gut health and disease. *Nat. Rev. Gastroenterol. Hepatol.* **2023**, *20*, 417–432. [CrossRef] [PubMed]
13. Zuo, L.; Kuo, W.-T.; Turner, J.R. Tight junctions as targets and effectors of mucosal immune homeostasis. *Cell. Mol. Gastroenterol. Hepatol.* **2020**, *10*, 327–340. [CrossRef]
14. Oami, T.; Yumoto, T.; Shimazui, T.; Sarmiento, S.; Klingensmith, N.J.; Chen, C.-W.; Otani, S.; Liang, Z.; Burd, E.M.; Mahdi, Z.K.; et al. Chronic ethanol use worsens gut permeability and alters tight junction expression in a murine sepsis model. *Shock* **2023**, *60*, 280–290. [CrossRef] [PubMed]
15. Suzuki, T. Regulation of intestinal epithelial permeability by tight junctions. *Cell Mol. Life Sci.* **2013**, *70*, 631–659. [CrossRef] [PubMed]
16. Buckley, A.; Turner, J.R. Cell biology of tight junction barrier regulation and mucosal disease. *Cold Spring Harb. Perspect. Biol.* **2018**, *10*, a029314. [CrossRef]
17. Lacy, B.E.; Wise, J.L.; Cangemi, D.J. Leaky gut syndrome: Myths and management. *Gastroenterol. Hepatol.* **2024**, *20*, 265.
18. Perez-Diaz-del-Campo, N.; Castelnuovo, G.; Ribaldone, D.G.; Caviglia, G.P. Fecal and circulating biomarkers for the non-invasive assessment of intestinal permeability. *Diagnostics* **2023**, *13*, 1976. [CrossRef]
19. Camilleri, M. Leaky gut: Mechanisms, measurement and clinical implications in humans. *Gut* **2019**, *68*, 1516–1526. [CrossRef]
20. Meyer, F.; Wendling, D.; Demougeot, C.; Prati, C.; Verhoeven, F. Cytokines and intestinal epithelial permeability: A systematic review. *Autoimmun. Rev.* **2023**, *22*, 103331. [CrossRef]
21. Camilleri, M.; Vella, A. What to do about the leaky gut. *Gut* **2022**, *71*, 424–435. [CrossRef] [PubMed]
22. Schoultz, I.; Keita, A.V. The intestinal barrier and current techniques for the assessment of gut permeability. *Cells* **2020**, *9*, 1909. [CrossRef] [PubMed]
23. Mahurkar-Joshi, S.; Chang, L. Epigenetic mechanisms in irritable bowel syndrome. *Front. Psychiatry* **2020**, *11*, 805. [CrossRef] [PubMed]

24. Wiley, J.W.; Zong, Y.; Zheng, G.; Zhu, S.; Hong, S. Histone H3K9 methylation regulates chronic stress and IL-6-induced colon epithelial permeability and visceral pain. *Neurogastroenterol. Motil.* **2020**, *32*, e13941. [CrossRef]
25. Zhou, Q.; Costinean, S.; Croce, C.M.; Brasier, A.R.; Merwat, S.; Larson, S.A.; Basra, S.; Verne, G.N. MicroRNA 29 targets nuclear factor-κB-repressing factor and Claudin 1 to increase intestinal permeability. *Gastroenterology* **2015**, *148*, 158–169.e8. [CrossRef]
26. Wiley, J.W.; Higgins, G.A.; Hong, S. Chronic psychological stress alters gene expression in rat colon epithelial cells promoting chromatin remodeling, barrier dysfunction and inflammation. *PeerJ* **2022**, *10*, e13287. [CrossRef]
27. Zhou, Q.; Souba, W.W.; Croce, C.M.; Verne, G.N. MicroRNA-29a regulates intestinal membrane permeability in patients with irritable bowel syndrome. *Gut* **2010**, *59*, 775–784. [CrossRef] [PubMed]
28. Chao, G.; Wang, Y.; Zhang, S.; Yang, W.; Ni, Z.; Zheng, X. MicroRNA-29a increased the intestinal membrane permeability of colonic epithelial cells in irritable bowel syndrome rats. *Oncotarget* **2017**, *8*, 85828–85837. [CrossRef]
29. Wohlfarth, C.; Schmitteckert, S.; Härtle, J.D.; Houghton, L.A.; Dweep, H.; Fortea, M.; Assadi, G.; Braun, A.; Mederer, T.; Pöhner, S.; et al. miR-16 and miR-103 impact 5-HT(4) receptor signalling and correlate with symptom profile in irritable bowel syndrome. *Sci. Rep.* **2017**, *7*, 14680. [CrossRef]
30. Martínez, C.; Rodiño-Janeiro, B.K.; Lobo, B.; Stanifer, M.L.; Klaus, B.; Granzow, M.; González-Castro, A.M.; Salvo-Romero, E.; Alonso-Cotoner, C.; Pigrau, M.; et al. miR-16 and miR-125b are involved in barrier function dysregulation through the modulation of claudin-2 and cingulin expression in the jejunum in IBS with diarrhoea. *Gut* **2017**, *66*, 1537–1538. [CrossRef]
31. Hou, Q.; Huang, Y.; Zhu, S.; Li, P.; Chen, X. MiR-144 increases intestinal permeability in IBS-D rats by targeting OCLN and ZO1. *Cell. Physiol. Biochem.* **2017**, *44*, 2256–2268. [CrossRef] [PubMed]
32. Fazio, A.; Bordoni, D.; Kuiper, J.W.P.; Weber-Stiehl, S.; Stengel, S.T.; Arnold, P.; Ellinghaus, D.; Ito, G.; Tran, F.; Messner, B.; et al. DNA methyltransferase 3A controls intestinal epithelial barrier function and regeneration in the colon. *Nat. Commun.* **2022**, *13*, 6266. [CrossRef] [PubMed]
33. Rawat, M.; Nighot, M.; Al-Sadi, R.; Gupta, Y.; Viszwapriva, D.; Yochum, G.; Koltun, W.; Ma, T.Y. IL1B increases intestinal tight junction permeability by up-regulation of MIR200C-3p which degrades occludin, m.R.N.A. *Gastroenterology* **2020**, *159*, 1375–1389. [CrossRef]
34. Bowes, M.M.; Casares-Marfil, D.; Sawalha, H. Intestinal permeability correlates with disease activity and DNA methylation changes in lupus patients. *Clin. Immunol.* **2024**, *262*, 110173. [CrossRef]
35. Higgins, G.A.; Hong, S.; Wiley, J.W. The role of epigenomic regulatory pathways in the gut-brain axis and visceral hyperalgesia. *Cell. Mol. Neurobiol.* **2022**, *42*, 361–376. [CrossRef]
36. Yuan, X.; Tan, Y.; Bajinka, O.; Jammeh, M.L.; Dukureh, A.; Obiegbusi, C.N.; Abdelhalim, K.A. The connection between epigenetics and gut microbiota-current perspective. *Cell Biochem. Funct.* **2024**, *42*, e3941. [CrossRef]
37. Wu, S.-E.; Hashimoto-Hill, S.; Woo, V.; Eshleman, E.M.; Whitt, J.; Engleman, L.; Karns, R.; Denson, L.A.; Haslam, D.B.; Alenghat, T. Microbiota-derived metabolite promotes HDAC3 activity in the gut. *Nature* **2020**, *586*, 108–112. [CrossRef] [PubMed]
38. Miousse, I.R.; Pathak, R.; Garg, S.; Skinner, C.M.; Melnyk, S.; Pavliv, O.; Hendrickson, H.; Landes, R.D.; Lumen, A.; Tackett, A.J.; et al. Short-term dietary methionine supplementation affects one-carbon metabolism and DNA methylation in the mouse gut and leads to altered microbiome profiles, barrier function, gene expression and histomorphology. *Genes Nutr.* **2017**, *12*, 22. [CrossRef]
39. Pepke, M.L.; Hansen, S.B.; Limborg, M.T. Unraveling host regulation of gut microbiota through the epigenome-microbiome axis. *Trends Microbiol.* **2024**. *Online ahead of print*. [CrossRef]
40. Speciale, A.; Molonia, M.S.; Muscarà, C.; Cristani, M.; Salamone, F.L.; Saija, A.; Cimino, F. An overview on the cellular mechanisms of anthocyanins in maintaining intestinal integrity and function. *Fitoterapia* **2024**, *175*, 105953. [CrossRef]
41. Jimenez-Rondan, F.R.; Ruggiero, C.H.; Lobean McKinley, K.; Koh, J.; Roberts, J.F.; Triplett, E.W.; Cousins, R.J. Enterocyte-specific deletion of metal transporter Zip14 (Slc39a14) alters intestinal homeostasis through epigenetic mechanisms. *Am. J. Physiol. Gastrointest. Liver Physiol.* **2023**, *324*, G159–G176. [CrossRef] [PubMed]
42. Khoshbin, K.; Camilleri, M. Effects of dietary components on intestinal permeability in health and disease. *Am. J. Physiol. Gastrointest. Liver Physiol.* **2020**, *319*, G589–G608. [CrossRef] [PubMed]
43. Amar, J.; Burcelin, R.; Ruidavets, J.B.; Cani, P.D.; Fauvel, J.; Alessi, M.C.; Chamontin, B.; Ferriéres, J. Energy intake is associated with endotoxemia in apparently healthy men. *Am. J. Clin. Nutr.* **2008**, *87*, 1219–1223. [CrossRef]
44. Leutner, M.; Göbl, C.; Wielandner, A.; Howorka, E.; Prünner, M.; Bozkurt, L.; Schlager, O.; Charwat-Resl, S.; Kautzky-Willer, A. Clinical and metabolic characteristics of treated hyperlipidemic patients additionally affected by subclinical hyperglycemia. *Lipids Health Dis.* **2016**, *15*, 10. [CrossRef]
45. Bowser, S.M.; McMillan, R.P.; Boutagy, N.E.; Tarpey, M.D.; Smithson, A.T.; Osterberg, K.L.; Neilson, A.P.; Davy, B.M.; Davy, K.P.; Hulver, M.W. Serum endotoxin, gut permeability and skeletal muscle metabolic adaptations following a short term high fat diet in humans. *Metabolism* **2020**, *103*, 154041. [CrossRef]
46. Roberts, C.L.; Keita, A.V.; Duncan, S.H.; O'Kennedy, N.; Söderholm, J.D.; Rhodes, J.M.; Campbell, B.J. Translocation of Crohns disease Escherichia coli across M-cells: Contrasting effects of soluble plant fibres and emulsifiers. *Gut* **2010**, *59*, 1331–1339. [CrossRef]
47. Mistry, R.H.; Liu, F.; Borewicz, K.; Lohuis, M.A.M.; Smidt, H.; Verkade, H.J.; Tietge, U.J.F. Long-term β-galacto-oligosaccharides supplementation decreases the development of obesity and insulin resistance in mice fed a western-type diet. *Mol. Nutr. Food Res.* **2020**, *64*, e1900922. [CrossRef]

48. Gondalia, S.V.; Wymond, B.; Benassi-Evans, B.; Berberzy, P.; Bird, A.R.; Belobrajdic, D.P. Substitution of refined conventional wheat flour with wheat high in resistant starch modulates the intestinal microbiota and fecal metabolites in healthy adults: A randomized, controlled trial. *J. Nutr.* **2022**, *152*, 1426–1437. [CrossRef]
49. Yamamoto, E.A.; Jørgensen, T.N. Relationships between vitamin D, gut microbiome, and systemic autoimmunity. *Front. Immunol.* **2020**, *10*, 499337. [CrossRef]
50. Thomas, R.L.; Jiang, L.; Adams, J.S.; Xu, Z.Z.; Shen, J.; Janssen, S.; Ackermann, G.; Vanderschueren, D.; Pauwels, S.; Knight, R.; et al. Vitamin D metabolites and the gut microbiome in older men. *Nat. Commun.* **2020**, *11*, 5997. [CrossRef]
51. Koren, O.; Tako, E. Chronic dietary zinc deficiency alters gut microbiota composition and function. *Proceedings* **2020**, *61*, 16. [CrossRef]
52. Skalny, A.V.; Aschner, M.; Lei, X.G.; Gritsenko, V.A.; Santamaria, A.; Alekseenko, S.I.; Prakash, N.T.; Chang, J.-S.; Sizova, E.A.; Chao, J.C.J.; et al. Gut microbiota as a mediator of essential and toxic effects of zinc in the intestines and other tissues. *Int. J. Mol. Sci.* **2021**, *22*, 13074. [CrossRef] [PubMed]
53. Abdulrahman, A.O.; Alzubaidi, M.Y.; Nadeem, M.S.; Khan, J.A.; Rather, I.A.; Khan, M.I. Effects of urolithins on obesity-associated gut dysbiosis in rats fed on a high-fat diet. *Int. J. Food Sci. Nutr.* **2021**, *72*, 923–934. [CrossRef] [PubMed]
54. Xu, B.; Yan, Y.; Yin, B.; Zhang, L.; Qin, W.; Niu, Y.; Tang, Y.; Zhou, S.; Yan, X.; Ma, L. Dietary glycyl-glutamine supplementation ameliorates intestinal integrity, inflammatory response, and oxidative status in association with the gut microbiota in LPS-challenged piglets. *Food Funct.* **2021**, *12*, 3539–3551. [CrossRef] [PubMed]
55. Xu, Q.; Hu, M.; Li, M.; Hou, J.; Zhang, X.; Gao, Y.; Chachar, B.; Li, X. Dietary bioactive peptide alanyl-glutamine attenuates dextran sodium sulfate-induced colitis by modulating gut microbiota. *Oxid. Med. Cell Longev.* **2021**, *2021*, 5543003. [CrossRef]
56. Tian, S.; Chu, Q.; Ma, S.; Ma, H.; Song, H. Dietary fiber and its potential role in obesity: A focus on modulating the gut microbiota. *J. Agric. Food Chem.* **2023**, *71*, 14853–14869. [CrossRef]
57. Rezende, E.S.V.; Lima, G.C.; Naves, M.M.V. Dietary fibers as beneficial microbiota modulators: A proposed classification by prebiotic categories. *Nutrition* **2021**, *89*, 111217. [CrossRef]
58. Ye, S.; Shah, B.R.; Li, J.; Liang, H.; Zhan, F.; Geng, F.; Li, B. A critical review on interplay between dietary fibers and gut microbiota. *Trends Food Sci. Technol.* **2022**, *124*, 237–249. [CrossRef]
59. Fusco, W.; Lorenzo, M.B.; Cintoni, M.; Porcari, S.; Rinninella, E.; Kaitsas, F.; Lener, E.; Mele, M.C.; Gasbarrini, A.; Collado, M.C.; et al. Short-chain fatty-acid-producing bacteria: Key components of the human gut microbiota. *Nutrients* **2023**, *15*, 2211. [CrossRef]
60. Blaak, E.E.; Canfora, E.E.; Theis, S.; Frost, G.; Groen, A.K.; Mithieux, G.; Nauta, A.; Scott, K.; Stahl, B.; van Harsselaar, J.; et al. Short chain fatty acids in human gut and metabolic health. *Benef. Microbes* **2020**, *11*, 411–455. [CrossRef]
61. Nogal, A.; Louca, P.; Zhang, X.; Wells, P.M.; Steves, C.J.; Spector, T.D.; Falchi, M.; Valdes, A.M.; Menni, C. Circulating levels of the short-chain fatty acid acetate mediate the effect of the gut microbiome on visceral fat. *Front. Microbiol.* **2021**, *12*, 711359. [CrossRef] [PubMed]
62. Liu, L.; Li, Q.; Yang, Y.; Guo, A. Biological function of short-chain fatty acids and its regulation on intestinal health of poultry. *Front. Vet. Sci.* **2021**, *8*, 736739. [CrossRef] [PubMed]
63. Lavefve, L.; Howard, L.R.; Carbonero, F. Berry polyphenols metabolism and impact on human gut microbiota and health. *Food Funct.* **2020**, *11*, 45–65. [CrossRef] [PubMed]
64. Aravind, S.M.; Wichienchot, S.; Tsao, R.; Ramakrishnan, S.; Chakkaravarthi, S. Role of dietary polyphenols on gut microbiota, their metabolites and health benefits. *Food Res. Int.* **2021**, *142*, 110189. [CrossRef]
65. Bouyahya, A.; El Omari, N.; El Hachlafi, N.; El Jemly, M.; Hakkour, M.; Balahbib, A.; El Menyiy, N.; Bakrim, S.; Mrabti, H.N.; Khouchlaa, A.; et al. Chemical compounds of berry-derived polyphenols and their effects on gut microbiota, inflammation, and cancer. *Molecules* **2022**, *27*, 3286. [CrossRef]
66. García-Villalba, R.; Tomás-Barberán, F.A.; Iglesias-Aguirre, C.E.; Giménez-Bastida, J.A.; González-Sarrías, A.; Selma, M.V.; Espín, J.C. Ellagitannins, urolithins, and neuroprotection: Human evidence and the possible link to the gut microbiota. *Mol. Asp. Med.* **2023**, *89*, 101109. [CrossRef]
67. García-Villalba, R.; Giménez-Bastida, J.A.; Cortés-Martín, A.; Ávila-Gálvez, M.A.; Tomás-Barberán, F.A.; Selma, M.V.; Espín, J.C.; González-Sarrías, A. Urolithins: A comprehensive update on their metabolism, bioactivity, and associated gut microbiota. *Mol. Nutr. Food Res.* **2022**, *66*, e2101019. [CrossRef]
68. Bellerba, F.; Muzio, V.; Gnagnarella, P.; Facciotti, F.; Chiocca, S.; Bossi, P.; Cortinovis, D.; Chiaradonna, F.; Serrano, D.; Raimondi, S.; et al. The association between vitamin D and gut microbiota: A systematic review of human studies. *Nutrients* **2021**, *13*, 3378. [CrossRef]
69. Chen, L.; Wang, Z.; Wang, P.; Yu, X.; Ding, H.; Wang, Z.; Feng, J. Effect of long-term and short-term imbalanced Zn manipulation on gut microbiota and screening for microbial markers sensitive to zinc status. *Microbiol. Spectr.* **2021**, *9*, e00483-21. [CrossRef]
70. Pajarillo, E.A.B.; Lee, E.; Kang, D.-K. Trace metals and animal health: Interplay of the gut microbiota with iron, manganese, zinc, and copper. *Anim. Nutr.* **2021**, *7*, 750–761. [CrossRef]
71. Ghosh, S.; Whitley, C.S.; Haribabu, B.; Jala, V.R. Regulation of intestinal barrier function by microbial metabolites. *Cell. Mol. Gastroenterol. Hepatol.* **2021**, *11*, 1463–1482. [CrossRef] [PubMed]
72. Levine, A.R.; Picoraro, J.A.; Dorfzaun, S.; LeLeiko, N.S. Emulsifiers and intestinal health: An introduction. *J. Pediatr. Gastroenterol. Nutr.* **2022**, *74*, 314–319. [CrossRef] [PubMed]

73. Naimi, S.; Viennois, E.; Gewirtz, A.T.; Chassaing, B. Direct impact of commonly used dietary emulsifiers on human gut Microbiota. *Microbiome* **2021**, *9*, 66. [CrossRef]
74. Bancil, A.S.; Sandall, A.M.; Rossi, M.; Chassaing, B.; Lindsay, J.O.; Whelan, K. Food additive emulsifiers and their impact on gut microbiome, permeability, and inflammation: Mechanistic insights in inflammatory bowel disease. *J. Crohns. Colitis* **2021**, *15*, 1068–1079. [CrossRef]
75. Ogulur, I.; Yazici, D.; Pat, Y.; Bingöl, E.N.; Babayev, H.; Ardicli, S.; Heider, A.; Rückert, B.; Sampath, V.; Dhir, R.; et al. Mechanisms of gut epithelial barrier impairment caused by food emulsifiers polysorbate 20 and polysorbate 80. *Allergy* **2023**, *78*, 2441–2455. [CrossRef] [PubMed]
76. Fitzpatrick, J.A.; Gibson, P.R.; Taylor, K.M.; Halmos, E.P. The effect of dietary emulsifiers and thickeners on intestinal barrier function and its response to acute stress in healthy adult humans: A randomised controlled feeding study. *Aliment. Pharmacol. Ther.* **2024**. *Online ahead of print*. [CrossRef]
77. Gibson, G.R.; Hutkins, R.; Sanders, M.E.; Prescott, S.L.; Reimer, R.A.; Salminen, S.J.; Scott, K.; Stanton, C.; Swanson, K.S.; Cani, P.D.; et al. Expert consensus document: The International Scientific Association for Probiotics and Prebiotics (ISAPP) consensus statement on the definition and scope of prebiotics. *Nat. Rev. Gastroenterol. Hepatol.* **2017**, *14*, 491–502. [CrossRef] [PubMed]
78. Makki, K.; Deehan, E.C.; Walter, J.; Bäckhed, F. The Impact of dietary fiber on gut microbiota in host health and disease. *Cell Host Microbe* **2018**, *23*, 705–715. [CrossRef]
79. Looijer-Van Langen, M.A.C.; Dieleman, L.A. Prebiotics in chronic intestinal inflammation. *Inflamm. Bowel Dis.* **2008**, *15*, 454–462. [CrossRef]
80. Francavilla, R.; Castellaneta, S.; Masciale, A.; Straziuso, S.; Polimeno, L.; Gagliardi, F.; Bohem, G.; Miniello, V. Intestinal permeability and faecal flora of infants fed with a prebiotic supplemented formula: A double blind placebo controlled study. *J. Pediatr. Gastroenterol. Nutr.* **2006**, *42*, E96–E97. [CrossRef]
81. Westerbeek, E.A.; van den Berg, J.P.; Lafeber, H.N.; Fetter, W.P.; Boehm, G.; Twisk, J.W.; van Elburg, R.M. Neutral and acidic oligosaccharides in preterm infants: A randomized, double-blind, placebo-controlled trial1234. *Am. J. Clin. Nutr.* **2010**, *91*, 679–686. [CrossRef] [PubMed]
82. Ho, J.; Nicolucci, A.C.; Virtanen, H.; Schick, A.; Meddings, J.; Reimer, R.A.; Huang, C. Effect of prebiotic on microbiota, intestinal permeability, and glycemic control in children with type 1 diabetes. *J. Clin. Endocrinol. Metab.* **2019**, *104*, 4427–4440. [CrossRef]
83. Olguin, F.; Araya, M.; Hirsch, S.; Brunser, O.; Ayala, V.; Rivera, R.; Gotteland, M. Prebiotic ingestion does not improve gastrointestinal barrier function in burn patients. *Burns* **2005**, *31*, 482–488. [CrossRef]
84. Russo, F.; Linsalata, M.; Clemente, C.; Chiloiro, M.; Orlando, A.; Marconi, E.; Chimienti, G.; Riezzo, G. Inulin-enriched pasta improves intestinal permeability and modifies the circulating levels of zonulin and glucagon-like peptide 2 in healthy young volunteers. *Nutr. Res.* **2012**, *32*, 940–946. [CrossRef] [PubMed]
85. Salden, B.N.; Troost, F.J.; Wilms, E.; Truchado, P.; Vilchez-Vargas, R.; Pieper, D.H.; Jáuregui, R.; Marzorati, M.; van de Wiele, T.; Possemiers, S.; et al. Reinforcement of intestinal epithelial barrier by arabinoxylans in overweight and obese subjects: A randomized controlled trial: Arabinoxylans in gut barrier. *Clin. Nutr.* **2018**, *37*, 471–480. [CrossRef] [PubMed]
86. Müller, M.; Hermes, G.D.A.; Emauel, E.C.; Holst, J.J.; Zoetendal, E.G.; Smidt, H.; Troost, F.; Schaap, F.G.; Damink, S.O.; Jocken, J.W.E.; et al. Effect of wheat bran derived prebiotic supplementation on gastrointestinal transit, gut microbiota, and metabolic health: A randomized controlled trial in healthy adults with a slow gut transit. *Gut Microbes* **2020**, *12*, 1704141. [CrossRef]
87. Ganda Mall, J.P.; Löfvendahl, L.; Lindqvist, C.M.; Brummer, R.J.; Keita, Å.V.; Schoultz, I. Differential effects of dietary fibres on colonic barrier function in elderly individuals with gastrointestinal symptoms. *Sci. Rep.* **2018**, *8*, 13404. [CrossRef]
88. Machado, A.M.; da Silva, N.B.M.; de Freitas, R.M.P.; de Freitas, M.B.D.; Chaves, J.B.P.; Oliveira, L.L.; Martino, H.S.D.; de Cássia Goncalves Alfenas, R. Effects of yacon flour associated with an energy restricted diet on intestinal permeability, fecal short chain fatty acids, oxidative stress and inflammation markers levels in adults with obesity or overweight: A randomized, double blind, placebo controlled clinical trial. *Arch. Endocrinol. Metab.* **2021**, *64*, 597–607.
89. Pedersen, C.; Gallagher, E.; Horton, F.; Ellis, R.J.; Ijaz, U.Z.; Wu, H.; Jaiyeola, E.; Diribe, O.; Duparc, T.; Cani, P.D.; et al. Host–microbiome interactions in human type 2 diabetes following prebiotic fibre (galacto-oligosaccharide) intake. *Br. J. Nutr.* **2016**, *116*, 1869–1877. [CrossRef]
90. Jain, P.K.; McNaught, C.E.; Anderson, A.D.G.; MacFie, J.; Mitchell, C.J. Influence of synbiotic containing Lactobacillus acidophilus La5, Bifidobacterium lactis Bb 12, Streptococcus thermophilus, Lactobacillus bulgaricus and oligofructose on gut barrier function and sepsis in critically ill patients: A randomised controlled trial. *Clin. Nutr.* **2004**, *23*, 467–475.
91. Cao, S.; Shaw, E.L.; Quarles, W.R.; Sasaki, G.Y.; Dey, P.; Hodges, J.K.; Pokala, A.; Zeng, M.; Bruno, R.S. Daily inclusion of resistant starch-containing potatoes in a dietary guidelines for Americans dietary pattern does not adversely affect cardiometabolic risk or intestinal permeability in adults with metabolic syndrome: A randomized controlled trial. *Nutrients* **2022**, *14*, 1545. [CrossRef] [PubMed]
92. Vaghef-Mehrabani, E.; Harouni, R.; Behrooz, M.; Ranjbar, F.; Asghari-Jafarabadi, M.; Ebrahimi-Mameghani, M. Effects of inulin supplementation on inflammatory biomarkers and clinical symptoms of women with obesity and depression on a calorie-restricted diet: A randomised controlled clinical trial. *Br. J. Nutr.* **2023**, *129*, 1897–1907. [CrossRef] [PubMed]
93. Hill, C.; Guarner, F.; Reid, G.; Gibson, G.R.; Merenstein, D.J.; Pot, B.; Morelli, L.; Canani, R.B.; Flint, H.J.; Salminen, S.; et al. Expert consensus document. The International Scientific Association for Probiotics and Prebiotics consensus statement on the scope and appropriate use of the term probiotic. *Nat. Rev. Gastroenterol. Hepatol.* **2014**, *11*, 506–514. [CrossRef]

94. Sanders, M.E.; Merenstein, D.J.; Reid, G.; Gibson, G.R.; Rastall, R.A. Probiotics and prebiotics in intestinal health and disease: From biology to the clinic. *Nat. Rev. Gastroenterol. Hepatol.* **2019**, *16*, 605–616. [CrossRef] [PubMed]
95. Gou, H.Z.; Zhang, Y.L.; Ren, L.F.; Li, Z.J.; Zhang, L. How do intestinal probiotics restore the intestinal barrier? *Front. Microbiol.* **2022**, *13*, 929346. [CrossRef]
96. Isolauri, E.; Majamaa, H.; Arvola, T.; Rantala, I.; Virtanen, E.; Arvilommi, H. Lactobacillus casei strain GG reverses increased intestinal permeability induced by cow milk in suckling rats. *Gastroenterology* **1993**, *105*, 1643–1650. [CrossRef]
97. Wang, Y.; Liu, Y.; Sidhu, A.; Ma, Z.; McClain, C.; Feng, W. Lactobacillus rhamnosus GG culture supernatant ameliorates acute alcohol-induced intestinal permeability and liver injury. *Am. J. Physiol. Gastrointest. Liver Physiol.* **2012**, *303*, G32–G41. [CrossRef]
98. Capurso, L. Thirty years of Lactobacillus rhamnosus GG: A review. *J. Clin. Gastroenterol.* **2019**, *53* (Suppl. 1), S1–S41. [CrossRef] [PubMed]
99. Ramezani Ahmadi, A.; Sadeghian, M.; Alipour, M.; Ahmadi Taheri, S.; Rahmani, S.; Abbasnezhad, A. The effects of probiotic/synbiotic on serum level of zonulin as a biomarker of intestinal permeability: A systematic review and meta-analysis. *Iran J. Public Health* **2020**, *49*, 1222–1231. [CrossRef]
100. Stratiki, Z.; Costalos, C.; Sevastiadou, S.; Kastanidou, O.; Skouroliakou, M.; Giakoumatou, A.; Petrohilou, V. The effect of a bifidobacter supplemented bovine milk on intestinal permeability of preterm infants. *Early Hum. Dev.* **2007**, *83*, 575–579. [CrossRef]
101. Sindhu, K.N.C.; Sowmyanarayanan, T.V.; Paul, A.; Babji, S.; Ajjampur, S.S.R.; Priyadarshini, S.; Sarkar, R.; Balasubramanian, K.A.; Wanke, C.A.; Ward, H.D.; et al. Immune response and intestinal permeability in children with acute gastroenteritis treated with Lactobacillus rhamnosus GG: A randomized, double-blind, placebo-controlled trial. *Clin. Infect. Dis.* **2014**, *58*, 1107–1115. [CrossRef] [PubMed]
102. Gupta, P.; Andrew, H.; Kirschner, B.S.; Guandalini, S. Is Lactobacillus GG helpful in children with Crohn's disease? Results of a preliminary, open-label study. *J. Pediatr. Gastroenterol. Nutr.* **2000**, *31*, 453–457.
103. Rosenfeldt, V.; Benfeldt, E.; Valerius, N.H.; Paerregaard, A.; Fleischer Michaelsen, K. Effect of probiotics on gastrointestinal symptoms and small intestinal permeability in children with atopic dermatitis. *J. Pediatr.* **2004**, *145*, 612–616. [CrossRef]
104. Sentongo, T.A.; Cohran, V.; Korff, S.; Sullivan, C.; Iyer, K.; Zheng, X. Intestinal permeability and effects of Lactobacillus rhamnosus therapy in children with short bowel syndrome. *J. Pediatr. Gastroenterol. Nutr.* **2008**, *46*, 41–47. [CrossRef]
105. Gotteland, M.; Cruchet, S.; Verbeke, S. Effect of Lactobacillus ingestion on the gastrointestinal mucosal barrier alterations induced by indometacin in humans. *Aliment. Pharmacol. Ther.* **2001**, *15*, 11–17. [CrossRef]
106. Montalto, M.; Gallo, A.; Curigliano, V.; D'Onofrio, F.; Santoro, L.; Covino, M.; Dalvai, S.; Gasbarrini, A.; Gasbrarrini, G. Clinical trial: The effects of a probiotic mixture on non-steroidal anti-inflammatory drug enteropathy—A randomized, double-blind, cross-over, placebo-controlled study. *Aliment. Pharmacol. Ther.* **2010**, *32*, 209–214. [CrossRef] [PubMed]
107. Akama, F.; Nishino, R.; Makino, S.; Kobayashi, K.; Kamikaseda, K.; Nagano, J.; Koga, Y. The effect of probiotics on gastric mucosal permeability in humans administered with aspirin. *Scand. J. Gastroenterol.* **2011**, *46*, 831–836. [CrossRef] [PubMed]
108. Judkins, T.C.; Solch-Ottaiano, R.J.; Ceretto-Clark, B.; Nieves, C., Jr.; Colee, J.; Wang, Y.; Tompkins, T.A.; Caballero-Calero, S.E.; Langkamp-Henken, B. The effect of an acute aspirin challenge on intestinal permeability in healthy adults with and without prophylactic probiotic consumption: A double-blind, placebo-controlled, randomized trial. *BMC Gastroenterol.* **2024**, *24*, 4. [CrossRef]
109. Garcia Vilela, E.; De Lourdes De Abreu Ferrari, M.; Da Gama Torres, H.O.; Gurerra Pinto, A.; Carneiro Aguirre, A.C.; Martins, F.P.; Andrade Goulart, E.M.; Da Cunha, A.S. Influence of Saccharomyces boulardii on the intestinal permeability of patients with Crohn's disease in remission. *Scand. J. Gastroenterol.* **2008**, *43*, 842–848. [CrossRef]
110. Wegh, C.A.M.; de Roos, N.M.; Hovenier, R.; Meijerink, J.; Besseling-van der Vaart, I.; van Hemert, S.; Witteman, B.J.M. Intestinal permeability measured by urinary sucrose excretion correlates with serum zonulin and faecal calprotectin concentrations in UC patients in remission. *J. Nutr. Metab.* **2019**, *2019*, 2472754. [CrossRef]
111. Zeng, J.; Li, Y.-Q.; Zuo, X.-L.; Zhen, Y.-B.; Yang, J.; Liu, C.-H. Clinical trial: Effect of active lactic acid bacteria on mucosal barrier function in patients with diarrhoea-predominant irritable bowel syndrome. *Aliment. Pharmacol. Ther.* **2008**, *28*, 994–1002. [CrossRef] [PubMed]
112. Bonfrate, L.; Di Palo, D.M.; Celano, G.; Algert, A.; Vitellio, P.; De Angelis, M.; Gobbetti, M.; Portincasa, P. Effects of *Bifidobacterium longum* BB536 and *Lactobacillus rhamnosus* HN001 in IBS patients. *Eur. J. Clin. Investig.* **2020**, *50*, e13201. [CrossRef] [PubMed]
113. Boonma, P.; Shapiro, J.M.; Hollister, E.B.; Badu, S.; Wu, Q.; Weidler, E.M.; Abraham, B.P.; Devaraj, S.; Luna, R.A.; Versalovic, J.; et al. Probiotic VSL#3 treatment reduces colonic permeability and abdominal pain symptoms in patients with irritable bowel syndrome. *Front. Pain Res.* **2021**, *2*, 691689.
114. Ait Abdellah, S.; Gal, C.; Laterza, L.; Velenza, V.; Settanni, C.R.; Napoli, M.; Schiavoni, E.; Mora, V.; Petito, V.; Gasbarrini, A. Effect of a multistrain probiotic on leaky gut in patients with diarrhea-predominant irritable bowel syndrome: A pilot study. *Dig. Dis.* **2023**, *41*, 489–499. [CrossRef]
115. Marchix, J.; Quénéhervé, L.; Bordron, P.; Aubert, P.; Durand, T.; Oullier, T.; Blondeau, C.; Ait Abdellah, S.; Bruley des Varannes, S.; Chaffron, S.; et al. Could the microbiota be a predictive factor for the clinical response to probiotic supplementation in IBS-D? A cohort study. *Microorganisms* **2023**, *11*, 277. [CrossRef]
116. Zhong, C.; Qu, C.; Wang, B.; Liang, S.; Zeng, B. Probiotics for preventing and treating small intestinal bacterial overgrowth: A meta-analysis and systematic review of current evidence. *J. Clin. Gastroenterol.* **2017**, *51*, 300–311. [CrossRef] [PubMed]

117. Leber, B.; Tripolt, N.J.; Bladdl, D.; Eder, M.; Wascher TCPieber, T.R.; Stauber, R.; Sourij, H.; Oettl, K.; Stadlbauer, V. The influence of probiotic supplementation on gut permeability in patients with metabolic syndrome: An open label, randomized pilot study. *Eur. J. Clin. Nutr.* **2012**, *66*, 1110–1115. [CrossRef]
118. DiMattia, Z.; Damani, J.J.; Van Syoc, E.; Rogers, C.J. Effect of probiotic supplementation on intestinal permeability in overweight and obesity: A systematic review of randomized controlled trials and animal studies. *Adv. Nutr.* **2024**, *15*, 100162. [CrossRef] [PubMed]
119. Tandon, P.; Moncrief, K.; Madsen, K.; Arrieta, M.C.; Owen, R.J.; Bain, V.G.; Wong, W.W.; Ma, M.M. Effects of probiotic therapy on portal pressure in patients with cirrhosis: A pilot study. *Liver Int.* **2009**, *29*, 1110–1115. [CrossRef]
120. Jayakumar, S.; Carbonneau, M.; Hotte, N.; Befus, A.D.; St Laurent, C.; Owen, R.; McCarthy, M.; Madsen, K.; Bailey, R.J.; Ma, M.; et al. VSL#3® probiotic therapy does not reduce portal pressures in patients with decompensated cirrhosis. *Liver Int.* **2013**, *33*, 1470–1477.
121. Kwak, D.S.; Jun, D.W.; Seo, J.G.; Chung WSPark, S.-E.; Lee, K.N.; Khalid-Saeed, W.; Lee, H.L.; Lee, O.Y.; Yoon, B.C.; Choi, H.S. Short-term probiotic therapy alleviates small intestinal bacterial overgrowth, but does not improve intestinal permeability in chronic liver disease. *Eur. J. Gastroenterol. Hepatol.* **2014**, *26*, 1353–1359. [CrossRef] [PubMed]
122. Horvath, A.; Leber, B.; Schmerboeck, B.; Tawdrous, M.; Zettel, G.; Hartl, A.; Madl, T.; Stryeck, S.; Fuchs, D.; Lemesch, S.; et al. Randomised clinical trial: The effects of a multispecies probiotic vs. placebo on innate immune function, bacterial translocation and gut permeability in patients with cirrhosis. *Aliment. Pharmacol. Ther.* **2016**, *44*, 926–935. [CrossRef] [PubMed]
123. Horvath, A.; Durdevic, M.; Leber, B.; di Vora, K.; Rainer, F.; Krones, E.; Douschan, P.; Spindelboeck, W.; Durchschein, F.; Zollner, G.; et al. Changes in the intestinal microbiome during a multispecies probiotic intervention in compensated cirrhosis. *Nutrients* **2020**, *12*, 1874. [CrossRef] [PubMed]
124. Ayob, N.; Nawawi, K.N.M.; Nor, M.H.M.; Ali, R.A.F.; Ahmad, H.F.; Oon, S.F.; Mokhtar, N.M. The effects of probiotics on small intestinal microbiota composition, inflammatory cytokines and intestinal permeability in patients with non-alcoholic fatty liver disease. *Biomedicines* **2023**, *11*, 640. [CrossRef]
125. Qin, H.-L.; Zheng, J.-J.; Tong, D.-N.; Chen, W.-X.; Fan, X.-B.; Hang, X.-M.; Jiang, Y.-Q. Effect of Lactobacillus plantarum enteral feeding on the gut permeability and septic complications in the patients with acute pancreatitis. *Eur. J. Clin. Nutr.* **2008**, *62*, 923–930. [CrossRef] [PubMed]
126. Besselink, M.G.; van Santvoort, H.C.; Renooij, W.; de Smet, M.B.; Boermeester, M.A.; Fischer, K.; Timmerman Hmali, U.A.; Cirkel, G.A.; Bollen, T.L.; van Ramshorst, B.; et al. Intestinal barrier dysfunction in a randomized trial of a specific probiotic composition in acute pancreatitis. *Ann. Surg.* **2009**, *250*, 712–719. [CrossRef]
127. McNaught, C.E.; Woodcock, N.P.; Anderson, A.D.G.; MacFie, J. A prospective randomised trial of probiotics in critically ill patients. *Clin. Nutr.* **2005**, *24*, 211–219. [CrossRef]
128. Alberda, C.; Gramlich, L.; Meddings, J.; Field, C.; McCargar, L.; Kutsogiannis, D.; Fedorak, R.; Madsen, K. Effects of probiotic therapy in critically ill patients: A randomized, double-blind, placebo-controlled trial. *Am. J. Clin. Nutr.* **2007**, *85*, 816–823. [CrossRef]
129. Presti, R.M.; Yeh, E.; Williams, B.; Landay, A.; Jacobson, J.M.; Wilson, C.; Fichtenbaum, C.J.; Utay, N.S.; Dube, M.P.; Klingman, K.L.; et al. A randomized, placebo-controlled trial assessing the effect of VISBIOME ES probiotic in people with HIV on antiretroviral therapy. *Open Forum Infect. Dis.* **2021**, *8*, ofab550. [CrossRef]
130. Mokkala, K.; Pussinen, P.; Houttu, N.; Koivuniemi, E.; Vahlberg, T.; Laitinen, K. The impact of probiotics and n-3 long-chain polyunsaturated fatty acids on intestinal permeability in pregnancy: A randomised clinical trial. *Benef. Microbes* **2018**, *9*, 199–208. [CrossRef]
131. Chaiyasut, C.; Sivamaruthi, B.S.; Lailerd, N.; Sirilun, S.; Khongtan, S.; Fukngoen, P.; Peerajan, S.; Saelee, M.; Chaiyasut, K.; Kesika, P.; et al. Probiotics supplementation improves intestinal permeability, obesity index and metabolic biomarkers in elderly Thai subjects: A randomized controlled trial. *Foods* **2022**, *11*, 268. [CrossRef] [PubMed]
132. de Roos, N.M.; van Hemert, S.; Rovers, J.M.P.; Smits, M.G.; Witteman, B.J.M. The effects of a multispecies probiotic on migraine and markers of intestinal permeability–results of a randomized placebo-controlled study. *Eur. J. Clin. Nutr.* **2017**, *71*, 1455–1462. [CrossRef] [PubMed]
133. Swanson, K.S.; Gibson, G.R.; Hutkins, R.; Reimer, R.A.; Reid, G.; Verbeke, K.; Scott KPHolscher, H.D.; Azad, M.B.; Delzenne, N.M.; Sanders, M.E. The International Scientific Association for Probiotics and Prebiotics (ISAPP) consensus statement on the definition and scope of synbiotics. *Nat. Rev. Gastroenterol. Hepatol.* **2020**, *17*, 687–701. [CrossRef]
134. Camilleri, M. Human intestinal barrier: Effects of stressors, diet, prebiotics, and probiotics. *Clin. Transl. Gastroenterol.* **2021**, *12*, e00308. [CrossRef] [PubMed]
135. Reddy, B.S.; Macfie, J.; Gatt, M.; Larsen, C.N.; Jensen, S.S.; Leser, T.D. Randomized clinical trial of effect of synbiotics, neomycin and mechanical bowel preparation on intestinal barrier function in patients undergoing colectomy. *Br. J. Surg.* **2007**, *94*, 546–554. [CrossRef]
136. Spindler-Vesel, A.; Bengmark, S.; Vovk, I.; Cerovic, O.; Kompan, L. Synbiotics, prebiotics, glutamine, or peptide in early enteral nutrition: A randomized study in trauma patients. *J. Parenter. Enter. Nutr.* **2007**, *31*, 119–126. [CrossRef]
137. Sharma, B.; Srivastava, A.; Singh, N.; Sachdev, V.; Kapur, S.; Saraya, A. Role of probiotics on gut permeability and endotoxemia in patients with acute pancreatitis: A double-blind randomized controlled trial. *J. Clin. Gastroenterol.* **2011**, *45*, 442–448. [CrossRef]

138. West, N.P.; Pyne, D.B.; Cripps, A.W.; Christophersen, C.T.; Conlon, M.A.; Fricker, P.A. Gut Balance, a synbiotic supplement, increases fecal Lactobacillus paracasei but has little effect on immunity in healthy physically active individuals. *Gut Microbes* **2012**, *3*, 221–227. [CrossRef]
139. Yokoyama, Y.; Nishigaki, E.; Abe, T.; Fukaya, M.; Asahara, T.; Nomoto, K.; Nagino, M. Randomized clinical trial of the effect of perioperative synbiotics versus no synbiotics on bacterial translocation after oesophagectomy. *Br. J. Surg.* **2014**, *101*, 189–199. [CrossRef]
140. Wilms, E.; Gerritsen, J.; Smidt, H.; Besseling-van der Vaart, I.; Rijkers, G.T.; Garcia Fuentes, A.R.; Masclee, A.A.M.; Troost, F.J. Effects of supplementation of the synbiotic Ecologic® 825/FOS P6 on intestinal barrier function in healthy humans: A randomized controlled trial. *PLoS ONE* **2016**, *11*, e0167775. [CrossRef]
141. Stenman, L.K.; Lehtinen, M.J.; Meland, N.; Christensen, J.E.; Yeung, N.; Saarinen, M.T.; Courtney, M.; Burcelin, R.; Lähdeaho, M.-L.; Linros, J.; et al. Probiotic with or without fiber controls body fat mass, associated with serum zonulin, in overweight and obese adults-randomized controlled trial. *EBioMedicine* **2016**, *13*, 190–200. [CrossRef] [PubMed]
142. Ferolla, S.M.; Couto, C.A.; Costa-Silva, L.; Armiliato, G.N.A.; Pereira, C.A.S.; Martins, F.S.; de Lourdes AFerrari, M.; Vilela, E.G.; Tores, H.O.G.; Cunha, A.S.; et al. Beneficial effect of synbiotic supplementation on hepatic steatosis and anthropometric parameters, but not on gut permeability in a population with nonalcoholic steatohepatitis. *Nutrients* **2016**, *8*, 397. [CrossRef] [PubMed]
143. Moser, A.M.; Spindelboeck, W.; Halwachs, B.; Strohmaier, H.; Kump, P.; Gorkiewicz, G.; Högenauer, C. Effects of an oral synbiotic on the gastrointestinal immune system and microbiota in patients with diarrhea-predominant irritable bowel syndrome. *Eur. J. Nutr.* **2019**, *58*, 2767–2778. [CrossRef] [PubMed]
144. Horvath, A.; Leber, B.; Feldbacher, N.; Steinwender, M.; Komarova, I.; Rainer, F.; Blesl, A.; Stadlbauer, V. The effects of a multispecies synbiotic on microbiome-related side effects of long-term proton pump inhibitor use: A pilot study. *Sci. Rep.* **2020**, *10*, 2723. [CrossRef]
145. Horvath, A.; Leber, B.; Feldbacher, N.; Tripolt, N.; Rainer, F.; Blesl, A.; Trieb, M.; Marsche, G.; Sourij, H.; Stadlbauer, V. Effects of a multispecies synbiotic on glucose metabolism, lipid marker, gut microbiome composition, gut permeability, and quality of life in diabesity: A randomized, double-blind, placebo-controlled pilot study. *Eur. J. Nutr.* **2020**, *59*, 2969–2983. [CrossRef]
146. Cosola, C.; Rocchetti, M.T.; di Bari, I.; Acquaviva, P.M.; Maranzano, V.; Corciulo, S.; Di Ciaula, A.; Di Palo, D.M.; La Forgia, F.M.; Fontana, S.; et al. An innovative synbiotic formulation decreases free serum indoxyl sulfate, small intestine permeability and ameliorates gastrointestinal symptoms in a randomized pilot trial in stage IIIb-IV CKD patients. *Toxins* **2021**, *13*, 334. [CrossRef]
147. Ghavami, A.; Khorvash, F.; Heidari, Z.; Khalesi, S.; Askari, G. Effect of synbiotic supplementation on migraine characteristics and inflammatory biomarkers in women with migraine: Results of a randomized controlled trial. *Pharmacol. Res.* **2021**, *169*, 105668. [CrossRef]
148. Liu, M.; Tandorost, A.; Moludi, J.; Dey, P. Prebiotics plus probiotics may favorably impact on gut permeability, endocannabinoid receptors, and inflammatory biomarkers in patients with coronary artery diseases: A clinical trial. *Food Sci. Nutr.* **2024**, *12*, 1207–1217. [CrossRef]

nutrients

MDPI

Review

Cosmeceuticals: A Review of Clinical Studies Claiming to Contain Specific, Well-Characterized Strains of Probiotics or Postbiotics

Ioannis M. Theodorou [1], Dorothea Kapoukranidou [2], Markos Theodorou [3], Joulia K. Tsetis [3], Alexandra Eleftheria Menni [4], Georgios Tzikos [4], Stella Bareka [4], Anne Shrewsbury [4], George Stavrou [5,†] and Katerina Kotzampassi [1,*,†]

1 Hellenic Institute for the Study of Sepsis (HISS), 11528 Athens, Greece; itheodorou@med.uoa.gr
2 Department of Physiology, Faculty of Medicine, Aristotle University of Thessaloniki, 54636 Thessaloniki, Greece; dkapoukr@gmail.com
3 Uni-Pharma S.A., 14564 Athens, Greece; theodor@uni-pharma.gr (M.T.); jtsetis@uni-pharma.gr (J.K.T.)
4 Department of Surgery, Aristotle University of Thessaloniki, 54636 Thessaloniki, Greece; alexmenn@auth.gr (A.E.M.); gtziko@auth.gr (G.T.); stella.mpareka@gmail.com (S.B.); a_shrewsbury@yahoo.com (A.S.)
5 Department of Surgery, Addenbrooke's Hospital, Cambridge CB2 2QQ, UK; stavgd@gmail.com
* Correspondence: kakothe@yahoo.com
† These authors contributed equally to this work.

Abstract: The skin serves as a critical barrier against external threats—dehydration, ultraviolet exposure, and infections—playing a significant role in internal homeostasis and moisture retention. Additionally, and equally importantly, it interacts dynamically with the complex microbiome resident in it, which is essential for maintaining skin health. Recent interest has focused on the use of probiotics and postbiotics, besides their ability to modulate the skin microbiome, to enhance barrier function, and exhibit anti-inflammatory properties, to be involved in skincare, by having the potential to improve skin hydration, elasticity, and overall appearance, as well as in reducing signs of aging, such as wrinkles and fine lines. The products—being a combination of a cosmetic regime plus probiotic[s] or postbiotic[s]—are named cosmeceuticals. However, to comply with the regulations for the characterization of a microorganism as a specific probiotic strain, the pro- or postbiotics incorporated into the cosmetic regime should be both genetically and phenotypically defined. Thus, in this review, we present 14 published clinical trials using such cosmetic products with specific, well-characterized strains of probiotics or postbiotics applied to volunteers with healthy skin. Looking at the results of these studies collectively, we can say that these genetically and phenotypically defined strains of either live or inanimate bacteria and/or their components seem to keep the treated skin at least fully hydrated, with intact epithelial tone, increased radiance, and with decreased wrinkle depth, while normalizing the commensal skin microbiota. Future advancements in personalized skin care may lead to genomic sequencing and metabolomics to tailor probiotic and postbiotic treatments to individual skin microbiomes, promising a new frontier in cosmeceuticals.

Keywords: cosmeceuticals; dermocosmetics; probiotics; postbiotics; skin health; topical use

1. Introduction

The skin, the body's largest and most complex organ, serves as the outermost protective barrier against external threats by playing a crucial role in internal homeostasis by means of exerting sensation, regulation, and protection from dehydration, external aggressions—such as ultraviolet exposure and temperature changes—as well as infections [1–3]. Additionally, the skin is a dynamic organ that closely interacts with a complex ecosystem of microorganisms, known as the skin microbiome. It houses, in a symbiotic relationship, up to one billion microbiota per square centimeter, including bacteria, fungi, viruses, and mites, which are absolutely essential for maintaining healthy skin by means of protecting against pathogenic microbes, modulating immune responses, and maintaining skin barrier function [4–7].

The diversity and abundance of these microbial taxa vary considerably between individuals, due to genetic factors, age, gender, diet, lifestyle, and between the different sites on an individual's skin surface, the latter being directly related to the skin type and location. Thus, we recognize moist, dry, and sebaceous or oily skin areas. Moist areas are mainly colonized by *Staphylococcus* and *Corynebacteria* species, as well as the fungus *Malassezia*, while the axilla is also colonized by Gram-positive bacteria of the genera *Micrococcus* and *Cutibacterium acnes* (formerly known as *Propionibacterium acnes*). Dry areas additionally host *Corynebacterium*, *Enhydrobacter*, and *Streptococcus*, while oily areas, house mainly the lipophilic *Cutibacterium* species, as well as *Staphylococcus* and *Malassezia* species [8–10].

Besides its contribution to restoring a balanced environment, the healthy microbiome produces metabolites that are crucial in maintaining skin moisture, elasticity, and resilience, such as organic acids, polysaccharides, and different proteins—mainly enzymes involved in the skin metabolic processes, such as hyaluronic acid production, ceramide synthesis through sphingomyelinase and the stimulation of melanocytes [4]. *Staphylococcus epidermidis*, a commensal bacterium, is probably the most typical example of this process, exhibiting interesting interactions with glycerol, which is a significant component of the skin's outermost layer of the epidermis, the stratum corneum. It metabolizes glycerol to by-products such as lactic acid, which can assist in maintaining an acidic skin environment, inhibiting the growth of pathogenic bacteria. Glycerol attracts water into the stratum corneum, thus enhancing its hydration and consecutively the preservation of the lipid matrix integrity in the stratum corneum, essential for avoiding trans-epidermal water loss, finally making the skin more flexible and less prone to cracking. Additionally, and more useful teleologically, by preserving skin hydration, it creates an environment that supports the multiplication of beneficial bacteria like *S. epidermidis*, which produce antimicrobial peptides that in turn inhibit the colonization of pathogenic bacteria such as *Staphylococcus aureus* [2,11–13]. Another ability of *S. epidermidis* is the stimulation of the production of ceramides in the skin, by producing the enzyme sphingomyelinase, which hydrolyzes the sphingomyelin present in the skin cell membranes, thus releasing ceramides, the outmost component of the lipid matrix of stratum corneum and plays a crucial role in maintaining the skin's osmotic barrier, thus improving hydration, and avoiding trans-epidermal water loss [14–17].

These few examples are informative of the inherent ability of commensal bacteria to keep the skin healthy. However, the skin is not in a "closed" laboratory, untouched by genetic and external factors. It not only reflects the general health status but mirrors physical aging, too—the two main types of which are natural aging, and photoaging. Natural or physical aging is in part genetically programmed, however, other internal components of the body, such as hormonal and immunological status, as well as psychological stress are strong additional endogenous factors that can also affect skin quality [1,18–20]. Beyond these, environmental factors such as smoking, lifestyle, changes in skin microbiota of whatever etiology, mechanical damage to tissue, and various other factors result in the already reduced number of fibroblasts producing fewer extracellular matrix components. The most significant of these is type I collagen, the reduced amount of which results in a thinner dermal matrix, reduced elasticity, and increased dehydration—most notably manifested by wrinkles and skin relaxation, laxity, and a rough-textured appearance [21–26]. At the same time, and supplementary to physical aging, the extent and frequency of ultraviolet radiation exposure speed up skin aging by means of the aberrant reactive oxygen species generation which leads to changes in the microbiome, raised skin pH, decreased collagen levels, and, mainly, an altered immune response [12,27].

Numerous experimental and ex vivo studies have shown that efforts to manipulate the skin bacterial inhabitants, replacing them with healthy ones, namely probiotics [28,29]—given either orally or topically—result in a degree of microbiome restoration, thus reducing inflammation, while enhancing immunomodulation and the epithelial barrier function through the upregulation of tight junction genes [6,30]. The same is also true for the use of non-viable bacteria, cell wall fragments, or their metabolites, now collectively named postbiotics [6,31–37].

Enhancement of barrier function, achieving a reduction in trans-epithelial water loss, increase in immunomodulatory properties, wound healing, and possible stimulation of collagen and ceramides production—otherwise recognized as "exerting skin-rejuvenating properties"—are each a good reason for applying probiotics and/or postbiotics to the skin and has attracted considerable attention from both scientific communities and dermo-cosmetic industry.

The US Federal Food, Drug, and Cosmetic Act defines cosmetics as *"articles intended to be… applied to the human body...for beautifying, promoting attractiveness, or altering the appearance"* [FD&C Act, sec. 201(i)], which definition was further clarified by the Modernization of Cosmetics Regulation Act of 2022 (MoCRA) and amended to include *"a preparation of cosmetic ingredients with a qualitatively and quantitatively set composition for use in a finished product"* [FD&C Act, sec. 361]. On the other hand, European Regulation No 1223/2009 defines cosmetics as "any substance or mixture intended to be placed in contact with the external parts of the human body… with a view exclusively or mainly to cleaning, perfuming, changing their appearance, protecting them, keeping them in good condition or correcting body odors". The same Regulation [improving the 1976 Directive 76/768/EC] strengthens the safety of cosmetic products by the introduction of the notion of "responsible person", having the obligation of reporting serious undesirable effects. Additionally [EU No 655/2013], underlines that the safety of a cosmetic product must be demonstrated and data on microbiological quality must be included in the Cosmetic Product Safety Report.

Although there are numerous products now marketed under the label "containing probiotics" or "containing probiotic lysate" there is reason for considerable caution. To comply with regulations for the characterization of a bacterium as a specific probiotic strain, both genetically and phenotypically, documented and peer-reviewed publications of experiments defining the rationale of their intended use are required [27,38,39]. Furthermore, a postbiotic must be derived from a well-defined microorganism or combination of microorganisms for which genomic sequences are known and prepared using a delineated technological process of biomass production and inactivation, which can be reliably reproduced [3,37,40]. The aim of this review is to select from a high volume of publications only the clinical studies fulfilling the above prerequisites—that is the microorganism used must be well characterized as a specific probiotic strain, live or inanimate [postbiotic], genetically and phenotypically identified, and its specific properties to have been documented experimentally first, the results having been published in peer-reviewed publications.

2. Searching the Literature and Findings

A detailed literature search was performed in PubMed; search terms included: topical use or application, cosmetics, cosmeceuticals, probiotics, postbiotics, skin or dermal, randomized clinical trials, clinical studies, and reviews. Preference was given to clinical trials; but all prior meta-analyses, reviews, or narrated reviews were used as possible data sources [Supplementary Materials, Flow Chart].

The trials finally used were only those that referred to cosmetic products [creams, shampoos, lotions] containing probiotics or postbiotics of a clearly identifiable strain [either single or multiple strains], which was applied to healthy-skin volunteers—all skin diseases needing pharmaceutics for systemic treatment were excluded. The final results of the trials—objected quantitative measurements—were compared with those of day 0 [baseline] for the same individual or the corresponding subjects of a placebo-treated group, as each clinical study had been designed by the researchers.

A total of 14 papers were found to fulfill the above criteria; 5 papers referred to the use of cosmetics incorporating probiotics and 9 papers referred to cosmetics incorporating postbiotics.

3. Cosmetics with Probiotics [Table 1]

3.1. *Lactiplantibacillus plantarum HY7714*

An early study from the Yakult Co., Yongin, Republic of Korea revealed that the orally taken probiotic formula with *L. plantarum* HY7714 exerts excellent protective effects on the skin of ultraviolet B-irradiated hairless mice against photoaging and dryness, thus achieving for the first time the characterization of a nutricosmetic formula [41,42].

In a double-blind, randomized, clinical study on 110 women aged between 41 and 59 years with Corneometer-confirmed dry skin and wrinkles [readings below 48 arbitrary units and crow's feet greater than grade 4], the *L. plantarum* HY7714 [10^{10} cfu/d] or placebo was given for 12 wks, the parameters of skin hydration, elasticity, gloss, and wrinkles being tested once per four weeks. The probiotic formulation isolated from the women's breast milk was found to exert multiple aesthetically beneficial effects: improved facial skin gloss and decreased wrinkle depth [assessed through a 3D skin imaging system] in week 12, with an increased elasticity of 13.2% in week 4 and 21.7% at the end of treatment. Trans-epidermal water loss was found significantly decreased, in parallel with an increase in the facial [$p < 0.01$] and forearm skin moisture content [$p < 0.05$] by week 12, all findings in relation to placebo. These results came following earlier extended experimentation by the authors' group on hairless mice, in which, among other things, they found that skin moisture content increased in association with ceramide levels—through the regulation of serine palmitoyl transferase and ceramidase expression in the skin—and that the procollagen expression also increased through a matrix metalloproteinase ((MMP)-1) [35].

3.2. *Nitrosomonas eutropha (D23)*

Lee NY et al. highlighted the anti-proliferative role of a purified strain of *N. eutropha* (D23)—an ammonia-oxidizing bacteria-generating nitrite and nitric oxide—on keratinocytes, reducing the hyperproliferative keratinization as well as the overall cutaneous inflammatory state and improving the skin xerosis-related pathologies, such as atopic dermatitis and keratosis pilaris [43]. Although two other clinical trials have further been conducted on skin diseases no publications exist, yet.

Notay et al. [44], based on the known beneficial effects of nitric oxide, such as reduced inflammation, increased vasodilation, and pathogenic bacteria killing, investigated the perspective of restoring aging parameters, that is facial wrinkle depth and severity, skin radiance, and pigmentation, after topical application of live *N. eutropha*, in aerosolized form.

Twenty-nine volunteers, after a washout week, received *N. eutropha* in buffer, twice daily, at a concentration of 1×10^9 cells/mL (the first 10 participants), and at a concentration of 8×10^9 cells/mL (the remaining participants). High-resolution facial photographs were obtained before and at treatment termination, only a week later. Facial wrinkles, quantified by means of algorithm-based modeling revealed a significant improvement in those who received the high-concentration product; radiance improved with both low and high concentrations, while there was no overall change in intensity of pigmentation. The authors reported a further schedule to evaluate possible facial microbiome changes, but the results have not yet been published.

3.3. *Lactiplantibacillus pentosus KCA1*

Onwuliri V, et al. [45] from Nnamdi Azikiwe University, Awka, Nigeria, having previously analyzed the most predominant genera of the human axilla in Nigerians [46], investigated the topical application of a cream containing the *L. pentosus* KCA1 to decrease the malodor volatile substances producing bacteria; the *Corynebacterium striatum*, *C. jeikeium* and *Staphylococcus haemolyticus*, *Staphylococcus hominis*, and *S. lugdunensis*, considered to be the most implicated.

Lyophilized *L. pentosus* KCA1, a probiotic of Nigerian origin [47], in a weight of 12 g was gently mixed with 75 g of an oil-based balm of coconut and lavender oil, plus cocoa and shea butter; this 87 g formula was used by each of the 25 young adult volunteers—13 females and

12 males—applied to the armpit twice daily for 14 days; skin swabs were collected on days 0 and 14. Although monitoring of physical activities as well as the use of antiseptic soap and deodorants and showers taken is impossible as it was based only on self-reporting, all participants reported an absence of axillary malodor during the treatment period.

The bacterial metabolic functional genes encoding pyridoxal phosphate-dependent enzymes revealed a significant down-regulation in the biotransformation of the odor precursor, after application of the *L. pentosus* KCA1 cream. Additionally, the application of this cream led to a significant decrease in the odor-producing *Corynebacterium* species, in both genders; *Corynebacteria* spp., as striatum and jeikeium were found significantly decreased by 96% and 73%, respectively, as also *S. hominis* by 20.8% in males. It is of interest that *C. acnes* also decreased by 46% in males and by over 77% in females, while *Lactobacillus* species generally increased in both diversity and abundance by over 385%.

3.4. *Lactiplantibacillus plantarum LB244R*

An oily texture, semi-solid formulation used as a tracer for the topical application of live *L. plantarum* LB244R® bacteria, at a concentration of 1×10^9 CFU/g [48]. *L. plantarum* LB244R® was selected due to its known antibacterial activity toward S. aureus clonal type 1 and its capacity to improve both atopic skin as well as aging skin [49], while the oily tracer included shea butter, refined oils of rapeseed, jojoba, and sunflower seed, hydrogenated olive oil, sunflower hybrid oil, and tocopherol. The probiotic regime was given a 24 mo shelf-life when kept refrigerated, and no preservatives were needed, due to the oily tracer.

This probiotic-containing ointment was tested on 21 postmenopausal women, aged 49 to 62 years with "normal" to dry skin [Fitzpatrick skin phototypes II to IV]. These women were instructed to apply the formula and massage until total absorption, on a cleaned facial skin, for 56 consecutive days, twice daily. The women were assessed by an experienced dermatologist on days 0, 28, and 56, to confirm the anti-aging potential of the probiotic ointment. Clinical evaluation, skin ultrasonography, and skin biomechanical property assessment, in relation to baseline, revealed an improvement in crow's feet, spot score, smoothness score, and complexion radiance, an increase in skin hydration, firmness and elasticity as well as dermal density and a decrease in the trans-epidermal water loss and the thickness of the sub-epidermal low echogenic band. However, there was no placebo-treatment group, this being a serious limitation of the study, since the other ingredients of the ointment, such as shea butter, seed oil, jojoba oil, olive oil, sunflower oil, and tocopherol are also known to exert hydration and anti-aging properties [48].

3.5. *Lactiplantibacillus plantarum LB244R*

A few months later, the same authors who had tested *L. plantarum* LB244R in an oily tracer including shea butter, refined oils of rapeseed, jojoba, and sunflower seed, hydrogenated olive oil, sunflower hybrid oil, and tocopherol with positive results, but without placebo group [48] performed a new study with a control group at that time [50].

In this newer study, they investigated the commercially available ointment containing 1×10^9 CFU/g live *L. plantarum* LB244R, isolated from fermented cabbage, in an oily tracer of Byturospermum parkii butter, Simmondsia chinensis seed oil, Brassica campestris seed oil, hydrogenated vegetable oil, Helianthus annuus hybrid oil, Prunus amygdalus dulcis oil, tocopherol, and Helianthus annuus seed oil or the vehicle ointment without bacteria as placebo. Forty-six postmenopausal females, having a mean age of 58.7 years, were randomly assigned to apply either the test ointment or placebo on previously cleaned skin of the face and periocular area, twice daily for 56 consecutive days. They were instructed to massage the product until complete absorption and come for assessment mid-period and at the end of the study.

The probiotic-containing ointment was found to bring significant improvement in relation to placebo to the subepidermal low echogenic band thickness and dermal density, assessed by ultrasonography; the skin firmness and elasticity, assessed by a dual-cutometer apparatus; the trans-epidermal water loss, skin hydration, and pH; the collagen fiber perimeter and density, assessed by confocal microscopy. Additionally, from the clinical evaluation, the crow's feet wrinkles, the spots, the skin smoothness, and the complexion radiance scores were found significantly improved in comparison to baseline. However, when comparing the final effects [day 56] of the test ointment versus placebo, the probiotic ointment was found to work significantly better in improving the subepidermal low echogenic band thickness, the dermal density, the skin hydration, and the crow's feet wrinkle score, only [50].

Table 1. Cosmetics with probiotics.

Live Bacteria	Applied on	Duration	Placebo Group	Findings	First Author [Reference]
L. plantarum HY7714 10^{10} cfu/d	Face	12 wks	Yes	Increased facial skin gloss and skin moisture content Decreased wrinkle depth Decreased TEWL	Lee DE [35]
N. eutropha (D23) 8×10^9 cells/mL	Face	1 wk	No	Increased facial radiance Decreased facial wrinkles Decreased the intensity of pigmentation	Notay M [44]
L. pentosus KCA1 lyophilized,12 g	Armpit	14 d	No	Absence of axillary malodor during the treatment Decrease in odor-producing Corynebacterium species	Onwuliri V [45]
L. plantarum LB244R 1×10^9 cfu/g	Face	56 d	No	Increased skin hydration, firmness, elasticity and density Increased smoothness score and complexion radiance Decreased in crow's feet, spot score and TEWL	Falholt-Elvebakken H [48]
L. plantarum LB244R 1×10^9 cfu/g	Face	56 d	Yes	Increased skin firmness, density, elasticity and smoothness Increased skin hydration, pH and complexion radiance score Decreased crow's feet wrinkles and TEWL	Elvebakken HF [50]

TEWL: trans-epithelial water loss.

4. Cosmetics with Postbiotics [Table 2]

4.1. *Streptococcus thermophilus S244, Dead by Sonication*

As early as 1999, Di Marzio et al. [51] revealed that bacteria of *S. thermophilus*, dead by sonication, when added to a keratinocytes culture were able to induce a significant increase in ceramide levels, in a time-dependent manner. The same result was confirmed after topical application of sonicated bacteria on the forearm skin of 17 healthy subjects for a 7-day period. These findings of increased ceramide levels in the stratum corneum, the outmost layer of the human epidermis, and thus of the clinical effect of increased hydration, were attributed to sphingomyelin hydrolysis, by means of the high levels of bacterial neutral sphingomyelinase from *S. thermophilus* S244; in turn, the increased ceramide levels could result in the enhancement of lipid barrier function and thus to stratum corneum flexibility, slowing down the skin aging process. For further documentation of the ability of *S. thermophilus* to induce a very significant increase in skin ceramide levels, a cream containing purified sphingomyelinase [Avant Garde, Sigma Tau, Pomezia, Rome, Italy] from *Bacillus cereus* [Sigma] was applied as a placebo; the results being comparable.

The same in vivo study was then later repeated with 20 healthy women in order to document improvement in skin hydration [52]. A sonicated *S. thermophilus* S244 bacteria-containing cream [Centro Ricerche YOMO, Italy] was topically applied twice daily to one forearm and the cream only to the other [control], daily for 15 consecutive days during the autumn [to avoid UV radiation exposure], on females over 60 years old, with a healthy skin. Trans-epidermal water loss was found unaffected between treated and controls, meaning that the normal permeability barrier still exists; but forearm skin hydration was found to significantly increase in the treated site in parallel with increased skin ceramides, findings actually related to the presence of S. thermophilus sphingomyelinase, which enabled maintenance of the dermal protective barrier and increase in resistance against age-related skin xerosis.

4.2. *Bifidobacterium longum Reuter Lysate*

Guéniche et al. [53], having already demonstrated, in both in vitro and in ex vivo human skin explant models, the beneficial effects of *B. longum* reuter lysate to improve sensitive skin, tested it as a cream formula containing 10% bacterium lysate, in a randomized double-blind study on the face, arms, and legs of 66 female volunteers, twice a day for two months. They had previously confirmed that the ultrasound-inactivated *B. longum* reuter lysate suspension of 5% in the aqueous medium led to an improvement in parameters relating to inflammation—a decrease in vasodilation, edema, mast cell degranulation, and TNF-alpha release—and more specifically of neurogenic inflammation, since it significantly inhibited capsaicin-induced CGRP release by neurons. The same regime, in a pilot clinical trial, was also found to lead to increased skin resistance to physical and chemical aggression in relation to controls. Given these anti-inflammatory properties, they tested this postbiotic in females with reactive skin, that is skin demonstrating excessive sensitivity to physical conditions like heat, cold, wind, or topically applied chemical products, resulting in a decrease in the skin's self-repair/rejuvenation ability.

Treated volunteers exhibited a significant improvement: increased skin resistance, that is a decrease in skin sensitivity assessed by stinging test [$p = 0.002$], and an improvement in skin barrier recovery [trans-epidermal water loss less than 15 g/cm^2/h, $p = 0.004$] assessed by repeated tape-stripping at the beginning, after a month and at the end of the 2nd month. Additionally, volunteers' self-assessment emphasized a decrease in skin roughness and dryness [$p = 0.03$], after just a month of treatment, versus controls. These new findings, in correlation with those previously reported, led the authors to conclude that the postbiotic *B. longum* reuter regime decreases skin sensitivity by reducing neuron reactivity.

4.3. *Lactobacillus brevis DSM17250*

The L. brevis DSM17250 was selected among several hundred Lactobacillus strains banked in the DSMZ [German Collection of Microorganisms and Cell Cultures (Braunschweig, Germany) with the criterion of being able to stimulate *S. epidermidis* growth in vitro. This specific bacterium, *L. brevis* DSM17250, was further found to exhibit an anti-inflammatory effect on human keratinocytes in vitro, as assessed by the secretion of the pro-inflammatory cytokine IL-1α, while acting specifically on commensal skin *S. epidermidis* DSM20044, enhancing the growth both in vitro and in vivo [54].

It was then used in a human study. Thirty volunteers, mainly females, with a mean age of 39 years, with skin xerosis at their lower legs [tibia], were allocated either to a standard hydrophilic ointment containing 0.88 mg/g of the *L. brevis* DSM17250 extract or to hydrophilic ointment alone, twice a day for a month. Treatment or the placebo ointment was applied to the skin corresponding to the right anterior tibia area, while the same skin area of the left side was left totally untreated, to serve as an internal control. All participants daily self-assessed regarding dryness, roughness, a feeling of tightness, itching, and burning in relation to the contralateral leg; and by the dermatologist on day 0 and then on days 7, 14, and 28, with respect to skin barrier function [trans-epidermal water loss], with clinical scores of redness, roughness, scaling and cracks/fissures; finally, an 8 cm^2 skin tape was thoroughly attached to the skin under study, to collect the bacteria adhering to it, for the assessment of differences over the course of treatment [54].

The postbiotic cream was found by self-evaluation test to significantly improve xerosis parameters—collectively by about 70% in relation to 57% in placebo—being parallel to the measurements of trans-epidermal water loss [8.98 $g/m^2/h$ in the treatment group versus 15.68 $g/m^2/h$ in placebo, on day 28]. Regarding skin microbiota, besides *S. epidermidis*, other commensals such as Micrococcus, *S. capitis*, and *S. xylosus* were also found, the total number of commensal skin bacteria being significantly increased, from 141 to 399 cfu in the 8 cm^2 area of stripping tape used [54].

4.4. Lactiplantibacillus plantarum-GMNL6—Heat-Killed

Tsai et al. [55] investigated whether heat-killed *L. plantarum*-GMNL6 interacts with skin microbiota resulting in improvement in skin health. Fifteen healthy volunteers applied a "base" cream containing heat-killed L. plantarum-GMNL6 [1×10^9 cells/g cream] to the right cheek and to the left, the cream only, twice a day for two months, after being subjected to skin quality, moisturizing, and color tests.

Skin hydration, assessed by either a Corneometer® CM 825 or a Skicon 200 EX®, was found to be significantly better than in the controls, as also occurred with facial skin quality, wrinkles, skin texture, tone, and UV spots, assessed by using Visia (Visia Complexion Analysis, Canfield, Parsippany, NJ, USA); skin erythema and melanin indexes, respectively, assessed by a Derma-Spectrometer were significantly reduced. Finally, the 16S rDNA sequencing used to analyze the bacterial abundance and the bacterial composition in the skin revealed that in the L. plantarum-treated right cheeks Cutibacterium was found to be significantly reduced, while Streptococcus and Staphylococcus showed a higher abundance in relation to the non-treated left cheeks [55].

4.5. Lacticaseibacillus paracasei GMNL-653—Heat-Killed

Two years later, they investigated the beneficial role of heat-killed *L. paracasei* GMNL-653 on human scalp health [56]. Twenty-two volunteers used a control shampoo for one month and for the next four months the same shampoo containing the *L. paracasei* GMNL-653 postbiotic. The scalp conditions, i.e., sebum secretion, dandruff formation, and hair growth were evaluated in 15-day intervals, while the scalp skin commensal Malassezia yeasts [*M. restricta* and *M. globose*]—etiologically related to pityriasis and seborrheic dermatitis—as well as the microbiota *C. acnes*, and *S. epidermidis*—known to reciprocally inhibit scalp bacteria—were detected by means of quantitative polymerase chain reaction [PCR], before and after application of control and postbiotic-containing shampoos.

Results showed that oil count and dandruff were significantly decreased, and hair volume statistically increased after treatment, but only in the subgroup of individuals with high levels and not in those with normal values at the beginning. In respect to microbiota, *C. acnes* was found statistically decreased and *M. globosa* increased after treatment in relation to the placebo, given in the first month. There was no correlation between *L. paracasei* and *S. epidermidis* or *M. restricta* in general. However, the presence of *L. paracasei* was positively correlated with *S. epidermidis* only, in the high dandruff subgroup, although *M. restricta* statistically decreased in this subgroup of high dandruff after the use of treatment shampoo.

It is clear that the beneficial effects on sebum secretion and dandruff achieved by shampoo containing the postbiotic *L. paracasei* GMNL-653 seem more significant for those with weak scalp conditions in relation to those with healthy scalps; the valuable role being attributable to the observed microbiota shift and more specifically to abundance changes occurring to C. *acnes* and *S. epidermidis* [56].

4.6. L. plantarum AN057, L. casei AN177, and S. thermophilus AN157 Metabolites

The probiotic strains *L. plantarum* AN057, *L. casei* AN177, and *S. thermophilus* AN157—first isolated from Balkanian fermented dairy products and then fully characterized by means of a genomic analysis—were subjected to co-fermentation, resulting in a postbiotic combination of metabolites, named CLS02021 [4]. The authors claim that the above strains were carefully selected, based on their potential to produce, through co-fermentation, specific metabolites, such as lipoteichoic acid, hyaluronic acid, lactic acid, and Sphingomyelinase and indeed in considerable quantities.

Fifty healthy adult females, up to 69 years of age, voluntarily participated in a double-blind, intra-individual, randomized split-face testing study [ClinicalTrials.gov: NCT05048121] lasting four weeks. They were instructed to apply the treatment cream CLS02021 and the placebo, twice daily, provided in blinded tubes having the only indications "Left" and "Right". Skin nourishment and elasticity, wrinkle depth, sebum production, melanin production, as well as skin sensitivity and cleanliness, were measured on days 0, 14, and 28, along with the safety profile.

A statistically significant improvement was reported between postbiotics and placebo groups regarding skin moisture and elasticity [$p < 0.0001$], pore size, and wrinkle depth [$p < 0.05$], while no difference was presented regarding sebum production, melanin, sensitivity, and cleanliness. The significant increase in skin moisture levels and elasticity is likely to be attributable to sphingomyelinase facilitating the production of ceramides, being the key components of skin barrier integrity maintenance [57], as well as to hyaluronic acid along with lactic acid, which, through their capacity to bind large water volumes, decrease the trans-epidermal water loss and rehydrate the skin, thereby filling in fine lines and reducing the appearance of wrinkles [58].

4.7. Epidermidibacterium Keratini (EPI-7) Ferment Filtrate

A novel, rod-shape, aerobic, Gram-positive bacterium of the *Actinobacterium phylum, E. keratini* (EPI-7), recently isolated from human epidermal keratinocytes from the cheeks of young females [59], was found to exhibit anti-aging properties in human dermal fibroblasts after being subjected to UV photo-aging. This occurs through the modulation of UV activity on matrix metalloproteinases [60], and through one of the EPI-7 ferment filtrates, orotic acid, known to be crucially involved in pyrimidines biosynthesis [61].

The authors [62] investigated the anti-aging efficacy and safety of the postbiotic EPI-7 ferment filtrate, applied topically for 3 weeks, in relation to the skin microbiome diversity. A total of 55 Korean women of different age groups, between 19 and 60+ years of age enrolled in this randomized, split-face clinical study showed highly significant improvements in skin barrier function, elasticity, and dermal density versus control treatment, possibly related to the restoration of commensal microbiota diversity observed.

Indeed, an increase in the abundance of the commensal bacteria of *Staphylococcus, Cutibacterium, Corynebacterium, Lawsonella, Streptococcus, Clostridium lactobacillus*, and *Prevotella* spp. was prominent, and more specifically, *Cutibacterium* was found significantly increased in parallel with *Clostridium*, and *Prevotella*. The authors consider that the enhancement of the normally distributed diversity of bacteria species without any alteration in the dominance of any specific microorganism in the skin microbiome is linked to the metabolite orotic acid action, however further analysis and clinical tests are required [62].

Additionally, application of the postbiotic EPI-7 resulted in no observable itching, pain, or erythema.

4.8. Lactiplantibacillus plantarum HDB Lysate

The postbiotic *L. plantarum* HDB [probiotic lysate], previously examined in human skin cells as to whether it improves the skin barrier [63], was tested twice a day for 2 weeks on the cheeks of 21 randomly assigned healthy females from Korea, voluntarily participating in this investigation—the other cheek served as control [64]. The skin-hydration parameters recorded before and after treatment or placebo application were then correlated with the skin microbiota of the participants, identified using 16s rRNA gene sequencing.

The postbiotic *L. plantarum* HDB, received from the HDB Cell Bank [Hyundai Bioland Co., Ltd., Ansan, Republic of Korea] named Dermabiotics HDB, was added to an essence cosmetic formula consisting of glycerin, butylene glycol, polyethylene glycol, oils, and preservatives, and this formula was also used as the control. The *L. plantarum* treatment was found to significantly enhance the moisture intensity of the keratin layer surface. Conversely, trans-epidermal water loss and skin redness were significantly reduced in relation to controls, as also seen with skin microbiome versus control: after *L. plantarum*

HDB treatment, the α-diversity analysis revealed a significantly decreased richness in species, although the composition of the skin microbiota was very diverse at the beginning, probably due to the range of women's ages [20–50 years old] [65].

After 2 weeks, the genera of the phylum Proteobacteria, known to dominate in the dry areas of the skin, was found to decrease, the level of decrease matching an improvement in skin condition in general; while the abundance of *Staphylococci* was related to the lowering of the hot flush level; however, from the genus *Lawsonella*, known as skin microbiota related to skin moisture content, *Lawsonella clevelandensis* showed a negative correlation with the keratin layer hydration, and Corynebacterium, a member of the same order, showed a positive correlation with the trans-epidermal water loss. The authors thus confirmed that the Dermabiotics HDB formula may be considered a potential skin microbiome-based cosmetic component [64].

4.9. Fermented lysates VHProbi® Mix R

A lotion made from fermented lysates of *Lacticaseibacillus rhamnosus* VHProbi® E06 (E06), *Lacticaseibacillus paracasei* VHProbi® E12 (E12), *Lactiplantibacillus plantarum* VHProbi® E15, and *Lactobacillus helveticus* VHProbi® Y21 was applied to investigate the possibility of enhancing the skin barrier [66].

Previous preliminary vitro studies have shown that the fermented cultures of *L. rhamnosus* VHProbi® E06 (E06) and *L. paracasei* VHProbi® E12 (E12) exerted an antioxidant effect, boosted the proliferation of HaCaT cells, and ameliorated the noxious effects of UV radiation, hydrogen peroxide and *S. aureus* ATCC 25,923 in the HaCaT cell models [66], while the fermented lysate from *L. plantarum* VHProbi® E15 (E15) improved the symptoms of acne [67].

Fifty-two adults with sensitive skin, defined as that based on a positive response to the lactic acid stinging test and having a score ≥ 8 in the Burden of Sensitive Skin [BoSS] questionnaire [66], were eligible to apply the lotion to their faces twice daily for a month. The 3% VHProbi® MixR was incorporated within 100 mL of aqua with propylene glycol, caprylic/capric triglyceride, mineral oil, cetearyl alcohol, PEG-100 glyceryl stearate, stearic acid, glyceryl stearate, 1,2-hexanediol, phenoxyethanol, xanthan gum, chlorophenesin, and L-arginine as preservatives, chelating agents, and thickeners in the lotion.

On day 30, a highly significant decrease [$p < 0.01$] in trans-epithelial water loss, skin redness, redness profile, and increased moisturization was found in relation to day 0. The BoSS questionnaire revealed an improvement of 24.3% from the baseline, while on self-assessment 75% of individuals reported a good or excellent drop in skin swelling, oozing, scabs, and rashes [66].

Table 2. Cosmetics with postbiotics.

Bacteria Used	Quantity/ Duration	Applied on	Placebo Group	Findings	Microbiome Modulation	First Author [Reference]
S. thermophilus S244 sonicated	— 15 d	Forearm	Yes	Increased skin hydration Increased skin ceramides	-	Di Marzio L [52]
B. longum reuter lysate	10% cream 2 mo	Face Arms Legs	Yes	Increased skin resistance and skin barrier Decreased skin sensitivity Decrease in skin roughness and dryness	-	Guéniche A [53]
L. brevis DSM17250 extract	0.88 mg/g ointment 28 d	Tibia	Internal Control	Decreased TEWL	Increase *S. epidermidis*	Holz C [54]
L. plantarum GMNL6 heat-killed	1×10^9 cells/g cream 2 mo	Face	Internal Control [split face]	Increased skin hydration Improvement of wrinkles, skin texture, tone and UV spots Decreased skin erythema and melanin indexes	Decreased *Cutibacterium* increased *Streptococcus Staphylococcus*	Tsai, WH [55]
L. paracasei GMNL-653 heat-killed	— Shampoo 4 mo	Scalp	Baseline	Decreased sebum secretion and dandruff Increased hair volume	Decreased *Cutibacterium acnes Malassezia globosa*	Tsai WH [56]
L. plantarum AN057, L. casei AN177, S. thermophilus AN157 co-fermented metabolites CLS02021	— 4 wks	Face	Internal Control [split face]	Increased skin moisture and elasticity Decreased skin pore size and wrinkle depth	-	Catic T [4]
E. keratini (EPI-7) fermented filtrate	— 3 wks	Face	Internal Control [split face]	Increased skin barrier function Increased elasticity, and dermal density	Increased *Cutibacterium, Clostridium, Prevotella*	Kim J [62]
L. plantarum HDB lysate	— 2 wks	Face	Internal Control [split face]	Increased skin moisture Decreased TEWL Decreased skin redness	Decreased *Proteobacteria, Staphylococcii, Lawsonella clevelandensis* increased *Corynebacterium acnes*	Kim KM [64]
L. rhamnosus VHProbi® E06 *L. paracasei VHProbi® E12* *L. plantarum VHProbi® E15* *L. helveticus VHProbi® Y21* fermented lysates *VHProbi®* Mix R	3% in aquatic solution 1 mo	Face	Baseline	Increase moisturization Increased Burden of Sensitive Skin Decreased TEWL Decreases skin redness, redness profile score Decreased skin swelling, oozing, scabs, rashes	-	Cui, H. [66]

5. Discussion

Cosmetic products serve to maintain youthful and healthy skin, as well as to address the signs of aging, by improving the skin's appearance and resilience. The main functions are [i] barrier repair and hydration, achievable through moisturizers and humectants. Moisturizers, such as hyaluronic acid, glycerin, and ceramides—and fatty acids in general—help to maintain or protect and/or repair skin epithelial barriers against environmental damage, to finally prevent dehydration. Humectants, such as urea and alpha hydroxy acids, attract water to the skin, keeping it moisturized [68,69]; [ii] tissue repair, through anti-aging ingredients promoting cell turnover and stimulating collagen production, thus improving the overall skin texture and the facial oval shape, as occur with retinol and various growth factors as well as stem cell technology, encouraging skin regeneration [70,71]; [iii] protection, against harmful UV radiation, and free radicals in general, causing skin damage and leading to premature aging [72]; [iv] brightening, as occurs with vitamin C, which reduces the appearance of dark spots and evens out skin tone; [v] firming, by different peptides, retinoids and plant extracts, which improve skin elasticity and reduce sagging; and [vi] cleansing, by means of gentle cleansers with balanced pH to remove dirt, oil, and impurities and maintain the skin's natural barrier. Additionally, there are exfoliation, anti-inflammatory and smoothing agents. Finally, there are products for special purposes or targeted products, such as serums with concentrated ingredients for specific skin concerns such as fine lines, hyperpigmentation, and dehydration; and masks, which provide intensive treatment for a short period, offering hydration, brightening, or soothing benefits [38,73–75].

However, the skin houses, in a symbiotic relationship, a complex ecosystem, the skin microbiome; the dynamic interaction with which is absolutely essential for many crucial functions for maintaining healthy skin [4–7]. Thus, our Greek grandmothers' secret receipt of full-fat sheep yogurt, mixed with a few drops of olive oil or lemon [depending on skin type] applied as a face mask on Saturday night after the weekly bath and before church on Sunday, is now being transformed into science and commerce. The starter for yogurt was initially the stomach contents of a newborn sheep killed for Easter. Almost a century later, we recognize this as a regime containing *S. thermophilus*, *Lactobacillus delbrueckii* subsp. bulgaricus and *L. casei* and, most probably, as a result of contamination, with other lactic acid bacteria, which produce lactic acid, decreasing pH and causing milk protein to coagulate [76,77].

In recent years, research at any complexity level [from cell cultures to genomic sequencing and metabolomics] has indicated that the incorporation of probiotics or their lysates or bacteria killed by heat, sonication, or other methods or merely cell wall fragments [altogether now called postbiotics] into cosmetic formulations can effectively modulate the skin microbiota, which has become a prominent therapeutic option for treating various skin disorders. Thus, topical applications have attracted considerable attention from scientific and industrial communities motivated by the human desire to be attractive, to fight the signs of age, and to tone down physical damage [53,78,79].

Hundreds of products advertised to protect the skin, mainly the face, or rebalance the skin microbiome and/or reported to enhance skin hydration, improve skin elasticity and radiance, and reduce the fine lines or the extent of wrinkles, are the new norm in the dermo-cosmetic field [9,34,35,80]. They are used worldwide in various "cosmeceutical" formulations such as creams, masks, lotions, serums, cleansers, and so on, and as anti-aging products due to their broad antimicrobial, anti-inflammatory, and antioxidant properties.

Thus, the term cosmeceuticals [as the word nutraceuticals used for orally taken probiotic regimes] means cosmetic products incorporate bioactive ingredients purported to have medical benefits. In early 2023, a publication by Yadav et al. [81] reported that 928 patents had been retrieved from the database after searching with the terms "probiotic" and "cosmetic" in 3 years, most applicants coming from the US, the Republic of China, and the Republic of Korea, but, at least for the US, there are no legal requirements to prove that these products live up to their claims. Thus, several cosmetic companies across the world have probiotic or postbiotic bacteria formulations commercially available, although the bacteria's origin and their clinical documentation are not always clear from the packaging or website.

However, it is well known from scientific research that not all *Lactobacilli* or *Bifidobacteria*, are considered to be probiotics, no that all have exactly the same probiotic properties. It is thus clear that the label "containing probiotics" or "containing probiotic lysate" says nothing at all. The microorganism used must be characterized as a specific probiotic strain, genetically and phenotypically identified, and its specific properties to have been documented experimentally first, the results having been published in peer-reviewed publications [27,37–39]. Furthermore, according to Telesetsky A et al. [82] the probiotic regime must have the same quantity of live bacteria used in the clinical trial, as the commercial product, to benefit the designated target site, and when people are the intended receivers, the delivery technique, dosage, and length of use should be determined through human studies [27,38,82].

In the present review, we selected those clinical studies on cosmeceuticals fulfilling all the above prerequisites. We thus found and analyzed only 14 studies: 5 incorporating probiotics, and 9 postbiotics [Tables 1 and 2]. The probiotics used were the species *L. plantarum* HY7714, *N. eutropha* (D23), and *L. plantarum* LB244R [two studies], applied to facial skin, and one clinical trial applied to the armpit [*L. pentosus* KCA1]. All four studies on facial skin revealed an improvement in skin appearance [wrinkle depth, skin radiance, and elasticity], while *L. plantarum* HY7714 and *L. plantarum* LB244R also significantly improved skin barrier function, decreasing the trans-epidermal water loss and increasing skin hydration. In the case of *L. pentosus* KCA1, applied to the armpit, it was found to decrease the odor-producing Corynebacterium species, thus achieving a significant improvement in axillary malodor during the treatment.

Nine preparations incorporated the postbiotics: Sonicated *S. thermophilus* S244, *Bifidobacterium longum* reuter lysate, heat-killed *L. plantarum*-GMNL6, the co-fermented *L. plantarum* AN057, *L. casei* AN177, and *S. thermophilus* AN157, E. keratini (EPI-7), *L. plantarum* HDB lysate, and a fermented lysate of *L. rhamnosus* VHProbi® E06, *L. paracasei* VHProbi® E12, *L. plantarum* VHProbi® E15, and *L. helveticus* VHProbi® Y21, all applied to facial skin or the forearm; another preparation, the heat-killed *L. paracasei* GMNL-653, used as a hair shampoo, exhibited positive results in decreasing sebum secretion and dandruff in parallel with a decrease in the abundance of *C. acnes* and *M. globose*, while there was an increase in hair volume. Finally, in the case of *L. brevis* DSM17250, applied on the skin of the tibia, the skin moisture was increased due to the strengthening of the skin barrier and the reduction of the trans-epithelial water loss, attributable to the modulation of commensal bacteria, and especially of *S. epidermidis*.

The 11 regimes for facial and forearm skin use were all found to keep the skin hydrated by strengthening the skin barrier, decreasing trans-epidermal water loss, and improving skin quality. No study directly referred to ceramide or collagen increase, while in five studies the skin microbiome remodeling was described: reduction of Proteobacteria and increase in the abundance of *Cutibacterium* and of *C. acnes*.

Considering the results of these studies collectively, we can say that these thoroughly studied probiotics, or the derived postbiotics, seem to keep the treated skin at least fully hydrated, with intact epithelial tone, positively affecting water loss; furthermore, they exert anti-inflammatory properties against various external attack [UV radiation, free radicals] thus delaying skin aging. Furthermore, some strains are involved in ceramide production as well as in boosting collagen synthesis, through fibroblast proliferation. In any case, a fully hydrated face shows improved elasticity, increased radiance, and decreased wrinkle depth. Most importantly, however, all these "genetically and phenotypically well-studied" cosmeceuticals can effectively regulate the skin microbiota towards a healthier one, their specialized action being absolutely species-specific [36,38].

However, these studies have several inherent drawbacks. First of all, those with the highest number of participants have a maximum of 55 subjects per study group—one on probiotics, with 55 subjects per arm, and 3 on postbiotics with 50, 55, and 52 subjects in total, while the remaining 10 have between 15 and 30 participants. The second drawback is that only three studies have a placebo group, two studies with probiotics, and one with postbiotics. Of the remaining 11, 4 with probiotics compare treatment results with baseline [before—after treatment], the treatment lasting 1 to 8 weeks [4 months for the shampoo study]. The seven studies use the corresponding half of the body for control. Finally, there are only four studies that report the ingredients of the formula used as a tracer. An initial study with probiotics reported a formula containing shea butter, seed oil, jojoba oil, olive oil, sunflower oil, and tocopherol plus the probiotic, the comparison being made before and after treatment. In the next study, the same authors used an oily tracer of *Byturospermum parkii* butter, *Simmondsia chinensis* seed oil, *Brassica campestris* seed oil, hydrogenated vegetable oil, *Helianthus annuus* hybrid oil, *Prunus amygdalus* dulcis oil, tocopherol, and *Helianthus annuus* seed oil, with or without the probiotic, the comparison made according to the split-face method. However, it is questionable as to how one can find differences between probiotics and placebo, the tracer having so many oils known for their beneficial effects on the skin. Finally, in two studies with postbiotics a detailed reference of the ingredients was also reported: glycerin, butylene glycol, polyethylene glycol, oils, and preservatives plus postbiotic was tested through the before-after comparison; and propylene glycol, caprylic/capric triglyceride, mineral oil, cetearyl alcohol, PEG-100 glyceryl stearate, stearic acid, glyceryl stearate, 1,2-hexanediol, phenoxyethanol, xanthan gum, chlorophenesin, L-arginine, chelating agents, and thickeners plus postbiotic or not, in a split-face study.

The skin reflects general health status and aging. As aging progresses, the fine lines become deep wrinkles, crow's feet, hooded eyelid, crepiness of the periorbital area, a double chin, etc., progressively appear. On the other hand, life expectancy is increasing, and since many people today do not have financial problems for survival, it is a very human reaction, not only for females, to look at their faces and bodies in the mirror and to desire to do something to counteract the effects of aging for themselves [73,80]. The use of beauty products, regardless of their origin, ingredients, manufacturers, and cost, is an integral part of daily care for many throughout the world, as well as a kind of psychotherapy [83,84]. The ongoing use of cosmeceuticals gives hope to the possibility of skin rejuvenation, the smoothing of wrinkles, and the freshening and firming of skin. Humans consent to pay for this—the timeless story of Goethe's Fausto—but consent to pay for reliable products, both in relation to their ingredients and their effectiveness.

6. Future Perspectives

The entrance of cosmeceuticals into the fight against dermo-aging is progressing rapidly, though it is still relatively early days. Probiotics and postbiotics are two distinct entities with a common origin, one from the other, both directly linked to a healthy skin microbiome. While the positive effects of specific probiotic strains on skin health are well-documented in cell line cultures and animal models, translating these findings to human studies presents significant challenges that will necessitate concerted and cooperative efforts involving robust clinical trials, on the part of researchers, industry, and regulatory bodies.

Over and above this, since everybody has a specific and individual microbiome, his "microbiota fingerprint", implicated in his dermal homeostasis, we believe that in the near future a prescription for personalized cosmeceutical products should be possible after a "rapid test" analysis of the skin microbiome. This would indeed be the new trend in dermo-cosmeceuticals.

Supplementary Materials: The following supporting information can be downloaded at: https://www.mdpi.com/article/10.3390/nu16152526/s1, Flow Chart.

Author Contributions: Conceptualization, K.K., I.M.T., and M.T.; methodology, K.K., I.M.T., and M.T.; validation, D.K. and J.K.T., formal analysis, K.K and G.T.; investigation, I.M.T. and S.D., resources, D.K.; data curation, A.E.M. and S.B.; writing—original draft preparation, I.M.T., G.S., and A.S.; writing—review and editing, A.S. and K.K.; visualization, G.S. and K.K.; supervision, G.S. and K.K.; project administration, M.T. and K.K. All authors have read and agreed to the published version of the manuscript.

Funding: This research received no external funding.

Conflicts of Interest: Authors Markos Theodorou and Joulia K. Tsetis were employed by the company Uni-Pharma S.A. The remaining authors declare that the research was conducted in the absence of any commercial or financial relationships that could be construed as a potential conflict of interest.

References

1. Guéniche, A.; Philippe, D.; Bastien, P.; Blum, S.; Buyukpamukcu, E.; Castiel-Higounenc, I. Probiotics for photoprotection. *Derm. Endocrinol.* **2009**, *1*, 275–279. [CrossRef] [PubMed]
2. Grice, E.A.; Segre, J.A. The skin microbiome. *Nat. Rev. Microbiol.* **2011**, *9*, 244–253. [CrossRef] [PubMed]
3. da Silva Vale, A.; de Melo Pereira, G.V.; de Oliveira, A.C.; de Carvalho Neto, D.P.; Herrmann, L.W.; Karp, S.G.; Soccol, V.T.; Soccol, C.R. Production, Formulation, and Application of Postbiotics in the Treatment of Skin Conditions. *Fermentation* **2023**, *9*, 264. [CrossRef]
4. Catic, T.; Pehlivanovic, B.; Pljakic, N.; Balicevac, A. The Moisturizing Efficacy of a Proprietary Dermo-Cosmetic Product (CLS02021) Versus Placebo in a 4-week Application Period. *Med. Arch.* **2022**, *76*, 108–114. [CrossRef]
5. Li, X.; Xing, L.; Lai, R.; Yuan, C.; Humbert, P. Literature mapping: Association of microscopic skin microflora and biomarkers with macroscopic skin health. *Clin. Exp. Dermatol.* **2021**, *46*, 21–27. [CrossRef] [PubMed]
6. Rawal, S.; Ali, S.A. Probiotics and postbiotics play a role in maintaining dermal health. *Food Funct.* **2023**, *14*, 3966–3981. [CrossRef] [PubMed]
7. Lolou, V.; Panayiotidis, M.I. Functional Role of Probiotics and Prebiotics on Skin Health and Disease. *Fermentation* **2019**, *5*, 41. [CrossRef]
8. Dréno, B.; Araviiskaia, E.; Berardesca, E.; Gontijo, G.; Sanchez Viera, M.; Xiang, L.F.; Martin, R.; Bieber, T. Microbiome in healthy skin, update for dermatologists. *J. Eur. Acad. Dermatol. Venereol.* **2016**, *30*, 2038–2047. [CrossRef] [PubMed]
9. Gueniche, A.; Perin, O.; Bouslimani, A.; Landemaine, L.; Misra, N.; Cupferman, S.; Aguilar, L.; Clavaud, C.; Chopra, T.; Khodr, A. Advances in Microbiome-Derived Solutions and Methodologies Are Founding a New Era in Skin Health and Care. *Pathogens* **2022**, *11*, 121. [CrossRef]
10. Egert, M.; Simmering, R. The Microbiota of the Human Skin. *Adv. Exp. Med. Biol.* **2016**, *902*, 61–81. [CrossRef]
11. Coppola, S.; Avagliano, C.; Sacchi, A.; Laneri, S.; Calignano, A.; Voto, L.; Luzzetti, A.; Berni Canani, R. Potential Clinical Applications of the Postbiotic Butyrate in Human Skin Diseases. *Molecules* **2022**, *27*, 1849. [CrossRef]
12. Keshari, S.; Balasubramaniam, A.; Myagmardoloonjin, B.; Herr, D.R.; Negari, I.P.; Huang, C.-M. Butyric Acid from Probiotic *Staphylococcus epidermidis* in the Skin Microbiome Down-Regulates the Ultraviolet-Induced Pro-Inflammatory IL-6 Cytokine via Short-Chain Fatty Acid Receptor. *Int. J. Mol. Sci.* **2019**, *20*, 4477. [CrossRef]
13. Fluhr, J.W.; Mao-Qiang, M.; Brown, B.E.; Wertz, P.W.; Crumrine, D.; Sundberg, J.P.; Feingold, K.R.; Elias, P.M. Glycerol regulates stratum corneum hydration in sebaceous gland deficient (asebia) mice. *J. Investig. Dermatol.* **2003**, *120*, 728–737. [CrossRef]
14. Imokawa, G.; Abe, A.; Jin, K.; Higaki, Y.; Kawashima, M.; Hidano, A. Decreased level of ceramides in stratum corneum of atopic dermatitis: An etiologic factor in atopic dry skin? *J. Investig. Dermatol.* **1991**, *96*, 523–526. [CrossRef]
15. Breiden, B.; Sandhoff, K. The role of sphingolipid metabolism in cutaneous permeability barrier formation. *Biochim. Biophys. Acta* **2014**, *1841*, 441–452. [CrossRef]
16. Rabionet, M.; Gorgas, K.; Sandhoff, R. Ceramide synthesis in the epidermis. *Biochim. Biophys. Acta* **2014**, *1841*, 422–434. [CrossRef]
17. Samadi, A.; Nasrollahi, S.A.; Rostami, M.N.; Rezagholi, Z.; Abolghasemi, F.; Firooz, A. Long-term effects of two 24-hour moisturizing products on skin barrier structure and function: A biometric and molecular study. *Health Sci. Rep.* **2021**, *4*, e308. [CrossRef]
18. Montagna, W.; Carlisle, K. Structural changes in aging human skin. *J. Investig. Dermatol.* **1979**, *73*, 47–53. [CrossRef]
19. Makrantonaki, E.; Bekou, V.; Zouboulis, C.C. Genetics and skin aging. *Derm.-Endocrinol.* **2012**, *4*, 280–284. [CrossRef]
20. Pageon, H.; Azouaoui, A.; Zucchi, H.; Ricois, S.; Tran, C.; Asselineau, D. Potentially beneficial effects of rhamnose on skin ageing: An in vitro and in vivo study. *Int. J. Cosmet. Sci.* **2019**, *41*, 213–220. [CrossRef]
21. Margolis, D.J.; Kruithof, E.K.; Barnard, M.; Howe, K.; Lazarus, G.S. Fibrinolytic abnormalities in two different cutaneous manifestations of venous disease. *J. Am. Acad. Dermatol.* **1996**, *34*, 204–208. [CrossRef]
22. Watson, R.E.; Griffiths, C.E.; Craven, N.M.; Shuttleworth, C.A.; Kielty, C.M. Fibrillin-rich microfibrils are reduced in photoaged skin. Distribution at the dermal-epidermal junction. *J. Investig. Dermatol.* **1999**, *112*, 782–787. [CrossRef]
23. Shuster, S.; Black, M.M.; McVitie, E. The influence of age and sex on skin thickness, skin collagen and density. *Br. J. Dermatol.* **1975**, *93*, 639–643. [CrossRef]
24. Russell-Goldman, E.; Murphy, G.F. The Pathobiology of Skin Aging: New Insights into an Old Dilemma. *Am. J. Pathol.* **2020**, *190*, 1356–1369. [CrossRef]
25. Zhang, S.; Duan, E. Fighting against Skin Aging: The Way from Bench to Bedside. *Cell Transplant.* **2018**, *27*, 729–738. [CrossRef]
26. Cole, M.A.; Quan, T.; Voorhees, J.J.; Fisher, G.J. Extracellular matrix regulation of fibroblast function: Redefining our perspective on skin aging. *J. Cell Commun. Signal.* **2018**, *12*, 35–43. [CrossRef]
27. Dou, J.; Feng, N.; Guo, F.; Chen, Z.; Liang, J.; Wang, T.; Guo, X.; Xu, Z. Applications of Probiotic Constituents in Cosmetics. *Molecules* **2023**, *28*, 6765. [CrossRef]
28. Hill, C.; Guarner, F.; Reid, G.; Gibson, G.R.; Merenstein, D.J.; Pot, B.; Morelli, L.; Canani, R.B.; Flint, H.J.; Salminen, S.; et al. Expert consensus document: The International Scientific Association for Probiotics and Prebiotics consensus statement on the scope and appropriate use of the term probiotic. *Nat. Rev. Gastroenterol. Hepatol.* **2014**, *11*, 506–514. [CrossRef]
29. Callewaert, C.; Knödlseder, N.; Karoglan, A.; Güell, M.; Paetzold, B. Skin microbiome transplantation and manipulation: Current state of the art. *Comput. Struct. Biotechnol. J.* **2021**, *19*, 624–631. [CrossRef]

30. Yu, X.; Wei, M.; Yang, D.; Wu, X.; Wei, H.; Xu, F. *Lactiplantibacillus plantarum* Strain FLPL05 Promotes Longevity in Mice by Improving Intestinal Barrier. *Probiotics Antimicrob. Proteins* **2023**, *15*, 1193–1205. [CrossRef]
31. Salminen, S.; Collado, M.C.; Endo, A.; Hill, C.; Lebeer, S.; Quigley, E.M.M.; Sanders, M.E.; Shamir, R.; Swann, J.R.; Szajewska, H.; et al. The International Scientific Association of Probiotics and Prebiotics (ISAPP) consensus statement on the definition and scope of postbiotics. *Nat. Rev. Gastroenterol. Hepatol.* **2021**, *18*, 649–667. [CrossRef]
32. Vinderola, G.; Druart, C.; Gosálbez, L.; Salminen, S.; Vinot, N.; Lebeer, S. Postbiotics in the medical field under the perspective of the ISAPP definition: Scientific, regulatory, and marketing considerations. *Front. Pharmacol.* **2023**, *14*, 1239745. [CrossRef] [PubMed]
33. Iordache, F.; Iordache, C.; Chifiriuc, M.; Bleotu, C.; Pavel, M.; Pelinescu, D.; Sasarman, E.; Lazar, V.; Bucur, M.; Dracea, O.; et al. Antimicrobial and immunomodulatory activity of some probiotic fractions with potential clinical application. *Arch. Zootech.* **2008**, *11*, 41–51.
34. Kimoto-Nira, H.; Aoki, R.; Sasaki, K.; Suzuki, C.; Mizumachi, K. Oral intake of heat-killed cells of *Lactococcus lactis* strain H61 promotes skin health in women. *J. Nutr. Sci.* **2012**, *1*, e18. [CrossRef]
35. Lee, D.E.; Huh, C.-S.; Ra, J.; Choi, I.-D.; Jeong, J.-W.; Kim, S.-H.; Ryu, J.H.; Seo, Y.K.; Koh, J.S.; Lee, J.-H.; et al. Clinical Evidence of Effects of Lactobacillus plantarum HY7714 on Skin Aging: A Randomized, Double Blind, Placebo-Controlled Study. *J. Microbiol. Biotechnol.* **2015**, *25*, 2160–2168. [CrossRef]
36. Duarte, M.; Oliveira, A.L.; Oliveira, C.; Pintado, M.; Amaro, A.; Madureira, A.R. Current postbiotics in the cosmetic market—An update and development opportunities. *Appl. Microbiol. Biotechnol.* **2022**, *106*, 5879–5891. [CrossRef]
37. Vinderola, G.; Sanders, M.E.; Salminen, S. The Concept of Postbiotics. *Foods* **2022**, *11*, 1077. [CrossRef]
38. Puebla-Barragan, S.; Reid, G. Probiotics in Cosmetic and Personal Care Products: Trends and Challenges. *Molecules* **2021**, *26*, 1249. [CrossRef]
39. Bermudez-Brito, M.; Plaza-Díaz, J.; Muñoz-Quezada, S.; Gómez-Llorente, C.; Gil, A. Probiotic mechanisms of action. *Ann. Nutr. Metab.* **2012**, *61*, 160–174. [CrossRef]
40. McFarland, L.V.; Evans, C.T.; Goldstein, E.J.C. Strain-Specificity and Disease-Specificity of Probiotic Efficacy: A Systematic Review and Meta-Analysis. *Front. Med.* **2018**, *5*, 124. [CrossRef]
41. Ra, J.; Lee, D.E.; Kim, S.H.; Jeong, J.-W.; Ku, H.K.; Kim, T.-Y.; Choi, I.-D.; Jeung, W.; Sim, J.-H.; Ahn, Y.-T. Effect of oral administration of Lactobacillus plantarum HY7714 on epidermal hydration in ultraviolet B-irradiated hairless mice. *J. Microbiol. Biotechnol.* **2014**, *24*, 1736–1743. [CrossRef] [PubMed]
42. Kim, H.M.; Lee, D.E.; Park, S.D.; Kim, Y.-T.; Kim, Y.J.; Jeong, J.W.; Jang, S.S.; Ahn, Y.-T.; Sim, J.-H.; Huh, C.-S.; et al. Oral administration of Lactobacillus plantarum HY7714 protects hairless mouse against ultraviolet B-induced photoaging. *J. Microbiol. Biotechnol.* **2014**, *24*, 1583–1591. [CrossRef] [PubMed]
43. Lee, N.Y.; Ibrahim, O.; Khetarpal, S.; Gaber, M.; Jamas, S.; Gryllos, I.; Dover, J.S. Dermal Microflora Restoration with Ammonia-Oxidizing Bacteria Nitrosomonas Eutropha in the Treatment of Keratosis Pilaris: A Randomized Clinical Trial. *J. Drugs Dermatol.* **2018**, *17*, 285–288. [PubMed]
44. Notay, M.; Saric-Bosanac, S.; Vaughn, A.R.; Dhaliwal, S.; Trivedi, M.; Reiter, P.N.; Rybak, I.; Li, C.C.; Weiss, L.B.; Ambrogio, L.; et al. The use of topical *Nitrosomonas eutropha* for cosmetic improvement of facial wrinkles. *J. Cosmet. Dermatol.* **2020**, *19*, 689–693. [CrossRef] [PubMed]
45. Onwuliri, V.; Agbakoba, N.R.; Anukam, K.C. Topical cream containing live lactobacilli decreases malodor-producing bacteria and downregulates genes encoding PLP-dependent enzymes on the axillary skin microbiome of healthy adult Nigerians. *J. Cosmet. Dermatol.* **2021**, *20*, 2989–2998. [CrossRef] [PubMed]
46. Natsch, A.; Schmid, J.; Flachsmann, F. Identification of odoriferous sulfanylalkanols in human axilla secretions and their formation through cleavage of cysteine precursors by a C-S lyase isolated from axilla bacteria. *Chem. Biodivers.* **2004**, *1*, 1058–1072. [CrossRef] [PubMed]
47. Anukam, K.C.; Macklaim, J.M.; Gloor, G.B.; Reid, G.; Boekhorst, J.; Renckens, B.; van Hijum, S.A.; Siezen, R.J. Genome sequence of Lactobacillus pentosus KCA1: Vaginal isolate from a healthy premenopausal woman. *PLoS ONE* **2013**, *8*, e59239. [CrossRef]
48. Falholt Elvebakken, H.; Bruntse, A.B.; Vedel, C.; Kjaerulff, S. Topical *Lactiplantibacillus plantarum* LB244R® ointment alleviates skin aging: An exploratory trial. *J. Cosmet. Dermatol.* **2023**, *22*, 1911–1918. [CrossRef] [PubMed]
49. Christensen, I.B.; Vedel, C.; Clausen, M.-L.; Kjærulff, S.; Agner, T.; Nielsen, D.S. Targeted Screening of Lactic Acid Bacteria with Antibacterial Activity toward *Staphylococcus aureus* Clonal Complex Type 1 Associated with Atopic Dermatitis. *Front. Microbiol.* **2021**, *12*, 733847. [CrossRef]
50. Elvebakken, H.F.; Christensen, I.B.; Vedel, C.; Kjærulff, S. A proof of concept: Clinical anti-aging efficacy and safety of *Lactiplantibacillus plantarum* LB244R® applied topically in a double-blinded placebo-controlled study. *J. Cosmet. Dermatol.* **2024**, *23*, 1233–1242. [CrossRef]
51. Di Marzio, L.; Cinque, B.; De Simone, C.; Cifone, M.G. Effect of the lactic acid bacterium *Streptococcus thermophilus* on ceramide levels in human keratinocytes in vitro and stratum corneum in vivo. *J. Investig. Dermatol.* **1999**, *113*, 98–106. [CrossRef] [PubMed]
52. Di Marzio, L.; Cinque, B.; Cupelli, F.; De Simone, C.; Cifone, M.G.; Giuliani, M. Increase of skin-ceramide levels in aged subjects following a short-term topical application of bacterial sphingomyelinase from Streptococcus thermophilus. *Int. J. Immunopathol. Pharmacol.* **2008**, *21*, 137–143. [CrossRef] [PubMed]

53. Guéniche, A.; Bastien, P.; Ovigne, J.M.; Kermici, M.; Courchay, G.; Chevalier, V.; Breton, L.; Castiel-Higounenc, I. *Bifidobacterium longum* lysate, a new ingredient for reactive skin. *Exp. Dermatol.* **2010**, *19*, e1–e8. [CrossRef] [PubMed]
54. Holz, C.; Benning, J.; Schaudt, M.; Heilmann, A.; Schultchen, J.; Goelling, D.; Lang, C. Novel bioactive from *Lactobacillus brevis* DSM17250 to stimulate the growth of *Staphylococcus epidermidis*: A pilot study. *Benef. Microbes* **2017**, *8*, 121–131. [CrossRef] [PubMed]
55. Tsai, W.-H.; Chou, C.-H.; Chiang, Y.-J.; Lin, C.-G.; Lee, C.-H. Regulatory effects of *Lactobacillus plantarum*-GMNL6 on human skin health by improving skin microbiome. *Int. J. Med. Sci.* **2021**, *18*, 1114–1120. [CrossRef] [PubMed]
56. Tsai, W.-H.; Fang, Y.-T.; Huang, T.-Y.; Chiang, Y.-J.; Lin, C.-G.; Chang, W.-W. Heat-killed *Lacticaseibacillus paracasei* GMNL-653 ameliorates human scalp health by regulating scalp microbiome. *BMC Microbiol.* **2023**, *23*, 121. [CrossRef]
57. Coderch, L.; López, O.; de la Maza, A.; Parra, J.L. Ceramides and skin function. *Am. J. Clin. Dermatol.* **2003**, *4*, 107–129. [CrossRef] [PubMed]
58. Juncan, A.M.; Moisă, D.G.; Santini, A.; Morgovan, C.; Rus, L.-L.; Vonica-Țincu, A.L.; Loghin, F. Advantages of Hyaluronic Acid and Its Combination with Other Bioactive Ingredients in Cosmeceuticals. *Molecules* **2021**, *26*, 4429. [CrossRef] [PubMed]
59. Lee, D.-G.; Trujillo, M.E.; Kang, S.; Nam, J.-J.; Kim, Y.-J. *Epidermidibacterium keratini* gen. nov., sp. nov., a member of the family Sporichthyaceae, isolated from keratin epidermis. *Int. J. Syst. Evol. Microbiol.* **2018**, *68*, 745–750. [CrossRef]
60. Lee, Y.-G.; Lee, D.-G.; Gwag, J.; Kim, M.; Kim, M.; Kim, H.-G.; Ko, J.-H.; Yeo, H.; Kang, S.; Baek, N.-I. A 1,1′-biuracil from *Epidermidibacterium keratini* EPI-7 shows anti-aging effects on human dermal fibroblasts. *Appl. Biol. Chem.* **2019**, *62*, 14. [CrossRef]
61. Brosnan, M.E.; Brosnan, J.T. Orotic acid excretion and arginine metabolism. *J. Nutr.* **2007**, *137*, 1656s–1661s. [CrossRef] [PubMed]
62. Kim, J.; Lee, Y.I.; Mun, S.; Jeong, J.; Lee, D.-G.; Kim, M.; Jo, H.; Lee, S.; Han, K.; Lee, J.H. Efficacy and Safety of Epidermidibacterium Keratini EPI-7 Derived Postbiotics in Skin Aging: A Prospective Clinical Study. *Int. J. Mol. Sci.* **2023**, *24*, 4634. [CrossRef] [PubMed]
63. Yang, S.-J.; Lee, C.-W.; Cha, S.Y.; Choi, J.-W.; Lee, S. Skin Barrier Enhancement of Ferment using Lava Seawater and *Lactobacillus plantarum* HDB1234 as a Novel Cosmetic Ingredient. *J. Korean Soc. Cosmetol.* **2021**, *27*, 356–363. [CrossRef]
64. Kim, K.M.; Song, J.-W.; Lee, C.-W.; Kim, D.-S.; Sohn, J.; Lee, S. Skin Barrier-Enhancing Effects of Dermabiotics HDB with Regulation of Skin Microbiota. *J. Microbiol. Biotechnol.* **2024**, *34*, 65–73. [CrossRef] [PubMed]
65. Kim, H.-J.; Oh, H.N.; Park, T.; Kim, H.; Lee, H.G.; An, S.; Sul, W.J. Aged related human skin microbiome and mycobiome in Korean women. *Sci. Rep.* **2022**, *12*, 2351. [CrossRef] [PubMed]
66. Cui, H.; Feng, C.; Zhang, T.; Martínez-Ríos, V.; Martorell, P.; Tortajada, M.; Cheng, S.; Cheng, S.; Duan, Z. Effects of a lotion containing probiotic ferment lysate as the main functional ingredient on enhancing skin barrier: A randomized, self-control study. *Sci. Rep.* **2023**, *13*, 16879. [CrossRef] [PubMed]
67. Cui, H.; Guo, C.; Wang, Q.; Feng, C.; Duan, Z. A pilot study on the efficacy of topical lotion containing anti-acne postbiotic in subjects with mild -to -moderate acne. *Front. Med.* **2022**, *9*, 1064460. [CrossRef] [PubMed]
68. Rawlings, A.V.; Harding, C.R. Moisturization and skin barrier function. *Dermatol. Ther.* **2004**, *17* (Suppl. S1), 43–48. [CrossRef] [PubMed]
69. Lodén, M. Role of topical emollients and moisturizers in the treatment of dry skin barrier disorders. *Am. J. Clin. Dermatol.* **2003**, *4*, 771–788. [CrossRef]
70. Huuskonen, L.; Anglenius, H.; Ahonen, I.; Tiihonen, K. Effects of Bacterial Lysates and Metabolites on Collagen Homeostasis in TNF-α-Challenged Human Dermal Fibroblasts. *Microorganisms* **2023**, *11*, 1465. [CrossRef]
71. Negari, I.P.; Keshari, S.; Huang, C.-M. Probiotic Activity of *Staphylococcus epidermidis* Induces Collagen Type I Production through FFaR2/p-ERK Signaling. *Int. J. Mol. Sci.* **2021**, *22*, 1414. [CrossRef] [PubMed]
72. Lee, J.-S.; Min, J.-W.; Gye, S.-B.; Kim, Y.-W.; Kang, H.-C.; Choi, Y.-S.; Seo, W.-S.; Lee, B.-Y. Suppression of UVB-Induced MMP-1 Expression in Human Skin Fibroblasts Using Lysate of *Lactobacillus iners* Derived from Korean Women's Skin in Their Twenties. *Curr. Issues Mol. Biol.* **2024**, *46*, 513–526. [CrossRef] [PubMed]
73. Lau, M.; Mineroff Gollogly, J.; Wang, J.Y.; Jagdeo, J. Cosmeceuticals for antiaging: A systematic review of safety and efficacy. *Arch. Dermatol. Res.* **2024**, *316*, 173. [CrossRef] [PubMed]
74. Han, J.H.; Kim, H.S. Skin Deep: The Potential of Microbiome Cosmetics. *J. Microbiol.* **2024**, *62*, 181–199. [CrossRef] [PubMed]
75. De Almeida, C.V.; Antiga, E.; Lulli, M. Oral and Topical Probiotics and Postbiotics in Skincare and Dermatological Therapy: A Concise Review. *Microorganisms* **2023**, *11*, 1420. [CrossRef] [PubMed]
76. Gkitsaki, I.; Potsaki, P.; Dimou, I.; Laskari, Z.; Koutelidakis, A.; Giaouris, E. Development of a functional Greek sheep yogurt incorporating a probiotic *Lacticaseibacillus rhamnosus* wild-type strain as adjunct starter culture. *Heliyon* **2024**, *10*, e24446. [CrossRef] [PubMed]
77. Ashraf, R.; Shah, N.P. Selective and differential enumerations of *Lactobacillus delbrueckii* subsp. bulgaricus, *Streptococcus thermophilus, Lactobacillus acidophilus, Lactobacillus casei* and *Bifidobacterium* spp. in yoghurt—A review. *Int. J. Food Microbiol.* **2011**, *149*, 194–208. [CrossRef] [PubMed]
78. Baldwin, H.E.; Bhatia, N.D.; Friedman, A.; Eng, R.M.; Seite, S. The Role of Cutaneous Microbiota Harmony in Maintaining a Functional Skin Barrier. *J. Drugs Dermatol.* **2017**, *16*, 12–18. [CrossRef] [PubMed]
79. Maisel, A.; Waldman, A.; Furlan, K.; Weil, A.; Sacotte, K.; Lazaroff, J.M.; Lin, K.; Aranzazu, D.; Avram, M.M.; Bell, A.; et al. Self-reported Patient Motivations for Seeking Cosmetic Procedures. *JAMA Dermatol.* **2018**, *154*, 1167–1174. [CrossRef]

80. Draelos, Z.; Bogdanowicz, P.; Saurat, J.H. Top weapons in skin aging and actives to target the consequences of skin cell senescence. *J. Eur. Acad. Dermatol. Venereol.* **2024**, *38* (Suppl. S4), 15–22. [CrossRef]
81. Yadav, N.; Ajmal, G.; Kumawat, D.M.; Diwan, A. Probiotic in Cosmetics: A Patents Landscape Study. *Int. J. Life Sci. Pharma Res.* **2023**, *13*, L48–L61. [CrossRef]
82. Telesetsky, A. *UN Food and Agriculture Organization: Exercising Legal Personality to Implement the UN Convention on the Law of the Sea*; Springer: Berlin/Heidelberg, Germany, 2020; pp. 203–220.
83. Nerini, A.; Matera, C.; Stefanile, C. Psychosocial predictors in consideration of cosmetic surgery among women. *Aesthetic Plast. Surg.* **2014**, *38*, 461–466. [CrossRef] [PubMed]
84. Ahluwalia, J.; Fabi, S.G. The psychological and aesthetic impact of age-related hair changes in females. *J. Cosmet. Dermatol.* **2019**, *18*, 1161–1169. [CrossRef] [PubMed]

MDPI AG
Grosspeteranlage 5
4052 Basel
Switzerland
Tel.: +41 61 683 77 34

Nutrients Editorial Office
E-mail: nutrients@mdpi.com
www.mdpi.com/journal/nutrients

www.ingramcontent.com/pod-product-compliance
Lightning Source LLC
Chambersburg PA
CBHW061800210926
51850CB00006B/605
* 9 7 8 3 7 2 5 8 7 6 3 5 8 *